DIABETES SOURCEBOOK

DIABETES SOURCEBOOK

Basic Information about Insulin-Dependent and Noninsulin-Dependent Diabetes Mellitus, Gestational Diabetes, and Diabetic Complications, Symptoms, Treatments, and Research Results, Including Statistics on Prevalence, Morbidity, and Mortality, Along With Source Listings for Further Help and Information.

Health Reference Series
Volume Three

Edited by
Karen Bellenir and
Peter D. Dresser

Omnigraphics, Inc. • *Penobscot Building* • *Detroit, MI 48226*

1994

BIBLIOGRAPHIC NOTE

This volume contains individual publications issued by the National Institutes of Health (NIH), its sister agencies, and subagencies. Numbered publications are: NIH 87-2946; 88-1587; 88-2177; 89-3016; 90-1585; 90-2098; 90-2904; 91-3185; 91-651; 92-1596; 92-241; 92-3235; 92-3422; 93-1587; 93-201; 93-2171; 93-2412; 93-2788; 93-3265; 93-3266; 93-3267; 93-3464; and EPA\530-SW-90-089. Unnumbered publications of the NIH, the Centers for Disease Control, the National Diabetes Information Clearing House, the National Eye Institute, the National Institute of Diabetes and Digestive and Kidney Disorders, and the National Institute of Dental Research, Indian Health Service, and the Library of Congress, and selected articles from the National Center for Research Resources *Reporter* are also included.

In addition, this volume contains unnumbered patient education fact sheets developed by the Michigan Diabetes Research and Training Center. These are used by permission.

Edited by
Karen Bellenir and
Peter D. Dresser

Omnigraphics, Inc.

* * *

Matthew P. Barbour, *Production Coordinator*
Laurie Lanzen Harris, *Vice President, Editorial*
Peter E. Ruffner, *Vice President, Administration*
James A. Sellgren, *Vice President, Operations and Finance*
Jane J. Steele, *Vice President, Research*

* * *

Frederick G. Ruffner, Jr., *Publisher*

Library of Congress Cataloging-in-Publication Data

Diabetes Sourcebook : basic information about insulin-dependent and noninsulin-dependent diabetes mellitus, gestational diabetes, and diabetic complications symptoms, treatments, and research results . . . / edited by Karen Bellenir and Peter D. Dresser.
p. cm. — (Health reference series ; v. 3)
Includes bibliographical references and index.
ISBN 1-55888-751-2
1. Diabetes—Popular works. I. Bellenir, Karen. II. Dresser, Peter D. III. Series.
RC660.4.D56 1994
616.4′62—dc20 94-39437
CIP

This book is printed on acid-free paper meeting the ANSI Z39.48 Standard. The infinity symbol that appears above indicates that the paper in this book meets that standard.

Printed in the United States

Contents

PART III: Complications of Diabetes

PART IV: Research in Diabetes

APPENDIX: Where to Go for More Help and Information

Preface

About this book

This volume is primarily comprised of documents published by the National Institutes of Health and its subagencies and sister agencies. Publications were selected to provide the layperson with basic information about insulin-dependent and noninsulin-dependent diabetes mellitus, gestational diabetes, and diabetic complications.

How to use this book

Part I—Defining Diabetes includes information about the disease called diabetes, its different forms, and its impact on the American population. To help the layperson overcome confusion about medical terms, it begins with *The Diabetes Dictionary*.

Part I also includes excerpts from the *1993 Diabetes Surveillance*, which was issued by the Centers for Disease Control and Prevention (CDC) in the Spring of 1994. The statistical highlights give an up-to-date snapshot of diabetes prevalence, morbidity, and mortality in the America and the impact of diabetes on various segments of the population. *Diabetes in the United States* provides information about the burden of diabetes in each of the 50 states.

Part II—Diabetes Management is directed to the patient with diabetes and his or her family and friends. Individual patient education sheets developed by the Michigan Diabetes Research and Training Center (DRTC) address some of the common concerns regarding self-care issues. The CDC-produced *Take Charge of Your Diabetes* includes advice to diabetics and offers "fill-in-the-blank" charts for recording important medical information. *Diabetes Translation*, from the National Diabetes Advisory Board's Long-Range Plan, describes the Federal government's efforts to communicate the results of on-going diabetes research to physicians and patients.

Part III - Complications of Diabetes describes some of the medical consequences of diabetes, their symptoms, treatments, and how to ameliorate their effects. Results of the Diabetes Control and Complications Trial (June 1993), which studied intensive insulin therapy, are also included.

Part IV - Research in Diabetes highlights the research accomplishments made during the 1980s and discusses areas of on-going study in the 1990s. Although some of the documents are more technical in nature than most patient materials, the information will be of interest to persons seeking an in-depth understanding of diabetes-related issues. Part IV also includes *Research Opportunities and Programs in the Division of Diabetes*, which describes various Federal programs that support current research.

The *Appendix* lists sources of further help and information. It includes a *Directory of Diabetes Organizations*, information about the National Diabetes Information Clearinghouse, a description of the work being done by the Diabetes Research and Training Centers, information about assistance for visually challenged diabetes patients, a bibliography of diabetic cookbooks, a Resource Guide for diabetes-related programs for black Americans and other minority populations, and a bibliography of materials available in Spanish and additional non-English languages.

Acknowledgements

The editor wishes to thank Margaret Mary Missar for her painstaking and thorough research; Peter Dresser for his assistance, guidance, and patience; and Bruce the Scanman, who made this book possible in more ways than one.

INTRODUCTION

Diabetes Overview

Almost everyone knows someone who has diabetes. Between 13 and 14 million people in the United States have diabetes mellitus, a serious, life-long disorder that is, as yet, incurable. Almost half of these people do not know they have diabetes and are not under medical care. Each year, 500,000 to 700,000 people are diagnosed with diabetes.

Although diabetes occurs most often in older adults, it is the second most common chronic disorder after cancer in U.S. children. Each year, 11,000 to 12,000 children and teenagers are diagnosed with diabetes.

What Is Diabetes?

Diabetes is a disorder of metabolism—the way the body uses digested food for growth and energy. Most of the food we eat is broken down by the digestive juices into chemicals including a simple sugar called glucose. After digestion, the glucose passes into the bloodstream where it is available for body cells to use for growth and energy.

For the glucose to get into the cells, insulin must be present. Insulin is a hormone produced by the pancreas.

When most people eat, the pancreas automatically produces the right amount of insulin to take care of the glucose. In people with diabetes, however, the pancreas either produces little or no insulin, or the body's cells do not respond to the insulin that is produced. As a result, glucose builds up in the blood, over flows into the urine, and passes out of the body. Thus, the

---

NIH Pub. No. 92-3235.

body loses its main source of fuel even though the blood contains large amounts.

There are two major types of diabetes. Type I, known as insulin-dependent diabetes (IDDM), is considered an autoimmune disease because the pancreatic cells that produce insulin, the beta cells, are destroyed by the body's own immune system. The pancreas then produces little or no insulin. To live, the person with IDDM needs daily injections of insulin. At present, scientists do not know exactly what causes the body's immune system to attack the beta cells, but they believe that both genetic factors and viruses may be involved. IDDM accounts for from 5 to 10 percent of diagnosed diabetes in the United States.

IDDM usually develops in children or young adults, although the disorder can appear at any age. Symptoms of IDDM usually develop over a short period, although beta cell destruction can begin months, or even years, earlier. Symptoms include increased thirst and urination, constant hunger, weight loss, blurred vision, and great tiredness. If not diagnosed and treated with insulin, the person can lapse into a life-threatening coma.

The most common form of diabetes is Type II, called noninsulin-dependent diabetes (NIDDM). Ninety to 95 percent of people with diabetes have NIDDM. This form of diabetes usually develops in adults over the age of 40, and it is most common among adults over 55. About 80 percent of people with NIDDM are overweight.

In NIDDM, the pancreas usually produces insulin, but for some reason, the body cannot use the insulin effectively. The end result is the same as for IDDM—an unhealthy buildup of glucose in the blood and an inability of the body to make efficient use of its main source of fuel.

The symptoms of NIDDM appear to develop gradually, and they tend to be vague and not as noticeable as in IDDM. Symptoms include feelings of tiredness or illness, frequent urination, especially at night, unusual thirst, weight loss, blurred vision, frequent infections, and slow healing of sores.

A third form of diabetes, called gestational diabetes, develops or is discovered during pregnancy. The diabetes usually disappears when the pregnancy is over, but women who have had gestational diabetes have an increased risk of developing NIDDM later in their lives.

Diabetes is not contagious. It cannot be "caught" from another person. However, having a family history of diabetes places a person at higher risk for diabetes, especially NIDDM. Other risk factors for NIDDM include being overweight, older, and of black, Hispanic, or Native American origin.

Scope and Impact of Diabetes

Diabetes is widely recognized as one of the leading causes of death and disability in the U.S. In 1986, diabetes caused or contributed to more than

187,000 deaths. The true toll is probably much higher because diabetes was not listed on half of the death certificates for people who had diabetes.

Diabetes is associated with long-term complications that affect almost every major part of the body. It can cause blindness, heart disease, strokes, kidney failure, amputations, nerve damage, and birth defects in babies born to women with diabetes.

In terms of medical care, treatment supplies, hospitalizations, time lost from work, disability payments, and premature death, diabetes costs this country over $40 billion annually.

Who Gets Diabetes?

Diabetes can develop in people of any age or ethnic background, although some groups appear to be at higher risk for certain types of diabetes. IDDM occurs equally among males and females, and it is more common in the white, non-Hispanic population.

Although worldwide statistics are not available, it appears that IDDM is unknown or rare in some ethnic groups, including some Asian, African, and Native American populations. On the other hand, some northern European countries, including Finland and Sweden, have very high rates of IDDM. The reasons for these differences are not known.

NIDDM is more common in older people, especially older women, and it occurs more often among black, Hispanic, and Native Americans. The prevalence of NIDDM in the U.S. black population is about 60 percent higher than in non-Hispanic whites. Compared with whites, Hispanic Americans have twice the rate of diabetes. Native Americans have the highest rates of diabetes in the world. In one tribe, the Pima Indians, half of all adults have NIDDM. The rate of diabetes is likely to increase because older people, Hispanics, and other minority people make up the fastest growing parts of the U.S. population.

Treatment of Diabetes

Before the discovery of insulin in 1921, all people with IDDM died within a few years of the onset of their disease. Although insulin is not considered a cure for diabetes, its discovery was the first major breakthrough in diabetes treatment. Today, daily injections of insulin are the basic therapy for IDDM. Insulin injections must be balanced with diet and mealtimes, exercise, and daily testing of blood glucose levels. Diet, exercise, and blood or urine testing for glucose also form the basis for management of NIDDM. In addition, some people with NIDDM take oral drugs or insulin to lower their blood glucose levels.

People with diabetes are responsible for their day-to-day care. They also should be under the general care of a doctor who monitors their diabetes control and checks for diabetes complications. Doctors that specialize in diabetes are called endocrinologists or diabetologists. In addition, people with diabetes often see other specialists such as ophthalmologists for eye examinations or podiatrists for foot care. People with diabetes often consult a dietitian for dietary guidance and a diabetes educator for instruction in day-to-day care.

The goal of diabetes treatment is to keep blood glucose levels as close to the normal (nondiabetic) range as possible. Most diabetes doctors believe that trying to keep blood glucose levels near the normal range will help prevent or delay the long-term complications of diabetes.

The National Institute of Diabetes and Digestive and Kidney Diseases (NIDDK), the Federal Government's lead agency for diabetes research at the National Institutes of Health (NIH), is conducting a major clinical study to help answer that question. The study, called the Diabetes Control and Complications Trial (DCCT), involves more than 1,400 people with IDDM and is being carried out at 29 centers nationwide. Results from the study are expected in 1994.

Research on Diabetes

The DCCT is one of many research programs being carried out by the Federal Government and by nongovernment organizations to improve the health and well-being of people with diabetes and to find ways to prevent and cure the disorder.

The NIDDK supports basic and clinical research in its own laboratories, in research centers, and at hospitals throughout the U.S. NIDDK also gathers and analyzes statistics about diabetes. Other NIH Institutes carry out research on diabetes-related eye diseases, heart and vascular complications, pregnancy, and dental problems. Other Government agencies that sponsor diabetes programs are the Centers for Disease Control, the Indian Health Service, the Health Resources and Services Administration, and the Department of Veterans Affairs.

Many organizations outside of the Government support diabetes research and education activities. These organizations include the American Diabetes Association, the Juvenile Diabetes Foundation International, the American Association of Diabetes Educators, the Joslin Diabetes Center, the International Diabetes Center, the Barbara Davis Center for Childhood Diabetes, drug companies that develop diabetes products, and many other groups. In the past 15 years, advances in diabetes research have led to better ways to manage diabetes and treat its complications. Major advances include:

- New forms of purified insulin, such as human insulin produced through genetic engineering.
- Development of better ways for doctors to monitor blood glucose levels and for people with diabetes to test their own blood glucose levels at home.
- Development of external and implantable insulin pumps that deliver appropriate amounts of insulin, replacing daily injections.
- The use of laser treatment for diabetic eye disease, reducing the risk of blindness.
- Successful transplantation of kidneys in people whose own kidneys failed because of diabetes.
- Better ways of managing diabetic pregnancies, improving chances of a successful outcome.
- Development of new drugs to treat NIDDM and better ways to manage this form of diabetes through weight control.

In the future, insulin may be administered through nasal sprays or taken in the form of a pill. Devices to "read" blood glucose levels without having to prick a finger to get a blood sample also are being developed.

Research also is ongoing to find the cause or causes of diabetes and ways to prevent and cure the disorder. Scientists are searching for genes that may be involved in NIDDM and IDDM. Some genetic markers for IDDM have been identified, and it is now possible to screen relatives of people with IDDM to see if they are at risk for diabetes. Studies now are under way using drugs that stop the immune system from attacking the beta cells to try to prevent IDDM from developing in people who are at high risk for the disorder.

Transplantation of the pancreas or insulin-producing beta cells offers the best hope of cure for people with IDDM. Some successful pancreas transplants have been performed. However, people who have transplants must take powerful drugs that prevent rejection of the transplanted organ. These drugs are costly and may eventually cause serious health problems. Scientists are working to develop less harmful drugs and better methods of transplanting pancreatic tissue to prevent rejection by the body.

For NIDDM, the focus is on ways to prevent diabetes. Preventive approaches include identifying people at high risk for the disorder and encouraging them to lose weight, exercise more, and follow a healthy diet.

PART ONE

DEFINING DIABETES

Chapter 1

The Diabetes Dictionary

Pronunciation Guide

The letters inside the parentheses give the reader a simple guide to how the word is said aloud.

The space between the letters shows the syllables.

The accent mark (´) shows which syllables to stress.

The hyphen follows syllables that should not be stressed.

A curved line above a letter (ă) gives it a "short" sound, and a straight line above a letter (ā) gives it a "long" sound.

For example: tes-tape (tĕs-tāp´). The word tes-tape has two syllables. The stress is on the last syllable-tape. The "e" has a short sound like the word bed or met. The "a" has a long sound like the word day.

The following examples show each marking used in this dictionary and some sample words that have the most common sounds for each marking.

ă as in cat, map
ā as in day, fade
ĕ as in bed, pet
ē as in bleed, meet
ĭ as in tip, fit
ī as in side, kite
ŏ as in stop, cot
ō as in toe, bone
ŭ as in cut, numb
ū as in glue, youth

NIH Pub. No. 89-3016

Introduction

This dictionary of diabetes terms defines words that are often used when talking or writing about diabetes. It is designed for people who have diabetes and their families and friends. It provides basic information about the disease, its long-term effects, and its care.

The words are listed in alphabetical order. Some words have many meanings; only those meanings that relate to diabetes are included. A term will refer the reader to another definition only when the second definition gives additional information about a topic that is directly related to the first term.

Prepared by:
National Diabetes Information Clearinghouse
National Institute of Diabetes and Digestive and Kidney Diseases
National Institutes of Health
Box NDIC
Bethesda, Maryland 20892

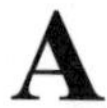

Acetohexamide
(as-ĕ´tŏ-heks´ah-mīd)

A pill taken to lower the level of glucose (sugar) in the blood. Only some people with noninsulin-dependent diabetes take these pills. *See also:* Oral hypoglycemic agents.

Acetone
(as´ĕ-tōn)

A chemical formed in the blood when the body uses fat instead of glucose (sugar) for energy. If acetone forms, it usually means that the cells do not have enough insulin, or cannot use the insulin that is in the blood, to use glucose for energy. Acetone passes through the body into the urine. Someone with a lot of acetone in the body can have breath that smells fruity and is called "acetone breath." *See also:* Ketone bodies.

Acidosis
(as´ĭ-dō´sĭs)

Too much acid in the body. For a person with diabetes, this can lead to diabetic ketoacidosis. *See also:* Diabetic ketoacidosis.

Acute
(ah-kyūt´)

Happens for a limited period of time; abrupt onset; sharp, severe.

Adrenal Glands
(ah-drē´năl glănds)
Two organs that sit on top of the kidneys and make and release hormones such as adrenalin (epinephrine). This and other hormones, including insulin, control the body's use of glucose (sugar).

Adult-Onset Diabetes
Former term for noninsulin-dependent or type II diabetes. *See also:* Noninsulin-dependent diabetes mellitus.

Adverse Effect
(ad´vĕrs ĕ-fĕkt´)
A harmful result.

Albuminuria
(al´bū-mĭ-nŭ´rē-ah)
More than normal amounts of a protein called albumin in the urine. Albuminuria may be a sign of kidney disease, a problem that can occur in people who have had diabetes for a long time.

Aldose Reductase Inhibitor
(ăl´dōs rĭ-dŭk´tās ĭn-hĭb´ĭt-ĭr)
A class of drugs being studied as a way to prevent eye and nerve damage in people with diabetes. Aldose reductase is an enzyme that is normally present in the eye and in many other parts of the body. It helps change glucose (sugar) into a sugar alcohol called sorbitol. Too much sorbitol trapped in eye and nerve cells can damage these cells, leading to retinopathy and neuropathy. Drugs that prevent or slow (inhibit) the action of aldose reductase are being studied as a way to prevent or delay these complications of diabetes.

Alpha Cell
(al´fah sĕl)
A type of cell in the pancreas (in areas called the islets of Langerhans). Alpha cells make and release a hormone called glucagon, which raises the level of glucose (sugar) in the blood.

Amino Acid
(ah-mē´nō as´ĭd)
The building blocks of proteins; the main material of the body's cells. Insulin is made of 51 amino acids joined together.

Angiopathy
(an-jē-ŏp´ah-thē)
Disease of the blood vessels (arteries, veins, and capillaries) that occurs when someone has diabetes for a long time. There are two types of angi-

opathy: macroangiopathy and microangiopathy. In macroangiopathy, fat and blood clots build up in the large blood vessels, stick to the vessel walls, and block the flow of blood. In microangiopathy the walls of the smaller blood vessels become so thick and weak that they bleed, leak protein, and slow the flow of blood through the body. Then the cells, for example, the ones in the center of the eye, do not get enough blood and may be damaged.

Antagonist

(an-tag´ah-nĭst)

One agent that opposes or fights the action of another. For example, insulin lowers the level of glucose (sugar) in the blood, whereas glucagon raises it; therefore, insulin and glucagon are antagonists.

Antibodies

(an´tē-bŏd´ēz)

Proteins that the body makes to protect itself from foreign substances. In diabetes, the body sometimes makes antibodies to work against pork or beef insulins because they are not exactly the same as human insulin or because they have impurities. The antibodies can keep the insulin from working well and may even cause the person with diabetes to have an allergic or bad reaction to the beef or pork insulins.

Antidiabetic Agent

(an´tĭ-dī´ah-bĕt´ĭc)

A substance that helps a person with diabetes control the level of glucose (sugar) in the blood so that the body works as it should. *See also:* Insulin; oral hypoglycemic agents.

Antiseptic

(an´tĭ-sĕp´tĭk)

An agent that kills bacteria. Alcohol is a common antiseptic. Before injecting insulin, many people use alcohol to clean their skin to avoid infection.

Arteriosclerosis

(ar-tĕ´rē-ō-sklĕ-rō´sĭs)

A group of diseases in which the walls of the arteries get thick and hard. In one type of arteriosclerosis, fat builds up inside the walls and slows the blood flow. (*See:* Atherosclerosis.) These diseases often occur in people who have had diabetes for a long time.

Artery

(ar´tĕr-ē)

A large blood vessel that carries blood from the heart to other parts of the body. Arteries are thicker and have walls that are stronger and more elastic than the walls of veins. *See also:* Blood vessels.

Artificial Endocrine Pancreas
(ar-tĭ-fĭ´shal ĕn´dō-krĭn pan´krē-ĕs)

A man-made device that constantly measures glucose (sugar) in the blood and, in response, releases the amount of insulin that the body needs at that time. This is a large, bedside machine that also goes by the name "artificial beta cell."

Aspartame
(ăs´păr-tām)

A man-made sweetener that people use in place of sugar because it has very few calories.

Aspiration
(ăs-pĭ-rā´shun)

The act of drawing back on a syringe to see if a needle has been injected into a blood vessel. A person giving an insulin injection may pull back on the plunger of the syringe slightly to check for blood before injecting the insulin.

Asymptomatic
(ā´sĭmp´tō-măt´ĭk)

No symptoms; no clear sign of disease present.

Atherosclerosis
(ath´ĕr-ō´ sklĕ-rō´sĭs)

One of many diseases in which fat builds up in the large- and medium-sized arteries. This buildup of fat may slow down or stop blood flow. This disease can happen to people who have had diabetes for a long time.

Autonomic Neuropathy
(aw-tō-nŏm´ik nyū-rŏp´ah-thē)

A disease of the nerves affecting mostly the internal organs such as the bladder muscles, the digestive tract, and the genital organs. These nerves are not under a person's conscious control and function automatically. *See also:* Neuropathy.

B

Beta Cell
(bā´tah sĕl)

A type of cell in the pancreas in areas called the islets of Langerhans. Beta cells make and release insulin, a hormone that controls the level of glucose (sugar) in the blood.

Beta Cell Transplantation

See: Islet cell transplantation.

Biosynthetic Human Insulin

(bī´ō´sĭn-thĕt´ĭk)

A man-made insulin that is very much like human insulin. *See also:* Human-insulin.

Biphasic Insulin

(bī-fāz´ĭk)

A type of insulin that is a mixture of 70 percent intermediate and 30 percent fast-acting insulin.

Blood Glucose

(blŭd glū´kōs)

The main sugar that the body makes from the three elements of food-proteins, fats, and carbohydrates—but mostly from carbohydrates. Glucose is the major source of energy for living cells and is carried to each cell though the bloodstream. However, the cells cannot use glucose without the help of insulin.

Blood Glucose Meter

(blŭd glū´kōs mē´tĕr)

A machine that helps test how much glucose (sugar) is in the blood. A specially coated strip containing a fresh sample of blood is inserted in a machine, which then calculates the correct level of glucose in the blood sample and shows the result in a digital display. Some meters have a memory that can store results from multiple tests.

Blood Glucose Monitoring

A way of testing how much glucose (sugar) is in the blood. A drop of blood from the tip of a finger or an earlobe is placed on the end of a special strip of paper. The paper strip has a chemical on it that makes it change color according to how much glucose is in the blood. A person can tell if the level of glucose is low, high, or normal in one of two ways. The first is visually by comparing the end of the paper strip to a color chart that is printed on the side of a test strip container.

Instead of comparing the strips to a color chart, some people use a machine (meter). They insert the strips into the meter and read the correct level of glucose in the blood.

Blood testing is often better than urine testing to monitor the levels of blood glucose.

Blood Pressure
(blŭd prĕsh´ŭr)
The force of the blood on the walls of arteries. Two levels of blood pressure are measured—the higher, or systolic, pressure, which occurs each time the heart pushes blood into the vessels, and the lower, or diastolic, pressure, which occurs when the heart rests. In a blood pressure reading of 120/80, for example, 120 is the systolic pressure and 80 is the diastolic pressure. A reading of 120/80 is said to be the normal range. Blood pressure that is too high can cause health problems such as heart attacks and strokes.

Blood-Sampling Devices
A small instrument for pricking the skin with a fine needle to obtain a sample of blood to test for glucose (sugar). *See also:* Blood glucose monitoring.

Blood Sugar
See: Blood glucose.

Blood Vessels
(blŭd vĕs´sĕls)
Tubes that act like a system of roads or canals to carry blood to and from all parts of the body. The three main types of blood vessels are arteries, veins, and capillaries. The heart pumps blood through these vessels so that the blood can carry with it oxygen and nutrients that the cells need or take away waste that the cells don't need.

Borderline Diabetes
(bŏr´dur-līn)
A term no longer used. *See:* Impaired glucose tolerance.

Brittle Diabetes
(brĭt´tul)
A term used when a person's blood glucose (sugar) level often swings very quickly from high to low and from low to high. Also called labile and unstable diabetes.

Bunion
(bŭnýŭn)
A bump or bulge on the first joint of the big toe caused by the swelling of a sac of fluid under the skin. Shoes that fit well can keep bunions from forming. Bunions can lead to other problems such as serious infections. *See also:* Foot care.

C

C.D.E.
(Certified Diabetes Educator)

A health care professional who is qualified by the American Association of Diabetes Educators to teach people with diabetes how to manage their condition.

C-Peptide
(sē pĕp´tīd)

A substance that the pancreas releases into the bloodstream in equal amounts to insulin. A test of C-peptide levels will show how much insulin the body is making.

Callus
(kăl´ŭs)

A small area of skin, usually on the foot, that has become thick and hard from rubbing or pressure. Calluses may lead to other problems such as serious infection. Shoes that fit well can keep calluses from forming. *See also:* Foot care.

Calorie
(kal´ŏ-rē)

Energy that comes from food. Some foods have more calories than others. Fats have many calories. Most vegetables have few. People with diabetes are advised to follow meal plans with suggested amounts of calories for each meal and/or snack. *See also:* Meal plan; exchange lists.

Capillary
(kap´ĭ-lar´ē)

The smallest of the body's blood vessels. Capillaries have walls so thin that oxygen and glucose can pass though them and enter the cells, and waste products such as carbon dioxide can pass back into the blood to be carried away and taken out of the body. Sometimes people who have had diabetes for a long time find that their capillaries become weak, especially those in the kidney and the retina of the eye. *See also:* Blood vessels.

Carbohydrate
(kar´bō-hī´drāt)

One of the three main classes of foods and a source of energy. Carbohydrates are mainly sugars and starches that the body breaks down into glucose (a simple sugar that the body can use to feed its cells). The body also uses carbohydrates to make a substance called glycogen that is stored in the liver and muscles for future use. If the body does not have enough insulin or cannot use the insulin it has, then the body will not be able to use carbohydrates for energy the way it should, and the condition is called diabetes. *See also:* Fats; protein.

Cardiologist
(kar-dē-ŏl´ō-jĭst)
A doctor who sees and takes care of people with heart disease; a heart specialist.

Cardiovascular
(kar´dē-ō-văs´kū-lăr)
Relating to the heart and blood vessels (arteries, veins, and capillaries); the circulatory system.

Chemical Diabetes
(khĕm´ĭ-kŭl)
A term no longer used. *See:* Impaired glucose tolerance.

Chlorpropamide
(klōr´prō´pah-mīd)
A pill taken to lower the level of glucose (sugar) in the blood. Only some people with noninsulin-dependent diabetes take these pills. *See also:* Oral hypoglycemic agents.

Cholesterol
(kŏ-lĕs´tĕr-ŏl)
A fat-like substance found in blood, muscle, liver, brain, and other tissues in people and animals. The body makes and needs some cholesterol. Too much cholesterol, however, may cause fat to build up in the artery walls and cause a disease that slows or stops the flow of blood. Butter and egg yolks are foods that have a lot of cholesterol.

Chronic
(krŏn´ĭk)
Present over a long period of time. Diabetes is an example of chronic disease.

Circulation
(ser´kyū-lā´shŭn)
The flow of blood through the heart and blood vessels of the body.

Coma
(kō´măh)
A sleep-like state; not conscious; can be due to a high or low level of glucose (sugar) in the blood. See also: Diabetic coma.

Comatose
(kō´măh-tōs)

In a coma; not conscious.

Complications of Diabetes
(kŏm-plĭ-kā´shŭns)

Harmful effects that may happen after a person has had diabetes for a long time. These include damage to the retina of the eye (retinopathy), the blood vessels (angiopathy), the nervous system (neuropathy), and the kidneys (nephropathy). Some experts believe that strict control of blood glucose levels may help reduce, delay, or prevent these problems.

Congenital Defects
(kŏn-jĕn´ĭ-tăl dē´feks)

Problems or conditions that are present at birth.

Congestive Heart Failure
(kŏn-jĕs´tĭv)

Heart failure from loss of pumping power by the heart, resulting in fluids collecting in the body. Congestive heart failure often develops gradually over several years, although it also can happen suddenly. It can be treated by drugs and in some cases, by surgery.

Contraindication
(kŏn´trăh-ĭn´dĭ-kā´shŭn)

A condition that makes a treatment not helpful or even harmful.

Controlled Disease

Taking care of oneself so that a disease has less of an effect on the body. People with diabetes can "control" the disease by staying on their diets, by exercising, and by taking medicine if it is needed. This care will help keep the glucose (sugar) level in the blood from becoming either too high or too low.

Coronary Disease
(kor´ŏ-nair-ē)

Damage to the heart. Not enough blood flows through the vessels because they are blocked with fat or have become thick and hard; this harms the muscles of the heart. People with diabetes are at a higher risk of coronary disease.

Coxsackie B4 Virus
(kok-săk´ē vī´rŭs)

An agent that has been shown to damage the beta cells of the pancreas in lab tests. This virus may be one cause of insulin-dependent diabetes.

Creatinine
(krē-ăt´ĭ-nĭn)

A chemical found in the blood and passed in the urine. A test of the amount of creatinine in blood or in blood and urine shows if the kidney is working right or if it is diseased. This is called the creatinine clearance test.

Cyclamate
(sī´klăh-māt)

A man-made chemical that people used instead of sugar. The Food and Drug Administration banned the sale of cyclamates in 1973 because lab tests showed that large amounts of cyclamates can cause bladder cancer in rats.

D

Dawn Phenomenon
(daun fĭ-năm´ĕ-nŏn)

A sudden rise in blood glucose levels in the early morning hours. This condition sometimes occurs in people with insulin-dependent diabetes and (rarely) in people with noninsulin-dependent diabetes. Unlike the Somogyi effect, it is not a result of an insulin reaction. People who have high levels of blood glucose in the mornings before eating may need to monitor their blood glucose during the night. If blood glucose levels are rising, adjustments in evening snacks or insulin dosages may be recommended. *See also:* Somogyi effect.

Debridement
(dă-brēd´mĭnt)

The removal of infected, hurt, or dead tissue.

Dehydration
(dē´hī-drā-shŭn)

Great loss of body water. If a person with diabetes has a very high level of glucose (sugar) in the urine, it causes loss of a great deal of water, and the person becomes very thirsty.

Delta Cell
(dĕl´tăh sĕl)

A type of cell in the pancreas (in areas called the islets of Langerhans). Delta cells make somatostatin, a hormone that is believed to control how the beta cells make and release insulin and how the alpha cells make and release glucagon.

Desensitization
(dē-sĕn´sĭ-tĭ-zā´shŭn)

A method to reduce or stop a response such as an allergic reaction to something. For instance, if a person with diabetes has a bad reaction to taking a full dose of beef insulin, the doctor gives the person a very small amount of the insulin at first. Over a period of time, larger doses are given until the person is taking the full dose. This is one way to help the body get used to the full dose and to avoid having the allergic reaction.

Dextrose
(dĕks´trōs)

A simple sugar found in the blood. It is the body's main source of energy. Also called glucose. See also: Blood glucose.

Diabetes Insipidus
(dī´ah-bē´tēz in-sĭp´ĭd-ŭs)

A disease of the pituitary gland; *not* diabetes mellltus. Diabetes insipidus is often called "water diabetes" to set it apart from "sugar diabetes." The cause and treatment are not the same as for diabetes mellitus. "Water diabetes" has diabetes in its name because people who have it show most of the same signs as someone with diabetes mellitus—they have to urinate often, get very thirsty and hungry, and feel weak. However, they do not have glucose (sugar) in their urine.

Diabetes Mellitus
(dī´ah-bē´tēz mĕl´ĭ-tĭs)

A disease that occurs when the body is not able to use sugar as it should. The body needs sugar for energy for daily activities. It gets sugar when it changes food into glucose (a form of sugar). Diabetes occurs when the body tries to use sugar in the blood for energy—but can't because the pancreas is not able to make enough of a hormone called insulin, or because the body cannot use the insulin it does have. The beta cells in areas of the pancreas called the islets of Langerhans usually make insulin.

There are two main types of diabetes mellitus: *insulin-dependent (type I)* and *noninsulin-dependent (type II)*. In *insulin-dependent* diabetes, the pancreas makes little or no insulin. This type usually appears suddenly, and the person must do three things daily to control the level of glucose in the blood: inject insulin, eat a planned diet, and exercise.

In *noninsulin-dependent* diabetes, the pancreas makes some insulin. A person with this type can sometimes control the disease by eating a planned diet and getting regular exercise. Others may need to take insulin or other medications plus eat a planned diet and exercise daily.

About 90 percent of the people who have diabetes have the *noninsulin-dependent* type. Many also weigh more than they should. Both types of diabetes appear in all age groups, but *noninsulin- dependent* diabetes usually occurs after the age of 40, and *insulin-dependent* usually occurs before age 30.

The signs of diabetes include having to urinate often, losing weight, getting very thirsty, and being hungry all the time. People with untreated diabetes are thirsty and have to urinate often because glucose builds to a high level in the bloodstream and the kidneys are working hard to flush out the extra amount. People with untreated diabetes often get hungry and tired because the body is not able to use food the way it should.

In *insulin-dependent* diabetes, if the level of insulin is too low for a long period of time, the body begins to break down its stores of fat. This causes the body to release acids (ketones) into the blood. The result is called ketoacidosis, a severe condition that may put a person into a coma if not treated right away.

The causes of diabetes are not known. Scientists think that *insulin-dependent* diabetes may be more than one disease and may have many causes. They are looking at heredity (whether or not the person has parents or other family members with the disease) and at factors both inside and outside the body, including viruses.

Noninsulin-dependent diabetes appears to be closely associated with obesity and with the body resisting the action of insulin.

Diabetic Amyotrophy
(ā-mē-ŏt´rō-fē)

A disease of the nerves leading to the muscles. This condition affects only one side of the body and occurs most often in older men with mild diabetes. See also: Neuropathy.

Diabetic Angiopathy
(an-jē-ŏp´ah-thē)

See: Angiopathy.

Diabetic Coma
(kō´măh)

A severe emergency in which a person is not conscious because the blood glucose (sugar) is too high and the body has too many ketones (acids). The person usually has a flushed face; dry skin and mouth; rapid and labored breathing; a fruity breath odor; a rapid, weak pulse; and low blood pressure. See also: Diabetic ketoacidosis.

Diabetic Ketoacidosis (DKA)
(kē´tō-as´ĭ-dō´sis)

Severe, out-of-control diabetes (high blood sugar) that needs emergency treatment. DKA happens when the blood does not have enough insulin because the person is ill, does not take a large enough dose of insulin, or gets too little exercise. The body starts using stored fat for energy, and ketone bodies (acids) build up in the blood.

Ketoacidosis starts slowly and builds up. The signs include nausea and vomiting, which can lead to loss of water from the body, stomach pain, and deep and rapid breathing. If the person is not given fluids and insulin right away, the ketoacidosis can lead to coma and even death.

Diabetic Nephropathy
(nĕ-frŏp´ah-thē)
See: Nephropathy

Diabetic Neuropathy
(nŭr-ŏp´ah-thē)
See: Neuropathy

Diabetic Retinopathy
(rĕt´ĭ-nŏp´ah-thē)

A disease of the small blood vessels of the retina of the eye. When it starts, the tiny blood vessels in the retina become larger, and they leak a little fluid into the center of the retina. The person's sight is blurred from this, and it is called *background retinopathy*. About 80 percent of the people with this leaking never have serious vision problems, and the disease never goes beyond this first stage.

However, at the next stage, the harm to sight can be more serious. Many new, tiny blood vessels grow out and across the eye. This is called *neovascularization*. The vessels may break and bleed into the clear gel that fills the center of the eye, and this blocks vision. Scar tissue may also form near the retina, pulling it away from the back of the eye. This stage is called *proliferative retinopathy*, and it can lead to impaired vision and even blindness. *See also:* Photocoagulation or vitrectomy for treatments.

Diabetologist
(dī´ah-bĕt´ŏl´ō-jĭst)

A doctor who sees and treats people with diabetes mellitus.

Diabetogenic
(dī´ah-bĕt´ŏ-jĕn´ĭk)

Causing diabetes. Certain drugs and some viruses may be diabetogenic.

Diagnosis
(dī´ăg-nō´sĭs)

The term used when a doctor finds that a person has a certain medical problem or disease.

Dialysis
(dī-ăl´ĭ-sĭs)

A method for removing waste such as urea from the blood when the kidneys can no longer do the job. There are two types of dialysis: *hemodialysis* and *peritoneal dialysis*. In *hemodialysis*, the person is connected to a machine (sometimes called an "artificial kidney") that cleans the person's blood by moving it slowly though a tubing system and a series of filters.

In *peritoneal dialysis*, a special solution is run through a tube into the peritoneum, a thin tissue that lines the cavity of the abdomen. The body's waste products are drawn out and removed. This is done in a hospital. A technique called *continuous ambulatory peritoneal dialysis* (commonly known as CAPD) allows this kind of dialysis to be done at home. Both types of dialysis may be used to treat people with diabetes who have a kidney disease.

Diastolic Blood Pressure
(dī´ah-stŏl´ĭk)

See: Blood pressure.

Diet Plan

See: Meal plan.

Dietitian
(dī-ĕ-tish´ăn)

An expert in nutrition who helps people plan the kinds and amounts of foods to eat for special health needs. A registered dietitian (R.D.) has special qualifications.

Diuretic
(dīúr-ĕt´ĭk)

A drug that increases the flow of urine to rid the body of extra fluid.

DNA (Deoxyribonucleic Acid)
(dē-ŏx´sē-rĭ´bō-nū-klā´ik as´ĭd)

A chemical substance in plant and animal cells that tells the cells what to do and when to do it. DNA is the information about what each person inherits from his or her parents.

Double-Voided Urine
(voi´dĭd ū´rĭn)

A sample of urine taken 30 minutes after a person has already emptied the bladder. The second sample is tested for the amount of glucose (sugar) present to check the level of control of diabetes closer to the time of the test. Also called second-voided urine.

E

Edema
(ĕ-dē´mah)

A swelling or puffiness of some part of the body such as the ankles. Water or other body fluids collect in the cells and cause the swelling.

Emergency Medical Identification

Cards, bracelets, or necklaces with a written message used by people with diabetes or other medical problems to alert others in case of a medical emergency such as coma.

Endocrine Glands
(ĕn´dō-krĭn)

Glands that release hormones into the bloodstream. They affect how the body uses food (metabolism). They also influence other body functions. One endocrine gland is the pancreas. It releases insulin so the body can use sugar for energy.

Endocrinologist
(ĕn´dŏ-krĭ-nŏl´ŏ-jist)

A doctor who treats people who have problems with their endocrine glands. The pancreas is an endocrine gland.

Endogenous
(ĕn-dŏj´ĕ-nŭs)

Grown or made inside the body. Insulin made by a person's own pancreas is endogenous insulin. Insulin that is made from beef or pork pancreas or derived from bacteria is exogenous because it comes from outside the body and must be injected.

Enzymes
(ĕn´zīmz)

A special type of protein. Enzymes help the body's chemistry work better and more quickly. Each enzyme usually has its own chemical job to do such as helping to change starch into glucose (sugar).

Epidemiology
(ĕp´ĭ-dē´mē-ŏl´ō-jē)

The study of a disease that deals with how many people have it, where they are, how many new cases are found, and how to control it.

Epinephrine
(ĕp´ĭ-nĕf´rĭn)

One of the secretions of the adrenal glands. It helps the liver release glucose (sugar) and limit the release of insulin. It also makes the heart beat faster and can raise blood pressure; also called adrenalin.

Etiology
(ĕ´tē-ŏl´ō-jē)

The study of what causes a disease; also the cause or causes of a certain disease.

Euglycemia
(ū´glĭ-sē´mē-ah)

A normal level of glucose (sugar) in the blood.

Exchange Lists

A grouping of foods to help people on special diets stay on the diet. Each group lists food in a serving size. A person can exchange, trade, or substitute a food serving in one group for another food serving in the same group. The lists put foods in six groups: (1) starch/bread, (2) meat, (3) vegetables, (4) fruit, (5) milk, and (6) fats. Within a food group, each serving has about the same amount of carbohydrate, protein, fat, and calories.

Exogenous
(eks-ŏj´ĕ-nŭs)

Grown or made outside the body; for instance, insulin made from pork or beef pancreas is exogenous insulin for people.

F

Fasting Blood Glucose Test

A method for finding out how much glucose (sugar) is in the blood. The test can show if a person has diabetes. In a lab or a doctor's office, a blood sample is taken (usually in the morning before breakfast because it is 8 hours or so after eating). If the blood glucose level is in the normal range, it will be from 70 to 110 mg/dL (depending on the type of blood that is tested). If the level is over 140 mg/dL, it usually means the person has diabetes (except for newborns and some pregnant women).

Fats

One of the three main classes of foods and a source of energy in the body. Fats help the body use some vitamins and keep the skin healthy. It is also the major way the body stores energy. In food, there are two types of fats: *saturated* and *unsaturated.*

Saturated fats are solid at room temperature and come chiefly from animal food products. Some examples are butter, lard, meat fat, solid shortening, palm oil, and coconut oil. They tend to raise the level of cholesterol, a fat-like substance in the blood.

Unsaturated fats, which include monounsaturated fats and polyunsaturated fats, are liquid at room temperature and come from plant oils such as olive, peanut, corn, cottonseed, sunflower, safflower, and soybean. These fats tend to lower the level of cholesterol in the blood. *See also:* Carbohydrate; protein.

Fatty Acids

A basic unit of fats. When insulin levels are too low or there is not enough glucose (sugar) to use for energy, the body burns fatty acids for energy. The body then makes ketone bodies, waste products that cause the acid level in the blood to become too high. This in turn may lead to ketoacidosis, a serious problem. *See also:* Diabetic ketoacidosis.

First-Voided Urine

(voi´dĭd ū´rĭn)

The first urine a person passes after a long period of time such as after sleeping.

Fluorescein Angiography

(flū-ŭh-rĕs´ē-ĭn ăn-jē-ŏg´răh-fē)

A method of taking a picture of the flow of blood in the vessels of the eye by tracing the progress of an injected dye.

Food Exchange

See: Exchange lists.

Foot Care

Taking special steps to avoid foot problems such as sores, cuts, bunions, and calluses. Good care includes bathing and looking closely at the feet, toes, and toenails daily and choosing shoes and socks or stockings that fit well. People with diabetes have to take special care of their feet because reduced blood flow sometimes means they will have less feeling in their feet than normal. They may not notice cuts and other problems as soon as they should.

Fractional Urine

(frăk´shŭn-ăl ū´rĭn)

Urine that a person collects for a certain period of time during 24 hours; usually from breakfast to lunch, from lunch to supper, from supper to bedtime, and from bedtime to rising. Also called "block urine."

Fructose
(frŭk´tōs)
A type of sugar found in many fruits and vegetables and in honey. Fructose is used to sweeten some diet foods.

Fundus of the Eye
(fŭn´dŭs)
The back or deep part of the eye, including the retina.

Funduscopy
(fŭn-dŭs´kō-pē)
Looking at the back area of the eye to see if there is any damage to the vessels that bring blood to the retina. The doctor uses a device called an ophthalmoscope to check the eye.

G

Galactose
(găh-lăk´tōs)
A type of sugar found in milk products and sugar beets that is also made by the body.

Gangrene
(gan´grēn)
The death of body tissues. It is most often caused by a loss of blood flow, especially in the legs and feet.

Gastroparesis
(găs-trō-pŭh-rē´sĭs)
A form of nerve damage that affects the stomach. Food is not digested properly and does not move though the stomach in a normal way, resulting in vomiting, nausea, or bloating and interfering with diabetes management. *See also:* Neuropathy.

Gene
(jēn)
A basic unit of heredity. Genes are made of DNA, a substance that tells cells what to do and when to do it. The information in the genes is passed from parent to child—for example, a gene might tell some cells to make the hair red or the eyes brown.

Genetic
(jĕ-nĕt´ĭk)
Relating to genes. *See also:* Gene; heredity.

Gestational Diabetes Mellitus (GDM)
(jĕs-tā´shŭn-ăl)

A type of diabetes mellitus that can occur when a woman is pregnant. In the second half of the pregnancy, the woman may have glucose (sugar) in the blood at a higher than normal level. However, when the pregnancy ends, the blood glucose levels return to normal in about 95 percent of all cases.

Gingivitis
(jĭn-jĭ-vī´tĭs)

An inflammation of the gums that if left untreated may lead to periodontal disease, a serious gum disorder. Signs of gingivitis are inflamed and bleeding gums. *See also:* Periodontal disease.

Gland

A group of special cells that make substances so that other parts of the body can work. For example, the pancreas is a gland that releases insulin so that the cells can use glucose (sugar) for energy. *See also:* Endocrine glands.

Glaucoma
(glăw-kō´măh)

An eye disease associated with increased pressure within the eye. Glaucoma can damage the optic nerve and cause impaired vision and blindness.

Glucagon
(glū´kă-gŏn)

A hormone that raises the level of glucose (sugar) in the blood. The alpha cells of the pancreas (in areas called the islets of Langerhans) make glucagon when the body needs to put more sugar into the blood.

Glucagon for injection is sometimes used when a person is in insulin shock. The glucagon is injected, and it helps raise the level of glucose in the blood. The cells react by using the extra insulin to make energy from the higher amount of glucose in the blood. Commercially available glucagon in the United States is manufactured by Eli Lilly and Company.

Glucose
(glū´kōs)

A simple sugar found in the blood. It is the body's main source of energy; also known as dextrose. *See also:* Blood glucose.

Glucose Tolerance Test
(glū´kōs tŏl´ĕr-ĕns)

A test to see if a person has diabetes. The test is given in a lab or doctor's office in the morning before the person has eaten. The person first gives a sample of blood. Then the person drinks a liquid that has glucose (sugar) in it. Every so often, the person gives a sample of blood again to see how the body deals with the glucose in the blood over time. The test will show if the person has diabetes.

Glycemic Response
(glī-sē´mĭk)
The effect of different foods on blood glucose (sugar) levels over a period of time. Researchers have discovered that some kinds of foods may raise blood glucose levels more than other foods containing the same amount of carbohydrates.

Glycogen
(glī´kŏ-jĕn)
A substance made up of sugars that is stored in the liver and muscles and releases glucose (sugar) into the blood when needed by cells. Glycogen is the chief source of stored fuel in the body.

Glycosuria
(glī´kō-sŭ´rē-ah)
Having glucose (sugar) in the urine.

Glycosylated Hemoglobin Test
(glī-kōs´ă-lā-tĭd hē´mĕ-glō´bĭn)
A blood test that measures a person's average blood glucose (sugar) level for the 2- to 3-month period before the test. *See:* Hemoglobin A_1C.

Gram
A unit of weight in the metric system. There are 28 grams in 1 ounce. In some diet plans for people with diabetes, the suggested amounts of food are given in grams.

H

Hemodialysis
(hē´mō-dī-ăl´ĭ-sĭs)
A mechanical method of cleaning the blood for people who have kidney disease. *See also:* Dialysis.

Hemoglobin A_1C (HbA_1C)
(hē´mĕ-glō´bĭn)
The substance of red blood cells that carries oxygen to the cells and sometimes joins with glucose (sugar). Because the glucose stays attached for the life of the cell, about 4 months, a test of hemoglobin A_1C shows the average blood glucose level for that period of time.

Heredity
(hĕ-rĕd´ĭ-tē)

The passing of a trait such as color of the eyes from parent to child (such as a child being born with blue eyes because one or both parents have blue eyes). A person "inherits" these traits through the genes.

High Blood Pressure

When the blood flows through the vessels at a greater than normal force. High blood pressure strains the heart; harms the arteries; and increases the risk of heart attack, stroke, and kidney problems. Also called hypertension.

Hives (Urticaria)
(ŭr-tĭ-că´rĭ-ah)

A skin reaction with slightly elevated patches that are redder or paler than the surrounding skin and often are accompanied by itching.

HLA Antigens
(an´tĭ-jĕnz)

Proteins on the outer part of the cell that help the body fight illness. These proteins vary from person to person. Scientists think that people with a certain type of HLA antigens are more likely to have insulin-dependent diabetes.

Home Blood Glucose Monitoring

A way a person can test how much glucose (sugar) is in the blood. Also called self monitoring of blood glucose. *See also:* Blood glucose monitoring.

Homeostasis
(hō´mē-ō-stā´sĭs)

When the body is working as it should because all of its systems are in balance.

Hormone
(hŏr´mōn)

A chemical released by special cells to tell other cells what to do. For instance, insulin is a hormone made by the beta cells in the pancreas, and when released, it tells other cells to use glucose (sugar) for energy.

Human Insulin
(hyū´mĕn ĭn´sŭ-lĭn)

Man-made insulins that are very similar to insulin produced by your own body. Human insulin has been available since October 1982.

Hyperglycemia
(hī´pĕr-glī-sē´mē-ah)

Too high a level of glucose (sugar) in the blood; a sign that diabetes is out of control. Many things can cause hyperglycemia. It occurs when the body does not have enough insulin or cannot use the insulin it does have to turn glucose into energy. Signs of hyperglycemia are a great thirst, a dry mouth, and a need to urinate often. For people with insulin-dependent diabetes, this may lead to diabetic ketoacidosis.

Hyperinsulinism
(hī´pĕr-ĭn´ sŭ-lĭn-ĭzm´)

Too high a level of insulin in the blood. This occurs when the body makes too much insulin on its own or when a person takes too much insulin. Too much insulin in the body may cause the blood glucose (sugar) level to go too low. People with this problem may feel shaky, nervous, weak, confused, or sweaty; have a headache; or feel hungry. *See also:* Hypoglycemia.

Hyperlipemia
(hī´pēr-lĭ-pĕ´mē-ah)

See: Hyperlipidemia.

Hyperlipidemia
(hī´pĕr-lĭp´ĭ-dē´mē-ah)

Too high a level of fats (lipids) in the blood.

Hyperosmolar Coma
(hī-pĕr-ŏz-mō´lăr kō´măh)

A coma (loss of consciousness) related to very high levels of glucose (sugar) in the blood and requiring emergency treatment. The person with this condition is usually older and very weak from loss of body fluids and weight. The person may or may not have a previous history of diabetes. Ketones (acids) are not present in the urine.

Hypertension
(hī´pĕr-tĕn´shŭn)

Blood pressure that is above the normal range. *See also:* High blood pressure.

Hypoglycemia
(hī´pō-glī-sē´mē-ah)

Too low a level of glucose (sugar) in the blood. This occurs when a person with diabetes has injected too much insulin, eaten too little food, or has exercised without extra food. A person with hypoglycemia may feel nervous, shaky, weak, or sweaty and have a headache, blurred vision, and hunger. Taking small amounts of sugar, juice, or food with sugar will usually help the person feel better within 10–15 minutes. *See also:* Insulin shock.

Hypotension
(hī-pō-tĕn´shŭn)

Low blood pressure or a sudden drop in blood pressure. A person rising quickly from a sitting or reclining position may have a sudden fall in blood pressure, causing dizziness or fainting.

I

Immunosuppressive Drugs
(ĭm-yū-nō-sŭ-prĕs´ĭv)

Drugs that block the body's ability to fight infection. A person receiving a kidney or pancreas transplant is given these drugs to stop the body from rejecting the new organ or tissue.

Impaired Glucose Tolerance (IGT)
(glū´kōs)

Blood glucose (sugar) levels higher than normal but below the level of someone with diabetes. Even though some persons may have a high level of glucose on the test, they may never develop true diabetes. This used to be called "borderline," "subclinical," "chemical," or "latent" diabetes.

Impotence
(ĭm´pō-tĕns)

The loss of a man's ability to have an erect penis and to emit semen. Some men may become impotent after having diabetes for a long time because the nerves have become damaged. Sometimes the problem has nothing to do with diabetes and may be treated with counseling.

Incidence
(ĭn´sĭ-dĕns)

How often a disease occurs; the number of new cases of a disease among a certain group of people for a certain period of time.

Ingestion
(ĭn-jĕs´chŭn)

Taking food, water, or medicines into the body by mouth.

Injection
(ĭn-jĕk´shŭn)

Putting liquid into the body with a needle and syringe. A person with diabetes injects insulin by putting the needle into the tissue under the skin (called subcutaneous). Other ways of giving an injection are to put the needle into a vein (intravenous) or into a muscle (intramuscular).

Injection Sites

Places on the body where people can inject insulin most easily. These are:

- The outer area of the upper arm.
- Just above and below the waist, except the area right around the navel (a 2-inch circle).
- The upper area of the buttock, just behind the hip bone.
- The front of the thigh, midway to the outer side, 4 inches below the top of the thigh to 4 inches above the knee.

These areas can vary with the size of the person.

Injection Site Rotation

Changing the areas on the body where a person injects insulin. The change keeps lumps or small dents in the skin from forming. These lumps or dents are called lipodystrophies. People who keep track of where they inject the needle can use a written record to chart the sites and can avoid lumps and skin dents by not using the same area too often.

Insulin

(ĭn´sŭ-lĭn)

A hormone that helps the body use glucose (sugar) for energy. The beta cells of the pancreas (in areas called the islets of Langerhans) make the insulin. When the body cannot make enough insulin on its own, a person with diabetes must inject insulin from other sources, i.e., beef, pork, human insulin (recombinant DNA origin), or human insulin (pork-derived, semisynthetic).

Insulin Allergy

(al´ĕr-jē)

When a person's body has an allergic or bad reaction to taking insulin made from pork or beef or from bacteria or because it is not exactly the same as human insulin or because it has impurities.

The allergy can be of two forms. Sometimes an area of skin becomes very red and itchy right around the place where the insulin is injected. This is called a local allergy.

In another form, a person's whole body can have a bad reaction. This is called a systemic allergy. The person can have hives or red patches all over the body or may feel changes in the heart rate and in the rate of breathing. A doctor may treat this allergy by prescribing purified insulins or by desensitization. *See also:* Desensitization.

Insulin Antagonist
(an-tag´ah-nist)

Something that opposes or fights the action of insulin. Insulin lowers the level of glucose (sugar) in the blood, whereas glucagon raises it; therefore, glucagon is an antagonist of insulin.

Insulin Binding

When insulin attaches itself to something else. This can occur in two ways. First, when a cell needs energy, insulin can bind with the outer part of the cell. The cell then brings glucose (sugar) inside and uses it for energy. With the help of insulin, the cell can do its work very well and very quickly. But sometimes the body acts against itself. In this second case, the insulin binds with the proteins that are supposed to protect the body from outside substances (antibodies). The body sees the pork or beef or bacterial insulin as an outside or "foreign" substance, and the insulin then binds with these proteins. When the insulin binds with the antibodies, it does not work as well as when it binds directly to the cell.

Insulin-Dependent Diabetes Mellitus (IDDM)

A chronic condition in which the pancreas makes little or no insulin. The body is then not able to use the glucose (blood sugar) for energy. IDDM usually starts abruptly. The signs of IDDM are a great thirst, hunger, a need to urinate often, and loss of weight. To treat the disease, the person must inject insulin, follow a diet plan, and exercise daily. IDDM usually occurs in children and adults who are under age 30. This type of diabetes used to be known as "juvenile diabetes," "juvenile-onset diabetes," and "ketosis-prone diabetes." It is also called type I diabetes mellitus.

Insulin-Induced Atrophy
(at´rō-fē)

Small dents that form on the skin when a person keeps injecting a needle in the same spot. They are harmless. *See also:* Lipoatrophy; injection site rotation.

Insulin-Induced Hypertrophy
(hĭ´pĕr-trō-fē)

Small lumps that form under the skin when a person keeps injecting a needle in the same spot. *See also:* Lipodystrophy; injection site rotation.

Insulin Pump

A man-made device that pumps insulin into the body all the time at a low (basal) rate. A plastic tube with a small needle inserted under the skin is attached to the body. The pump keeps the level of insulin steady between meals. At mealtimes, the person enters the mealtime dose (bolus) of insulin by pressing the appropriate keys prior to eating. The pump runs on batteries. It is used by people with insulin-dependent diabetes.

Insulin Reaction
(rē-ăk´shŭn)

Too low a level of glucose (sugar) in the blood (hypoglycemia). This occurs when a person with diabetes has injected too much insulin, eaten too little food, or has exercised without extra food. The person may feel hungry, nauseated, weak, nervous, shaky, confused, and sweaty. Taking small amounts of sugar, juice, or food with sugar will usually help the person feel better within 10–15 minutes. ***See also:*** Hypoglycemia; insulin shock.

Insulin Receptors
(rē-sĕp´tŏrz)

Areas on the outer part of a cell that allow the cell to join or bind with insulin that is in the blood. When the cell and insulin bind together, the cell can take glucose (sugar) from the blood and use it for energy.

Insulin Resistance
(rē-zĭs´tăns)

When a person's body will not allow insulin to do what it is supposed to do. The person may take very high daily doses of insulin (200 units or more) or change to a different, more purified insulin to bring the level of blood glucose (sugar) back to normal. Also called "insulin insensitivity." The condition can occur when a person weighs too much and often improves if the person loses weight.

Insulin Shock
(shŏk)

A severe condition that occurs when the level of blood glucose (sugar) drops quickly. The signs are shaking, sweating, dizziness, double vision, convulsions, and collapse. Insulin shock may occur when an insulin reaction is not treated quickly enough. *See also:* Hypoglycemia; insulin reaction.

Insulinoma
(ĭn´sŭ-lĭn-ō´mah)

A tumor of the beta cells in areas of the pancreas called the islets of Langerhans. Although not usually cancerous, such tumors may cause the body to make extra insulin and may lead to a blood glucose (sugar) level that is too low.

Intermittent Claudication
(ĭn´tĭr-mĭt´ĕnt klaw-dĭ-kā´shŭn)

Pain in the muscles of the leg that occurs off and on, usually while walking or exercising, and results in lameness (claudication). The pain results from a narrowing of the blood vessels feeding the muscle. Drugs are available to treat this condition.

Intramuscular Injection
(in´trăh-mŭs´kū-lar)
Putting a fluid into a muscle with a needle and syringe.

Intravenous Injection
(in´trăh-vē´nŭs)
Putting a fluid into a vein with a needle and syringe.

Islet Cell Transplantation
(ī´let sel trans-plan-tā´shŭn)
Moving the beta (islet) cells from a donor pancreas and putting them into a person whose pancreas has stopped producing insulin. The beta cells make the insulin that the body needs to use glucose (sugar) for energy. Although transplanting islet cells may one day help people with diabetes, the procedure is still in the research stage.

Islets of Langerhans
(lang´ĕr-hănz)
Special groups of cells in the pancreas. They make and secrete hormones that help the body break down and use food. Named after Paul Langerhans, the German scientist who discovered them in 1869, these cells sit in clusters in the pancreas. There are five types of cells in an islet: beta cells, which make insulin; alpha cells, which make glucagon; delta cells, which make somatostatin; and PP cells and D cells, about which little is known.

J

Jet Injector
A device that uses high pressure to propel insulin through the skin and into the tissue.

Juvenile-Onset Diabetes
(jōō´veh-nīle ŏn´sĕt dī´ah-bē´tēz)
Former term for insulin-dependent or type I diabetes. *See:* Insulin-dependent diabetes mellitus.

K

Ketoacidosis
(kē´tō-as´ĭ-dō´sĭs)
See: Diabetic ketoacidosis.

Ketone Bodies
(kē´tōn)

Chemicals that the body makes when there is not enough insulin in the blood and it must break down fat for its energy. Ketone bodies can poison and even kill body cells. When the body does not have the help of insulin, the ketones build up in the blood and then "spill" over into the urine so that the body can get rid of them. The body can also rid itself of one type of ketone, called acetone, through the lungs. This gives the breath a fruity odor. Ketones that build up in the body for a long time lead to serious illness and coma. *See also:* Diabetic ketoacidosis.

Ketonuria
(kē´tō-nŭ´rē-ah)

Having ketone bodies in the urine; a warning sign of diabetic ketoacidosis (DKA).

Ketosis
(kē-tō´sĭs)

A condition of having ketone bodies build up in body tissues and fluids. The signs of ketosis are nausea, vomiting, and stomach pain. Ketosis can lead to ketoacidosis.

Kidney Disease
(kĭd´nē)

Any one of several chonic conditions that are caused by damage to the cells of the kidney. People who have had diabetes for a long time may have kidney damage. Also called nephopathy.

Kidneys
(kĭd´nēz)

Two organs in the lower back that clean waste and poisons from the blood. The kidneys are shaped like two large beans, and they act as the body's filter. They also control the level of some chemicals in the blood such as hydrogen, sodium, potassium, and phosphate.

Kidney Threshold

The point at which the blood is holding too much of a substance such as glucose (sugar) and the kidneys "spill" the excess sugar into the urine. *See also:* Renal threshold.

Kussmaul Breathing
(koos´mowl)

The rapid, deep, and labored breathing of people who have ketoacidosis or who are in a diabetic coma. Kussmaul breathing is named for Adolph

Kussmaul, the 19th century German doctor who first noted it. Also called "air hunger."

L

Labile Diabetes

(lā´bīl)

A term used to indicate when a person's blood glucose (sugar) level often swings very quickly from high to low and from low to high. Also called brittle diabetes.

Lactic Acidosis

(lăk´tĭk as´ĭ-dō´sĭs)

The buildup of lactic acid in the body. The cells make lactic acid when they use glucose (sugar) for energy. If too much lactic acid stays in the body, the balance tips and the person begins to feel ill. The signs of lactic acidosis are deep and rapid breathing, vomiting, and abdominal pain. Lactic acidosis may be caused by diabetic ketoacidosis or liver or kidney disease.

Lactose

(lăk´tōs)

A type of sugar found in milk and milk products (cheese, butter, etc.).

Lancet

(lan´sĕt)

A fine, sharp-pointed blade or needle for pricking the skin.

Latent Diabetes

(lā´tĕnt)

Former term for impaired glucose tolerance. *See also:* Impaired glucose tolerance.

Laser Treatment

(lā´zŭr)

Using a special, strong beam of light (laser) to heal a damaged area. A person with diabetes might be treated with a laser beam to heal blood vessels in the eye. *See also:* Photocoagulation.

Lente Insulin

(lĕn´tē)

A type of insulin that is intermediate-acting.

Lipid
(lĭp´ĭd)

A term for fat. The body stores fat as energy for future use just like a car that has a reserve fuel tank. When the body needs energy, it can break down the lipids into fatty acids and burn them like glucose (sugar).

Lipoatrophy
(lĭp´ō-ă-trŏ-fē)

Small dents in the skin that form when a person keeps injecting the needle in the same spot. *See also:* Lipodystrophy.

Lipodystrophy
(lĭp´ŏ-dĭs´trō-fē)

Lumps or small dents in the skin that form when a person keeps injecting the needle in the same spot. Lipodystrophies are harmless. People who want to avoid them can do so by changing (rotating) the places where they inject their insulin. The new, purified insulins may also help. *See also:* Injection site rotation.

M

Macroangiopathy
(mak´rō-ăn´jē-ŏp´ah-thē)

See: Angiopathy.

Macrovascular Disease
(mak´rō-văs´kū-lar)

A disease of the large blood vessels that occurs when someone has had diabetes for a long time. Fat and blood clots build up in the large blood vessels and stick to the vessel walls.

Macular Edema
(măk´ū-lĭr ĕ-dē´măh)

A swelling (edema) in the macula, an area near the center of the retina of the eye that is responsible for fine or reading vision. Macular edema is a common complication associated with diabetic retinopathy. *See also:* Diabetic retinopathy; retina.

Maturity-Onset Diabetes
(măh-tyoor´ĭ-tē ŏn´sĕt dī´ah-bē´tēz)

Former term for noninsulin-dependent or type II diabetes. *See:* Noninsulin-dependent diabetes mellitus.

Meal Plan

A guide for controlling the amount of calories, carbohydrates, proteins, and fats a person eats. People with diabetes can use such plans as the Exchange Lists or the Point System to help them plan their meals so that they can keep their diabetes under control. *See also:* Exchange lists; point system.

Metabolism

(mĕ-tăb´ĕ-lĭzm)

The term for the way the cells chemically change food so that it can be used to keep the body alive. It is a two-part process. One part is called *catabolism*—when the body uses food for energy. The other is called *anabolism*—when the body uses food to build or mend cells.

Mg/dL

Milligrams per deciliter. Term used to describe how much glucose (sugar) is in a specific amount of blood. In self monitoring of blood glucose, test results are given as the amount of glucose in milligrams per deciliter of blood. A fasting reading of 70 to 110 mg/dL is considered in the normal range.

Microaneurysm

(mī´krō-an´yĕ-rĭzm)

A very small swelling that forms on the side of tiny blood vessels. These small swellings may break and bleed into nearby tissue. People with diabetes sometimes get microaneurysms in the retina of the eye.

Microangiopathy

(mī´krō-ăn´jē-ŏp´ah-thē)

See: Angiopathy.

Microvascular Disease

(mī´krō-văs´kyū-lar)

A disease of the smallest blood vessels that sometimes occurs when someone has had diabetes for a long time. The walls of the vessels become abnormally thick but weak, and therefore they bleed, leak protein, and slow the flow of blood through the body. Then some cells, for example, the ones in the center of the eye, may not get enough blood and may be damaged.

Mixed Dose

Combining two kinds of insulin in one injection. A mixed dose commonly combines regular insulin, which is fast acting, with a longer acting insulin such as NPH. A mixed dose insulin schedule may be prescribed to provide both short-term and long-term coverage.

Mononeuropathy

(mŏn´ō-nyū-rŏp´ah-thē)

A form of diabetic neuropathy affecting a single nerve. The eye is a common site for this form of nerve damage. *See also:* Neuropathy.

Morbidity Rate
(mŏr-bĭd´ĭ-tē)
The sickness rate; the number of people who are sick or have a disease compared with the number who are well.

Mortality Rate
(mŏr-tăl´ĭ-tē)
The death rate; the number of people who die of a certain disease compared with the total number of people. Mortality is most often stated as deaths per 1,000, per 10,000, or per 100,000 persons.

Myocardial Infarction
(mī´ō-kŏr´dē-ŭl ĭn-fărk´shŭn)
Also called a heart attack; results from permanent damage to an area of the heart muscle. This happens when the blood supply to the area is interrupted because of narrowed or blocked blood vessels.

N

Necrobiosis Lipoidica Diabeticorum
(nĕk´rō-bī-ō´sĭs lĭ-pōy´dĭk-ah dī´ah-bĕt-ĭ-kōr´ŭm)
A skin condition usually on the lower part of the legs. The lesions can be small or extend over a large area. They are usually raised, yellow, and waxy in appearance and often have a purple border. Young women are most often affected. This condition occurs in people with diabetes, or it may be a sign of diabetes. It also occurs in people who do not have diabetes.

Neovascularization
(nē´ō-văs´kū-lar-ĭ-zā´shŭn)
The term used when new, tiny blood vessels grow in a new place, for example, out from the retina. *See also:* Diabetic retinopathy.

Nephrologist
(nĕ-frŏl´ō-jĭst)
A doctor who sees and treats people with kidney diseases.

Nephropathy
(nĕ-frŏp´ah-thē)
Disease of the kidneys caused by damage to the small blood vessels or to the units in the kidneys that clean the blood. People who have had diabetes for a long time may have kidney damage.

Neurologist
(nyū-rŏl´ō-jĭst)

A doctor who sees and treats people with problems of the nervous system.

Neuropathy
(nyū-rŏp´ah-thē)

Disease of the nervous system. Many people who have had diabetes for a long time have nerve damage. Although nerve damage can affect many parts of the body, it is very common for people with diabetes to have pain in their feet and legs or for those areas to tingle or feel numb. (This is called peripheral neuropathy.) Other forms of nerve damage cause double vision, diarrhea, paralysis of the bladder, and loss of feeling or response during sexual activity for both men and women.

Noninsulin-Dependent Diabetes Mellitus (NIDDM)

The most common form of diabetes mellitus; about 90 percent of the people with diabetes have this kind. Unlike the insulin- dependent type of diabetes, in which the pancreas makes no insulin, people with the noninsulin-dependent type usually have a pancreas that will make some insulin even though it may not be enough. Yet, because some insulin is made, people who have NIDDM can often control it by diet and exercise. If not, they may need to combine insulin or a pill with diet and exercise. Also, some persons with NIDDM make large amounts of insulin but are resistant to its action. Generally, NIDDM occurs in people who are over age 40. Most of the people who have this type are overweight. Noninsulin-dependent diabetes mellitus used to be called "adult-onset diabetes," "maturity-onset diabetes," "ketosis-resistant diabetes," and "stable diabetes." It is also called type II diabetes mellitus.

Nonketotic Coma
(nŏn-kē-tŏt´ĭk kō´măh)

A type of coma caused by not enough insulin. A nonketotic crisis means: (1) very high levels of glucose (sugar) in the blood; (2) absence of ketoacidosis; (3) great loss of body fluid; and (4) a sleepy, confused, or comatose state. Nonketotic coma often results from some other problem such as a severe infection or kidney failure.

NPH Insulin

A type of insulin that is intermediate-acting.

Nutrition
(nū-trĭsh´ūn)

The process by which the body draws nutrients from food and uses them to make or mend its cells.

Nutritionist
(nū-trĭsh´ŭn-ĭst)
See: Dietitian.

Obesity
(ō-bēs´ĭ-tē)
When people have 20 percent (or more) extra body fat for their age, height, sex, and bone structure. Fat works against the action of insulin. Extra body fat is thought to be a risk factor for diabetes.

Obstetrician
(ŏb´stĕ-trĭsh´ŭn)
A doctor who sees and gives care to pregnant women and delivers babies.

OGTT
See: Oral glucose tolerance test.

Ophthalmologist
(ŏph´thăl-mŏl´ō-jĭst)
A doctor who sees and treats people with eye problems or diseases.

Optometrist
(ŏp-tŏm´ĕ-trĭst)
A person professionally trained to test the eyes and to detect and treat eye problems and some diseases by prescribing and adapting corrective lenses and other optical aids and by suggesting eye exercise programs.

Oral Glucose Tolerance Test (OGTT)
Checking to see if a person has diabetes. *See:* Glucose tolerance test.

Oral Hypoglycemic Agents
(hī´pō-glī-sē´mĭk)
Pills or capsules that people take to lower the level of glucose (sugar) in the blood. They work for some people whose pancreas still makes some insulin. The pills can help the body in several ways such as causing the cells in the pancreas to release more insulin.

Six types of these pills are for sale in the United States. Four, known as "first-generation" drugs, have been in use for some time. Two types are called "second-generation" drugs. These drugs have been developed recently. They are stronger than first generation drugs and have fewer side effects. All oral hypoglycemic agents belong to a class of drugs known as sulfonylureas. Each type of pill is sold under two names: one is the generic name as listed by the Food and Drug Administration; the other is the trade name given by the manufacturer. They are:

First-Generation Agents:
Generic Name: Tolbutamide
Trade Name: Orinase
Generic Name: Acetohexamide
Trade Name: Dymelor
Generic Name: Tolazamide
Trade Name: Tolinase
Generic Name: Chlorpropamide
Trade Name: Diabinese

Second-Generation Agents:
Generic Name: Glipizide
Trade Name: Glucotrol
Generic Name: Glyburide
Trade Name: Diabeta, Micronase

Overt Diabetes
(ō-vĕrt´)

Diabetes in the person who shows clear signs of the disease such as a great thirst and the need to urinate often.

P

Pancreas
(păn´krē-us)

An organ behind the lower part of the stomach that is about the size of a hand. It makes insulin so that the body can use glucose (sugar) for energy. It also makes enzymes that help the body digest food. Spread all over the pancreas are areas called the islets of Langerhans. The cells in these areas each have a special purpose. The alpha cells make glucagon, which raises the level of glucose in the blood; the beta cells make insulin; the delta cells make somatostatin. There are also the PP cells and the D_1 cells, about which little is known.

Pancreatectomy
(păn´krē-ah-tĕk´tŏ-mē)

A procedure in which a surgeon takes out the pancreas.

Pancreatic Transplant
(păn-krē-ă´tĭk)

An experimental procedure that involves replacing the pancreas of a person who has diabetes with a healthy pancreas that can make insulin. The healthy pancreas comes from a donor who has just died or from a living relative who can donate half a pancreas and still have enough to take care of his or her own needs.

Pancreatitis
(păn-krē-ah-tī´tĭs)

Inflammation (pain, tenderness) of the pancreas; it can make the pancreas stop working. It is caused by drinking too much alcohol, by disease in the gallbladder, or by a virus.

Peak Action

The time period when the effect of something is as strong as it can be such as when insulin is having the most effect on the glucose (sugar) in the blood.

Pediatric Endocrinologist
(pē´dē-at´rĭk en´dō-krĭ-nŏl´ō-jĭst)

A doctor who sees and treats children with problems of the endocrine glands; the pancreas is an endocrine gland.

Periodontal Disease
(per´ē-ō-dŏn´tal)

Damage to the gums. People who have diabetes are more likely to have gum disease than people who do not have diabetes.

Periodontist
(pĕr´ē-ō-dŏn´tĭst)

A specialist in the treatment of diseases of the gums.

Peripheral Neuropathy
(pĕ-rĭf´ĕr-ăl nyū-rŏp´ ah-thē)

See: Neuropathy.

Peripheral Vascular Disease (PVD)
(pĕ-rĭf´ĕr-ăl văs´kyū-lăr)

Disease in the blood vessels of the arms, legs, and feet. People who have had diabetes for a long time may get this because their arms, legs, and feet do not receive enough blood. The signs of PVD are aching pains in the arms, legs, and feet (especially when walking) and foot sores that heal slowly. Although people with diabetes cannot always avoid PVD, doctors say they have a better chance of avoiding it if they take good care of their feet, don't smoke, and keep both their blood pressure and diabetes under good control.

Peritoneal Dialysis
(pĕr´ĭ-tĕ-nē´ăl dī-ăl´ĭ-sĭs)

A way to clean the blood for people who have kidney disease. *See also:* Dialysis.

Pharmacist
(făhr´măh-sĭst)

A person trained to prepare and distribute drugs and to give information about them.

Photocoagulation
(fō´tō-kō-ag´ū-lā´shŭn)

Using a special, strong beam of light (laser) to seal off bleeding blood vessels such as in the eye. This can also burn away blood vessels that should not have grown in the eye. This is the main treatment for diabetic retinopathy.

Pituitary Gland
(pĭ-tū´ĭ-tair´ē)

An endocrine gland in the small, bony cavity at the base of the brain. Often called "the master gland," the pituitary serves the body in many ways—in growth, in food use, and in reproduction.

Podiatrist
(păh-dī´ah-trĭst)

A doctor who treats and takes care of people's feet.

Podiatry
(păh-dī´ah-trē)

The care and treatment of human feet in health and disease.

Point System

A way to plan meals that uses points to rate foods. The foods are placed in four classes: calories, carbohydrates, proteins, and fats. Each food is given a point value within its class. A person with a planned diet for the day can choose foods in the same class that have the same point values for meals and snacks.

Polydipsia
(pŏl´ē-dĭp´sē-ah)

A great thirst that lasts for long periods of time; a sign of diabetes.

Polyphagia
(pŏl´ē-fā´jē-ah)

Very great hunger; a sign of diabetes. People with this great hunger often lose weight.

Polyunsaturated Fats
(pŏl´ē-ŭn-sătch´ĕr-ā-tĕd)

A type of fat that comes from vegetables. *See also:* Fats.

Polyuria
(pŏl´ē-ŭr´ē-ah)
Having to urinate often; a common sign of diabetes.

Postprandial Blood Glucose
(pōst-prăn´dē-ăl)
Blood taken 1–2 hours after eating to see the amount of glucose (sugar) in the blood.

Preeclampsia
(prē-ĕ-klămp´sē-ah)
A condition that some women with diabetes have during the late stages of pregnancy. Two signs of this condition are high blood pressure and swelling because the body cells are holding extra water.

Prevalence
(prĕv´ah-lĕns)
The number of people in a given group or population who are reported to have a disease.

Previous Abnormality of Glucose Tolerance (PrevAGT)
A term for people who have had above-normal levels of blood glucose (sugar) when tested for diabetes in the past but who show as normal on a current test. PrevAGT used to be called either "latent diabetes" or "pre-diabetes."

Prognosis
(prŏg-nō´sĭs)
Telling a person now what is likely to happen in the future because of having a disease.

Proinsulin
(prō-ĭn´sŭ-lĭn)
The substance made first in the pancreas that is then made into insulin. When insulin is purified from the pancreas of pork or beef, all the proinsulin is not fully removed. When some people use these insulins, the proinsulin can cause the body to react with a rash, to resist the insulin, or even to make dents or lumps in the skin at the place where the insulin is injected. The purified insulins have less proinsulin and other impurities than the other types of insulins.

Proliferative Retinopathy
(prō-lĭf´ĕr-ă-tĭv rĕt´ĭ-nŏp´ah-thē)
A disease of the small blood vessels of the retina of the eye. *See also:* Diabetic retinopathy.

Prosthesis
(prŏs-thē´sĭs)
A man-made substitute for a missing body part such as an arm or a leg; also an implant such as for the hip.

Protein
(prō´tēn)
One of the three main classes of food. Proteins are made of amino acids, which are called the building blocks of the cells. The cells need proteins to grow and to mend themselves. Protein is found in many foods such as meat, fish, poultry, and eggs. *See also:* Carbohydrate; fats.

Proteinuria
(prō´tē-in-ŭ´rē-ah)
Too much protein in the urine. This may be a sign of kidney damage.

Purified Insulins
Insulins with much less of the impure proinsulin. It is thought that the use of purified insulins may help avoid or reduce some of the problems of people with diabetes such as allergic reactions.

PZI (Protamine Zinc Insulin)
(prōt´ah-mēn)
A type of insulin that is long acting.

R

Reagents
(rē-ā´jĕnts)
Strips or tablets that people use to test the level of glucose (sugar) in their blood and urine or the level of acetone in their urine. These reagents are treated with chemicals that change color during the test. Each type of reagent has its own color code to show how much glucose or acetone there is at the time of the test.

Rebound
(rē´bownd)
A swing to a high level of glucose (sugar) in the blood after having a low level. *See also:* Somogyi effect.

Receptors
(rē-sĕp´tŏrz)
Areas on the outer part of a cell that allow the cell to join or bind with insulin that is in the blood. *See also:* Insulin receptors.

Regular Insulin

A type of insulin that is fast acting.

Renal

(rē´năl)

A term that means having something to do with the kidneys.

Renal Threshold

When the blood is holding so much of a substance such as glucose (sugar) that the kidneys allow the excess to spill into the urine. This is also called "kidney threshold," "spilling point," and "leak point."

Retina

(rĕt´ĭ-nah)

The center part of the back lining of the eye that senses light. It has many small blood vessels that are sometimes harmed when a person has had diabetes for a long time.

Retinopathy

(rĕt´ĭ-nŏp´ah-thē)

A disease of the small blood vessels in the retina of the eye. *See also:* Diabetic retinopathy.

Risk Factor

Anything that raises the chance that a person will get a disease. With noninsulin-dependent diabetes, people have a greater risk of getting the disease if they weigh a lot more (20 percent or more) than they should.

S

Saccharin

(săk´ah-rĭn)

A man-made sweetener that people use in place of sugar because it has no calories.

Saturated Fat

(sătch´ĕ-rā´tĕd)

A type of fat that comes from animals. *See also:* Fats.

Second-Voided Urine

(voi´dĭd ū´rĭn)

A sample of urine taken 30 minutes after a person has already emptied the bladder. Also called "double-voided urine."

Secondary Diabetes

When a person gets diabetes because of another disease or because of taking certain drugs or chemicals.

Secrete

(sĕ-krēt´)

To make and give off such as when the beta cells make insulin and then put it out into the blood so that the other cells in the body can use it to turn glucose (sugar) into energy.

Segmental Transplantation

(sĕg-mĕn´tŭl)

A surgical procedure in which a part of a pancreas that contains insulin-producing cells is placed in a person whose pancreas has stopped making insulin.

Self Monitoring of Blood Glucose

A way a person can test how much glucose (sugar) is in the blood. Also called home blood glucose monitoring. *See also:* Blood glucose monitoring.

Semilente Insulin

(sĕm´ĕ-lĕn´tē)

A type of insulin that is fast acting.

Shock

A severe condition that disturbs the body. A person with diabetes can go into shock when the level of blood glucose (sugar) drops suddenly. *See also:* Insulin shock.

Somatostatin

(sō´măh-tō-stă´tĭn)

A hormone made by the delta cells of the pancreas (in areas called the islets of Langerhans). Scientists think it may control how the body secretes two other hormones, insulin and glucagon.

Somogyi Effect

(săh´mō-gē)

A swing to a high level of glucose (sugar) in the blood from an extremely low level, usually occurring after an untreated insulin reaction during the night. The swing is caused by the release of stress hormones to counter low glucose levels. People who experience high levels of blood glucose in the morning may need to test their blood glucose levels in the middle of the night. If blood glucose levels are falling or low, adjustments in evening snacks or insulin doses may be recommended. This condition is named after Dr. Michael Somogyi, the man who first wrote about it. Also called rebound.

Sorbitol
(sŏr´bĭ-tŏl)

A sugar alcohol the body uses slowly. It is a sweetener used in diet foods. It is called a nutritive sweetener because it has four calories in every gram, just like table sugar and starch.

Sorbitol is also produced by the body. Too much sorbitol in cells can cause damage. Diabetic retinopathy and neuropathy may be related to too much sorbitol in the cells of the eyes and nerves.

Spilling Point

When the blood is holding so much of a substance such as glucose (sugar) that the kidneys allow the excess to spill into the urine. *See also:* Renal theshold.

Split Dose

Division of a prescribed daily dose of insulin into two or more injections given over the course of a day. Also may be referred to as multiple injections. Many people who use insulin feel that split doses offer more consistent control over blood glucose (sugar) levels.

Subclinical Diabetes
(sŭb-klĭn´ĭ-kăl)

A term no longer used. *See:* Impaired glucose tolerance.

Subcutaneous Injection
(sŭb´kū-tā´nē-ŭs)

Putting a fluid into the tissue under the skin with a needle and syringe. *See also:* Injection.

Sucrose
(sū´krōs)

Table sugar; a form of sugar that the body must break down into a more simple form before the blood can absorb it and take it to the cells.

Sugar

A class of carbohydrates that taste sweet. Sugar is a quick and easy fuel for the body to use. Types of sugar are lactose, glucose, fructose, and sucrose.

Sulfonylureas
(sŭl´fŏ-nĭl-yŭ-rē´ahs)

Pills or capsules that people take to lower the level of glucose (sugar) in the blood. *See also:* Oral hypoglycemic agents.

Symptom
(sĭmp´tŭm)

A sign of disease. Having to urinate often is a symptom of diabetes.

Syndrome
(sĭn´drōm)

A set of signs or a series of events that alert a person to a health problem.

Syringe
(sĭ-rĭnj´)

A device used to inject liquids into body tissues. The syringe for insulin has a hollow plastic or glass tube (barrel) with a plunger inside. The plunger forces the insulin through the needle into the body. Most insulin syringes now come with a needle attached. The side of the syringe has markings to show how much insulin is being injected.

Systolic Blood Pressure
(sĭs-tŏl´ĭk)

See: Blood pressure.

T

Thrush

An infection of the mouth. In people with diabetes, this infection may be caused by high levels of glucose (sugar) in mouth fluids, which helps the growth of fungus that causes the infection. Patches of whitish-colored skin in the mouth are signs of this disease.

Tolazamide
(tŏl-ăz´ăh-mīd)

A pill taken to lower the level of glucose (sugar) in the blood. Only some people with noninsulin-dependent diabetes take these pills. *See also:* Oral hypoglycemic agents.

Tolbutamide
(tŏl-bū´tăh-mīd)

A pill taken to lower the level of glucose (sugar) in the blood. Only some people with noninsulin-dependent diabetes take these pills. *See also:* Oral hypoglycemic agents.

Toxemia of Pregnancy
(tŏk-sē´mē-ah)

A condition in which poisons such as the body's own waste products build up in the body of a pregnant woman and may cause harm to both the mother and baby. The first signs of toxemia are swelling near the eyes and ankles (edema), headache, high blood pressure, and weight gain that the mother might confuse with the normal weight gain of being pregnant. The mother may have both glucose (sugar) and acetone in her urine. The mother should tell the doctor about these signs at once.

Toxic
(tŏk´sĭk)
Harmful; having to do with poison.

Trauma
(traw´mah)
A wound, hurt, or injury to the body. Trauma can also be mental such as when a person feels great stress.

Triglyceride
(trī-glĭs´ĕr-īd)
A type of blood fat. The body needs insulin to remove this type of fat from the blood. When diabetes is under control and a person's weight is what it should be, the level of triglycerides in the blood is usually about what it should be.

Twenty-Four Hour Urine
The total amount of a person's urine for a 24-hour period.

Type I Diabetes Mellitus
See: Insulin-dependent diabetes mellitus.

Type II Diabetes Mellitus
See: Noninsulin-dependent diabetes mellitus.

U

U-40, U-100
See: Unit of insulin.

Ulcer
(ŭl´sĭr)
A break in the skin; a deep sore. People with diabetes may get ulcers from minor scrapes on the feet or legs, from cuts that heal slowly, or from the rubbing of shoes that don't fit well. Ulcers can become infected.

Ultralente Insulin
(ŭl´trăh-lĕn´tē)
A type of insulin that is long acting.

Unit of Insulin

The basic measure of insulin. U-40 insulin means 40 units of insulin in one (1) milliliter (mL) or cubic centimeter (cc) of solution. U-100 insulin means 100 units of insulin per milliliter or cubic centimeter of solution.

Unsaturated Fats
(ŭn-săt˘u-rāt´ĕd)

A type of fat. *See also:* Fats.

Unstable Diabetes
(ŭn-stā´bĕl)

A type of diabetes when a person's blood glucose (sugar) level often swings very quickly from high to low and from low to high. Also called brittle diabetes or labile diabetes.

Urea
(yū-rē´ah)

One of the chief waste products of the body. When the body breaks down food, it uses what it needs and throws the rest away as waste. The kidneys flush the waste from the body in the form of urea, which is in the urine.

Urine Testing
(ū´rĭn)

Checking urine to see if it contains glucose (sugar) and ketones. Special strips of paper or tablets (called reagents) are put into a small amount of urine or urine plus water. Changes in the color of the strip show the amount of glucose or ketones in the urine. Urine testing is the only way to check for the presence of ketones, a sign of serious illness. However, urine testing is less desirable than blood testing for monitoring the level of glucose in the body. *See also:* Blood glucose monitoring; reagents.

Urologist
(yŭ´rŏl´ŏ-jĭst)

A doctor who sees men and women for treatment of the urinary tract and men for treatment of the genital organs.

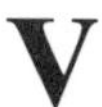

Vaginitus
(văj´ĭ-nī´tĭs)

An infection of the vagina usually caused by a fungus. A woman with this condition may have itching or burning and may notice a discharge.

Women who have diabetes may develop vaginitus more often than women who do not have diabetes.

Vascular
(văs´kyū-lĕr)
Relating to the body's blood vessels (arteries, veins, and capillaries).

Vein
(vān)
A blood vessel that carries blood to the heart. *See also:* Blood vessels.

Vitrectomy
(vĭt-rĕk´tŏ-mē)
Removing the gel from the center of the eyeball because it has blood and scar tissue in it that blocks sight. An eye surgeon replaces the clouded gel with a clear fluid. *See also:* Diabetic retinopathy.

Vitreous Humor
(vit´rē-ŭs hū-mŏr)
The clear jelly (gel) that fills the center of the eye.

Void
To empty the bladder voluntarily in order to obtain a urine sample for testing.

Chapter 2

Diabetes Surveillance

Overview of the Burden of Diabetes Mellitus

Introduction

Diabetes mellitus is a major cause of morbidity and premature mortality in the United States. Diabetes is the most frequent cause of blindness among working-age adults, the major cause of nontraumatic lower-extremity amputation and end-stage renal disease. It is a major cause of congenital malformations, perinatal mortality, premature mortality, disability, and health-care costs. In addition, diabetes is an important risk factor of many chronic conditions, including stroke, ischemic heart disease, and peripheral vascular disease. Uncontrolled diabetes is associated with diabetic ketoacidosis. The disease burden of diabetes and its complications is large, disproportionately affects minority populations, and is likely to increase as minority populations grow and the total population becomes older.

Public health surveillance of diabetes and it complications is critical to increasing the recognition of the burden of diabetes, formulating health care policy, identifying high-risk groups, developing strategies to reduce the burden of this disease, and evaluating progress in disease prevention and

---

Excerpts from *Diabetes Surveillance 1993.* U.S. Department of Health and Human Services, Public Health Service, Centers for Disease Control, 1993. For a complete copy of this report write to: Technical Information Services Branch, National Center for Chronic Disease Prevention and Health Promotion, Rhodes Bldg—Rm 1113, MS-K13, Centers for Disease Control and Prevention, 4770 Buford Highway, N.E., Atlanta, GA 30341–3724.

control. An ongoing surveillance system that systematically collects, analyzes, and disseminates national data on diabetes and its complications has been established by the Centers for Disease Control and Prevention (CDC). This surveillance system uses data sources providing periodic and representative data about the burden of diabetes in the United States. These data sources include vital statistics, the National Health Interview Survey, the National Hospital Discharge Survey, and Medicare claims data for end-stage renal disease.

Unfortunately, the periodic and representative data provided by these sources are insufficient for analyzing national trends in diabetes and its complications among most minority populations. The absence of periodic and nationally representative data with which to monitor trends among these groups is unfortunate because data from special surveys and studies of minority populations reveal that the burden of diabetes among these populations is large. For example, the 1982–1984 age-adjusted prevalence of diabetes among Puerto Ricans in the New York City area and Mexican Americans in the southwest was over twice that for non-Hispanic whites. Age-specific diabetes prevalence for these groups are presented in [Figure 2–1]. Additionally, the age-adjusted prevalence of diagnosed diabetes among Indian Health Service patients was 2.8 times that for the U.S. population. The prevalence of diabetes among American Indians varies by tribe, and the Pima Indians of Arizona have the highest recorded prevalence (approximately 50% of adults ≥35 years of age). Furthermore, not only are racial and ethnic minority populations more likely to have developed diabetes, they are also at greater risk for many of the complications of diabetes.

Data Analysis

This report presents data from CDC's diabetes surveillance system. It contains figures and tables on diabetes prevalence and incidence, mortality, hospitalizations, cardiovascular disease, nontraumatic lower extremity amputation, diabetic ketoacidosis, end-stage renal disease, and disability. In each [instance], the data displayed were limited to specific demographic subgroups for which relatively stable estimates could be obtained. Where possible, we examined trends in diabetes and its complications by age, sex, and race. To improve the precision and reliability of some estimates, more than one year of data was used for some estimates. Typically, these estimates were based on three-year moving averages, where three years of data were used to provide an estimate for the middle year. Also, where possible, estimates were provided by region of the country or by state.

We examined the disease burden of diabetes by using two different methods for calculating rates. First, we calculated rates useful for describing

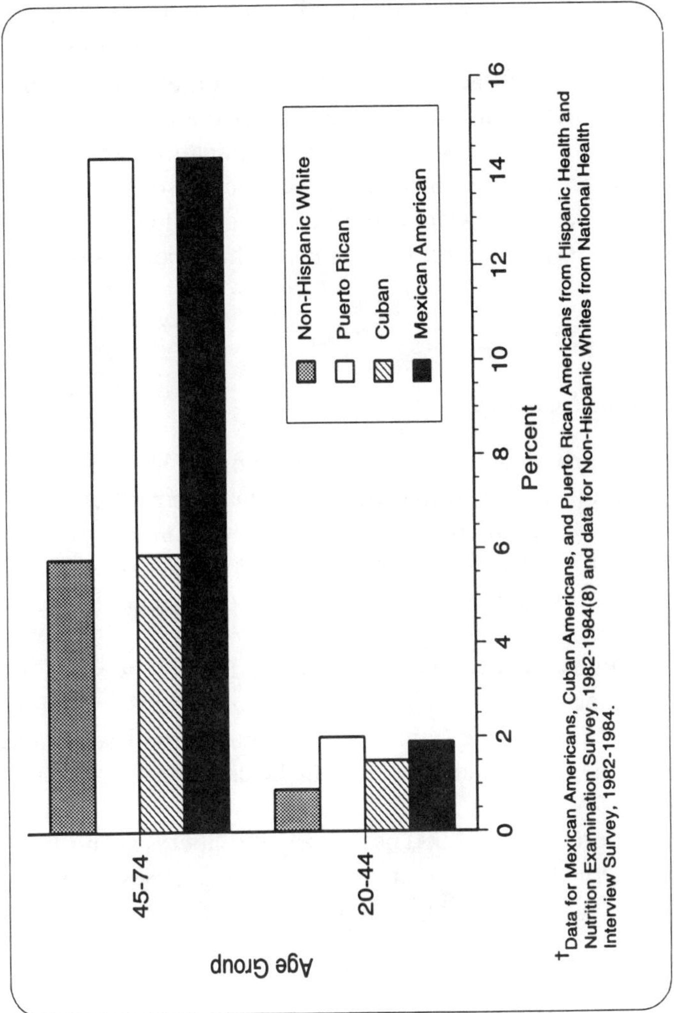

Figure 2.1

Prevalence of Diagnosed Diabetes Per 100 Population by Hispanic Origin,† United States, 1982-1984

the disease burden of diabetes among the U.S. population by using estimates of the resident population of the United States as the denominator. These rates were age-adjusted according to the direct method, and the 1980 U.S. population was the standard. Second, we calculated rates useful for comparing the risk of mortality and diabetic complications among subgroups of persons with diabetes by using estimates of the persons with diabetes as the denominator. These rates were age-adjusted according to the direct method, and the 1980 U.S. population of persons with diabetes was the standard.

Results

Prevalence and Incidence

In 1990, approximately 6.5 million persons in the United States (2.6% of the population) reported that they had diabetes mellitus [see Table 2–1 following the text of this report] and a similar number probably had this disabling chronic disease without being aware of it. Although the prevalence of diabetes has increased since 1959, the rate of increase leveled off during the last decade.

The age-adjusted prevalence of known diabetes was almost twice as great among blacks as whites in 1990, and black females aged 65–74 years had the highest prevalence (almost 21%). During the last decade, the age-adjusted prevalence of diabetes among black males increased 13% [see Tables 2–2; 2–3; 2–4; 2–5].

In 1990, there were 607,000 new cases of diabetes in the United States. The incidence of diabetes increased in the early 1980s, leveled off in the middle of the decade, and then decreased in 1989 and 1990.

Mortality

Mortality in the general population. The annual number of deaths for which diabetes is the underlying cause increased from 34,851 in 1980 to 46,833 in 1990 [See Table 2–6]. Between 1980 and 1988, age-adjusted diabetes mortality rates in the United States remained relatively constant for whites, but increased among blacks. In 1989, age-adjusted diabetes mortality increased 14%. A recent analysis found the large increase in 1989 to be strongly associated with the implementation of the revised 1989 U.S. Standard Certificate of Death and the magnitude of the increase to be associated with the adoption of two revisions to the death certificate designed to improve cause-of-death recording. These revisions were increasing the number of lines on which to report causes of death in Part I from 3 to 4 lines and incorporating instructions or examples for completing the cause-of-death sections (including the use of diabetes as an example of a contributing cause of death to illustrate the proper completion of a death certificate). Although this analysis suggests that the recent increase in diabetes mortality may be due, in large part, to changing cause-of-death certification practices resulting from the implementation of the 1989 U.S. Standard Certificate, data from population-based cohort studies are needed to confirm this hypothesis.

The annual number of deaths for which diabetes was listed as any cause of mortality (diabetes-related deaths) increased from 135,931 in 1980 to 160,848 in 1989. Race-sex temporal trends in age-adjusted diabetes-related mortality were similar to those for diabetes as an underlying cause; rates remained relatively constant for whites but, increased among blacks.

Between 1980 and 1989, diabetes-related mortality rates and mortality rates for diabetes as an underlying cause of death increased with age; the highest rates occurred among persons ≥85 years of age.

Mortality in the diabetic population. Diabetes mortality rates for the general population are affected by differences in diabetes prevalence among demographic groups. Rates using the population reporting to have diabetes in the denominator are useful for comparing the risk of mortality among subgroups of persons with diabetes. When estimates of the diabetic population are used in calculating diabetes mortality rates, racial disparities in mortality for diabetes as an underlying cause of death and as any listed cause of death substantially decrease [see Figure 2–2]. This decrease indicates that these racial disparities resulted from, in large part, the greater prevalence of diabetes among blacks. Mortality due to diabetes as an underlying cause among blacks, however, remained higher than among whites, and black males have the highest rates.

Hospitalizations

In 1990, there were 2.8 million diabetes-related hospital discharges (i.e., discharges listing diabetes as one of the discharge diagnoses), accounting for 24.5 million days of hospital stay. The most frequently listed primary diagnosis among diabetes-related discharges was diseases of the circulatory system (33% of discharges), followed by diabetes (15% of discharges) [see Table 2–7].

In 1990, diabetes as a primary discharge diagnosis accounted for approximately 420,000 hospital discharges, for an average length of stay (LOS) of 7.8 days. Age-adjusted hospital discharge rates with diabetes as a primary diagnosis and the LOS of these discharges have decreased since 1983, the year Medicare's prospective reimbursement system was implemented. Between 1983 and 1990, the decrease in discharge rates per 1,000 diabetic population was greater among whites (50%) than among blacks

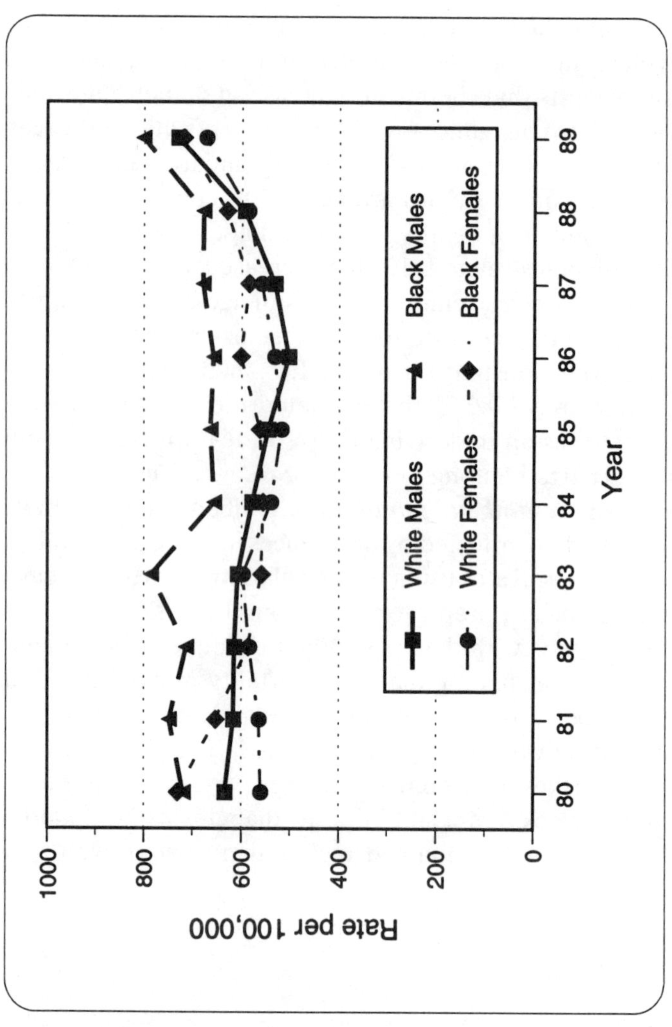

Figure 2.2

Age-standardized Mortality Rates for Diabetes as Underlying Cause of Death per 100,000 Diabetic Population, by Race, Sex, and Year, United States,1980-1989

(30%) and was greater among white females (57%) than among white males (40%).

Although the age-specific rate of diabetes as primary diagnosis per 1,000 persons with diabetes was highest among persons <45 years of age, rates of hospital discharge with diabetes as any listed discharge diagnosis (diabetes-related discharges) increased with age. Temporal trends in the age-adjusted rates of diabetes-related discharges were also different; rates increased in the early eighties, decreased slightly in 1985, and then increased once again. White females were the exception to this trend; they were the only race-sex group whose rates were lower in 1990 than in 1980 [see Figure 2–3].

Cardiovascular Disease

In 1989, about 48% of all diabetes-related deaths had major cardiovascular disease (CVD) listed as the underlying cause of death (n=77,137). Of the deaths attributed to CVD, 62% (n=47,551) were caused by ischemic heart disease (IHD), and 15% (n=11,224) were caused by stroke [see Table 2–8]. Age-specific rates for these diseases increased dramatically with age.

Between 1980 and 1989, age-adjusted mortality rates for stroke decreased 25% (from 220.9 to 165.6 per 100,000 diabetic population). Most of the decrease occurred during the first half of the decade. Between 1982 and 1986, age-adjusted mortality rates decreased 14% for CVD and 16% for IHD and then leveled off. All declines in mortality rates from CVD, IHD, and stroke were apparent among persons with diabetes who were ≥65 years of age. Trends in those younger were less clear.

Of the four race-sex groups examined, white males had the highest age-adjusted mortality rates for CVD and IHD. However, CVD and IHD mortality rates for black males exceeded those for white males among diabetic males <65 years of age, and rates for black females exceeded those for white females among diabetic females <65 years of age. Although age-adjusted mortality rates for stroke displayed less disparity by race and sex, age-specific rates were higher for blacks <65 years of age.

In 1990, about 32% of all diabetes-related hospital discharges had CVD as the primary discharge diagnosis (n=896,000). Age-adjusted rates of hospital discharge for CVD, IHD, and stroke increased between 1980 and 1990, and stroke had the largest increase, 45%. The rate of increase in age-adjusted rates of hospital discharge for CVD and IHD were greater among blacks than among whites, and black females displayed the greatest increase. Although age-specific rates for CVD, IHD and stroke increased with age, the rate of increase among CVD and IHD was greatest among persons <45 years of age.

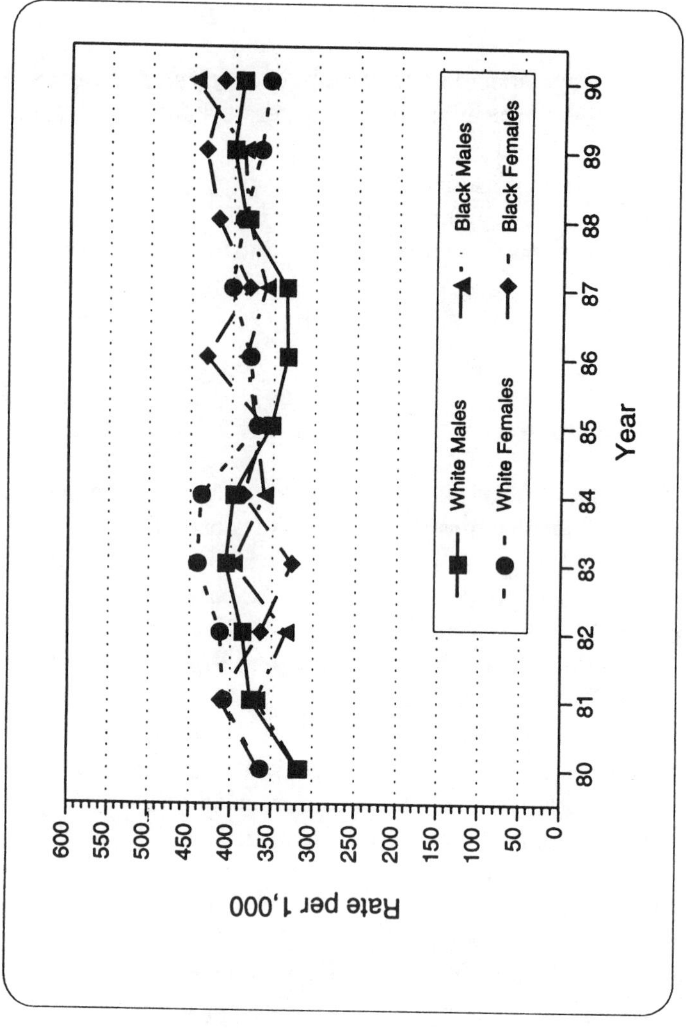

Figure 2.3

Age-standardized Rates of Hospital Discharges with Diabetes as Any Listed Diagnosis per 1,000 Diabetic Population, by Race, Sex, and Year, United States, 1980-1990

Nontraumatic Lower Extremity Amputation

In 1990, there were approximately 54,000 diabetes-related hospital discharges with lower extremity amputation (LEA) as a reported procedure [see Table 2–9]. These discharges accounted for 1.1 million days of hospital stay, for an average LOS of 21 days. The average LOS of LEA discharges decreased through the mid 1980s and then leveled off. The rate of hospital discharge with LEA was relatively stable from 1980 to 1982, increased 44% in 1983, and then leveled off. LEA rates increased with age and were higher among males than females and higher among blacks than among whites [see Tables 2–10; 2–11].

Diabetic Ketoacidosis

In 1990, diabetic ketoacidosis (DKA) was the primary diagnosis for 82,000 hospital discharges and a listed diagnosis on 104,000 hospital discharges. The average LOS for a primary diagnosis of DKA increased with age and averaged 6 days [see Table 2–12]. Hospital discharge rates for DKA as primary diagnosis, however, decreased with age, and diabetic persons <45 years of age had more than 16 times the rate of those ≥65 years of age.

Among the race-sex groups examined, rates were highest among black males, followed by black females, white females, and white males [see Table 2–13]. Age-adjusted DKA rates increased among black males during the latter part of the 1980s, and 1990 rate for black males was more than 3 times the rate for white males (33.7 vs 10.4 per 1,000 diabetic population).

In 1989, DKA was the underlying cause of death for 1,858 deaths. Between 1980–1987, the age-adjusted rates of DKA mortality declined from 30.7 to 24.2 per 100,000 diabetic population and then increased to 28.4 in 1989. The highest DKA mortality rates were among persons ≥75 years of age, followed by persons <45 years of age [see Figure 2–4]. Among the race-sex groups examined, rates were highest among black males, followed by black females and then by whites. In 1990, the age-adjusted DKA mortality rate for black males was nearly twice that for white males (53.2 vs 27.1 per 100,000 diabetic population).

End-Stage Renal Disease

The number of new cases of end-stage renal disease attributable to diabetes (ESRD-DM) increased from 2,220 in 1980 to 13,332 in 1989 [see Table 2–14]. Between 1980 and 1989, the age-adjusted incidence of ESRD-DM among persons with diabetes increased dramatically from 38.51 to 210.43 per 100,000 diabetic population. Age differences decreased during

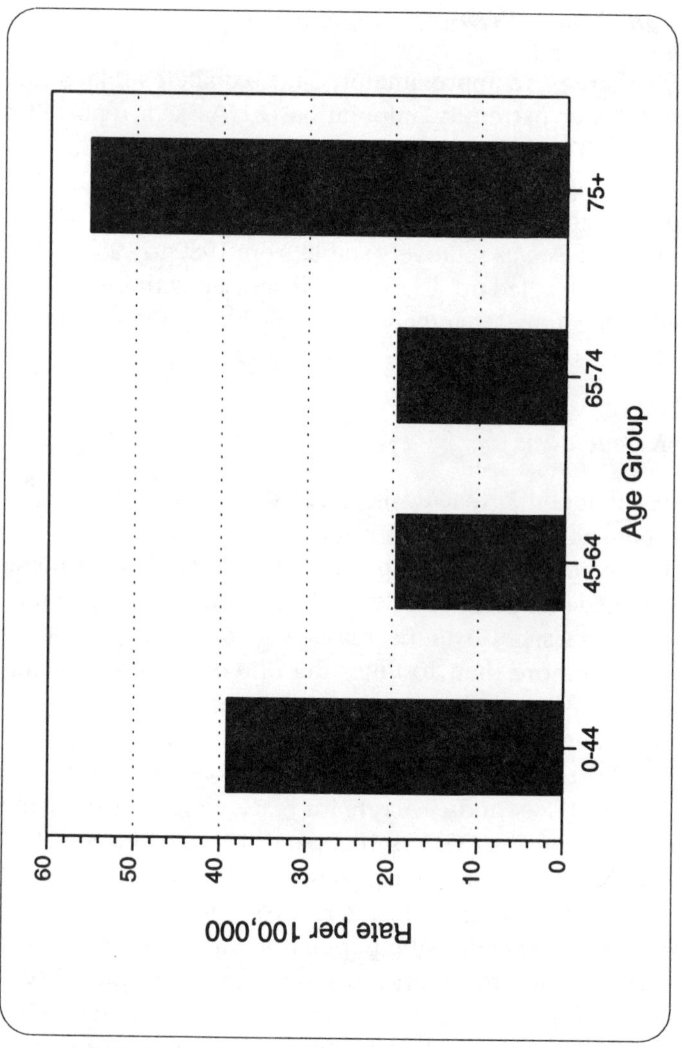

Figure 2.4

Mortality Rates per 100,000 Diabetic Population for DKA as Underlying of Death, by Age, United States, 1989

this decade because incidence increased at a greater rate among the older age groups.

The age-adjusted incidence of ESRD-DM was greater for blacks with diabetes than for whites with diabetes and highest for black females with diabetes. In 1989, the age-adjusted ESRD-DM incidence for black males was 1.6 times that for white males (324.9 vs 199.0 per 100,000 persons with diabetes), and the ESRD-DM incidence for black females was 2.2 times that for white females (356.6 vs 161.1 per 100,000 persons with diabetes).

Disability

Approximately half of all persons with diabetes reported that they were limited in activity (3.3 million in 1990) and about 60% attributed their limitation to diabetes. The proportion reporting that they were limited in activity increased with increasing age, and this proportion tended to level off after age 64 [see Table 2–16]. In general, age-adjusted rates of being limited in activity were higher for blacks than for whites and higher for females than for males [see Figure 2–5].

Between 1983 and 1990, the number of restricted-activity days among persons with diabetes averaged 34 days per year; and half of these days were bed days. The average number of restricted-activity days and bed-rest days were greater among blacks than among whites [see Figure 2–6].

Conclusions

The number of persons known to have diabetes increased by more than 700,000 from 1980 to 1990. The overall rate of increase in diabetes prevalence slowed and reached a plateau in the 1980s. Because the prevalence of diabetes increases with age, the number of persons with diabetes is likely to increase as the population grows older, even if age-specific prevalence were to remain constant. Because non-insulin-dependent diabetes (NIDDM) accounts for 95% of all prevalent cases of diabetes, effective intervention strategies are urgently needed for the primary prevention of NIDDM. These strategies should focus on promoting healthful behaviors such as improved diet, exercise, and weight control among groups at high risk for developing diabetes, including blacks, Hispanics, American Indians, and other minority groups.

Almost half of all diabetes-related deaths and about one third of all diabetes-related hospitalizations were due to major CVD. Thus, reducing CVD risk factors among persons with diabetes could have a major impact on morbidity and mortality. Although no one has studied the effectiveness of CVD risk-factor reduction among diabetic persons, studies have shown

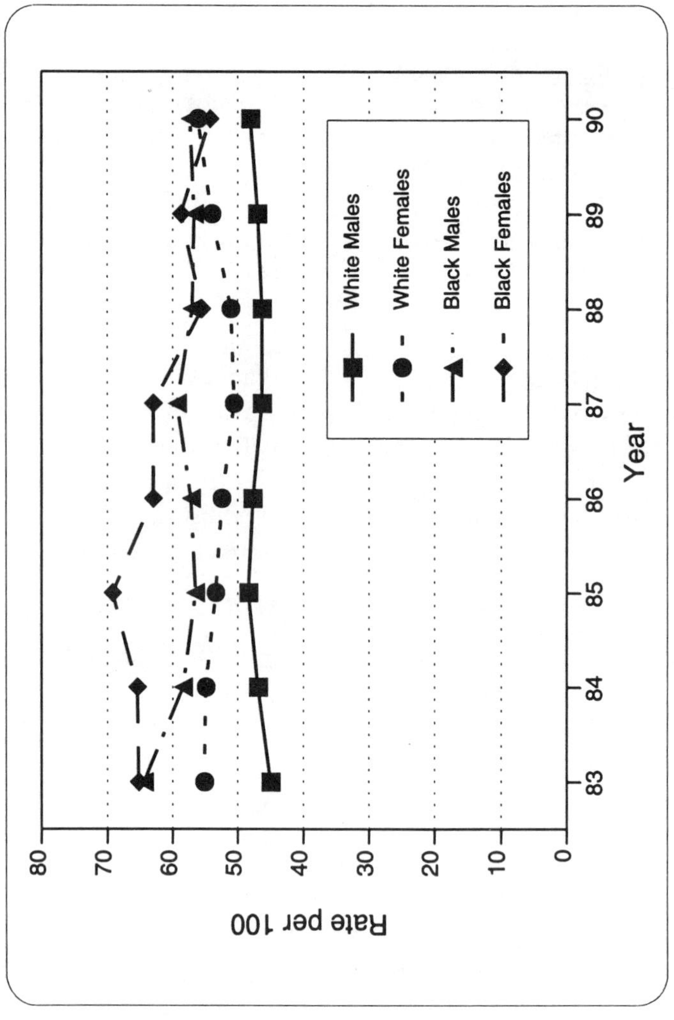

Figure 2.5

Age-adjusted Prevalence of Being Limited in Activity Among Persons with Diabetes per 100 Diabetic Population, by Race and Sex, United States Civilian Noninstitutionalized Population, 1983-1990

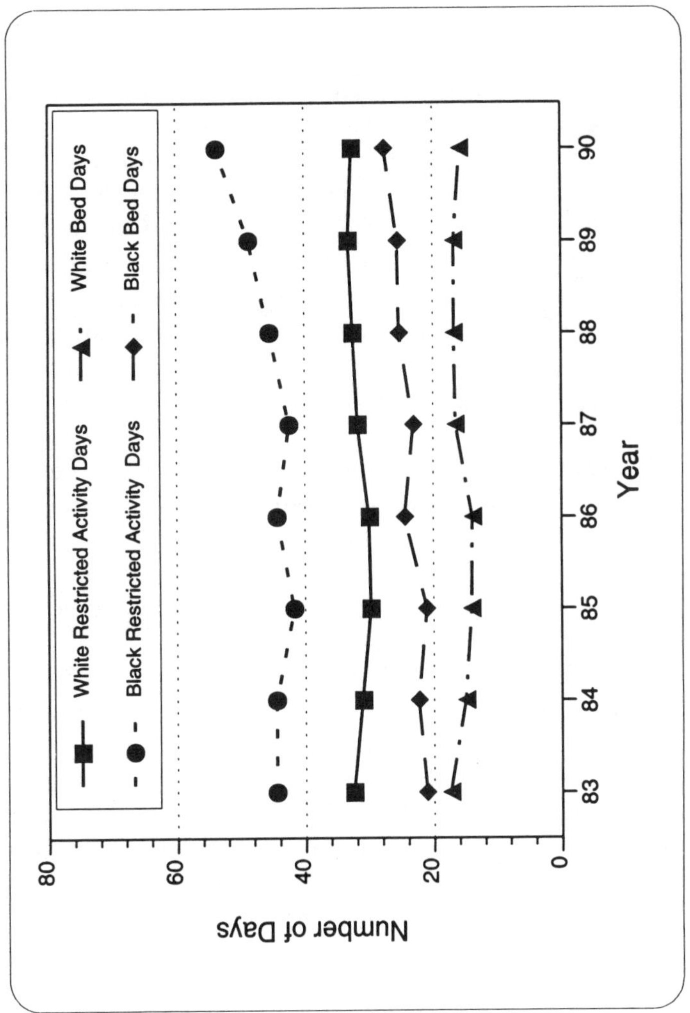

Figure 2.6

Age-adjusted Number of Restricted Activity Days and Bed Days Due to Acute and Chronic Conditions per Diabetic Person, by Race, United States Civilian Noninstitutionalized Population, 1983-1990

CVD risk factors are essentially the same for diabetic and nondiabetic populations. Thus, prevention efforts should promote exercise, weight control, smoking prevention and cessation, hypertension prevention and blood pressure control, and lipid and glycemic control. Diabetes is the leading cause of ESRD in the United States. Our surveillance data indicate the incidence of ESRD-DM has increased dramatically in the 1980s. This increase may be due to increased incidence of disease, increased recognition of the etiologic role of diabetes in ESRD, increased use of treatment, or a combination of these factors. Efforts to prevent and slow the progression of ESRD-DM among persons with diabetes should include controlling hyperglycemia, annual monitoring for early markers of renal disease, controlling hypertension, and identifying and eliminating barriers to preventive care and treatment.

Our surveillance data indicate that the prevalence of disability among persons with diabetes is high. In addition to previously mentioned efforts to reduce risk factors for CVD and kidney disease, efforts to prevent disability should include promoting healthy lifestyles, educating patients and professionals, and incorporating consensus standards of care into health-care delivery systems.

Not only are blacks and other racial/ethnic minorities more likely to develop diabetes, they are also at greater risk for many of the complications of diabetes. Compared to whites, blacks have higher rates of diabetes mortality, DKA mortality, hospital discharges with diabetes and DKA as the primary diagnoses, LEA, ESRD-DM incidence, and disability. For cardiovascular disease, where mortality and hospital discharge rates for whites tended to exceed those for blacks, rates were higher among blacks than whites in the younger age groups. Whether this increased risk of mortality and complications among blacks reflects more severe disease, barriers to health care services (including preventive care services), or a combination of these and other factors remains undetermined. Our surveillance data and other data sources highlight the need to intensify prevention efforts among blacks, Hispanics, American Indians, and other minorities who disproportionately suffer from the burden of diabetes and its complications.

Table 2.1: Prevalence of Diabetes, by Age and Year, United States, 1980–1990

Age Group		1980	1981	1982	1983	1984	1985	1986	1987	1988	1989	1990
0-44	Number[a]	975	981	979	993	1010	1025	1148	1165	1223	1141	1171
	Rate[b]	6.2	6.2	6.1	6.1	6.2	6.2	6.9	6.9	7.2	6.7	6.8
45-64	Number	2466	2497	2561	2496	2415	2494	2551	2584	2546	2472	2498
	Rate	55.4	56.1	57.6	56.1	54.2	56.0	57.2	57.7	56.0	53.9	54.1
65-74	Number	1431	1467	1392	1522	1624	1715	1695	1647	1653	1710	1733
	Rate	91.4	92.4	86.3	92.8	97.8	101.8	99.0	94.5	93.8	95.8	96.0
75+	Number	893	872	878	926	1023	1159	1194	1193	1128	1079	1077
	Rate	88.9	84.5	82.6	84.7	91.0	100.5	100.8	98.0	90.5	84.3	82.6
Total	Number	5765	5817	5810	5936	6072	6392	6588	6590	6550	6402	6478
	Rate	25.4	25.3	25.1	25.4	25.7	26.9	27.4	27.2	26.8	25.9	26.0
Age-adjusted Rate		25.4	25.4	25.1	25.4	25.7	26.7	27.2	26.9	26.4	25.5	25.6

[a] In thousands, three year moving average. [b] Per 1,000 persons, three year moving average.

Table 2.2: Prevalence of Diabetes, by Age and Year, White Males, United States, 1980–1990

Age Group		1980	1981	1982	1983	1984	1985	1986	1987	1988	1989	1990
0-44	Number[a]	339	355	387	382	384	348	423	453	491	432	408
	Rate[b]	5.1	5.3	5.7	5.6	5.6	5.0	6.0	6.4	6.9	6.1	5.7
45-64	Number	968	970	969	900	865	969	1046	1063	1015	940	947
	Rate	51.2	51.3	51.4	47.8	46.0	51.5	55.6	56.3	53.0	48.6	48.7
65-74	Number	569	524	463	475	555	621	657	618	585	602	632
	Rate	92.8	84.3	73.3	73.9	85.1	93.8	97.4	89.8	84.0	85.3	88.7
75+	Number	239	261	285	317	333	359	390	402	353	321	292
	Rate	73.7	78.8	84.0	91.0	93.4	98.1	104.0	104.3	89.1	78.9	70.2
Total	Number	2114	2110	2105	2074	2137	2297	2516	2536	2443	2295	2280
	Rate	22.2	22.0	21.8	21.3	21.8	23.3	25.3	25.3	24.2	22.6	22.3
Age-adjusted Rate		23.2	23.0	22.8	22.3	22.8	26.3	26.4	26.3	24.9	23.1	22.7

[a] In thousands, three year moving average. [b] Per 1,000 persons, three year moving average.

Table 2.3: Prevalence of Diabetes, by Age and Year, White Females, United States, 1980–1990

Age Group		1980	1981	1982	1983	1984	1985	1986	1987	1988	1989	1990
0-44	Number[a]	446	456	432	438	446	508	532	483	468	462	518
	Rate[b]	6.8	6.9	6.5	6.5	6.6	7.5	7.8	7.1	6.8	6.7	7.5
45-64	Number	990	987	1019	1033	1008	1003	972	971	966	971	1002
	Rate	48.1	48.1	49.9	50.7	49.6	49.5	48.1	48.0	47.2	47.2	48.5
65-74	Number	678	716	677	740	772	787	768	751	790	815	811
	Rate	84.9	88.5	82.5	88.8	91.6	92.3	88.8	85.5	89.1	90.9	89.7
75+	Number	550	513	494	494	551	625	607	581	568	570	600
	Rate	92.5	83.8	78.3	76.0	82.5	91.3	86.3	80.5	76.9	75.4	78.1
Total	Number	2663	2672	2622	2704	2777	2924	2878	2785	2792	2819	2931
	Rate	26.6	26.5	25.9	26.5	27.0	28.3	27.7	26.6	26.5	26.6	27.5
Age-adjusted Rate		24.1	24.0	23.4	23.9	24.3	25.3	24.7	23.7	23.5	23.5	24.3

[a] In thousands, three year moving average. [b] Per 1,000 persons, three year moving average.

Table 2.4: Prevalence of Diabetes, by Age and Year, Black Males, United States, 1980–1990

Age Group		1980	1981	1982	1983	1984	1985	1986	1987	1988	1989	1990
0-44	Number[a]	73	64	62	37	55	62	82	90	80	76	52
	Rate[b]	7.4	6.4	6.0	3.5	5.2	5.9	7.6	8.2	7.2	6.7	4.6
45-64	Number	186	184	178	201	210	216	197	201	236	239	248
	Rate	98.7	97.2	93.2	104.2	108.3	110.1	99.8	100.9	116.8	117.3	120.9
65-74	Number	62	67	69	82	84	93	84	96	77	71	49
	Rate	108.1	116.8	120.1	142.7	145.0	159.2	143.3	160.5	128.6	116.7	79.9
75+	Number	29	23	25	24	35	34	39	34	50	54	67
	Rate	103.6	79.3	83.7	79.8	111.6	107.3	119.5	104.4	150.9	159.4	195.0
Total	Number	350	338	333	344	384	405	402	421	443	440	417
	Rate	27.6	26.4	25.6	26.1	28.8	30.0	29.3	30.3	31.5	30.8	28.9
Age-adjusted Rate		36.4	35.0	34.4	36.2	39.7	41.3	40.0	41.1	43.4	42.7	41.0

[a] In thousands, three year moving average. [b] Per 1,000 persons, three year moving average.

Table 2.5: Prevalence of Diabetes, by Age and Year, Black Females, United States, 1980–1990

Age Group		1980	1981	1982	1983	1984	1985	1986	1987	1988	1989	1990
0-44	Number[a]	112	97	86	116	108	91	87	108	134	132	145
	Rate[b]	10.6	9.0	7.9	10.5	9.7	8.1	7.6	9.4	11.4	11.2	12.1
45-64	Number	251	282	319	297	277	254	273	272	235	227	203
	Rate	108.2	120.8	135.6	124.9	115.4	104.8	112.0	110.2	94.2	89.8	79.6
65-74	Number	103	136	159	198	184	180	141	139	151	175	185
	Rate	132.5	172.3	197.9	243.6	224.0	216.6	167.8	163.5	174.6	199.4	208.8
75+	Number	71	71	68	84	93	119	128	149	143	122	105
	Rate	151.2	144.9	134.1	160.1	170.6	211.6	219.7	247.1	230.1	190.6	161.9
Total	Number	538	586	632	695	662	644	629	668	663	655	638
	Rate	38.1	41.0	43.5	47.3	44.5	42.7	41.2	43.2	42.3	41.2	39.7
Age-adjusted Rate		44.3	48.2	51.6	55.6	52.3	50.4	48.4	50.2	48.6	47.5	45.5

[a] In thousands, three year moving average. [b] Per 1,000 persons, three year moving average.

Table 2.6: Number of Deaths with Diabetes as Underlying Cause and Mortality Rates per 100,000 Population, by Age and Year, United States, 1980–1989

Age Group		1980	1981	1982	1983	1984	1985	1986	1987	1988	1989
0-14	Number	53	46	63	51	36	44	36	41	40	53
	Rate	0.1	0.1	0.1	0.1	0.1	0.1	0.1	0.1	0.1	0.1
15-24	Number	128	149	134	129	119	121	140	119	119	136
	Rate	0.3	0.4	0.3	0.3	0.3	0.3	0.4	0.3	0.3	0.4
25-34	Number	572	554	533	584	578	537	634	618	656	687
	Rate	1.5	1.4	1.4	1.5	1.4	1.3	1.5	1.4	1.5	1.6
35-44	Number	900	916	922	1064	1072	1165	1174	1203	1395	1432
	Rate	3.5	3.5	3.3	3.6	3.5	3.7	3.6	3.5	4.0	3.9
45-54	Number	2188	2167	2060	2078	2005	1991	2158	2258	2502	2784
	Rate	9.6	9.6	9.2	9.3	9.0	8.9	9.5	9.8	10.5	11.3

55-64	Number	5789	5620	5643	5900	5495	5819	5780	5914	6109	6942
	Rate	26.6	25.7	25.6	26.7	24.8	26.3	26.3	27.2	28.4	32.7
65-74	Number	10111	9841	9711	10185	9934	10159	10269	10789	11092	13168
	Rate	64.6	62.0	60.2	62.1	59.8	60.3	60.0	61.9	62.9	73.7
75-84	Number	10134	10221	10339	10923	10857	11308	11048	11470	11907	14160
	Rate	130.3	128.1	126.1	129.7	125.6	127.4	121.3	122.6	124.1	143.9
85+	Number	4971	5120	5170	5328	5690	5817	5939	6118	6548	7470
	Rate	219.0	218.5	212.6	212.2	219.9	218.6	217.1	217.4	227.5	252.6
Total	Number	34851	34642	34583	36246	35787	36969	37184	38532	40368	46833
	Rate	15.3	15.1	14.9	15.5	15.2	15.5	15.5	15.9	16.5	19.0
Age-adjusted Rate		15.3	15.0	14.6	15.1	14.6	14.8	14.7	14.9	15.4	17.6

Table 2.7: Distribution of Primary Diagnoses Among All Hospital Discharges with Diabetes as Any Listed Diagnosis, United States, 1990

Primary Diagnosis *(ICD-9-CM Codes)*	**Percent**
Diseases of the Circulatory System *(390-459)*	32.6
Diabetes *(250)*	14.8
Diseases of the Digestive System *(520-579)*	8.6
Diseases of the Respiratory System *(460-519)*	8.5
Diseases of the Genitourinary System *(580-629)*	5.9
Injury and Poisoning *(800-999)*	5.8
Neoplasms *(140-239)*	4.8
Diseases of the Musculoskeletal System and Connective Tissue *(710-739)*	3.7
Other Endocrine, Nutritional, and Metabolic Diseases and Immunity Disorders *(240-279, not 250)*	3.4
Diseases of the Skin and Subcutaneous Tissue *(680-709)*	3.0
Infectious and Parasitic Diseases *(001-139)*	2.2
Mental Disorders *(290-319)*	2.1
Diseases of the Nervous System and Sense Organs *(320-389)*	1.9
Complications of Pregnancy, Childbirth, and the Puerperium *(630-676)*	1.1
Other	1.6

Table 2.8: Number of Deaths with Major Cardiovascular Disease as Underlying Cause and Mortality Rates per 100,000 Diabetic Population, by Age and Year, United States, 1980–1989

Age Group		1980	1981	1982	1983	1984	1985	1986	1987	1988	1989
0-44	Number	834	860	859	955	1057	995	1110	1139	1120	1039
	Rate	85.6	87.6	87.7	96.2	104.6	97.1	96.7	97.7	91.6	91.0
45-64	Number	14931	15201	14875	15248	15246	15317	15205	15100	14813	13958
	Rate	605.5	608.9	580.8	611.0	631.3	614.2	596.0	584.3	581.8	564.7
65-74	Number	23024	22775	22905	23656	23880	24379	23910	24527	24221	23057
	Rate	1608.7	1552.9	1645.0	1554.7	1470.1	1421.8	1410.6	1489.0	1465.7	1348.1
75+	Number	36802	36206	37002	38527	38812	39322	39895	39885	40716	39078
	Rate	4121.3	4151.3	4215.3	4161.7	3795.4	3392.4	3342.5	3343.9	3609.1	3622.4
Total	Number	75594	75044	75657	78397	78999	80023	80129	80658	80876	77137
	Rate	1311.3	1290.2	1302.1	1320.8	1301.0	1251.8	1216.4	1224.0	1234.8	1204.8
Age-adjusted Rate		1311.2	1303.8	1324.6	1308.2	1240.6	1240.6	1139.2	1154.1	1187.2	1152.7

Table 2.9: Number of Nontraumatic Lower Extremity Amputation Hospital Length of Stay (LOS) for Discharges with Diabetes as a Listed Diagnosis, by Age and Year, United States, 1980–1990

Age Group		1980	1981	1982	1983	1984	1985	1986	1987	1988	1989	1990
	Discharges[a]	13	11	12	19	19	23	18	18	22	20	23
0-64	Days[a]	486	368	353	578	549	557	406	385	444	398	468
	Average LOS	37.5	33.2	30.3	31.1	28.5	23.8	22.7	21.7	19.9	20.2	20.6
	Discharges	12	9	9	17	14	16	17	20	13	19	15
65-74	Days	385	335	277	545	395	396	376	416	290	357	265
	Average LOS	33.3	38.3	30.3	31.9	28.1	25.0	22.4	20.4	22.7	19.0	17.3
	Discharges	12	10	10	12	14	14	13	18	20	14	16
75+	Days	423	330	346	414	384	355	272	328	358	249	375
	Average LOS	36.3	33.1	33.8	35.8	27.4	25.9	20.7	18.6	18.2	18.2	23.7
	Discharges	36	30	31	47	47	53	48	56	55	52	54
Total	Days	1295	1033	975	1536	1328	1308	1054	1129	1092	1004	1108
	Average LOS	35.8	34.6	31.4	32.5	28.1	24.7	22.0	20.3	19.9	19.3	20.6

[a] In thousands

Table 2.10: Hospital Discharge Rate for Nontraumatic Lower Extremity Amputation with Diabetes as a Listed Diagnosis per 10,000 Population, by Sex and Year, United States, 1980–1990

Sex		1980	1981	1982	1983	1984	1985	1986	1987	1988	1989	1990
Male	Rate	1.8	1.3	1.3	2.0	1.9	2.1	2.3	2.4	3.0	2.5	2.4
	Age-adjusted Rate	2.0	1.5	1.5	2.2	2.1	2.2	2.5	2.5	3.2	2.6	2.5
Female	Rate	1.4	1.3	1.3	2.0	2.1	2.4	1.7	2.2	1.6	1.8	2.0
	Age-adjusted Rate	1.3	1.2	1.2	1.8	1.9	2.1	1.5	1.9	1.3	1.5	1.7
Total	Rate	1.6	1.3	1.3	2.0	2.0	2.2	2.0	2.3	2.2	2.1	2.2
	Age-adjusted Rate	1.6	1.3	1.3	2.0	2.0	2.2	1.9	2.2	2.1	2.0	2.0

Table 2.11: Hospital Discharge Rate for Nontraumatic Lower Extremity Amputation with Diabetes as a Listed Diagnosis per 10,000 Population, by Race and Year, United States, 1980–1990

Race		1980	1981	1982	1983	1984	1985	1986	1987	1988	1989	1990
White	Rate	1.2	1.2	1.2	1.8	1.6	1.6	1.4	1.7	1.8	1.7	1.7
	Age-adjusted Rate	1.1	1.2	1.1	1.7	1.5	1.5	1.3	1.6	1.7	1.5	1.6
Black	Rate	3.0	2.1	1.6	2.8	3.4	4.6	4.2	3.3	3.1	4.0	2.8
	Age-adjusted Rate	3.9	2.7	1.9	3.6	4.2	5.6	5.2	4.1	3.7	4.6	3.2
Total	Rate	1.6	1.3	1.3	2.0	2.0	2.2	2.0	2.3	2.2	2.1	2.2
	Age-adjusted Rate	1.6	1.3	1.3	2.0	2.0	2.2	1.9	2.2	2.1	2.0	2.0

Table 2.12: Number of Hospital Discharges with Diabetic Ketoacidosis as Primary Diagnosis, Length of Stay (LOS), by Age and Year, United States, 1980–1990

Age Group		1980	1981	1982	1983	1984	1985	1986	1987	1988	1989	1990
0-19	Discharges[a]	16	15	16	20	21	21	21	29	25	21	20
	Days[a]	99	72	71	109	105	98	80	144	111	82	76
	Average LOS	6.2	4.9	4.4	5.3	5.0	4.6	3.8	5.0	4.4	3.9	3.9
20-44	Discharges	21	23	24	31	37	32	37	39	39	35	39
	Days	132	177	151	197	188	184	192	174	199	173	222
	Average LOS	6.3	7.6	6.4	6.3	5.0	5.7	5.2	4.4	5.1	5.0	5.8
45-64	Discharges	12	18	15	12	16	16	16	13	9	12	16
	Days	116	152	206	126	140	119	105	116	93	93	97
	Average LOS	9.4	8.4	14.2	10.8	8.5	7.4	6.5	8.7	10.0	7.9	6.1
65+	Discharges	10	8	6	9	10	11	11	11	10	8	8
	Days	106	127	63	94	97	95	100	77	82	71	96
	Average LOS	10.4	15.4	10.6	11.0	9.4	8.5	8.8	6.8	8.3	8.7	11.4
Total	Discharges	59	64	60	72	85	81	85	93	84	75	82
	Days	452	528	492	526	530	496	477	511	485	418	491
	Average LOS	7.6	8.2	8.2	7.3	6.2	6.1	5.6	5.5	5.8	5.6	6.0

[a] In thousands.

Table 2.13: Number of Discharges with Diabetic Ketoacidosis as Primary Diagnosis and Hospital Discharge Rate per 10,000 Population, by Race, Sex, and Year, United States, 1980–1990

Race, Sex		1980	1981	1982	1983	1984	1985	1986	1987	1988	1989	1990
White Males	Number[a]	16	18	18	17	23	24	23	28	21	16	25
	Rate	1.6	1.8	1.9	1.8	2.3	2.4	2.3	2.8	2.1	1.6	2.4
	Age-adjusted Rate	1.7	1.8	1.8	1.8	2.3	2.4	2.3	2.8	2.0	1.6	2.4
White Females	Number	27	29	24	33	35	32	32	34	28	29	27
	Rate	2.7	2.9	2.4	3.3	3.4	3.1	3.0	3.2	2.7	2.8	2.5
	Age-adjusted Rate	2.7	2.8	2.4	3.3	3.4	3.1	3.0	3.2	2.7	2.8	2.5
Black Males	Number	5	6	6	8	12	6	10	10	12	11	11
	Rate	4.2	4.9	4.3	6.2	9.1	4.8	7.3	7.4	8.8	7.9	8.0
	Age-adjusted Rate	4.8	5.7	4.6	6.1	9.9	4.6	7.5	7.9	8.6	7.9	8.2
Black Females	Number	7	10	7	8	7	11	12	8	11	10	9
	Rate	4.8	6.8	4.6	5.5	4.7	7.1	7.7	5.3	6.9	6.1	5.7
	Age-adjusted Rate	5.0	7.2	4.9	5.7	5.2	7.5	8.1	5.7	6.8	6.0	5.8
Total	Number	59	64	60	72	85	81	85	93	84	75	82
	Rate	2.6	2.8	2.6	3.1	3.6	3.4	3.6	3.8	3.4	3.1	3.3
	Age-adjusted Rate	2.6	2.8	2.6	3.1	3.6	3.4	3.5	3.8	3.4	3.0	3.3

[a] In thousands.

Table 2.14: Number of Persons Initiating Treatment for ESRD Related to Diabetes and Rate per 1,000,000 Population, by Age and Year, United States, 1980–1989

Age Group		1980	1981	1982	1983	1984	1985	1986	1987	1988	1989
0-34	Number	415	615	798	824	950	1053	1080	1077	1018	1204
	Rate	3.2	4.6	6.0	6.2	7.1	7.9	8.1	8.1	7.6	9.0
35-44	Number	334	523	673	808	979	1066	1199	1233	1316	1499
	Rate	12.9	19.8	24.0	27.6	32.1	33.6	36.4	36.0	37.4	41.2
45-54	Number	421	653	919	1042	1179	1401	1553	1683	1897	2245
	Rate	18.5	28.9	41.0	46.6	52.7	62.4	68.6	73.0	79.3	91.2
55-64	Number	598	1017	1430	1703	2044	2282	2527	2859	3142	3593
	Rate	27.5	46.4	64.9	77.0	92.3	103.1	114.9	131.5	146.0	169.1
65-74	Number	375	679	903	1169	1456	1779	2221	2512	2975	3619
	Rate	24.0	42.8	56.0	71.3	87.7	105.7	129.7	144.2	168.8	202.6
75+	Number	77	96	200	250	360	479	576	745	832	1172
	Rate	7.7	9.3	18.8	22.9	32.0	41.5	48.6	61.2	66.7	91.6
Total	Number	2220	3583	4923	5796	6968	8060	9156	10109	11180	13332
	Rate	9.8	15.6	21.3	24.8	29.5	33.9	38.1	41.7	45.7	54.0
Age-adjusted Rate		9.8	15.6	21.2	24.7	29.3	33.6	37.8	41.3	45.1	53.2

Table 2.15: Number of Persons Undergoing Treatment for End-Stage Renal Disease (ESRD) Related to Diabetes, by Race, Sex, and Year, United States, 1980–1989

Race and Sex	1980	1981	1982	1983	1984	1985	1986	1987	1988	1989
White Males	2361	3189	4423	5649	7074	8567	10079	11494	12978	14965
White Females	1767	2620	3748	4939	6135	7425	8816	10260	11737	13669
Black Males	631	915	1275	1725	2148	2777	3341	3818	4457	5090
Black Females	909	1318	1943	2609	3379	4142	4886	5773	6564	7608
Other Race Males	15	41	106	187	268	349	436	541	658	787
Other Race Females	21	57	143	231	312	439	566	655	816	988
Total	6044	8550	11967	15614	19549	23916	28366	32817	37510	43446

Table 2.16: Prevalence of Being Limited in Activity Among Persons with Diabetes by Age and Year, United States Civilian Noninstitutionalized Population, 1983–1990

Age Group		1983	1984	1985	1986	1987	1988	1989	1990
0-44	Number[a]	360	363	376	379	388	389	390	388
	Rate	36.7	36.5	37.3	33.6	33.8	32.2	34.6	33.6
45-64	Number	1252	1256	1329	1358	1354	1299	1312	1341
	Rate	51.1	52.2	53.4	53.1	52.1	50.9	52.8	53.5
65-74	Number	919	972	997	987	914	896	937	975
	Rate	61.7	60.8	58.8	58.7	55.9	54.4	54.9	56.6
75+	Number	572	583	646	604	582	560	577	596
	Rate	64.5	63.3	62.1	56.6	54.8	55.7	60.1	62.5
Total	Number	3103	3174	3348	3328	3239	3144	3217	3301
	Rate	53.4	53.6	53.7	51.7	50.3	49.0	51.2	52.1
Age-adjusted Rate		53.4	53.4	53.4	51.7	50.4	49.4	51.4	52.3

[a] In thousands; three-year moving average

Chapter 3

Diabetes in the United States: A Strategy for Prevention

Foreword

As we better realize the potential that public health offers for improving both the longevity and quality of life, we must also acknowledge how far many Americans, especially those with low incomes, are from achieving that potential. The aging of our society, the prohibitive costs of many of the technologies developed for diagnosing and treating disease, and the ecologic consequences of industrialization and population growth contribute to the magnitude of the challenge we face. To meet such challenges, we can rely in great measure on what we already know about preventing disease and promoting health.

Healthy People 2000: National Health Promotion and Disease Prevention Objectives provides a plan for significantly reducing preventable death and disability, enhancing quality of life, and greatly reducing disparities in the health status of populations within our society. The health of the nation will be measured by the extent to which these indicators are accomplished for all of its people.

Chronic and disabling conditions have a profound effect not only on mortality rates, but also on quality of life. Diabetes imposes a major burden of preventable illness, premature mortality, and excessive financial cost upon persons with diabetes and on the United States as a whole; moreover, it

---

Excerpts from: *Diabetes in the United States: A Strategy for Prevention*, U.S. Department of Health & Human Services, Public Health Service, Centers for Disease Control and Prevention, National Center for Chronic Disease Prevention and Health Promotion, Division of Diabetes Translation, 1993.

imposes a disproportionate and needless burden upon minorities and the elderly.

The Burden of Diabetes in the United States

About 13 million Americans have diabetes, of whom about 6.5 million (about 2.6% of the population) have been diagnosed.

Each year about 651,000 new cases of diabetes are identified.

In 1989, diabetes contributed to more than 160,000 deaths and ranked seventh among leading causes of death in the United States.

Americans with diabetes not only face a shortened life span, but also suffer from many preventable diabetes-related complications each year:

- 54,000 lower-extremity amputations
- 13,332 new cases of end-stage renal disease
- 15,000–39,000 new cases of blindness
- 3.3 million persons with long-term reduction in normal activity
- 2.8 million hospitalizations among persons with diabetes, including 896,000 hospitalizations due to cardiovascular disease.

In 1990, a conservative estimate of about $25.7 billion in direct medical costs and costs resulting from lost productivity was attributed to diabetes.

The Burden of Diabetes Among African Americans

More than 2.1 million African Americans have diabetes, of whom about 1.1 million (about 3.5% of the African American population) have been diagnosed.

The annual number of new cases of diabetes among African Americans is currently unknown.

In 1989, diabetes contributed to more than 23,000 deaths and was the seventh among leading cause of death among African Americans.

African Americans with diabetes not only face a shortened life span, but also suffer from many preventable diabetes-related complications each year:

- 9,000 lower extremity amputations
- 3,625 new cases of end-stage renal disease
- 2,400–6,300 new cases of blindness
- 681,000 persons with long-term reduction in normal activity

- 408,000 hospitalizations among persons with diabetes, including 115,000 hospitalizations due to cardiovascular disease.

The Burden of Diabetes Among Hispanic Americans

In 1989, diabetes was the seventh leading cause of death among Hispanic Americans.

The percentage of Hispanic Americans diagnosed with diabetes varies by subgroup:

- Puerto Rican Americans—5.5%
- Mexican Americans—5.4%
- Cuban Americans—3.6%

The annual number of new cases of diabetes among Hispanic Americans is currently unknown. Additional data are needed.

Hispanic Americans with diabetes not only face a shortened life span, but also suffer from many preventable diabetes-related complications each year. However, reliable national estimates of these conditions are not currently available.

The Burden of Diabetes Among American Indians

About 6.3% of all American Indians 15 years of age and over have diagnosed diabetes. However, this percentage varies widely by tribe. Pima Indians have the highest rate of diabetes ever recorded (34%).

In 1987, diabetes contributed to the deaths of 52 out of every 1,000 American Indians with diabetes.

A reliable estimate of the annual number of diabetes-related hospitalizations among American Indians is unknown. Additional data are needed.

The rate of end-stage renal disease in American Indians with diabetes is at least 2.8 times that for diabetic white Americans.

The Burden of Diabetes Among Elderly Americans

More than 2.8 million Americans, 65 years of age and older (about 9% of this population) have been diagnosed with diabetes.

Between 1985 and 1990, the annual number of new cases of diabetes among Americans 65 years of age and older averaged more than 181,000 new cases each year.

In 1989, diabetes contributed to more than 125,000 deaths and was the fifth leading cause of death among Americans 65 years of age and older.

Elderly Americans with diabetes not only face a shortened life span, but also suffer from many preventable diabetes-related complications each year:

- 31,000 lower-extremity amputations
- 4,791 new cases of end-stage renal disease
- 8,800–22,700 new cases of blindness
- 1.5 million persons with long-term reduction in activity
- 1.6 million hospitalizations among persons with diabetes, including 591,000 hospitalizations due to cardiovascular disease.

A National Strategy for Prevention

Since 1977, the Centers for Disease Control and Prevention (CDC), in response to a congressional mandate, has supported state-based diabetes control programs to prevent and control complications of diabetes. Currently, these funds support efforts in 26 states and one territory.

In 1988, Congress broadened the mandate related to the health burden of diabetes by designating CDC the lead agency for translating and coordinating diabetes research findings into widespread clinical and public health practice. These activities are coordinated by the Division of Diabetes Translation in the National Center for Chronic Disease Prevention and Health Promotion. CDC seeks to reduce the burden of diabetes by targeting four areas:

- Defining the burden of diabetes
- Developing new approaches to reduce the burden of diabetes
- Conducting programs for reducing the burden of diabetes
- Coordinating the translation of diabetes research into practice.

Defining the Burden of Diabetes

National health objectives for the year 2000 have been formulated for diabetes and its complications. To monitor the progress toward achieving these and other indices, a systematic diabetes surveillance system must be established to provide both national and state-based data on the nature and distribution of the burden of diabetes and its complications, including its impact on disability and quality of life. Further, it is necessary to understand why certain segments of our society are particularly at risk for consequences of diabetes.

The ongoing collection and analysis of public health data are critical in formulating policy, identifying high-risk groups, targeting interventions, and evaluating progress in disease prevention and control. Although information related to diabetes morbidity and mortality are contained in several sources and surveys, no nationally unified surveillance system for diabetes and its complications exists.

CDC has begun to identify sources of data and publishes both an annual national surveillance report and summary data on diabetes for individual states. CDC also intends to work with various states and territories to study the feasibility of establishing surveillance systems that will systematically compile, analyze, and interpret national data on diabetes and its complications.

Developing New Approaches for Reducing the Burden of Diabetes

The burden of diabetes affects all ethnic and socioeconomic populations across the United States. Efforts to reduce the burden require not only scientific investigation but also education, and training among persons with diabetes and health professionals who deliver diabetes care. In addition, it is important to establish an equitable and efficient system wherein clinical, public health, and environmental activities can occur to reduce the burden of diabetes. Developing new and transferable programs, approaches, and materials is critical in attempting to reduce the burden of diabetes.

Within the past three years, CDC has taken the lead in developing and disseminating major consensus documents and education materials to promote clinical and public health practice. Recent publications include THE PREVENTION AND TREATMENT OF COMPLICATIONS OF DIABETES: A GUIDE FOR PRIMARY CARE PRACTITIONERS and its companion publication, TAKE CHARGE OF YOUR DIABETES: A GUIDE FOR CARE, which is written in nontechnical language and features illustrations representing various cultural groups and also imparts positive self-care behaviors [For your convenience both these publications are reproduced in this volume; see Chapters 35 and 15.]. TAKE CHARGE OF YOUR DIABETES: A GUIDE FOR CARE has been successfully tested nationally and will be revised to include qualitative evaluation with targeted focus groups. In 1993, we will conduct geographically distinct focus groups of Spanish-speaking persons with diabetes to evaluate and revise a Spanish version of A GUIDE FOR CARE.

CDC has also developed and tested Diabetes Today, a training course for building skills in planning and conducting community-based programs for persons with diabetes. The course will help prepare health professionals, community leaders, and other diabetes advocates to serve as catalysts for mobilizing their resources to reduce the burden of diabetes.

In an effort to focus on economic issues and concerns so relevant to the prevention and treatment of diabetes CDC will attempt to launch pilot projects such as the Comprehensive Financing and Case Management for Medicaid Eligible Persons with Diabetes. This project will focus on comprehensive approaches to financing and delivering health care to persons with diabetes through such mechanisms as prospective reimbursement.

Project DIRECT (Diabetes Intervention: Reaching and Educating Communities Together), formerly known as Community Health Care Models for Diabetes Prevention and Control is an important community-based intervention trial project currently under way in Wake County, North Carolina. Its goal is to demonstrate the effectiveness of community-based public health approaches in reducing the burden, risk factors, and preventable complications of diabetes in communities with large African American populations. Expected to continue for about 10 years, Project DIRECT represents a broad-based, multidisciplinary, multiple agency approach that will define future directions in the prevention and control of diabetes for the CDC and its constituents.

Developing New Approaches for Reducing the Burden of Diabetes

The National Diabetes Advisory Board in its recent annual report to Congress identified this community initiative as an important opportunity for translating diabetes research into public health practice.

As additional resources become available, new education and training programs will be developed and shared with public, private, state and local organizations.

Conducting Programs to Reduce the Burden of Diabetes

CDC's efforts to reduce the burden of diabetes have traditionally focused on treatment of the disease and its complications. CDC recognizes that this focus must expand to include programs targeting the prevention of diabetes and its related complications, while also providing resources and other assistance to additional states and territories attempting to reduce morbidity and mortality associated with diabetes.

CDC has established formal partnerships with state and territorial health agencies to conduct diabetes control programs (DCPs). These state-based DCPs have demonstrated that applying public health interventions at the community level can impact on needless and preventable complications associated with diabetes, both for individuals and entire communities. DCPs provide the basic tools communities need to develop and conduct local programs that address a community' s unique mix of problems, needs and resources. These programs are currently funded at an average level of about $173,000 annually and they remain highly localized within individual states. The DCPs are established in 26 states and one territory. Funding for CDC's state-based programs was last increased in 1985.

All DCPs currently address diabetic eye disease—the single greatest cause of blindness in working-age Americans. At least 60% of all new cases of blindness could be prevented each year through early detection and treatment of diabetes-related eye disease simply by using technology available. Research shows that providing appropriate eye care to persons with diabetes can save more than $165 million annually in federal budgetary outlays. However, CDC's state-based programs are currently reaching fewer than five percent of persons at risk for blindness from diabetic eye disease.

Most DCPs address diabetic lower extremity disease—which causes 54,000 leg, foot, and toe amputations each year among adult Americans. Limb amputations are responsible not only for increased mortality but also for reduced mobility, productivity and quality of life. More than half of these amputations could be prevented with tools already available, thus saving more than $600 million in hospitalizations alone.

Several DCPs also focus programs on prevention of adverse outcomes of pregnancy. In addition, activities to reduce risk factors for diabetes associated cardiovascular disease have been developed by DCPs.

A national public health response to reducing the burden of diabetes would require an expanded network of programs in additional states and territories. The foundation created by the existing DCPs places CDC in a good position to develop and manage that network.

Coordinating the Translation of Diabetes Research into Practice

In 1987, the National Diabetes Advisory Board (NDAB) recommended that the Centers for Disease Control and Prevention (CDC) serve as the lead federal agency for diabetes translation. This leadership role involves maintaining CDC linkages with respected public and private agencies, developing new diabetes control programs, expanding existing ones, coordinating diabetes translation initiatives, developing guidelines for diabetes care, and measuring progress in achieving those guidelines. The Diabetes Mellitus Interagency Coordinating Committee (DMICC), in its responsibilities for translating the results of the National Institutes of Health's Diabetes Control and Complications Trial (DCCT), is an example of how the CDC fulfills the recommendations of the NDAB.

CDC has begun to coordinate diabetes surveillance; assess clinical practice behaviors; analyze data to help identify cost-effective care practices; and understand the relationship between diabetes, disability, and the quality of life.

CDC is pursuing "partnerships" with various organizations throughout the public health community. CDC will continue to nurture partnerships with leading public health organizations such as the American Diabetes Association, the Juvenile Diabetes Foundation, the American Academy of Ophthalmology, the American Association of Diabetes Educators, the American Dietetic Association, and the American Optometric Association. Other efforts to build on existing partnerships will include other state and federal agencies and groups such as CDC's own Technical Advisory Committee, the Association of State and Territorial Health Officials, the American Public Health Association, the Association of State and Territorial Chronic Disease Program Directors, the U.S. Conference of Local Health Officers, the National Association of County Health Officials, Diabetes Research and Training Centers, the Agency for Health Care Policy and Research, the Office of Minority Health, the Indian Health Service, and the National Eye Institute.

CDC has led in the development and distribution of practice guidelines for practitioners, patients, and communities. Further, recognizing the importance of cost implications and economic considerations in chronic disease such as diabetes, CDC will continue to provide leadership for the Finance Coordinating Committee in addressing vital economic issues relevant to diabetes care.

Surveillance data on diabetes clearly indicate that diabetes and its complications disproportionately affect specific segments of the U.S. population. Therefore, CDC will strive to form new partnerships with individuals, agencies, and organizations representing populations at highest risk of diabetes. These will include national organizations and agencies such as the American Association of Retired Persons, the National Congress of Black Churches, the Asian American Health Forum and others.

The Burden of Diabetes for the Individual States

Diabetes imposes a significant health and economic burden on every state and territory throughout the nation.

THE BURDEN OF Diabetes in Alabama

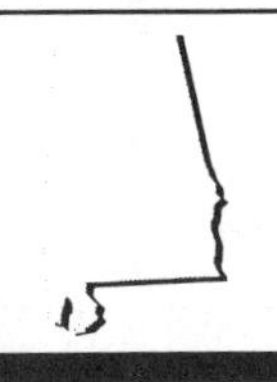

More than 234,000 residents are estimated to have diabetes, only half of whom have been diagnosed.

Number of Persons with Diagnosed Diabetes

Age	*Number*
0-44	19,583
45-64	45,407
65-74	30,870
75+	21,411
Total	***117,271***

Race	*Number*
White	77,579
African American	38,627
Other	1,065

Sex	*Number*
Male	48,558
Female	68,713

Diabetes contributed to the deaths of more than 2,100 residents.

Number of Deaths Due to Diabetes as Underlying or Contributory Cause

Age	*Number*
0-44	71
45-64	426
65-74	605
75+	1,009
Total	***2,111***

Race	*Number*
White	1,368
African American	742
Other	1

Sex	*Number*
Male	836
Female	1,275

Residents with diabetes face not only a shortened life span, but also suffer from many preventable diabetes-related complications each year.

Diabetes-related Conditions per Year

990	lower extremity amputations
234	new cases of end-stage renal disease
282-702	new cases of blindness
59,193	residents with long-term reduction in activity
52,258	hospitalizations
16,628	hospitalizations due to cardiovascular disease among persons with diabetes

In 1990, the direct (medical care) and indirect (lost productivity) cost of diabetes in Alabama was about $458,000,000.

THE BURDEN OF Diabetes in Alaska

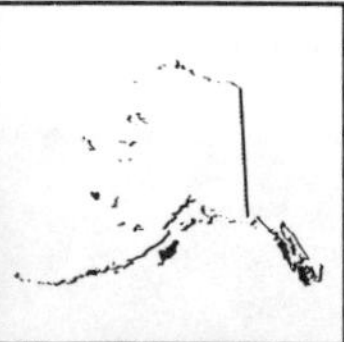

More than 20,000 residents are estimated to have diabetes, only half of whom have been diagnosed.

Number of Persons with Diagnosed Diabetes

Age	*Number*
0-44	3,100
45-64	4,812
65-74	1,587
75+	692
Total	***10,191***

Race	*Number*
White	6,872
African American	430
Other	2,889

Sex	*Number*
Male	4,967
Female	5,224

Diabetes contributed to the deaths of more than 90 residents.

Number of Deaths Due to Diabetes as Underlying or Contributory Cause

Age	*Number*
0-44	7
45-64	24
65-74	34
75+	28
Total	***93***

Race	*Number*
White	75
African American	6
Other	12

Sex	*Number*
Male	46
Female	47

Residents with diabetes face not only a shortened life span, but also suffer from many preventable diabetes-related complications each year.

Diabetes-related Conditions per Year

70	lower extremity amputations
17	new cases of end-stage renal disease
20-61	new cases of blindness
4,801	residents with long-term reduction in activity
3,830	hospitalizations
1,074	hospitalizations due to cardiovascular disease among persons with diabetes

In 1990, the direct (medical care) and indirect (lost productivity) cost of diabetes in Alaska was about $40,000,000.

THE BURDEN OF Diabetes in Arizona

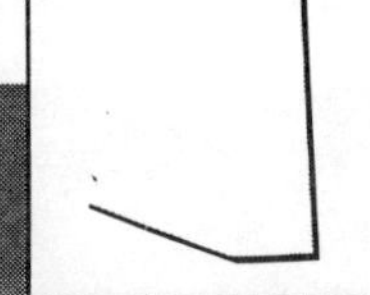

More than 184,000 residents are estimated to have diabetes, only half of whom have been diagnosed.

Number of Persons with Diagnosed Diabetes

Age	*Number*
0-44	17,290
45-64	33,839
65-74	26,529
75+	14,801
Total	***92,459***

Race	*Number*
White	81,832
African American	3,336
Other	7,291

Sex	*Number*
Male	41,139
Female	51,320

Diabetes contributed to the deaths of more than 1,500 residents.

Number of Deaths Due to Diabetes as Underlying or Contributory Cause

Age	*Number*
0-44	69
45-64	345
65-74	478
75+	656
Total	***1,548***

Race	*Number*
White	1,363
African American	55
Other	130

Sex	*Number*
Male	775
Female	773

Residents with diabetes face not only a shortened life span, but also suffer from many preventable diabetes-related complications each year.

Diabetes-related Conditions per Year

762	lower extremity amputations
271	new cases of end-stage renal disease
222-554	new cases of blindness
46,210	residents with long-term reduction in activity
40,531	hospitalizations
12,766	hospitalizations due to cardiovascular disease among persons with diabetes

In 1990, the direct (medical care) and indirect (lost productivity) cost of diabetes in Arizona was about $361,000,000.

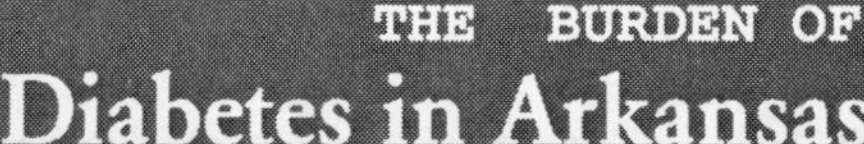

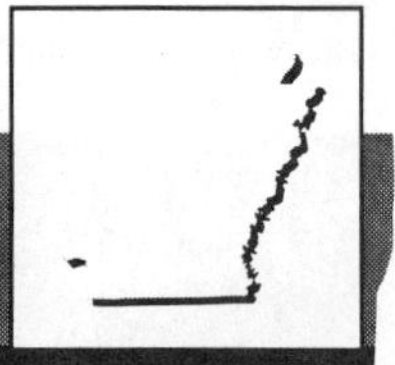

THE BURDEN OF Diabetes in Arkansas

More than 136,000 residents are estimated to have diabetes, only half of whom have been diagnosed.

Number of Persons with Diagnosed Diabetes

Age	*Number*
0-44	10,771
45-64	24,698
65-74	18,937
75+	13,635
Total	***68,041***

Race	*Number*
White	53,161
African American	14,081
Other	799

Sex	*Number*
Male	28,947
Female	39,094

Diabetes contributed to the deaths of more than 1,400 residents.

Number of Deaths Due to Diabetes as Underlying or Contributory Cause

Age	*Number*
0-44	46
45-64	278
65-74	401
75+	723
Total	***1,448***

Race	*Number*
White	1,146
African American	301
Other	1

Sex	*Number*
Male	609
Female	839

Residents with diabetes face not only a shortened life span, but also suffer from many preventable diabetes-related complications each year.

Diabetes-related Conditions per Year

587	lower extremity amputations
115	new cases of end-stage renal disease
167-407	new cases of blindness
34,563	residents with long-term reduction in activity
31,006	hospitalizations
9,957	hospitalizations due to cardiovascular disease among persons with diabetes

In 1990, the direct (medical care) and indirect (lost productivity) cost of diabetes in Arkansas was about $266,000,000.

THE BURDEN OF Diabetes in California

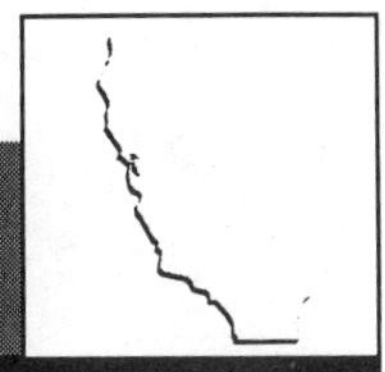

More than 1,456,000 residents are estimated to have diabetes, only half of whom have been diagnosed.

Number of Persons with Diagnosed Diabetes

Age	Number
0-44	148,991
45-64	291,043
65-74	180,250
75+	108,427
Total	***728,711***

Race	Number
White	547,654
African American	74,329
Other	106,728

Sex	Number
Male	322,373
Female	406,338

Diabetes contributed to the deaths of more than 16,500 residents.

Number of Deaths Due to Diabetes as Underlying or Contributory Cause

Age	Number
0-44	479
45-64	3,385
65-74	4,940
75+	7,782
Total	***16,587***

Race	Number
White	13,811
African American	1,871
Other	905

Sex	Number
Male	7,746
Female	8,841

Residents with diabetes face not only a shortened life span, but also suffer from many preventable diabetes-related complications each year.

Diabetes-related Conditions per Year

5,856	lower extremity amputations
1,696	new cases of end-stage renal disease
1688-4364	new cases of blindness
361,078	residents with long-term reduction in activity
311,412	hospitalizations
96,416	hospitalizations due to cardiovascular disease among persons with diabetes

In 1990, the direct (medical care) and indirect (lost productivity) cost of diabetes in California was about $2,849,000,000.

THE BURDEN OF

Diabetes in Colorado

More than 148,000 residents are estimated to have diabetes, only half of whom have been diagnosed.

Number of Persons with Diagnosed Diabetes

Age	Number
0-44	15,989
45-64	30,096
65-74	17,830
75+	10,493
Total	***74,408***

Race	Number
White	67,782
African American	4,000
Other	2,626

Sex	Number
Male	33,130
Female	41,278

Diabetes contributed to the deaths of more than 1,300 residents.

Number of Deaths Due to Diabetes as Underlying or Contributory Cause

Age	Number
0-44	34
45-64	242
65-74	367
75+	746
Total	***1,389***

Race	Number
White	1,304
African American	70
Other	15

Sex	Number
Male	647
Female	742

Residents with diabetes face not only a shortened life span, but also suffer from many preventable diabetes-related complications each year.

Diabetes-related Conditions per Year

590	lower extremity amputations
159	new cases of end-stage renal disease
170-446	new cases of blindness
36,686	residents with long-term reduction in activity
31,438	hospitalizations
9,652	hospitalizations due to cardiovascular disease among persons with diabetes

In 1990, the direct (medical care) and indirect (lost productivity) cost of diabetes in Colorado was about $291,000,000.

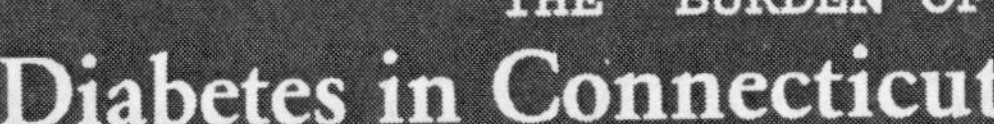

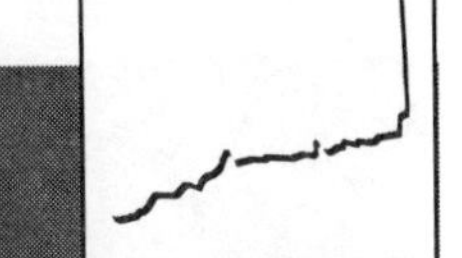

THE BURDEN OF Diabetes in Connecticut

More than 174,000 residents are estimated to have diabetes, only half of whom have been diagnosed.

Number of Persons with Diagnosed Diabetes

Age	*Number*
0-44	14,961
45-64	34,080
65-74	23,624
75+	14,834
Total	***87,499***

Race	*Number*
White	77,080
African American	8,846
Other	1,573

Sex	*Number*
Male	37,698
Female	49,801

Diabetes contributed to the deaths of more than 2,400 residents.

Number of Deaths Due to Diabetes as Underlying or Contributory Cause

Age	*Number*
0-44	57
45-64	444
65-74	685
75+	1,221
Total	***2,407***

Race	*Number*
White	2,208
African American	187
Other	12

Sex	*Number*
Male	1,148
Female	1,259

Residents with diabetes face not only a shortened life span, but also suffer from many preventable diabetes-related complications each year.

Diabetes-related Conditions per Year

730	lower extremity amputations
166	new cases of end-stage renal disease
209-524	new cases of blindness
44,011	residents with long-term reduction in activity
38,571	hospitalizations
12,231	hospitalizations due to cardiovascular disease among persons with diabetes

In 1990, the direct (medical care) and indirect (lost productivity) cost of diabetes in Connecticut was about $342,000,000.

THE BURDEN OF Diabetes in Delaware

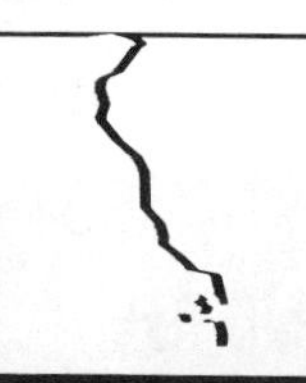

More than 34,000 residents are estimated to have diabetes, only half of whom have been diagnosed.

Number of Persons with Diagnosed Diabetes

Age	*Number*
0-44	3,204
45-64	7,154
65-74	4,780
75+	2,661
Total	***17,799***

Race	*Number*
White	13,619
African American	3,830
Other	350

Sex	*Number*
Male	7,702
Female	10,097

Diabetes contributed to the deaths of more than 620 residents.

Number of Deaths Due to Diabetes as Underlying or Contributory Cause

Age	*Number*
0-44	17
45-64	139
65-74	208
75+	263
Total	***627***

Race	*Number*
White	483
African American	142
Other	2

Sex	*Number*
Male	274
Female	353

Residents with diabetes face not only a shortened life span, but also suffer from many preventable diabetes-related complications each year.

Diabetes-related Conditions per Year

145	lower extremity amputations
53	new cases of end-stage renal disease
42-107	new cases of blindness
8,894	residents with long-term reduction in activity
7,683	hospitalizations
2,415	hospitalizations due to cardiovascular disease among persons with diabetes

In 1990, the direct (medical care) and indirect (lost productivity) cost of diabetes in Delaware was about $70,000,000.

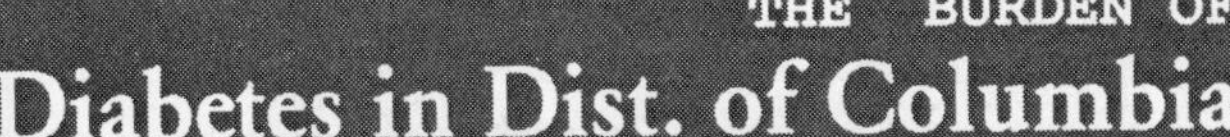
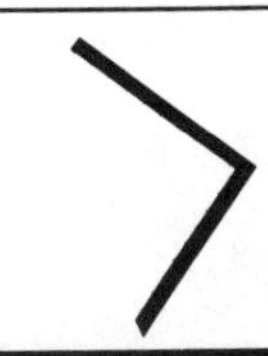

THE BURDEN OF

Diabetes in Dist. of Columbia

More than 46,000 residents are estimated to have diabetes, only half of whom have been diagnosed.

Number of Persons with Diagnosed Diabetes

Age	*Number*
0-44	3,301
45-64	9,310
65-74	6,183
75+	4,465
Total	***23,259***

Race	*Number*
White	4,522
African American	18,281
Other	456

Sex	*Number*
Male	9,023
Female	14,236

Diabetes contributed to the deaths of more than 490 residents.

Number of Deaths Due to Diabetes as Underlying or Contributory Cause

Age	*Number*
0-44	15
45-64	123
65-74	159
75+	191
Total	***490***

Race	*Number*
White	99
African American	389
Other	2

Sex	*Number*
Male	219
Female	271

Residents with diabetes face not only a shortened life span, but also suffer from many preventable diabetes-related complications each year.

Diabetes-related Conditions per Year

200	lower extremity amputations
59	new cases of end-stage renal disease
57-139	new cases of blindness
11,853	residents with long-term reduction in activity
10,493	hospitalizations
3,383	hospitalizations due to cardiovascular disease among persons with diabetes.

In 1990, the direct (medical care) and indirect (lost productivity) cost of diabetes in Dist. of Columbia was about $91,000,000.

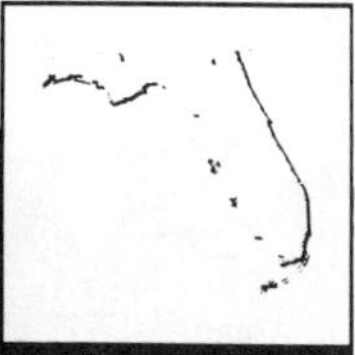

THE BURDEN OF Diabetes in Florida

More than 802,000 residents are estimated to have diabetes, only half of whom have been diagnosed.

Number of Persons with Diagnosed Diabetes

Age	*Number*
0-44	55,732
45-64	138,422
65-74	127,278
75+	79,579
Total	***401,011***

Race	*Number*
White	337,190
African American	58,006
Other	5,815

Sex	*Number*
Male	174,234
Female	226,777

Diabetes contributed to the deaths of more than 8,000 residents.

Number of Deaths Due to Diabetes as Underlying or Contributory Cause

Age	*Number*
0-44	218
45-64	1,437
65-74	2,363
75+	4,042
Total	***8,061***

Race	*Number*
White	6,867
African American	1,171
Other	23

Sex	*Number*
Male	3,976
Female	4,085

Residents with diabetes face not only a shortened life span, but also suffer from many preventable diabetes-related complications each year.

Diabetes-related Conditions per Year

3,506	lower extremity amputations
605	new cases of end-stage renal disease
1010-2402	new cases of blindness
205,039	residents with long-term reduction in activity
184,898	hospitalizations
60,187	hospitalizations due to cardiovascular disease among persons with diabetes

In 1990, the direct (medical care) and indirect (lost productivity) cost of diabetes in Florida was about $1,568,000,000.

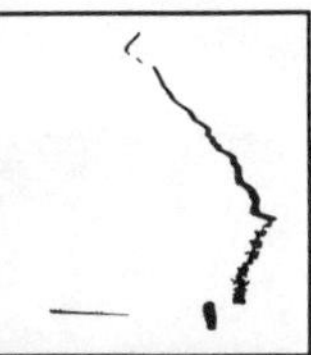

THE BURDEN OF Diabetes in Georgia

More than 334,000 residents are estimated to have diabetes, only half of whom have been diagnosed.

Number of Persons with Diagnosed Diabetes

Age	*Number*	*Race*	*Number*
0-44	33,479	White	108,611
45-64	68,715	African American	56,677
65-74	39,897	Other	2,324
75+	25,521		
Total	***167,612***	***Sex***	***Number***
		Male	70,155
		Female	97,457

Diabetes contributed to the deaths of more than 3,200 residents.

Number of Deaths Due to Diabetes as Underlying or Contributory Cause

Age	*Number*	*Race*	*Number*
0-44	152	White	2,190
45-64	761	African American	1,097
65-74	984	Other	8
75+	1,398		
Total	***3,295***	***Sex***	***Number***
		Male	1,379
		Female	1,916

Residents with diabetes face not only a shortened life span, but also suffer from many preventable diabetes-related complications each year.

Diabetes-related Conditions per Year

1,352	lower extremity amputations
390	new cases of end-stage renal disease
387-1004	new cases of blindness
83,212	residents with long-term reduction in activity
71,698	hospitalizations
22,233	hospitalizations due to cardiovascular disease among persons with diabetes

In 1990, the direct (medical care) and indirect (lost productivity) cost of diabetes in Georgia was about $655,000,000.

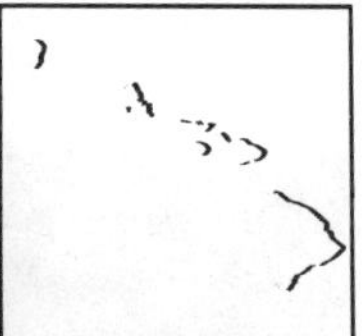

THE BURDEN OF Diabetes in Hawaii

More than 78,000 residents are estimated to have diabetes, only half of whom have been diagnosed.

Number of Persons with Diagnosed Diabetes

Age	*Number*
0-44	5,993
45-64	16,802
65-74	10,289
75+	6,821
Total	***39,905***

Race	*Number*
White	7,754
African American	398
Other	31,753

Sex	*Number*
Male	18,061
Female	21,844

Diabetes contributed to the deaths of more than 630 residents.

Number of Deaths Due to Diabetes as Underlying or Contributory Cause

Age	*Number*
0-44	15
45-64	152
65-74	171
75+	296
Total	***634***

Race	*Number*
White	128
African American	1
Other	505

Sex	*Number*
Male	323
Female	311

Residents with diabetes face not only a shortened life span, but also suffer from many preventable diabetes-related complications each year.

Diabetes-related Conditions per Year

336	lower extremity amputations
98	new cases of end-stage renal disease
96-239	new cases of blindness
20,203	residents with long-term reduction in activity
17,587	hospitalizations
5,621	hospitalizations due to cardiovascular disease among persons with diabetes

In 1990, the direct (medical care) and indirect (lost productivity) cost of diabetes in Hawaii was about $156,000,000.

THE BURDEN OF

Diabetes in Idaho

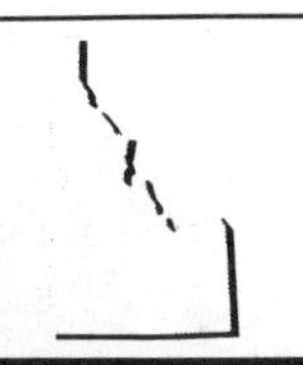

More than 46,000 residents are estimated to have diabetes, only half of whom have been diagnosed.

Number of Persons with Diagnosed Diabetes

Age	*Number*
0-44	4,709
45-64	8,741
65-74	6,262
75+	3,896
Total	***23,608***

Race	*Number*
White	22,848
African American	77
Other	683

Sex	*Number*
Male	10,731
Female	12,877

Diabetes contributed to the deaths of more than 470 residents.

Number of Deaths Due to Diabetes as Underlying or Contributory Cause

Age	*Number*
0-44	13
45-64	67
65-74	123
75+	267
Total	***470***

Race	*Number*
White	461
African American	0
Other	9

Sex	*Number*
Male	230
Female	240

Residents with diabetes face not only a shortened life span, but also suffer from many preventable diabetes-related complications each year.

Diabetes-related Conditions per Year

193	lower extremity amputations
44	new cases of end-stage renal disease
56-141	new cases of blindness
11,757	residents with long-term reduction in activity
10,316	hospitalizations
3,223	hospitalizations due to cardiovascular disease among persons with diabetes

In 1990, the direct (medical care) and indirect (lost productivity) cost of diabetes in Idaho was about $92,000,000.

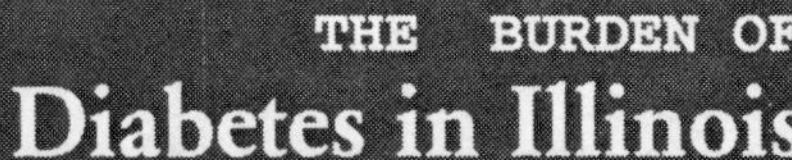
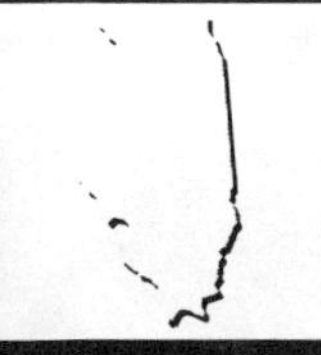

THE BURDEN OF Diabetes in Illinois

More than 610,000 residents are estimated to have diabetes, only half of whom have been diagnosed.

Number of Persons with Diagnosed Diabetes

Age	*Number*	*Race*	*Number*
0-44	54,711	White	235,998
45-64	119,818	African American	59,363
65-74	79,365	Other	9,922
75+	51,389		
Total	***305,283***	***Sex***	***Number***
		Male	130,152
		Female	175,131

Diabetes contributed to the deaths of more than 8,000 residents.

Number of Deaths Due to Diabetes as Underlying or Contributory Cause

Age	*Number*	*Race*	*Number*
0-44	217	White	6,802
45-64	1,530	African American	1,150
65-74	2,362	Other	51
75+	3,894		
Total	***8,003***	***Sex***	***Number***
		Male	3,527
		Female	4,476

Residents with diabetes face not only a shortened life span, but also suffer from many preventable diabetes-related complications each year.

Diabetes-related Conditions per Year

2,530	lower extremity amputations
548	new cases of end-stage renal disease
725-1828	new cases of blindness
153,087	residents with long-term reduction in activity
133,883	hospitalizations
42,220	hospitalizations due to cardiovascular disease among persons with diabetes

In 1990, the direct (medical care) and indirect (lost productivity) cost of diabetes in Illinois was about $1,193,000,000.

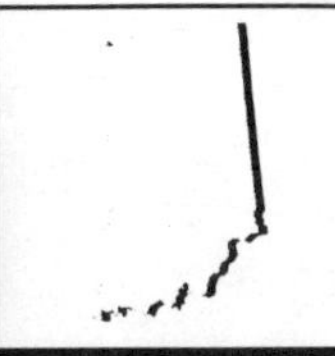

THE BURDEN OF Diabetes in Indiana

More than 282,000 residents are estimated to have diabetes, only half of whom have been diagnosed.

Number of Persons with Diagnosed Diabetes

Age	*Number*	*Race*	*Number*
0-44	25,746	White	124,530
45-64	54,807	African American	15,580
65-74	37,372	Other	1,412
75+	23,597		
Total	***141,522***	***Sex***	***Number***
		Male	60,808
		Female	80,714

Diabetes contributed to the deaths of more than 3,900 residents.

Number of Deaths Due to Diabetes as Underlying or Contributory Cause

Age	*Number*	*Race*	*Number*
0-44	85	White	3,542
45-64	708	African American	378
65-74	1,148	Other	0
75+	1,979		
Total	***3,920***	***Sex***	***Number***
		Male	1,692
		Female	2,228

Residents with diabetes face not only a shortened life span, but also suffer from many preventable diabetes-related complications each year.

Diabetes-related Conditions per Year

1,171	lower extremity amputations
219	new cases of end-stage renal disease
336-848	new cases of blindness
70,893	residents with long-term reduction in activity
62,030	hospitalizations
19,543	hospitalizations due to cardiovascular disease among persons with diabetes

In 1990, the direct (medical care) and indirect (lost productivity) cost of diabetes in Indiana was about $553,000,000.

THE BURDEN OF

Diabetes in Iowa

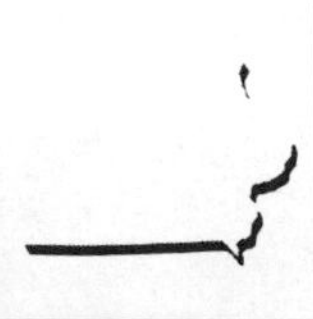

More than 146,000 residents are estimated to have diabetes, only half of whom have been diagnosed.

Number of Persons with Diagnosed Diabetes

Age	*Number*	*Race*	*Number*
0-44	12,163	White	71,432
45-64	25,907	African American	1,458
65-74	20,415	Other	737
75+	15,142		
Total	***73,627***	***Sex***	***Number***
		Male	31,651
		Female	41,976

Diabetes contributed to the deaths of more than 1,900 residents.

Number of Deaths Due to Diabetes as Underlying or Contributory Cause

Age	*Number*	*Race*	*Number*
0-44	42	White	1,877
45-64	277	African American	36
65-74	463	Other	8
75+	1,139		
Total	***1,921***	***Sex***	***Number***
		Male	845
		Female	1,076

Residents with diabetes face not only a shortened life span, but also suffer from many preventable diabetes-related complications each year.

Diabetes-related Conditions per Year

637	lower extremity amputations
124	new cases of end-stage renal disease
181-441	new cases of blindness
37,355	residents with long-term reduction in activity
33,682	hospitalizations
10,793	hospitalizations due to cardiovascular disease among persons with diabetes

In 1990, the direct (medical care) and indirect (lost productivity) cost of diabetes in Iowa was about $288,000,000.

THE BURDEN OF

Diabetes in Kansas

More than 126,000 residents are estimated to have diabetes, only half of whom have been diagnosed.

Number of Persons with Diagnosed Diabetes

Age	*Number*
0-44	11,410
45-64	22,829
65-74	16,974
75+	12,404
Total	***63,617***

Race	*Number*
White	57,555
African American	4,613
Other	1,449

Sex	*Number*
Male	27,480
Female	36,137

Diabetes contributed to the deaths of more than 1,500 residents.

Number of Deaths Due to Diabetes as Underlying or Contributory Cause

Age	*Number*
0-44	31
45-64	239
65-74	392
75+	850
Total	***1,512***

Race	*Number*
White	1,406
African American	92
Other	14

Sex	*Number*
Male	673
Female	839

Residents with diabetes face not only a shortened life span, but also suffer from many preventable diabetes-related complications each year.

Diabetes-related Conditions per Year

540	lower extremity amputations
100	new cases of end-stage renal disease
154-381	new cases of blindness
32,063	residents with long-term reduction in activity
28,681	hospitalizations
9,101	hospitalizations due to cardiovascular disease among persons with diabetes

In 1990, the direct (medical care) and indirect (lost productivity) cost of diabetes in Kansas was about $249,000,000.

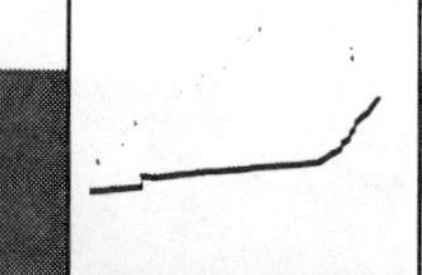

THE BURDEN OF Diabetes in Kentucky

More than 188,000 residents are estimated to have diabetes, only half of whom have been diagnosed.

Number of Persons with Diagnosed Diabetes

Age	*Number*
0-44	16,991
45-64	36,275
65-74	24,896
75+	16,068
Total	***94,230***

Race	*Number*
White	83,748
African American	9,810
Other	672

Sex	*Number*
Male	40,410
Female	53,820

Diabetes contributed to the deaths of more than 2,300 residents.

Number of Deaths Due to Diabetes as Underlying or Contributory Cause

Age	*Number*
0-44	65
45-64	445
65-74	696
75+	1,144
Total	***2,350***

Race	*Number*
White	2,132
African American	216
Other	2

Sex	*Number*
Male	986
Female	1,364

Residents with diabetes face not only a shortened life span, but also suffer from many preventable diabetes-related complications each year.

Diabetes-related Conditions per Year

783	lower extremity amputations
142	new cases of end-stage renal disease
225-564	new cases of blindness
47,261	residents with long-term reduction in activity
41,462	hospitalizations
13,082	hospitalizations due to cardiovascular disease among persons with diabetes

In 1990, the direct (medical care) and indirect (lost productivity) cost of diabetes in Kentucky was about $368,000,000.

THE BURDEN OF Diabetes in Louisiana

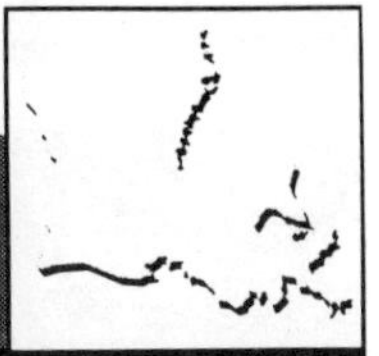

More than 230,000 residents are estimated to have diabetes, only half of whom have been diagnosed.

Number of Persons with Diagnosed Diabetes

Age	Number
0-44	21,825
45-64	45,641
65-74	28,795
75+	19,247
Total	**115,508**

Race	Number
White	69,351
African American	44,544
Other	1,613

Sex	Number
Male	48,195
Female	67,313

Diabetes contributed to the deaths of more than 2,900 residents.

Number of Deaths Due to Diabetes as Underlying or Contributory Cause

Age	Number
0-44	74
45-64	664
65-74	893
75+	1,316
Total	**2,947**

Race	Number
White	1,755
African American	1,178
Other	14

Sex	Number
Male	1,108
Female	1,839

Residents with diabetes face not only a shortened life span, but also suffer from many preventable diabetes-related complications each year.

Diabetes-related Conditions per Year

950	lower extremity amputations
317	new cases of end-stage renal disease
272-692	new cases of blindness
57,712	residents with long-term reduction in activity
50,352	hospitalizations
15,774	hospitalizations due to cardiovascular disease among persons with diabetes

In 1990, the direct (medical care) and indirect (lost productivity) cost of diabetes in Louisiana was about $452,000,000.

THE BURDEN OF

Diabetes in Maine

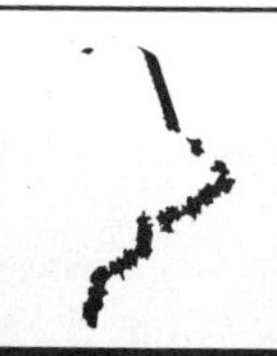

More than 60,000 residents are estimated to have diabetes, only half of whom have been diagnosed.

Number of Persons with Diagnosed Diabetes

Age	Number
0-44	5,516
45-64	11,396
65-74	8,199
75+	5,396
Total	***30,507***

Race	Number
White	30,073
African American	106
Other	328

Sex	Number
Male	13,291
Female	17,216

Diabetes contributed to the deaths of more than 900 residents.

Number of Deaths Due to Diabetes as Underlying or Contributory Cause

Age	Number
0-44	25
45-64	158
65-74	260
75+	460
Total	***903***

Race	Number
White	897
African American	0
Other	6

Sex	Number
Male	414
Female	489

Residents with diabetes face not only a shortened life span, but also suffer from many preventable diabetes-related complications each year.

Diabetes-related Conditions per Year

254	lower extremity amputations
33	new cases of end-stage renal disease
73-183	new cases of blindness
15,317	residents with long-term reduction in activity
13,525	hospitalizations
4,275	hospitalizations due to cardiovascular disease among persons with diabetes

In 1990, the direct (medical care) and indirect (lost productivity) cost of diabetes in Maine was about $119,000,000.

THE BURDEN OF Diabetes in Maryland

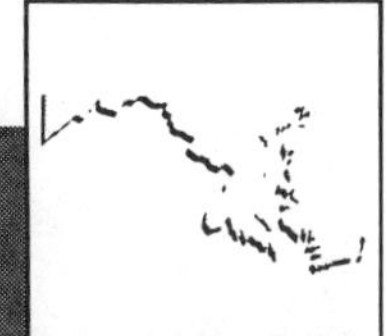

More than 258,000 residents are estimated to have diabetes, only half of whom have been diagnosed.

Number of Persons with Diagnosed Diabetes

Age	*Number*
0-44	24,067
45-64	55,547
65-74	31,540
75+	18,228
Total	***129,382***

Race	*Number*
White	84,824
African American	39,653
Other	4,905

Sex	*Number*
Male	55,917
Female	73,465

Diabetes contributed to the deaths of more than 3,100 residents.

Number of Deaths Due to Diabetes as Underlying or Contributory Cause

Age	*Number*
0-44	109
45-64	653
65-74	1,018
75+	1,406
Total	***3,188***

Race	*Number*
White	2,329
African American	840
Other	19

Sex	*Number*
Male	1,414
Female	1,774

Residents with diabetes face not only a shortened life span, but also suffer from many preventable diabetes-related complications each year.

Diabetes-related Conditions per Year

1,040	lower extremity amputations
270	new cases of end-stage renal disease
299-775	new cases of blindness
64,386	residents with long-term reduction in activity
54,900	hospitalizations
17,111	hospitalizations due to cardiovascular disease among persons with diabetes

In 1990, the direct (medical care) and indirect (lost productivity) cost of diabetes in Maryland was about $506,000,000.

THE BURDEN OF

Diabetes in Massachusetts

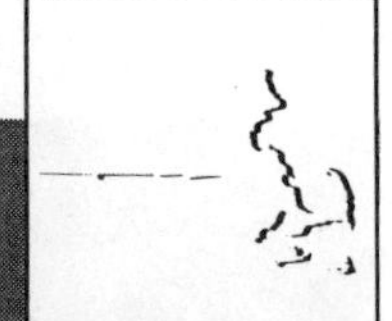

More than 308,000 residents are estimated to have diabetes, only half of whom have been diagnosed.

Number of Persons with Diagnosed Diabetes

Age	*Number*	*Race*	*Number*
0-44	27,701	White	140,897
45-64	57,192	African American	9,701
65-74	42,011	Other	4,131
75+	27,825		
Total	***154,729***	***Sex***	***Number***
		Male	65,236
		Female	89,493

Diabetes contributed to the deaths of more than 4,400 residents.

Number of Deaths Due to Diabetes as Underlying or Contributory Cause

Age	*Number*	*Race*	*Number*
0-44	83	White	4,211
45-64	696	African American	177
65-74	1,314	Other	25
75+	2,320		
Total	***4,413***	***Sex***	***Number***
		Male	2,011
		Female	2,402

Residents with diabetes face not only a shortened life span, but also suffer from many preventable diabetes-related complications each year.

Diabetes-related Conditions per Year

1,299	lower extremity amputations
245	new cases of end-stage renal disease
391-927	new cases of blindness
77,781	residents with long-term reduction in activity
68,862	hospitalizations
21,807	hospitalizations due to cardiovascular disease among persons with diabetes

In 1990, the direct (medical care) and indirect (lost productivity) cost of diabetes in Massachusetts was about $605,000,000.

THE BURDEN OF

Diabetes in Michigan

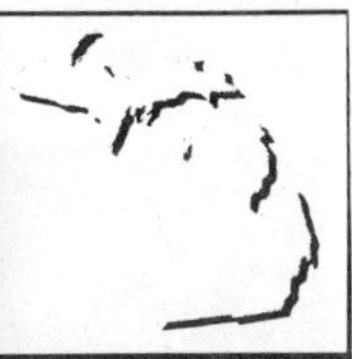

More than 482,000 residents are estimated to have diabetes, only half of whom have been diagnosed.

Number of Persons with Diagnosed Diabetes

Age	*Number*
0-44	44,681
45-64	95,546
65-74	63,130
75+	38,257
Total	***241,614***

Race	*Number*
White	191,177
African American	45,928
Other	4,509

Sex	*Number*
Male	104,302
Female	137,312

Diabetes contributed to the deaths of more than 6,700 residents.

Number of Deaths Due to Diabetes as Underlying or Contributory Cause

Age	*Number*
0-44	222
45-64	1,309
65-74	2,076
75+	3,190
Total	***6,797***

Race	*Number*
White	5,686
African American	1,054
Other	57

Sex	*Number*
Male	2,960
Female	3,837

Residents with diabetes face not only a shortened life span, but also suffer from many preventable diabetes-related complications each year.

Diabetes-related Conditions per Year

1,980	lower extremity amputations
548	new cases of end-stage renal disease
570-1447	new cases of blindness
120,720	residents with long-term reduction in activity
104,911	hospitalizations
32,934	hospitalizations due to cardiovascular disease among persons with diabetes

In 1990, the direct (medical care) and indirect (lost productivity) cost of diabetes in Michigan was about $945,000,000.

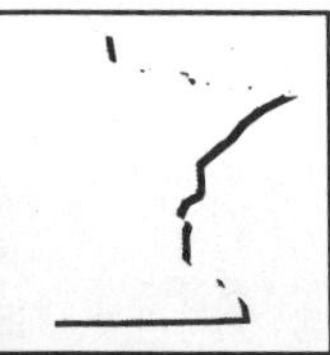

THE BURDEN OF Diabetes in Minnesota

More than 208,000 residents are estimated to have diabetes, only half of whom have been diagnosed.

Number of Persons with Diagnosed Diabetes

Age	Number
0-44	20,495
45-64	38,624
65-74	26,600
75+	19,207
Total	***104,926***

Race	Number
White	99,766
African American	2,239
Other	2,921

Sex	Number
Male	46,050
Female	58,876

Diabetes contributed to the deaths of more than 2,500 residents.

Number of Deaths Due to Diabetes as Underlying or Contributory Cause

Age	Number
0-44	67
45-64	377
65-74	639
75+	1,478
Total	***2,561***

Race	Number
White	2,497
African American	31
Other	33

Sex	Number
Male	1,184
Female	1,377

Residents with diabetes face not only a shortened life span, but also suffer from many preventable diabetes-related complications each year.

Diabetes-related Conditions per Year

874	lower extremity amputations
198	new cases of end-stage renal disease
249-628	new cases of blindness
52,485	residents with long-term reduction in activity
46,504	hospitalizations
14,584	hospitalizations due to cardiovascular disease among persons with diabetes

In 1990, the direct (medical care) and indirect (lost productivity) cost of diabetes in Minnesota was about $410,000,000.

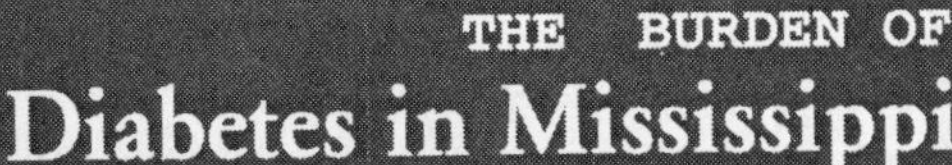

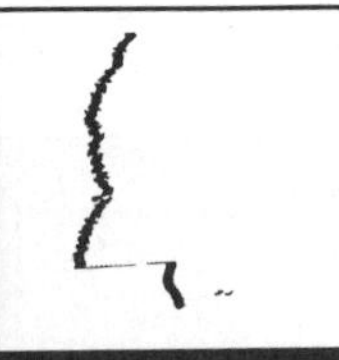

THE BURDEN OF Diabetes in Mississippi

More than 150,000 residents are estimated to have diabetes, only half of whom have been diagnosed.

Number of Persons with Diagnosed Diabetes

Age	*Number*
0-44	13,205
45-64	28,274
65-74	19,260
75+	14,812
Total	***75,551***

Race	*Number*
White	42,583
African American	32,386
Other	582

Sex	*Number*
Male	30,961
Female	44,590

Diabetes contributed to the deaths of more than 1,700 residents.

Number of Deaths Due to Diabetes as Underlying or Contributory Cause

Age	*Number*
0-44	52
45-64	381
65-74	492
75+	859
Total	***1,784***

Race	*Number*
White	1,018
African American	749
Other	17

Sex	*Number*
Male	691
Female	1,093

Residents with diabetes face not only a shortened life span, but also suffer from many preventable diabetes-related complications each year.

Diabetes-related Conditions per Year

642	lower extremity amputations
147	new cases of end-stage renal disease
182-452	new cases of blindness
38,128	residents with long-term reduction in activity
33,990	hospitalizations
10,791	hospitalizations due to cardiovascular disease among persons with diabetes

In 1990, the direct (medical care) and indirect (lost productivity) cost of diabetes in Mississippi was about $295,000,000.

THE BURDEN OF

Diabetes in Missouri

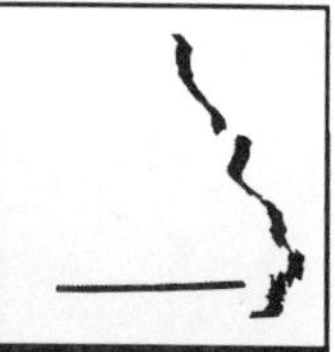

More than 278,000 residents are estimated to have diabetes, only half of whom have been diagnosed.

Number of Persons with Diagnosed Diabetes

Age	*Number*
0-44	23,448
45-64	52,182
65-74	37,155
75+	26,444
Total	***139,229***

Race	*Number*
White	117,467
African American	19,936
Other	1,826

Sex	*Number*
Male	59,057
Female	80,172

Diabetes contributed to the deaths of more than 3,500 residents.

Number of Deaths Due to Diabetes as Underlying or Contributory Cause

Age	*Number*
0-44	80
45-64	591
65-74	928
75+	1,922
Total	***3,521***

Race	*Number*
White	3,013
African American	500
Other	8

Sex	*Number*
Male	1,499
Female	2,022

Residents with diabetes face not only a shortened life span, but also suffer from many preventable diabetes-related complications each year.

Diabetes-related Conditions per Year

1,184	lower extremity amputations
263	new cases of end-stage renal disease
337-834	new cases of blindness
70,346	residents with long-term reduction in activity
62,541	hospitalizations
19,925	hospitalizations due to cardiovascular disease among persons with diabetes

In 1990, the direct (medical care) and indirect (lost productivity) cost of diabetes in Missouri was about $544,000,000.

THE BURDEN OF Diabetes in Montana

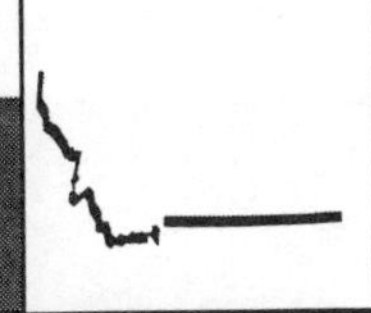

More than 40,000 residents are estimated to have diabetes, only half of whom have been diagnosed.

Number of Persons with Diagnosed Diabetes

Age	***Number***
0-44	3,656
45-64	7,632
65-74	5,523
75+	3,498
Total	***20,309***

Race	***Number***
White	18,858
African American	54
Other	1,397

Sex	***Number***
Male	9,195
Female	11,114

Diabetes contributed to the deaths of more than 430 residents.

Number of Deaths Due to Diabetes as Underlying or Contributory Cause

Age	***Number***
0-44	13
45-64	61
65-74	121
75+	244
Total	***439***

Race	***Number***
White	401
African American	0
Other	38

Sex	***Number***
Male	182
Female	257

Residents with diabetes face not only a shortened life span, but also suffer from many preventable diabetes-related complications each year.

Diabetes-related Conditions per Year

170	lower extremity amputations
49	new cases of end-stage renal disease
49-122	new cases of blindness
10,193	residents with long-term reduction in activity
8,972	hospitalizations
2,835	hospitalizations due to cardiovascular disease among persons with diabetes

In 1990, the direct (medical care) and indirect (lost productivity) cost of diabetes in Montana was about $79,000,000.

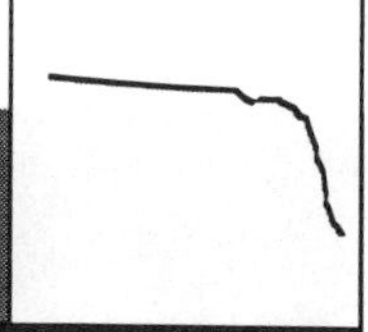

THE BURDEN OF Diabetes in Nebraska

More than 80,000 residents are estimated to have diabetes, only half of whom have been diagnosed.

Number of Persons with Diagnosed Diabetes

Age	*Number*
0-44	7,187
45-64	14,317
65-74	10,679
75+	8,095
Total	***40,278***

Race	*Number*
White	37,905
African American	1,750
Other	623

Sex	*Number*
Male	17,445
Female	22,833

Diabetes contributed to the deaths of more than 1,000 residents.

Number of Deaths Due to Diabetes as Underlying or Contributory Cause

Age	*Number*
0-44	22
45-64	141
65-74	260
75+	612
Total	***1,035***

Race	*Number*
White	990
African American	32
Other	13

Sex	*Number*
Male	474
Female	561

Residents with diabetes face not only a shortened life span, but also suffer from many preventable diabetes-related complications each year.

Diabetes-related Conditions per Year

345	lower extremity amputations
83	new cases of end-stage renal disease
97-241	new cases of blindness
20,327	residents with long-term reduction in activity
18,254	hospitalizations
5,800	hospitalizations due to cardiovascular disease among persons with diabetes

In 1990, the direct (medical care) and indirect (lost productivity) cost of diabetes in Nebraska was about $157,000,000.

THE BURDEN OF Diabetes in Nevada

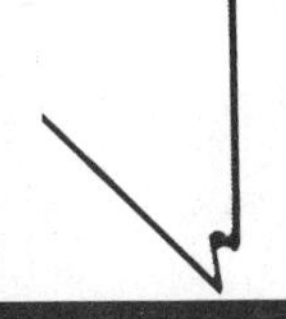

More than 58,000 residents are estimated to have diabetes, only half of whom have been diagnosed.

Number of Persons with Diagnosed Diabetes

Age	*Number*	*Race*	*Number*
0-44	5,666	White	25,563
45-64	12,901	African American	2,285
65-74	7,891	Other	1,924
75+	3,314		
Total	***29,772***	***Sex***	***Number***
		Male	14,102
		Female	15,670

Diabetes contributed to the deaths of more than 480 residents.

Number of Deaths Due to Diabetes as Underlying or Contributory Cause

Age	*Number*	*Race*	*Number*
0-44	14	White	424
45-64	132	African American	43
65-74	165	Other	14
75+	170		
Total	***481***	***Sex***	***Number***
		Male	251
		Female	230

Residents with diabetes face not only a shortened life span, but also suffer from many preventable diabetes-related complications each year.

Diabetes-related Conditions per Year

233	lower extremity amputations
55	new cases of end-stage renal disease
69-178	new cases of blindness
14,721	residents with long-term reduction in activity
12,340	hospitalizations
3,825	hospitalizations due to cardiovascular disease among persons with diabetes

In 1990, the direct (medical care) and indirect (lost productivity) cost of diabetes in Nevada was about $116,000,000.

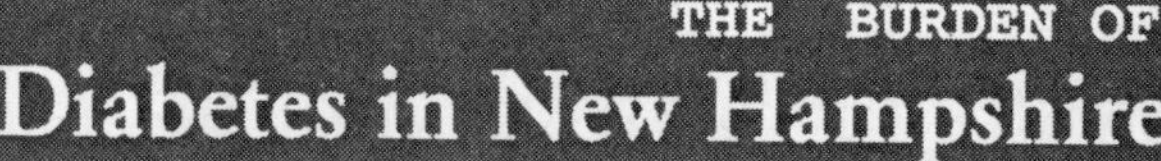

THE BURDEN OF Diabetes in New Hampshire

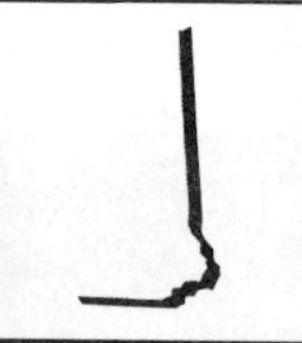

More than 50,000 residents are estimated to have diabetes, only half of whom have been diagnosed.

Number of Persons with Diagnosed Diabetes

Age	*Number*
0-44	5,204
45-64	9,818
65-74	6,385
75+	4,038
Total	***25,445***

Race	*Number*
White	24,988
African American	175
Other	282

Sex	*Number*
Male	11,234
Female	14,211

Diabetes contributed to the deaths of more than 710 residents.

Number of Deaths Due to Diabetes as Underlying or Contributory Cause

Age	*Number*
0-44	16
45-64	117
65-74	206
75+	379
Total	***718***

Race	*Number*
White	717
African American	0
Other	1

Sex	*Number*
Male	331
Female	387

Residents with diabetes face not only a shortened life span, but also suffer from many preventable diabetes-related complications each year.

Diabetes-related Conditions per Year

206	lower extremity amputations
39	new cases of end-stage renal disease
60-152	new cases of blindness
12,632	residents with long-term reduction in activity
10,994	hospitalizations
3,412	hospitalizations due to cardiovascular disease among persons with diabetes

In 1990, the direct (medical care) and indirect (lost productivity) cost of diabetes in New Hampshire was about $99,000,000.

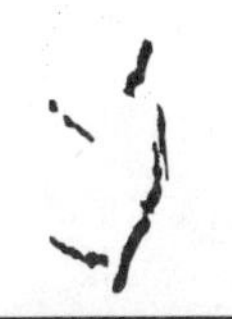

THE BURDEN OF

Diabetes in New Jersey

More than 430,000 residents are estimated to have diabetes, only half of whom have been diagnosed.

Number of Persons with Diagnosed Diabetes

Age	*Number*
0-44	35,859
45-64	86,993
65-74	58,100
75+	34,529
Total	***215,481***

Race	*Number*
White	169,656
African American	37,120
Other	8,705

Sex	*Number*
Male	92,508
Female	122,973

Diabetes contributed to the deaths of more than 6,500 residents.

Number of Deaths Due to Diabetes as Underlying or Contributory Cause

Age	*Number*
0-44	138
45-64	1,265
65-74	1,993
75+	3,122
Total	***6,519***

Race	*Number*
White	5,603
African American	879
Other	37

Sex	*Number*
Male	2,885
Female	3,634

Residents with diabetes face not only a shortened life span, but also suffer from many preventable diabetes-related complications each year.

Diabetes-related Conditions per Year

1,787	lower extremity amputations
425	new cases of end-stage renal disease
514-1290	new cases of blindness
108,353	residents with long-term reduction in activity
94,166	hospitalizations
29,870	hospitalizations due to cardiovascular disease among persons with diabetes

In 1990, the direct (medical care) and indirect (lost productivity) cost of diabetes in New Jersey was about $842,000,000.

THE BURDEN OF

Diabetes in New Mexico

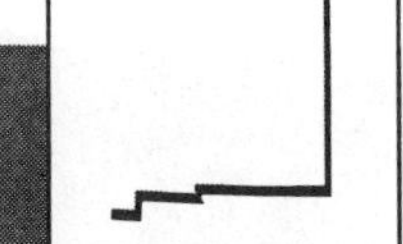

More than 70,000 residents are estimated to have diabetes, only half of whom have been diagnosed.

Number of Persons with Diagnosed Diabetes

Age	Number
0-44	7,426
45-64	14,158
65-74	9,022
75+	5,278
Total	***35,884***

Race	Number
White	30,739
African American	976
Other	4,169

Sex	Number
Male	15,998
Female	19,886

Diabetes contributed to the deaths of more than 680 residents.

Number of Deaths Due to Diabetes as Underlying or Contributory Cause

Age	Number
0-44	35
45-64	143
65-74	206
75+	298
Total	***682***

Race	Number
White	603
African American	13
Other	66

Sex	Number
Male	343
Female	339

Residents with diabetes face not only a shortened life span, but also suffer from many preventable diabetes-related complications each year.

Diabetes-related Conditions per Year

287	lower extremity amputations
102	new cases of end-stage renal disease
83-215	new cases of blindness
17,763	residents with long-term reduction in activity
15,324	hospitalizations
4,740	hospitalizations due to cardiovascular disease among persons with diabetes

In 1990, the direct (medical care) and indirect (lost productivity) cost of diabetes in New Mexico was about $140,000,000.

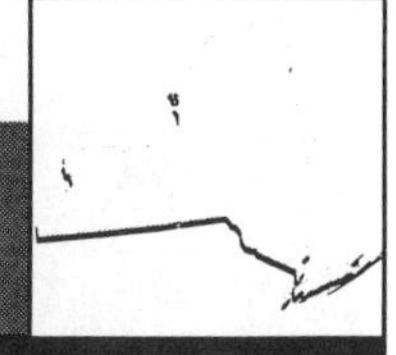

THE BURDEN OF Diabetes in New York

More than 1,010,000 residents are estimated to have diabetes, only half of whom have been diagnosed.

Number of Persons with Diagnosed Diabetes

Age	*Number*
0-44	85,295
45-64	204,057
65-74	131,577
75+	84,851
Total	***505,780***

Race	*Number*
White	372,340
African American	108,459
Other	24,981

Sex	*Number*
Male	212,434
Female	293,346

Diabetes contributed to the deaths of more than 11,600 residents.

Number of Deaths Due to Diabetes as Underlying or Contributory Cause

Age	*Number*
0-44	304
45-64	2,299
65-74	3,365
75+	5,709
Total	***11,677***

Race	*Number*
White	9,711
African American	1,857
Other	109

Sex	*Number*
Male	5,161
Female	6,516

Residents with diabetes face not only a shortened life span, but also suffer from many preventable diabetes-related complications each year.

Diabetes-related Conditions per Year

4,211	lower extremity amputations
866	new cases of end-stage renal disease
1205-3029	new cases of blindness
254,447	residents with long-term reduction in activity
221,944	hospitalizations
70,334	hospitalizations due to cardiovascular disease among persons with diabetes

In 1990, the direct (medical care) and indirect (lost productivity) cost of diabetes in New York was about $1,977,000,000.

THE BURDEN OF Diabetes in North Carolina

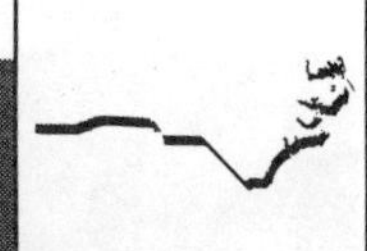

More than 368,000 residents are estimated to have diabetes, only half of whom have been diagnosed.

Number of Persons with Diagnosed Diabetes

Age	*Number*
0-44	32,203
45-64	73,858
65-74	48,809
75+	29,711
Total	***184,581***

Race	*Number*
White	127,669
African American	53,064
Other	3,848

Sex	*Number*
Male	77,411
Female	107,170

Diabetes contributed to the deaths of more than 4,900 residents.

Number of Deaths Due to Diabetes as Underlying or Contributory Cause

Age	*Number*
0-44	173
45-64	1,119
65-74	1,550
75+	2,153
Total	***4,995***

Race	*Number*
White	3,452
African American	1,478
Other	65

Sex	*Number*
Male	2,215
Female	2,780

Residents with diabetes face not only a shortened life span, but also suffer from many preventable diabetes-related complications each year.

Diabetes-related Conditions per Year

1,525	lower extremity amputations
383	new cases of end-stage renal disease
439-1105	new cases of blindness
92,581	residents with long-term reduction in activity
80,521	hospitalizations
25,429	hospitalizations due to cardiovascular disease among persons with diabetes

In 1990, the direct (medical care) and indirect (lost productivity) cost of diabetes in North Carolina was about $722,000,000.

THE BURDEN OF

Diabetes in North Dakota

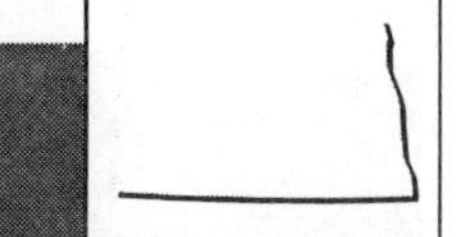

More than 32,000 residents are estimated to have diabetes, only half of whom have been diagnosed.

Number of Persons with Diagnosed Diabetes

Age	*Number*
0-44	2,926
45-64	5,522
65-74	4,289
75+	3,302
Total	***16,039***

Race	*Number*
White	15,279
African American	44
Other	716

Sex	*Number*
Male	7,167
Female	8,872

Diabetes contributed to the deaths of more than 420 residents.

Number of Deaths Due to Diabetes as Underlying or Contributory Cause

Age	*Number*
0-44	11
45-64	55
65-74	90
75+	266
Total	***422***

Race	*Number*
White	401
African American	0
Other	21

Sex	*Number*
Male	189
Female	233

Residents with diabetes face not only a shortened life span, but also suffer from many preventable diabetes-related complications each year.

Diabetes-related Conditions per Year

138	lower extremity amputations
47	new cases of end-stage renal disease
40-96	new cases of blindness
8,092	residents with long-term reduction in activity
7,304	hospitalizations
2,320	hospitalizations due to cardiovascular disease among persons with diabetes

In 1990, the direct (medical care) and indirect (lost productivity) cost of diabetes in North Dakota was about $63,000,000.

THE BURDEN OF

Diabetes in Ohio

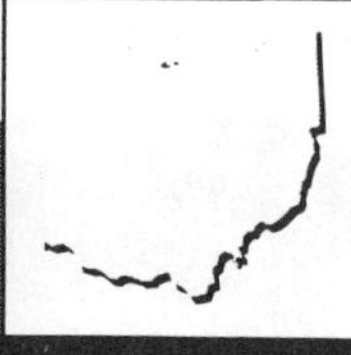

More than 576,000 residents are estimated to have diabetes, only half of whom have been diagnosed.

Number of Persons with Diagnosed Diabetes

Age	*Number*
0-44	50,313
45-64	111,938
65-74	78,316
75+	47,526
Total	***288,093***

Race	*Number*
White	241,344
African American	43,475
Other	3,274

Sex	*Number*
Male	122,921
Female	165,172

Diabetes contributed to the deaths of more than 9,300 residents.

Number of Deaths Due to Diabetes as Underlying or Contributory Cause

Age	*Number*
0-44	178
45-64	1,715
65-74	2,904
75+	4,579
Total	***9,376***

Race	*Number*
White	8,229
African American	1,127
Other	20

Sex	*Number*
Male	4,134
Female	5,242

Residents with diabetes face not only a shortened life span, but also suffer from many preventable diabetes-related complications each year.

Diabetes-related Conditions per Year

2,391	lower extremity amputations
550	new cases of end-stage renal disease
688-1725	new cases of blindness
144,625	residents with long-term reduction in activity
126,459	hospitalizations
40,011	hospitalizations due to cardiovascular disease among persons with diabetes

In 1990, the direct (medical care) and indirect (lost productivity) cost of diabetes in Ohio was about $1,126,000,000.

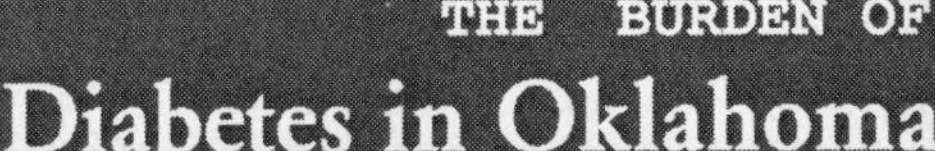

THE BURDEN OF Diabetes in Oklahoma

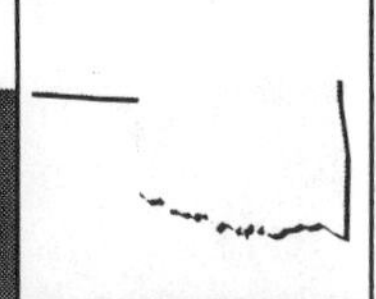

More than 170,000 residents are estimated to have diabetes, only half of whom have been diagnosed.

Number of Persons with Diagnosed Diabetes

Age	*Number*
0-44	14,709
45-64	32,798
65-74	22,524
75+	15,938
Total	***85,969***

Race	*Number*
White	68,452
African American	7,834
Other	9,683

Sex	*Number*
Male	36,876
Female	49,093

Diabetes contributed to the deaths of more than 1,900 residents.

Number of Deaths Due to Diabetes as Underlying or Contributory Cause

Age	*Number*
0-44	57
45-64	386
65-74	503
75+	980
Total	***1,926***

Race	*Number*
White	1,567
African American	193
Other	166

Sex	*Number*
Male	787
Female	1,139

Residents with diabetes face not only a shortened life span, but also suffer from many preventable diabetes-related complications each year.

Diabetes-related Conditions per Year

725	lower extremity amputations
179	new cases of end-stage renal disease
207-515	new cases of blindness
43,359	residents with long-term reduction in activity
38,384	hospitalizations
12,194	hospitalizations due to cardiovascular disease among persons with diabetes

In 1990, the direct (medical care) and indirect (lost productivity) cost of diabetes in Oklahoma was about $336,000,000.

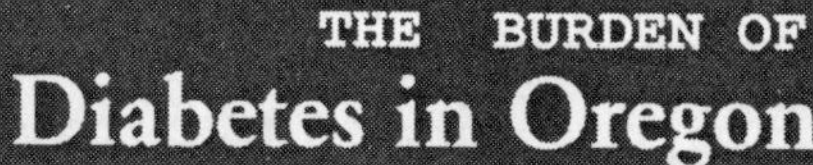

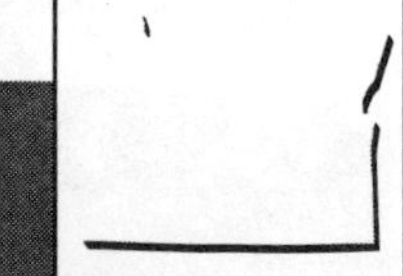

THE BURDEN OF Diabetes in Oregon

More than 144,000 residents are estimated to have diabetes, only half of whom have been diagnosed.

Number of Persons with Diagnosed Diabetes

Age	Number
0-44	12,881
45-64	26,870
65-74	20,345
75+	12,762
Total	***72,858***

Race	Number
White	68,279
African American	1,428
Other	3,151

Sex	Number
Male	32,414
Female	40,444

Diabetes contributed to the deaths of more than 1,700 residents.

Number of Deaths Due to Diabetes as Underlying or Contributory Cause

Age	Number
0-44	49
45-64	286
65-74	508
75+	901
Total	***1,744***

Race	Number
White	1,678
African American	35
Other	31

Sex	Number
Male	803
Female	941

Residents with diabetes face not only a shortened life span, but also suffer from many preventable diabetes-related complications each year.

Diabetes-related Conditions per Year

611	lower extremity amputations
126	new cases of end-stage renal disease
176-436	new cases of blindness
36,626	residents with long-term reduction in activity
32,364	hospitalizations
10,263	hospitalizations due to cardiovascular disease among persons with diabetes

In 1990, the direct (medical care) and indirect (lost productivity) cost of diabetes in Oregon was about $285,000,000.

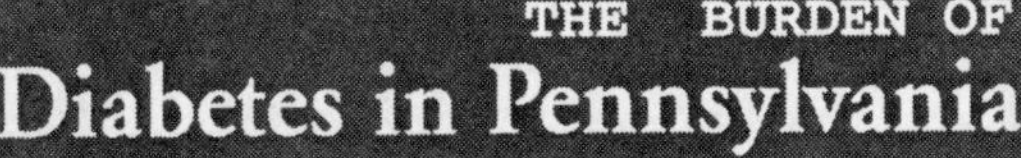

THE BURDEN OF Diabetes in Pennsylvania

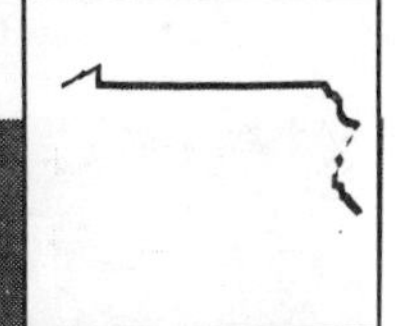

More than 678,000 residents are estimated to have diabetes, only half of whom have been diagnosed.

Number of Persons with Diagnosed Diabetes

Age	*Number*
0-44	52,437
45-64	125,477
65-74	100,337
75+	61,185
Total	***339,436***

Race	*Number*
White	291,495
African American	43,480
Other	4,461

Sex	*Number*
Male	143,137
Female	196,299

Diabetes contributed to the deaths of more than 11,500 residents.

Number of Deaths Due to Diabetes as Underlying or Contributory Cause

Age	*Number*
0-44	205
45-64	1,872
65-74	3,557
75+	5,906
Total	***11,540***

Race	*Number*
White	10,470
African American	1,049
Other	21

Sex	*Number*
Male	4,957
Female	6,583

Residents with diabetes face not only a shortened life span, but also suffer from many preventable diabetes-related complications each year.

Diabetes-related Conditions per Year

2,892	lower extremity amputations
659	new cases of end-stage renal disease
834-2033	new cases of blindness
172,061	residents with long-term reduction in activity
152,622	hospitalizations
49,047	hospitalizations due to cardiovascular disease among persons with diabetes

In 1990, the direct (medical care) and indirect (lost productivity) cost of diabetes in Pennsylvania was about $1,327,000,000.

THE BURDEN OF Diabetes in Rhode Island

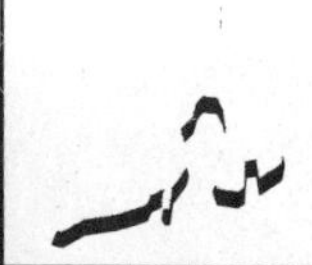

More than 52,000 residents are estimated to have diabetes, only half of whom have been diagnosed.

Number of Persons with Diagnosed Diabetes

Age	*Number*
0-44	4,503
45-64	9,403
65-74	7,757
75+	4,979
Total	***26,642***

Race	*Number*
White	24,838
African American	1,216
Other	588

Sex	*Number*
Male	11,171
Female	15,471

Diabetes contributed to the deaths of more than 830 residents.

Number of Deaths Due to Diabetes as Underlying or Contributory Cause

Age	*Number*
0-44	13
45-64	128
65-74	229
75+	469
Total	***839***

Race	*Number*
White	806
African American	28
Other	5

Sex	*Number*
Male	388
Female	451

Residents with diabetes face not only a shortened life span, but also suffer from many preventable diabetes-related complications each year.

Diabetes-related Conditions per Year

227	lower extremity amputations
42	new cases of end-stage renal disease
66-160	new cases of blindness
13,459	residents with long-term reduction in activity
12,020	hospitalizations
3,839	hospitalizations due to cardiovascular disease among persons with diabetes

In 1990, the direct (medical care) and indirect (lost productivity) cost of diabetes in Rhode Island was about $104,000,000.

THE BURDEN OF Diabetes in South Carolina

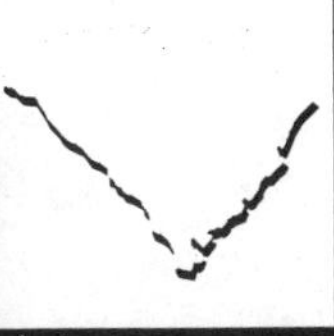

More than 194,000 residents are estimated to have diabetes, only half of whom have been diagnosed.

Number of Persons with Diagnosed Diabetes

Age	*Number*
0-44	17,675
45-64	38,842
65-74	25,757
75+	14,810
Total	***97,084***

Race	*Number*
White	59,911
African American	36,316
Other	857

Sex	*Number*
Male	40,429
Female	56,655

Diabetes contributed to the deaths of More than 2,200 residents.

Number of Deaths Due to Diabetes as Underlying or Contributory Cause

Age	*Number*
0-44	68
45-64	533
65-74	726
75+	904
Total	***2,231***

Race	*Number*
White	1,389
African American	838
Other	4

Sex	*Number*
Male	945
Female	1,286

Residents with diabetes face not only a shortened life span, but also suffer from many preventable diabetes-related complications each year.

Diabetes-related Conditions per Year

794	lower extremity amputations
241	new cases of end-stage renal disease
229-581	new cases of blindness
48,503	residents with long-term reduction in activity
41,981	hospitalizations
13,189	hospitalizations due to cardiovascular disease among persons with diabetes

In 1990, the direct (medical care) and indirect (lost productivity) cost of diabetes in South Carolina was about $380,000,000.

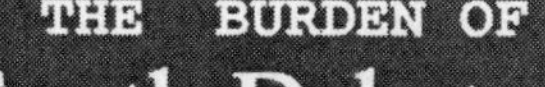

THE BURDEN OF Diabetes in South Dakota

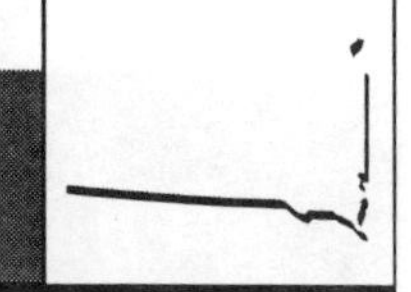

More than 36,000 residents are estimated to have diabetes, only half of whom have been diagnosed.

Number of Persons with Diagnosed Diabetes

Age	Number
0-44	3,189
45-64	6,251
65-74	4,958
75+	3,678
Total	***18,076***

Race	Number
White	16,646
African American	57
Other	1,373

Sex	Number
Male	7,976
Female	10,100

Diabetes contributed to the deaths of more than 460 residents.

Number of Deaths Due to Diabetes as Underlying or Contributory Cause

Age	Number
0-44	14
45-64	67
65-74	123
75+	259
Total	***463***

Race	Number
White	414
African American	0
Other	49

Sex	Number
Male	223
Female	240

Residents with diabetes face not only a shortened life span, but also suffer from many preventable diabetes-related complications each year.

Diabetes-related Conditions per Year

156	lower extremity amputations
28	new cases of end-stage renal disease
44-108	new cases of blindness
9,135	residents with long-term reduction in activity
8,236	hospitalizations
2,625	hospitalizations due to cardiovascular disease among persons with diabetes

In 1990, the direct (medical care) and indirect (lost productivity) cost of diabetes in South Dakota was about $71,000,000.

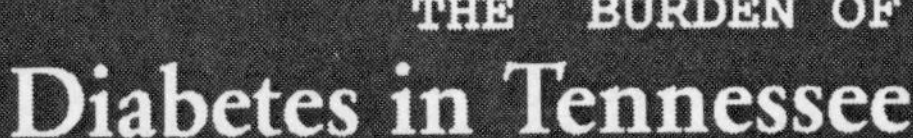

THE BURDEN OF Diabetes in Tennessee

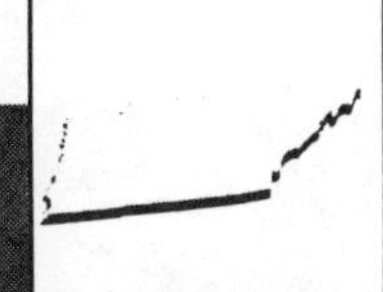

More than 264,000 residents are estimated to have diabetes, only half of whom have been diagnosed.

Number of Persons with Diagnosed Diabetes

Age	*Number*
0-44	22,974
45-64	52,236
65-74	34,602
75+	22,832
Total	***132,644***

Race	*Number*
White	103,668
African American	27,792
Other	1,184

Sex	*Number*
Male	55,996
Female	76,648

Diabetes contributed to the deaths of more than 3,000 residents.

Number of Deaths Due to Diabetes as Underlying or Contributory Cause

Age	*Number*
0-44	94
45-64	564
65-74	892
75+	1,475
Total	***3,025***

Race	*Number*
White	2,379
African American	635
Other	11

Sex	*Number*
Male	1,216
Female	1,809

Residents with diabetes face not only a shortened life span, but also suffer from many preventable diabetes-related complications each year.

Diabetes-related Conditions per Year

1,106	lower extremity amputations
254	new cases of end-stage renal disease
316-794	new cases of blindness
66,691	residents with long-term reduction in activity
58,438	hospitalizations
18,497	hospitalizations due to cardiovascular disease among persons with diabetes

In 1990, the direct (medical care) and indirect (lost productivity) cost of diabetes in Tennessee was about $519,000,000.

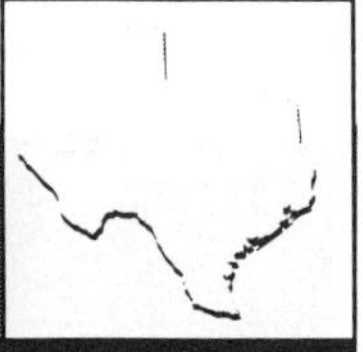

THE BURDEN OF Diabetes in Texas

More than 798,000 residents are estimated to have diabetes, only half of whom have been diagnosed.

Number of Persons with Diagnosed Diabetes

Age	*Number*	*Race*	*Number*
0-44	84,955	White	321,504
45-64	158,128	African American	67,000
65-74	95,260	Other	10,662
75+	60,823		
Total	***399,166***	***Sex***	***Number***
		Male	173,880
		Female	225,286

Diabetes contributed to the deaths of more than 7,700 residents.

Number of Deaths Due to Diabetes as Underlying or Contributory Cause

Age	*Number*	*Race*	*Number*
0-44	264	White	6,542
45-64	1,682	African American	1,211
65-74	2,253	Other	33
75+	3,587		
Total	***7,786***	***Sex***	***Number***
		Male	3,372
		Female	4,414

Residents with diabetes face not only a shortened life span, but also suffer from many preventable diabetes-related complications each year.

Diabetes-related Conditions per Year

3,200	lower extremity amputations
1,169	new cases of end-stage renal disease
920-2391	new cases of blindness
197,350	residents with long-term reduction in activity
170,564	hospitalizations
52,557	hospitalizations due to cardiovascular disease among persons with diabetes

In 1990, the direct (medical care) and indirect (lost productivity) cost of diabetes in Texas was about $1,560,000,000.

THE BURDEN OF Diabetes in Utah

More than 66,000 residents are estimated to have diabetes, only half of whom have been diagnosed.

Number of Persons with Diagnosed Diabetes

Age	*Number*
0-44	8,858
45-64	12,266
65-74	7,967
75+	4,715
Total	***33,806***

Race	*Number*
White	32,115
African American	300
Other	1,391

Sex	*Number*
Male	15,164
Female	18,642

Diabetes contributed to the deaths of more than 680 residents.

Number of Deaths Due to Diabetes as Underlying or Contributory Cause

Age	*Number*
0-44	40
45-64	95
65-74	194
75+	358
Total	***687***

Race	*Number*
White	671
African American	3
Other	13

Sex	*Number*
Male	283
Female	404

Residents with diabetes face not only a shortened life span, but also suffer from many preventable diabetes-related complications each year.

Diabetes-related Conditions per Year

262	lower extremity amputations
62	new cases of end-stage renal disease
76-202	new cases of blindness
16,410	residents with long-term reduction in activity
14,169	hospitalizations
4,243	hospitalizations due to cardiovascular disease among persons with diabetes

In 1990, the direct (medical care) and indirect (lost productivity) cost of diabetes in Utah was about $132,000,000.

THE BURDEN OF

Diabetes in Vermont

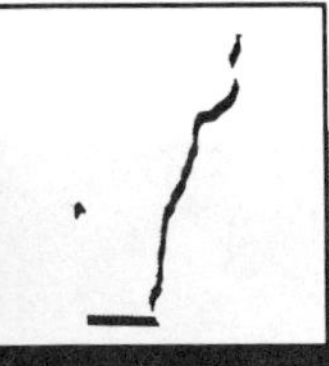

More than 26,000 residents are estimated to have diabetes, only half of whom have been diagnosed.

Number of Persons with Diagnosed Diabetes

Age	*Number*
0-44	2,612
45-64	5,005
65-74	3,308
75+	2,187
Total	***13,112***

Race	*Number*
White	12,955
African American	43
Other	114

Sex	*Number*
Male	5,773
Female	7,339

Diabetes contributed to the deaths of more than 380 residents.

Number of Deaths Due to Diabetes as Underlying or Contributory Cause

Age	*Number*
0-44	12
45-64	53
65-74	101
75+	220
Total	***386***

Race	*Number*
White	383
African American	2
Other	1

Sex	*Number*
Male	184
Female	202

Residents with diabetes face not only a shortened life span, but also suffer from many preventable diabetes-related complications each year.

Diabetes-related Conditions per Year

108	lower extremity amputations
22	new cases of end-stage renal disease
31-79	new cases of blindness
6,531	residents with long-term reduction in activity
5,716	hospitalizations
1,784	hospitalizations due to cardiovascular disease among persons with diabetes

In 1990, the direct (medical care) and indirect (lost productivity) cost of diabetes in Vermont was about $51,000,000.

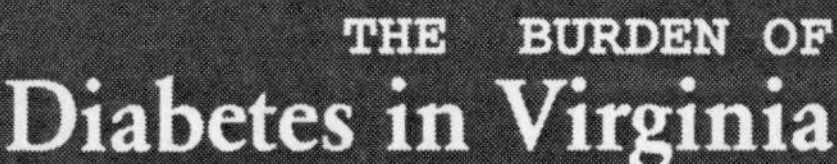

THE BURDEN OF Diabetes in Virginia

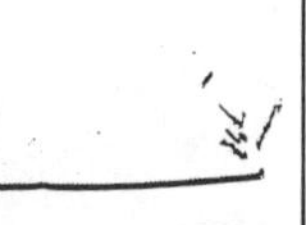

More than 322,000 residents are estimated to have diabetes, only half of whom have been diagnosed.

Number of Persons with Diagnosed Diabetes

Age	*Number*	*Race*	*Number*
0-44	30,596	White	114,224
45-64	66,834	African American	42,300
65-74	40,173	Other	5,100
75+	24,021		
Total	***161,624***	***Sex***	***Number***
		Male	69,617
		Female	92,007

Diabetes contributed to the deaths of more than 3,200 residents.

Number of Deaths Due to Diabetes as Underlying or Contributory Cause

Age	*Number*	*Race*	*Number*
0-44	100	White	2,334
45-64	698	African American	897
65-74	1,002	Other	16
75+	1,447		
Total	***3,247***	***Sex***	***Number***
		Male	1,418
		Female	1,829

Residents with diabetes face not only a shortened life span, but also suffer from many preventable diabetes-related complications each year.

Diabetes-related Conditions per Year

1,308	lower extremity amputations
315	new cases of end-stage renal disease
376-968	new cases of blindness
80,471	residents with long-term reduction in activity
69,195	hospitalizations
21,587	hospitalizations due to cardiovascular disease among persons with diabetes

In 1990, the direct (medical care) and indirect (lost productivity) cost of diabetes in Virginia was about $632,000,000.

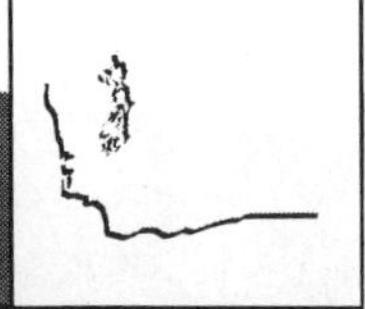

THE BURDEN OF Diabetes in Washington

More than 236,000 residents are estimated to have diabetes, only half of whom have been diagnosed.

Number of Persons with Diagnosed Diabetes

Age	*Number*
0-44	23,122
45-64	45,853
65-74	30,952
75+	18,690
Total	***118,617***

Race	*Number*
White	105,346
African American	4,174
Other	9,097

Sex	*Number*
Male	53,193
Female	65,424

Diabetes contributed to the deaths of more than 2,300 residents.

Number of Deaths Due to Diabetes as Underlying or Contributory Cause

Age	*Number*
0-44	71
45-64	391
65-74	707
75+	1,190
Total	***2,359***

Race	*Number*
White	2,222
African American	67
Other	70

Sex	*Number*
Male	1,082
Female	1,277

Residents with diabetes face not only a shortened life span, but also suffer from many preventable diabetes-related complications each year.

Diabetes-related Conditions per Year

968	lower extremity amputations
213	new cases of end-stage renal disease
279-710	new cases of blindness
59,070	residents with long-term reduction in activity
51,406	hospitalizations
16,057	hospitalizations due to cardiovascular disease among persons with diabetes

In 1990, the direct (medical care) and indirect (lost productivity) cost of diabetes in Washington was about $464,000,000.

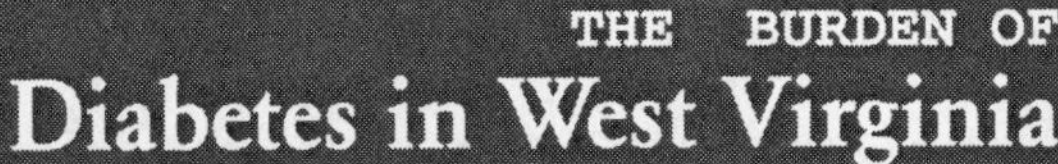

THE BURDEN OF Diabetes in West Virginia

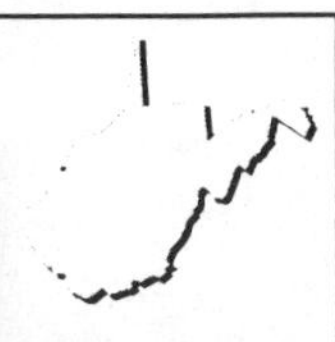

More than 98,000 residents are estimated to have diabetes, only half of whom have been diagnosed.

Number of Persons with Diagnosed Diabetes

Age	*Number*
0-44	7,727
45-64	18,367
65-74	14,205
75+	8,881
Total	***49,180***

Race	*Number*
White	46,243
African American	2,610
Other	327

Sex	*Number*
Male	21,041
Female	28,139

Diabetes contributed to the deaths of more than 1,800 residents.

Number of Deaths Due to Diabetes as Underlying or Contributory Cause

Age	*Number*
0-44	45
45-64	345
65-74	547
75+	875
Total	***1,812***

Race	*Number*
White	1,714
African American	96
Other	2

Sex	*Number*
Male	753
Female	1,059

Residents with diabetes face not only a shortened life span, but also suffer from many preventable diabetes-related complications each year.

Diabetes-related Conditions per Year

419	lower extremity amputations
90	new cases of end-stage renal disease
120-295	new cases of blindness
24,907	residents with long-term reduction in activity
22,068	hospitalizations
7,078	hospitalizations due to cardiovascular disease among persons with diabetes

In 1990, the direct (medical care) and indirect (lost productivity) cost of diabetes in West Virginia was about $192,000,000.

THE BURDEN OF
Diabetes in Wisconsin

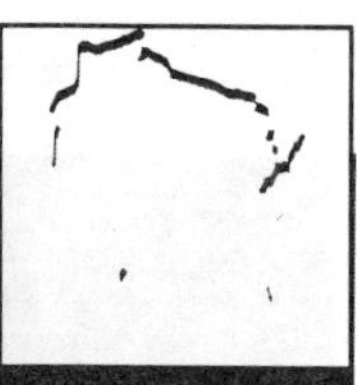

More than 244,000 residents are estimated to have diabetes, only half of whom have been diagnosed.

Number of Persons with Diagnosed Diabetes

Age	*Number*
0-44	22,614
45-64	45,272
65-74	32,596
75+	22,434
Total	***122,916***

Race	*Number*
White	114,242
African American	6,366
Other	2,308

Sex	*Number*
Male	53,768
Female	69,148

Diabetes contributed to the deaths of more than 3,300 residents.

Number of Deaths Due to Diabetes as Underlying or Contributory Cause

Age	*Number*
0-44	64
45-64	483
65-74	857
75+	1,905
Total	***3,309***

Race	*Number*
White	3,167
African American	108
Other	34

Sex	*Number*
Male	1,523
Female	1,786

Residents with diabetes face not only a shortened life span, but also suffer from many preventable diabetes-related complications each year.

Diabetes-related Conditions per Year

1,031	lower extremity amputations
253	new cases of end-stage renal disease
294-736	new cases of blindness
61,715	residents with long-term reduction in activity
54,709	hospitalizations
17,278	hospitalizations due to cardiovascular disease among persons with diabetes

In 1990, the direct (medical care) and indirect (lost productivity) cost of diabetes in Wisconsin was about $481,000,000.

THE BURDEN OF Diabetes in Wyoming

More than 20,000 residents are estimated to have diabetes, only half of whom have been diagnosed.

Number of Persons with Diagnosed Diabetes

Age	*Number*
0-44	2,169
45-64	4,027
65-74	2,500
75+	1,475
Total	***10,171***

Race	*Number*
White	9,725
African American	103
Other	343

Sex	*Number*
Male	4,648
Female	5,523

Diabetes contributed to the deaths of more than 170 residents.

Number of Deaths Due to Diabetes as Underlying or Contributory Cause

Age	*Number*
0-44	4
45-64	33
65-74	48
75+	85
Total	***170***

Race	*Number*
White	160
African American	2
Other	8

Sex	*Number*
Male	71
Female	99

Residents with diabetes face not only a shortened life span, but also suffer from many preventable diabetes-related complications each year.

Diabetes-related Conditions per Year

81	lower extremity amputations
19	new cases of end-stage renal disease
24-61	new cases of blindness
5,023	residents with long-term reduction in activity
4,324	hospitalizations
1,332	hospitalizations due to cardiovascular disease among persons with diabetes

In 1990, the direct (medical care) and indirect (lost productivity) cost of diabetes in Wyoming was about $40,000,000.

Chapter 4

Diabetes in Adults

Introduction

Several factors motivated this information booklet on adult-onset diabetes. First, although the illness is a major health problem, striking between 10 and 11 million Americans, diabetes often goes undiagnosed. As many as half the people with the disorder don't know they have it. Second, we now have made major advances in understanding the causes of this disease. Third—and most importantly—these advances have provided new strategies for preventing and treating diabetes.

Background

Diabetes is the seventh leading cause of death in the United States and the single leading cause of kidney disease. More than 250,000 Americans die each year from causes directly related to the illness. The disorder is also the leading cause of blindness and, aside from traumatic injury, the chief cause of amputations in the United States. Diabetics have doubled the risk of the general population for heart attack and stroke. Moreover, diabetics also are less likely to recover from these injuries.

But the good news is that many of the complications of diabetes, as well as the defects underlying the illness, can be controlled and treated—particularly the type of diabetes that develops in adults.

There are actually two forms of diabetes. Type I diabetes affects only

---

NIH Pub. No. 90–2904.

about five to 10 percent of the 10 million people with the disease, and it occurs predominantly in children. Type I illness often begins suddenly and can be life-threatening. If medical treatment, including insulin, is not begun very quickly, the child may die. For this reason, Type I diabetes is referred to as insulin-dependent diabetes (IDDM).

This booklet focuses on Type II diabetes, which affects the other 90 to 95 percent of the diabetic population. In addition to primarily affecting adults, it differs from Type I disease in other significant ways. For example, although some Type II diabetics take insulin, these people do not run the risk of becoming acutely and profoundly ill if they stop using the medication. For this reason, Type II diabetes is also known as noninsulin-dependent diabetes (NIDDM).

Defining the Illness

Whenever one eats a meal, digested sugar, or glucose, leaves the stomach through tiny blood vessels, passing to the liver and pancreas, and from there to the general circulation. The pancreas responds to the influx of glucose by producing the hormone known as insulin. Insulin influences the liver to store excess glucose. It also enables the body's cells to incorporate glucose—a vital source of energy—from the blood. Muscle cells use glucose as fuel, while fat cells store the compound, converting it into lipids or fat particles that can easily be tapped for energy as the body needs it.

People with Type I diabetes do not produce enough insulin for these life-sustaining processes to continue as needed. Researchers have documented that among Type I patients, the pancreatic cells that normally produce the hormone have virtually all been killed—apparently due to a misguided attack by the body's immune system.

Among Type II patients, the underlying problem is different, but the end result is the same: an unhealthy buildup of glucose in the blood and an inability for the body's cells to properly use the compound. Type II individuals have their normal amount of insulin-secreting pancreatic cells—known as the islets—and these cells still produce a reasonable amount and sometimes even greater than normal amount of insulin. But for unknown reasons, the muscle and fat cells in these patients appear insensitive to insulin secretion. Researchers believe the insensitivity results from an apparent defect in the insulin receptors found on the surface of muscle and fat cells. The defect prevents the cells from locking onto insulin in the blood stream, stopping the cells from properly using blood glucose.

Scientists know that most overweight people have some insulin resistance—a cellular insensitivity to the action of glucose. In fact, the fatter they are, the more insulin resistance they develop. But the pancreas of most of these and other insulin-resistant individuals can compensate for the insensitivity by producing sufficiently large amounts of insulin. These people do not have Type II diabetes, although they may be at risk for the disorder. But in some people, the pancreas cannot make enough insulin to overcome the resistance problem. These individuals develop Type II disease.

In summary, Type II, or noninsulin-dependent, diabetes occurs due to a combination of two problems: resistance by the body's tissues to insulin activity, and an inability of islet cells to overcome this resistance by producing extra amounts of the hormone.

Symptoms

Diabetes—both Type I and Type II—is an insidious disease. There often are no obvious warning signs that a person either cannot secrete enough insulin or cannot properly use the hormone to break down glucose stored in the blood. Yet once diabetes is suspected, simple and inexpensive blood and urine tests can easily identify the problem. Thus, the ability to identify symptoms that may signal diabetes onset becomes crucial to controlling this disease.

One of the first signs of something wrong is insatiable thirst, often associated with excessive urination. Both symptoms occur because the body attempts to rid itself of unusually high levels of blood sugar through constant excretion of fluids, leaving the individual in constant need of fluid replacement. In turn, massive fluid intake and urination can alternately swell and shrink body tissues, causing other symptoms, such as blurry vision. Such blurriness may prompt people to see a doctor long before other diabetes-related symptoms become apparent. Effective treatment of the diabetes tends to alleviate this visual problem.

As time goes on, diabetic patients—particularly those whose other symptoms have not triggered them to seek medical treatment—may suffer even more serious eye problems. Some may have a progressive, permanent loss of vision before the diagnosis of diabetes is made.

People who develop diabetes often have sensory nerve damage, losing the ability to feel appropriate pain and the sense of touch, especially in the feet. Sometimes, one of the first signs of disease is numbness or tingling in the feet or lower leg. Alternatively, nerve damage may cause unprovoked excruciating pain again usually in the legs and feet that can incapacitate a person, preventing him or her from walking, sleeping or performing other routine functions of daily living.

In those people unable to feel pain, such everyday occurrences as blisters can go unchecked, leading to cuts, bruises, ulcers and other serious injuries of the lower extremities. Ulcers may lead to serious infections that prompt a doctor's visit. Only then is the patient diagnosed as diabetic.

Over time, diabetes can also damage the involuntary nervous system, causing such problems as sexual impotence. Diabetics also have increased atherosclerosis—hardening of the arteries, or the buildup of plaque and fatty material inside blood vessel walls. Often, physicians do not detect this problem—other diabetes symptoms have not tipped them off to look for it—until after a heart attack or stroke.

Some people later found to have diabetes often report feelings of fatigue, malaise and a general lack of energy. Individuals may blame such feelings on aging, depression or their poor physical shape. But when these people do see a doctor, they are found to have diabetes—and are likely to have had it for some years.

Those at Risk

Because the symptoms of Type II diabetes are both varied and elusive, it is imperative to identify those people at highest risk for the disease. These individuals might regularly undergo a thorough medical checkup for diabetes, helping to catch the disorder early on, before extensive damage occurs.

We now know that obese people carry an unusually high risk for developing Type II diabetes. Physicians estimate that 60 to 90 percent of people with this form of diabetes are overweight. Studies show that among the Pima Indians of the southwestern United States, the ethnic group with the highest known incidence of noninsulin-dependent diabetes in the world, obesity is a major health problem.

The risk for Type II diabetes for both sexes also increases with age. As the body ages, its ability to efficiently use insulin for glucose metabolism begins to deteriorate. Heredity is another risk factor. If one or both parents developed noninsulin-dependent diabetes, a person's chances of having the disease is increased. The risk is increased approximately two-fold for each parent with Type II diabetes. If both parents are affected then the risk is four-fold higher. If one of two identical twins develops Type II diabetes, researchers calculate that the second twin has nearly a 90 percent chance of developing the illness within five to 10 years.

In the United States, certain minority populations have a higher-than-normal rate of Type II diabetes. Among blacks, the illness occurs about 1.5 times as frequently as in the general population. Hispanics and Oriental Americans have a rate about twice that of the general population. We've already mentioned the plight of the Pimas. Half of the tribe members over age 35 now develop the disorder. Up until about 40 years ago, the Pimas did not have this high rate. Through about 1940, the Pimas survived mainly on desert foods, dining mostly on vegetables, grains and subsistence crops. As western, high-fat, high-calorie foods became increasingly available to the Pimas, they began to develop widespread obesity. Combined with a possible genetic predisposition for insulin resistance, researchers believe that obesity has triggered the high incidence of Type II diabetes in the Pimas.

Treatment

The chief way to treat or control Type II diabetes is to eat an appropriate calorie diet and begin regular exercise under a doctor's supervision. Both of these lifestyle changes, which can improve cardiovascular fitness, have an added benefit among Type II diabetics. They help people lose weight, which in some cases can reverse or reduce insulin resistance, one of the underlying causes of the disease. Researchers have found that losing weight sometimes increases the body's sensitivity to insulin. In fact, some formerly obese Type II diabetics no longer have the disease after shedding pounds, even if they have not lost enough to attain their ideal body weight. Losing weight, however, does not guarantee elimination of the disease.

Among other lifestyle changes, diabetics should avoid alcohol. Not only is alcohol high in calories and low in nutrients, it can damage the liver and pancreas organs already under stress in diabetes.

Diabetics who smoke should make every effort to stop. Known to raise the risk of heart attack and stroke in the general population, smoking can be particularly dangerous for diabetics, who already have a higher risk for developing cardiovascular problems.

In addition and in conjunction with these behavioral changes, drug therapy may also help the Type II diabetic. About one-third of Type II patients take insulin injections because the drug gives them optimum control of the disease.

Physicians also prescribe other drugs that seem to stimulate the pancreas to make more insulin and to increase the sensitivity of muscle and fat cells to the hormone. The exact action of these medications, available in pill form, is not well understood. There are a variety of such medications but all are in the same basic class of drugs called sulfonylureas. Their generic names include tolbutamide, chlorpropamide, tolazamide, acetohexamide, glipizide and glyburide. Many Type II patients may benefit from these drugs but many do not respond sufficiently and need to take insulin injections for optimal treatment.

Aside from these considerations, patients can help maintain and even improve their condition by becoming active members of the health care team. For example, daily self-inspections of the feet can help spot early signs of infection that might otherwise go unnoticed, given the nerve damage and lack of pain sensation common among diabetics. And individuals also can perform a simple home test to monitor their body's ability to control blood sugar. The test involves pricking a finger with a sterile needle stick and measuring blood levels with a glucose meter now available at drug stores. Such monitoring can supplement, but not replace, more sensitive tests regularly performed by a physician.

While the combination of diet, exercise, drugs and self-monitoring has greatly increased the survival and well being of diabetics, we are far from the end of the journey in controlling, and ultimately preventing, this disease.But with the recent discovery of separate genetic factors that may play a role in Type I and Type II diabetes, it is hopeful that by the year 2000 we will have genetic markers to aid us in improved diagnosis, treatment and prevention of this disease.

Questions and Answers

Q. Can an obese person with Type II diabetes completely eliminate the disease by losing weight through diet and exercise?

A. Yes. For some people, that's exactly the case. In fact, certain individuals don't even have to reach normal weight. It appears that if an obese person who recently developed diabetes begins to lose pounds, their sensitivity to insulin increases even before they attain ideal weight. Unfortunately, this phenomenon does not always occur in the same patients as time goes on. If the disease has persisted for many years, shedding pounds may not be sufficient to overcome it.

Q. Do people of normal weight who have a low-fat, low-calorie diet still have a higher risk for developing diabetes if one of their parents had the disease?

A. Yes. But it is worthwhile for those with a strong family history of diabetes to be extra vigilant about their diet and cardiovascular fitness. It may reduce their elevated risk for developing diabetes, or it may delay onset of the disease.

Q. At what point should a Type II diabetic begin taking insulin supplements?

A. That's a difficult question and there doesn't seem to be a consensus on this. We have no rule that says blood sugar level X means someone requires insulin. Clearly, a patient is a candidate for insulin when other treatment has failed and there's reason to believe the drug may help. But the patient should understand the risks and benefits of insulin therapy, and the decision to go ahead with this treatment should involve all members of the health care team.

Biography

Robert Silverman, M.D., Ph.D.
Chief, Diabetes Programs Branch
National Institute of Diabetes and Digestive and Kidney
Diseases National Institutes of Health

Robert Silverman received both a medical degree and a doctorate in biochemistry from the Washington University School of Medicine in St. Louis. He joined the National Institutes of Health in 1981, serving as a medical staff fellow in the National Institute of Diabetes and Digestive and Kidney Diseases. Since 1984, Dr. Silverman has headed the Diabetes Programs Branch, which supports more than $100 million in diabetes research each year.

Chapter 5

Diabetes in Black Americans

Diabetes mellitus is a major health problem in black Americans. In 1986, the Task Force on Black and Minority Health, appointed by the secretary of the Department of Health and Human Services (DHHS) cited diabetes as one of six health problems responsible for excess mortality among U.S. minority populations.

In 1990, black Americans comprised 12.1 percent of the U.S. population, according to the U.S. Bureau of the Census. Almost 30 million Americans are black, 13.2 percent more than in 1980. Census figures document that blacks have higher rates of poverty and unemployment than do whites. They also have a prevalence of noninsulin-dependent diabetes mellitus (NIDDM) that is 60 percent higher than in whites.

Relatively uncommon among black Americans at the beginning of this century, diabetes is now the fourth leading cause of death by disease among black women and the sixth among black men. A report issued by the National Center for Health Statistics (NCHS) in 1987 noted that the prevalence of diagnosed diabetes in black Americans has increased fourfold in just over two decades, from 228,000 in 1963 to approximately 1 million in 1985. This is almost double the rate of increase among white, non-Hispanic Americans. Another 1 million blacks are estimated to have undiagnosed diabetes.

Blacks have higher rates of diabetes at all adult age levels, and among those 65 to 74 years of age, one in four has diabetes. Among black women diabetes can almost be termed epidemic: One in four black women older than 55 has diabetes—double the rate in white women.

NIH Pub. No. 93–3266.

Black Americans also experience higher rates of at least three of the serious complications of diabetes: blindness, amputations, and end-stage renal disease (ESRD). Rates of severe visual impairment are 40 percent higher in black patients with diabetes than in white patients. Compared to whites, black women are three times more likely to be blind as a result of diabetes and black men have 30 percent higher rates of blindness. Black patients undergo twice as many amputations as do whites, and studies in Michigan and Texas found that the rate of ESRD was at least four times higher in blacks with diabetes.

Government surveys indicate that the higher diabetes rate in blacks prevails across all major sociodemographic parameters—age, sex, educational level, marital status, living arrangement, and regional category. The prevalence of diabetes among blacks is highest in women, older people, the less educated, and persons in families with low incomes.

The 1989 National Health Interview Survey (NHIS) queried 600 black Americans and 1,585 white, non-Hispanic Americans with diabetes about various aspects of their diabetes care. Findings reveal that compared to whites, blacks tended to weigh more, were more likely to use insulin and to have received diabetes education, had seen a doctor slightly more often in the past year, and had had their blood pressure and feet checked more often in the past 6 months. In terms of self monitoring, black patients performed more urine tests each week but fewer blood tests, and they were less likely to have heard of hemoglobin A1c testing.

The NHIS survey also revealed that, compared to whites, a larger percentage of black diabetes patients had seen a dietitian in the past 12 months, and slightly more blacks reported seeing a podiatrist or cardiologist in the past year. Both groups appeared to be comparable in terms of eye care however. Among both black and white patients, only about 44 percent had seen an ophthalmologist in the past 12 months, although almost 80 percent of both black and white patients reported having an eye examination in the past 2 years. Finally, although black patients were more likely to smoke, they smoked fewer cigarettes per day than did white patients.

Defining the Problem

The U.S. Government has cosponsored two national conferences, one in 1988 and one in 1989, to examine the problem of diabetes in blacks and to define issues and priority areas for activities to reduce the impact of diabetes on black Americans. Both conferences were chaired by Dr. Louis W. Sullivan, secretary of DHHS. The first conference focused on epidemiological and research findings relevant to diabetes and its complications in blacks, and the second on ways to increase diabetes awareness within the professional and black lay communities.

Some major findings noted at the first conference were:

- Black people have a higher prevalence of obesity, a strong risk factor for NIDDM. Among people with diagnosed diabetes, 83 percent of adult black women are obese compared with 62 percent of white women and 45 percent of black men are obese compared with 39 percent of white men.
- Black Americans are known to have a high prevalence of hypertension, which is associated with retinopathy and kidney complications, major complications in black patients. Studies are needed to elucidate the disease processes involved in these conditions in black patients and to develop better methods of prevention and treatment.
- Studies of dietary habits of black Americans indicate that they consume less fiber and more cholesterol-rich foods than do whites, although their total intake of calories and fat is lower.
- Black people tend to have less access to financial, social, health, and educational resources that would improve their health status and health awareness.
- Educational resources, including materials and programs, oriented to black patients are needed that take into account black lifestyles, interests, and cultural and economic considerations.

The second conference targeted two critical audiences for diabetes awareness activities: health professionals and the black community itself. Speakers at the conference called for increased physician awareness of diabetes as a serious disease; increased screening activities, especially among high-risk minority patients; and increased education of black patients in modern diabetes management techniques. The need to involve the black community in health promotion activities, especially among black women, was stressed.

The National Diabetes Information Clearinghouse has compiled a directory of programs and other resources to help health educators, public health officials, community leaders, and others in developing educational programs to foster awareness of diabetes and its management among black Americans. The directory, *Diabetes-Related Programs for Black Americans: A Resource Guide,* includes descriptions of diabetes-related programs that are targeted to black people or that serve communities with substantial black populations.

Single copies of the directory are available free from:

National Diabetes Information Clearinghouse
Box NDIC
9000 Rockville Pike
Bethesda, MD 20892
(301) 468–2162

[NOTE: For your convenience, the directory has been included in the appendix.]

Chapter 6

Diabetes in Hispanics

The rate of diabetes among Hispanic Americans, one of the fastest growing minorities in the United States, far exceeds that of white, non-Hispanic Americans. Data from the Hispanic Health and Nutrition Examination Survey (HHANES) of 1982–84 have confirmed what earlier studies have indicated: Diabetes is a major health problem among American Latinos.

Analysis of HHANES data indicates that 1.3 million Hispanics over 21 years of age have diabetes, almost 10 percent of the adult Hispanic population. Compared with whites, rates of diabetes (diagnosed and undiagnosed) are 50 to 60 percent higher in Cubans and 110 to 120 percent higher in Mexican-Americans and Puerto Ricans.

The most common form of diabetes in Hispanics is noninsulin-dependent (Type II) diabetes, which usually develops in adults over the age of 40. In the 45 to 74 age group, 26.1 percent of Puerto Ricans, 23.9 percent of Mexican-Americans, and 15.8 percent of Cubans have diabetes. One-third of Hispanics 65 to 74 years old have diabetes, compared with 17 percent of non-Hispanic whites in this age group.

Impaired glucose tolerance (IGT), probably the most significant risk factor for diabetes, also is prevalent among older Hispanics. About one-half of Mexican-Americans and Puerto Ricans over the age of 55 have either diabetes or IGT, according to HHANES data. Between the ages of 65 and 74, Hispanics are more likely to have abnormal levels of glucose tolerance than normal levels.

NIH Pub. No. 93–3265.

Severely overweight Hispanics appear to be at higher risk for diabetes than their non-Hispanic counterparts. Findings from the HHANES study indicate that obese Hispanics, with the exception of Cubans at the highest weight level, are more likely to have diabetes than are obese non-Hispanic whites and blacks. The study also found that among Mexican-Americans, 39 percent of the women and 30 percent of the men are overweight. Among Puerto Ricans, the rates are 37 percent in women and 25 percent in men; among Cubans, the rates are 34 percent in women and 29 percent in men.

The HHANES is the most comprehensive national survey to date of the health status of Hispanics living on the U.S. mainland. The survey, conducted by the National Center for Health Statistics, included Mexican-Americans in five southwestern states, Cubans in the Miami area, and Puerto Ricans in the New York City area.

Other studies in Texas and California indicate that Mexican-Americans have higher death rates from diabetes and are more vulnerable to some of the severe complications of diabetes than are non-Hispanics. In a study conducted in San Antonio, Mexican-American diabetes patients had higher rates of severe retinopathy than non-Hispanic patients in that area. These data are confirmed in preliminary findings from the 1988 National Health and Nutrition Examination Survey. Other reports suggest that Mexican-Americans are six times more likely than non-Hispanics to develop end-stage renal disease, they are more subject to severe hyperglycemia, and Mexican-American women have high rates of gestational diabetes and resulting birth complications. Yet, a study of Texas border counties found that 60 percent of diabetes-caused blindness could have been prevented with proper treatment, as could 51 percent of kidney failures and 67 percent of diabetes-related amputations of feet and legs.

The severity of the diabetes problem in Hispanic Americans is compounded by limited access to health care. According to the Current Population Survey of 1989, one-third of Hispanics lack health insurance of any kind, compared with 12 percent of non-Hispanic whites, about 19 percent of non-Hispanic blacks, and 18 percent of other ethnic minorities. Some 37 percent of Mexican-Americans are uninsured, as well as more than 20 percent of Cubans and 15.5 percent of Puerto Ricans. Findings from HHANES indicate that uninsured rates among Puerto Ricans and Cubans may be as high as 22 and 28.6 percent, respectively. Fewer Puerto Ricans are uninsured because they are more likely to be covered under state Medicaid programs.

The HHANES findings suggest that lack of health insurance may translate into lack of medical care for many Hispanics. The survey shows that uninsured Hispanics were less likely to have seen a physician within the past year and more likely never to have had a physical examination. A study in San Antonio found that uninsured Mexican-American diabetes patients had higher rates of microvascular complications.

These findings pose new problems and considerations for public health programs. Hispanics are currently the second largest minority group in the United States with a population of more than 22 million in 1990. Approximately two-thirds of Hispanics are of Mexican-American origin. Between 1980 and 1990, the Hispanic population grew 40 percent. By the year 2000, Hispanics may be the largest minority group, with a projected population of 31 million; and by 2080, their numbers may increase an additional 200 percent (40 million persons).

Hispanics are also a "young" population group, with a median age of about 26 years compared with 34 for the U.S. population as a whole. However, like other population groups, Hispanics are experiencing an increase in life expectancy and their elderly population has increased by 75 percent since 1980. As the Hispanic elderly population continues to increase, health problems such as noninsulin-dependent diabetes, which is associated with aging, can be expected to have an even greater effect on this community.

Meeting the Challenge: NIDDK Targets Programs for Hispanics

The National Institute of Diabetes and Digestive and Kidney Diseases (NIDDK), the U.S. Government's primary agency for diabetes research, has taken several steps to address the burden of diabetes in Hispanic Americans. In May 1988, Dr. Phillip Gorden, NIDDK director, convened a 2-day symposium that brought together leading researchers in the fields of diabetes and Hispanic health care. Speakers discussed characteristics of diabetes and its complications in Hispanics, as well as genetic and nongenetic factors that may account for the higher prevalence of diabetes in this population. Researchers noted that among Mexican-Americans in Texas, the risk for diabetes appears to be positively correlated with the degree of Native American ancestry. Other similarities to diabetes in Native Americans were suggested, including the influence of obesity, particularly upper-body obesity, a westernized lifestyle, and the presence of hyperinsulinism.

The NIDDK supports research projects concerned with diabetes in Hispanics, including projects that address complications of the disorder in this population and projects that focus on primary prevention of diabetes. The National Eye Institute and the National Heart, Lung, and Blood Institute of the National Institutes of Health have funded research studies in Puerto Rico and Texas on eye and cardiovascular complications of diabetes.

In addition, the NIDDK's National Diabetes Data Group (NDDG) has collaborated with the National Center for Health Statistics in several epidemiological surveys that included Hispanic populations: HHANES, the 1989 National Health Interview Survey, and the 1988–91 National Health and Nutrition Examination Survey. Analysis of data from these surveys is helping NDDG to define more clearly the extent of the diabetes problem in U.S. Hispanics.

The NIDDK has collaborated with the National Coalition of Hispanic Health and Human Service Organizations (COSSMHO) in several projects, including organizing workshops on diabetes for the Sixth Biennial National Hispanic Conference on Health and Human Services and helping to develop an independently funded diabetes research grant program. The Diabetes Research and Training Center at the Albert Einstein School of Medicine in New York City, an NIDDK-funded center, is working with COSSMHO in developing materials for non-Hispanic physicians who care for Hispanic patients.

The National Diabetes Information Clearinghouse, a service of NIDDK, distributes a listing of Spanish-language diabetes education materials available from a variety of sources. In addition, the NDIC offers a number of Spanish-language publications, including a dictionary of diabetes-related terms and brochures about periodontal disease and diabetes. These materials are available from: National Diabetes Information Clearinghouse, Box NDIC, 9000 Rockville Pike, Rockville, MD 20892 (301) 468–2162

[For your convenience, a copy of *Diabetes Educational Materials in Spanish and Other Languages* is reproduced in the Appendix of this volume.]

Additional Reading

Journal of the American Medical Association (JAMA), vol. 265, no. 2, January 9, 1991. This issue summarizes data from HHANES and other studies, presenting a comprehensive look at the health of Hispanic Americans.

American Journal of Public Health, supplement, vol. 80, December 1990. This special supplement present the results of HHANES, focusing on findings related to health status and health care needs in the Hispanic-American community.

Diabetes Care, supplement, vol. 14, no. 7, suppl. 3, July 1991. This issue reports the proceedings of the NIDDK-sponsored symposium, "Diabetes in Hispanic Americans," held in May 1988.

"Race and Hispanic Origin," *1990 Census Profile,* Number 2, June 1991. Published by the U.S. Department of Commerce, Economics and Statistics Administration, Bureau of the Census. Contact Customer Services, U.S. Bureau of the Census, Washington, DC 20233; telephone (301) 763–4100.

"Statement of Eleanor Chelimsky, Assistant Comptroller General, Before the House Select Committee on Aging and the Congressional Hispanic Caucus, September 19, 1991," in *Hispanic Access to Health Care, Report to Congressional Requesters,* January 1992. Available from the U.S. General Accounting Office, Washington, DC 20548; telephone (202) 275–6241.

Chapter 7

Diabetes in Japanese Americans

A complex interaction of environmental and genetic factors appears to cause the high incidence of noninsulin-dependent, or type II, diabetes mellitus and abnormal glucose tolerance in second-generation Japanese-American men, say researchers at the University of Washington in Seattle. These factors, which may be key disease determinants in other populations as well, include intra-abdominal obesity, diet, and sociocultural stress.

"Because Japanese Americans have retained much racial homogeneity, they provide a unique opportunity to examine the effects of sociocultural and economic change in the etiology of a common chronic disease such as diabetes," notes Dr. Wilfred Fujimoto, professor of medicine at the University of Washington School of Medicine and associate program director of the General Clinical Research Center at the University of Washington Medical Center.

Testing of more than 200 second-generation Japanese-American men 45 to 74 years old from the Seattle area showed that 31 percent had abnormal glucose tolerance, which is higher than the prevalence of abnormal glucose tolerance in Caucasian Americans. The investigators also found that 34 percent of the Japanese-American men in the study had type II diabetes, a mild form of the disease caused by insulin resistance, an inability of the liver and skeletal muscle to properly respond to insulin. Most people with insulin resistance react by producing an abnormally high level of blood insulin, hyperinsulinemia. Type II diabetes often develops in overweight people who are more than 40 years old, according to the researchers.

Research Resources Reporter, October 1990.

The Seattle investigators have particularly focused on the link between obesity and glucose intolerance. A critical factor appears to be intra-abdominal obesity, a marker for increased fat deposits among the visceral organs.

"Japanese-American men are clearly heavier than native Japanese, but the degree of obesity in Japanese-American men is less than in the Caucasian population in the United States," says Dr. Fujimoto. What seems to distinguish Japanese-American men from their Caucasian neighbors is that they may be more susceptible to the adverse consequences of increased fat in the abdomen.

Abdominal fat has been traditionally measured using skin fold measurements and approximated by a person's waist to hip ratio, but computed tomography (CT, a procedure to record internal body images) provides the most definitive assessment. "CT is the only reliable way to measure visceral fat deposits," says Dr. Fujimoto. "But it's expensive and involves radiation exposure." To minimize cost and radiation exposure, Dr. Fujimoto has limited CT fat analyses to three "slices" through a person's body at the chest, mid-abdomen, and mid-thigh. "This is obviously a very limited examination, so we've also tried to relate these measures to skinfold thicknesses at various other body sites," he explains.

The results of these studies showed that many Japanese-American men have intra-abdominal obesity. Serial study findings also indicate that among Japanese Americans, men with greater amounts of visceral fat are more likely to develop type II diabetes. Insulin resistance is another characteristic that seems to predict the eventual onset of type II diabetes in these men.

"Which comes first, insulin resistance or abdominal obesity, remains an important question," notes Dr. Fujimoto. "One hypothesis is that intra-abdominal fat occurs first. When this fat is catabolized it generates free fatty acids that directly enter the liver and may cause insulin resistance. But," he cautions, "this has not yet been proven." Although this scheme of cause and effect exists in animals, it's very difficult to make similar measurements in people.

The Seattle researchers are also exploring the possible causes of intra-abdominal obesity in Japanese Americans. One factor may be sociocultural stress, which they have documented in this population using interviews and by measuring blood levels of the catecholamine stress hormones such as epinephrine and norepinephrine. "There seems to be an association between visceral adiposity and levels of catecholamines," says Dr. Fujimoto. Diet is probably another determinant of visceral fat. "The typical Japanese-American diet is significantly higher in animal fat than is the typical Japanese diet," he notes.

The role of genetics in this process remains murky. "Type II diabetes clearly has a strong hereditary component, but Japanese-American men with no family history of the disease show a much stronger relationship between visceral fat and diabetes. What we don't know," adds Dr. Fujimoto, "is whether the propensity to deposit fat viscerally is genetically determined. If it is, it would mean that people with this predisposition may deposit visceral fat especially under extenuating circumstances like stress or diet."

The insulin resistance and subsequent hyperinsulinemia that Dr. Fujimoto believes results from intra-abdominal fat may do more than just cause type II diabetes. "We see a strong association of intra-abdominal obesity and hyperinsulinemia with high plasma triglycerides, low plasma high-density lipoprotein (HDL)-cholesterol, and coronary artery disease," he says. Research findings by other investigators suggest that hyperinsulinemia may elevate plasma triglyceride levels and reduce plasma HDL-cholesterol, effects that are conducive to development of atherosclerosis and could lead to coronary artery disease.

Researchers have also linked hyperinsulinemia to the development of hypertension in several study populations, but this relationship is not clearly apparent in Japanese Americans. "Perhaps that's because their hypertension is strongly related to other factors, such as salt consumption," says Dr. Fujimoto.

To extend the findings, the Seattle team has begun examining the prevalence of diabetes and coronary artery disease in Japanese-American women. "We found that the prevalence of diabetes and impaired glucose tolerance is considerably elevated in these women compared to native Japanese women," says Dr. Fujimoto. Studies now in progress will try to determine whether the higher prevalence correlates with visceral obesity and insulin resistance.

Another research avenue is taking the Seattle investigators to Sao Paulo, Brazil, home to a sizeable group of expatriate Japanese. "A preliminary analysis shows that the incidence of diabetes in Japanese-Brazilian men is, surprisingly, almost the same as in Japanese-American men," says Dr. Fujimoto. "This is an important clue, because whatever is important in causing type II diabetes in Japanese men must be common to both the Sao Paulo and Seattle populations."

—Mitchel Zoler, Ph.D.

Additional reading:

1. Bergstrom, R. W., Newell-Morris, L. L., Leonetti, D. L., Shuman, W. P., Wahl, P. W., and Fujimoto W. Y., Association of elevated fasting C-Peptide level and increased intra-abdominal fat distribution with development of NIDDM in Japanese-American men. *Diabetes* 39:104–111, 1990.

2. Fujimoto, W. Y., Bergstrom, R. W., Newell-Morris, L., and Leonetti, D. L., Nature and nurture in the etiology of type II diabetes mellitus in Japanese Americans. *Diabetes/Metabolism Reviews* 5:607–625, 1989.

3. Newell-Morris, L., Treder, R. P., Shulman, W. P., and Fujimoto, W. Y., Fatness, fat distribution, and glucose tolerance in second-generation Japanese-American (Nisei) men. *American Journal of Clinical Nutrition* 50:9–18, 1989.

4. Shulman, W. P., Newell-Morris, L., Leonetti, D. L., Wahl, P. W., Moceri, V. M., Moss, A. A., and Fujimoto, W. Y. Abnormal body fat distribution detected by computed tomography in diabetic men. *Investigative Radiology* 21:483–487, 1986.

The research described in this article was supported by the General Clinical Research Centers Program of the National Center for Research Resources, the National Institute of Diabetes and Digestive and Kidney Diseases, the Diabetes Endocrinology Research Center, the Northwest Lipid Research Center Lipoprotein Laboratory, and the National Science Foundation.

Chapter 8

Insulin-Dependent Diabetes

Insulin-dependent diabetes (IDDM) is a chronic disease that usually begins in childhood. It is not the most common form of diabetes—IDDM accounts for only 5 percent or less of diabetes in this country. Often, though, IDDM has a much greater impact on a person's life than the more common adult-onset form of diabetes, known as noninsulin-dependent diabetes (NIDDM). The onset of IDDM is usually more swift and severe than that of NIDDM. A child with IDDM can become sick very quickly. If treatment does not begin shortly after the first symptoms, the child may need to be hospitalized. Once the diagnosis is made, a person with IDDM needs daily injections of the hormone insulin to survive.

Insulin, discovered in the 1920's, has literally made the difference between life and death for thousands of people with IDDM. Insulin is not a cure for diabetes, however. Even with careful insulin treatment, people who have had diabetes for years are at greater than average risk of developing problems that involve the heart, blood vessels, eyes, kidneys, and nerves. While most of those with IDDM can lead physically active and professionally challenging lives, they do not have the luxury of taking their health for granted.

Research is adding rapidly to our knowledge of diabetes. Besides searching for a cure, scientists are learning how to help people with diabetes enjoy a longer life with fewer health problems.

NIH Pub. No. 90–2098.

What Is Diabetes?

Diabetes mellitus impairs the way the body uses digested food for energy. The sugars and starches (carbohydrates) in the food we eat are broken down by digestive juices into a simple sugar called glucose. Glucose circulates in the blood as the major energy source for the body. For cells in muscles and other tissues to use glucose for energy, the hormone insulin must be present. Insulin is produced by the pancreas gland located behind the stomach. When the right amount of insulin is present, glucose is either used as fuel for energy or stored in the liver for future use.

In diabetes, however, the pancreas may not make enough insulin, or the body does not respond to the insulin that is present. Sometimes, a person with diabetes can have both these problems. As a result, glucose builds up in the blood and tissues, overflows into the urine, and is excreted. Thus, the body loses its main source of fuel.

In IDDM the pancreas makes little or no natural insulin, and a person with IDDM needs daily injections of the hormone to stay alive. IDDM generally occurs in children and adolescents, though it can appear at any age. An estimated 300,000 to 500,000 persons in the United States have IDDM. International statistics on IDDM are unreliable. In general, however, IDDM is unknown or rare in some ethnic groups, including the Japanese, Chinese, American Indians, Polynesians, and South African blacks. On the other hand, Sweden and Finland have very high rates: in Sweden it is estimated that 3 children in 1,000 have IDDM versus 1.6 in 1,000 in the United States. The reasons for these differences are not yet known.

NIDDM is the more common form of diabetes. Of the 11 million Americans who have diabetes, over 95 percent have NIDDM. Fully half of those with NIDDM don't know they have it. NIDDM usually occurs after age 40. In NIDDM, the pancreas can produce insulin, but the body does not use it efficiently. For this reason, most people with NIDDM can control their diabetes with careful dieting and regular exercise. When diet and exercise fail to control NIDDM, insulin or oral drugs can be used to help control the condition.

Effective treatment exists for both IDDM and NIDDM. Even with treatment, however, both types of diabetes can cause long-term damage to the eyes, nerves, heart, and kidneys. These complications can lead to blindness, heart attack, stroke, kidney disease, and serious infections that may require limb amputation. In IDDM, episodes of very high or low blood sugar can cause a coma. Careful treatment of diabetes is the most effective way to minimize the chances of complications.

Symptoms

The symptoms of IDDM can be sudden and severe. They may include frequent urination, extreme thirst, constant hunger, blurred vision, and extreme fatigue. Because people with IDDM lack insulin, glucose builds up in the blood. The kidneys, trying to remove the excess sugar, excrete large amounts of water and essential body elements, causing frequent urination and thirst.

Because the body cannot use glucose, its first source of energy, it turns to stored fat and protein for fuel. As the body uses fat and protein, weight is lost. Breakdown products of fat collect in blood and raise its acid content. If levels of these products are high enough, a critical condition called ketoacidosis can develop, requiring prompt treatment.

How Is Diabetes Treated?

A person with IDDM must have insulin injections to survive. Without insulin, symptoms worsen until the patient loses consciousness and slips into a coma. With daily insulin shots and a careful diet, however, most people with IDDM can lead active lives with the same ambitions and challenges as those without diabetes.

Treatment for IDDM includes a daily routine of insulin shots or use of an insulin pump. Following a doctor's instructions, a person with IDDM buys insulin and syringes and injects himself or herself daily. (The parent of a young child with IDDM can do this for the child.) More and more people are also using home blood glucose monitoring devices to measure their blood glucose during the day. In this way, they can tailor the insulin dose more closely to changes in their hour-to-hour blood glucose. Blood glucose monitoring is a more accurate way to monitor diabetes treatment than urine testing.

Eating the right foods at the right time is an important part of treatment. A person with IDDM needs to time meals with insulin doses to keep blood glucose from getting too high or low. The foods you choose can play a role in controlling blood glucose levels, too. Increasing the proportion of fiber and complex carbohydrates in your diet and avoiding refined sugar may aid in reducing drastic changes in blood glucose and may, in some people, permit lowering of insulin dose. Foods containing fiber include beans, whole grains, and some fruits, while complex carbohydrates, or starches, include potatoes, rice, and pasta.

Reducing fats and cholesterol can help reduce the risk of heart disease, which affects people with diabetes more often than those with normal glucose metabolism.

Exercise, like diet, can help reduce the risk of heart disease. Being fit can also bring a sense of well-being and strength that has special meaning for someone with a chronic illness like diabetes.

Exercise carefully, though. Strenuous exercise increases the muscles' use of glucose, so it can lower glucose in the blood. At the same time, exercise also stimulates the body to release glucose and fats for use as energy. This stimulus can have the effect of raising blood glucose. In order to exercise safely, you should balance insulin dose, meals, and the timing of exercise to keep blood glucose levels from getting too high or too low.

What Causes Diabetes?

No one knows exactly what causes IDDM. What is clear is that the body's own immune or disease-fighting system for some reason turns against the body's own tissues. Certain substances formed by the immune system attack the beta cells of the pancreas, destroying their ability to make insulin.

Research shows that most, if not all, people with IDDM may inherit traits that put them at risk for IDDM. However, not everyone who inherits these traits develops IDDM. One or more factors in the environment are believed to trigger the immune system to destroy the insulin-producing cells. In some cases, the trigger may be a viral infection. Scientists have, in a few cases, been able to link the onset of diabetes with a virus. In most cases, however, the trigger for diabetes is unknown.

Complications of Diabetes

The discovery of insulin in 1921 lengthened the lives of people with IDDM from weeks or months to decades. In spite of insulin's life-preserving effects, diabetes remains a deadly disease. This fact is largely due to the complications of diabetes that develop over many years of insulin treatment. The complications affect the heart, eyes, kidneys, and nerves. Much of the damage done to these organs involves changes in small blood vessels throughout the body. Research is under way to determine whether very careful control of blood glucose can prevent or delay diabetic complications. Studies are also under way to determine why some people with IDDM have trouble with complications while others live long, relatively healthy lives.

Until the answers to these questions are known, it is wise for people with IDDM to follow their doctor's advice in controlling blood glucose and to be aware of the signs and risk factors for complications of diabetes.

Acute Complications

The acute complications of diabetes are the rapid effects that can occur when blood glucose levels climb too high or fall too low. If an insulin injection is missed, for example, blood glucose rises, and the person affected may start to feel weak and hungry, and may urinate frequently. Since the body can't use glucose for energy, it shifts to using fats and protein. The products of fat and protein metabolism, substances called ketones, are toxic when they reach high enough levels. This condition is called ketoacidosis, and it can cause coma and death if untreated. Ketoacidosis can develop slowly over several days. The warning symptoms may include abdominal pain, nausea and vomiting, rapid breathing and a fruity odor on the person's breath, and drowsiness.

Glucose can also fall too low in diabetes. Going too long without a meal, engaging in strenuous exercise, or taking too large a dose of insulin can cause glucose to drop, a condition called hypoglycemia, or insulin shock. Common symptoms of hypoglycemia include trembling, nervousness, sweating, hunger, headache, nausea, drowsiness, or a feeling similar to drunkenness. Like ketoacidosis, hypoglycemia can cause coma and death if untreated. A quick, sugar-rich snack or drink such as orange juice or an injection of glucagon, a hormone that raises glucose levels, can restore normal glucose levels.

Long-Term Complications

In young people, acute complications pose the greatest threat to survival for people with IDDM. As people grow older, the long-term complications become more important. Diabetes can damage many organs through its effects on blood vessels. How this occurs is not well understood, but the damage can lead to kidney, heart, eye, and nerve disease.

Kidney Disease

Kidney disease is the greatest threat to life in adults with IDDM. The kidneys have a complex network of small blood vessels that filter impurities from blood for excretion in urine. Diabetes can damage these small blood vessels so that the kidneys cannot perform their waste-filtering work. The kidneys are essential to life. People can live without one kidney, but those who lose both must have their blood cleansed by a dialysis machine or have a kidney transplant.

High blood pressure can increase the chances that someone will develop kidney disease, so keeping blood pressure under control is especially important for someone with IDDM.

Heart Disease

Diabetes doubles the risk of heart disease. For reasons not yet well understood, fat and cholesterol collect more rapidly in the arteries of people with diabetes than in those without diabetes. These fatty deposits reduce the supply of blood to the heart and can lead to a heart attack.

Other risk factors for heart disease include hypertension or high blood pressure, obesity, high amounts of fats and cholesterol in blood, and cigarette smoking. The more these factors can be eliminated, the more a person reduces the risk of heart disease.

Eye Disease

The major threat to vision from diabetes is diabetic retinopathy. Retinopathy means disease of the retina, the light-sensing tissue at the back of the eye. Diabetes causes changes in the tiny vessels that supply the retina with blood. The blood vessels may swell and leak fluid. When retinopathy is more severe, new blood vessels may grow from the back of the eye and bleed into the clear gel, or vitreous, that fills the eye.

A yearly eye examination enables an eye doctor to detect chances before vision is affected and eye disease becomes harder to treat. Scientists have found that laser treatment for diabetic retinopathy can help prevent loss of vision and can, in some cases, restore vision lost as a result of this disease. A yearly eye exam by an eye doctor is the best way to make sure that changes in eyesight are diagnosed early and that effective treatment is carried out when it can be most helpful.

Diabetic Nerve Disease

Nerve damage from diabetes (diabetic neuropathy) can dull sensation in the feet, legs, and fingertips. When this happens, bruises or sores may go unnoticed until they become open or infected. Reduced blood flow caused by diabetes' effects on the blood vessels (peripheral vascular disease) can slow healing of foot sores. Because of diabetic neuropathy and peripheral vascular disease, people with diabetes are at increased risk of needing amputation when leg and foot sores become gravely infected.

Severe pain in the legs and feet sometimes comes with diabetic neuropathy. Pain-killing drugs and sometimes antidepressant drugs are used to treat painful neuropathy. In most cases, the pain subsides on its own with time.

Diabetic neuropathy can also affect body functions such as digestion. A doctor may prescribe drugs to relieve these symptoms. In addition, diabetes can, over time, affect the nerves that control erection in men. A doctor can find out whether impotence is the result of emotional or physical changes, such as diabetes, and then suggest treatment or counseling.

Pregnancy

With insulin treatment available, IDDM no longer poses the threat it once did to the health of the pregnant mother. The infant of a mother with IDDM does, however, have a higher than average risk of birth defects, stillbirth, respiratory distress, and other problems at birth. A mother's careful control of her glucose is essential to the health and life of her baby. With careful diabetes control, beginning before conception if possible, it is likely that the child will be healthy in every way.

Does Diabetes Run in Families?

A susceptibility to diabetes can be inherited. The brothers and sisters of a child with diabetes have a higher than average risk of developing IDDM. However, their risk remains small—only about 1 in 20 children with a diabetic sibling will develop IDDM. In fact, an identical twin of a child with IDDM has less than a 50 percent chance of developing the disease. Scientists are still doing research to determine how and why certain factors—both inherited and environmental—sometimes lead to diabetes.

Illness and Surgery

Illness, such as influenza, and stress, such as personal losses or conflicts, can affect the body's use of glucose. During times of illness and stress, a person needs to be even more careful about keeping glucose in control.

Surgery also places unusual stress on the body. Surgical teams take special precautions when doing surgery on a person with IDDM. The best way to ensure that doctors are aware of a patient's diabetes is to tell them.

Research in Diabetes

Diabetes research is the best hope that one day a means of curing and possibly preventing diabetes will be found. In the last 10 years, diabetes researchers have made great strides in understanding this disease. Critical to this effort has been the technology developed in genetics, microbiology, immunology, and other disciplines that have given diabetes researchers the tools they need to examine at the cell level what happens in diabetes.

The National Institute of Diabetes and Digestive and Kidney Diseases (NIDDK) was established by Congress in 1950 as an institute of the National Institutes of Health (NIH), whose mission is to improve human health through biomedical research. The NIH is the research arm of the Public Health Service under the U.S. Department of Health and Human Services.

The NIDDK conducts and supports a variety of research in diabetes and its complications. In the past several years, scientists have identified the genetic factors that are associated with both IDDM and NIDDM. A major goal of future research will be to clarify how inherited factors affect the immune or disease-fighting system to result in IDDM. Already, scientists have identified immune factors circulating in blood that indicate increased risk of developing IDDM. This information may lead to early identification of IDDM cases and will help pave the way to understanding why the immune system goes awry in IDDM.

Scientists also have a better understanding of how insulin works in glucose metabolism. For example, groups of researchers at Memorial Sloan-Kettering Cancer Center, New York; the University of California, San Francisco; Mt. Zion Hospital and Medical Center, San Francisco; and Stanford University, Stanford, California, recently cloned and analyzed the structure of the insulin receptor, a molecule on cell surfaces to which insulin must attach in order to act. Defects in receptor function have been linked to abnormalities in glucose metabolism.

Human insulin made by recombinant DNA techniques is commercially available, as are externally worn pumps that can be programmed by the wearer to deliver insulin through a catheter in the abdomen. Research is continuing on internally implantable pumps, and clinical trials on at least one such pump have been undertaken.

New treatments are being developed for the complications of diabetes. Laser photocoagulation therapy has been shown to reduce the risk of blindness in people with diabetic retinopathy. Preventive measures and medications are available to help control high blood pressure, to avoid lower extremity amputations, and to reduce the risk of tooth loss from periodontal (gum) disease. Understanding how maternal diabetes can affect the unborn child is increasing, and with it, strategies to improve the chances that such a child will be born normal and healthy.

Research on transplantation of the insulin-producing cells of the pancreas is ongoing. The aim of this research is to provide a means of transplanting insulin-producing cells into someone with diabetes without the need to suppress the immune system to prevent rejection. If successful, the procedure would eliminate the need for daily injections of insulin.

Clinical Trials

Clinical trials are one means to test new approaches to treatment that emerge from basic research. In a clinical trial, new and existing treatments are compared with each other or with no treatment.

The NIDDK is supporting and planning clinical trials that are designed to weigh the benefits and risks of various approaches to treatment of diabetes and its complications. For information about NIDDK-supported clinical trials, contact the National Institute of Diabetes and Digestive and Kidney Diseases, National Institutes of Health, Building 31, Room 9A04, Bethesda, Maryland 20892.

Chapter 9

Noninsulin-Dependent Diabetes

This booklet is about *noninsulin-dependent diabetes.* The word "diabetes" in the text of this booklet refers to noninsulin-dependent diabetes unless otherwise specified.

Introduction

Of the estimated 13 to 14 million people in the United States with diabetes, between 90 and 95 percent have **noninsulin-dependent or type II diabetes.** Formerly called adult-onset, this form of diabetes usually begins in adults over age 40, and is most common after age 55. Nearly half of people with diabetes don't know it because the symptoms often develop gradually and are hard to identify at first. The person may feel tired or ill without knowing why. Diabetes can cause problems that damage the heart, blood vessels, eyes, kidneys, and nerves.

Although there is no cure for diabetes yet, daily treatment helps control blood sugar, and may reduce the risk of complications. Under a doctor's supervision, treatment usually involves a combination of weight loss, exercise and medication.

This booklet isn't a guide to treatment and it doesn't replace the advice of a doctor. It's one of many sources of extra information about diabetes. Local diabetes groups and clinics sponsor meetings and educational programs about diabetes that also can be helpful. At the end of this book is a list of groups that have information on diabetes programs.

NIH Pub. No. 92–241.

What is Diabetes?

The two types of diabetes, insulin-dependent and noninsulin-dependent, are different disorders. While the causes, short-term effects, and treatments for the two types differ, both can cause the same long-term health problems. Both types also affect the body's ability to use digested food for energy. Diabetes doesn't interfere with digestion, but it does prevent the body from using an important product of digestion, glucose (commonly known as sugar), for energy.

After a meal the digestive system breaks some food down into glucose. The blood carries the glucose or sugar throughout the body, causing blood glucose levels to rise. In response to this rise the hormone insulin is released into the bloodstream to signal the body tissues to metabolize or burn the glucose for fuel, causing blood glucose levels to return to normal. A gland called the pancreas, found just behind the stomach, makes insulin. Glucose the body doesn't use right away goes to the liver, muscle or fat for storage.

In someone with diabetes, this process doesn't work correctly. In people with insulin-dependent diabetes, the pancreas doesn't produce insulin. This condition usually begins in childhood and is also known as type I (formerly called juvenile-onset) diabetes. People with this kind of diabetes must have daily insulin injections to survive.

In people with noninsulin-dependent diabetes the pancreas usually produces some insulin, but the body's tissue don't respond very well to the insulin signal and, therefore, don't metabolize the glucose properly, a condition called insulin resistance. Insulin resistance is an important factor in noninsulin-dependent diabetes.

Symptoms

The symptoms of diabetes may begin gradually and can be hard to identify at first. They may include fatigue, a sick feeling, frequent urination, especially at night, and excessive thirst. When there is extra glucose in blood, one way the body gets rid of it is through frequent urination. This loss of fluids causes extreme thirst. Other symptoms may include sudden weight loss, blurred vision, and slow healing of skin, gum and urinary tract infections. Women may notice genital itching.

A doctor also may suspect a patient has diabetes if the person has health problems related to diabetes. For instance, heart disease, changes in vision, numbness in the feet and legs or sores that are slow to heal, may prompt a doctor to check for diabetes. These symptoms do not mean a person has diabetes, but anyone who has these problems should see a doctor.

What Causes Noninsulin-Dependent Diabetes?

There is no simple answer to what causes noninsulin-dependent diabetes. While eating sugar, for example, doesn't cause diabetes, eating large amounts of sugar and other rich, fatty foods, can cause weight gain. Most people who develop diabetes are overweight. Scientists do not fully understand why obesity increases someone's chances of developing diabetes, but they believe obesity is a major factor leading to noninsulin-dependent diabetes. Current research should help explain why the disorder occurs and why obesity is such an important risk factor.

A major cause of diabetes is insulin resistance. Scientists are still searching for the causes of insulin resistance, but they have identified two possibilities. The first could be a defect in insulin receptors on cells. Like an appliance that needs to be plugged into an electrical outlet, insulin has to bind to a receptor to function. Several things can go wrong with receptors. There may not be enough receptors for insulin to bind to, or a defect in the receptors may prevent insulin from binding.

A second possible cause involves the process that occurs after insulin plugs into the receptor. Insulin may bind to the receptor, but the cells don't read the signal to metabolize the glucose. Scientists are studying cells to see why this might happen.

Who Develops Noninsulin-Dependent Diabetes?

Age, sex, weight, physical activity, diet, lifestyle, and family health history all affect someone's chances of developing diabetes. The chances that someone will develop diabetes increase if the person's parents or siblings have the disease. Experts now know that diabetes is more common in African Americans, Hispanics, Native Americans and Native Hawaiians than whites. They believe this is the result of both heredity and environmental factors, such as diet and lifestyle. The highest rate of diabetes in the world is in an Arizona community of American Indians called the Pimas. While the chances of developing diabetes increase with age, gender isn't a risk factor, although African American women are more likely to develop diabetes than African American men.

While people can't change family history, age, or race, it is possible to control weight and physical fitness. A doctor can decide if someone is at risk for developing diabetes and offer advice on reducing that risk.

Diagnosing Diabetes

A doctor can diagnose diabetes by checking for symptoms such as excessive thirst and frequent urination and by testing for glucose in blood or urine. When blood glucose rises above a certain point, the kidneys pass the extra glucose in the urine. However, a urine test alone is not sufficient to diagnose diabetes.

A second method for testing glucose is a blood test usually done in the morning before breakfast (fasting glucose test) or after a meal (postprandial glucose test).

The oral glucose tolerance test is a second type of blood test used to check for diabetes. Sometimes it can detect diabetes when a simple blood test does not. In this test, blood glucose is measured before and after a person has consumed a thick, sweet drink of glucose and other sugars. Normally, the glucose in a person's blood rises quickly after the drink and then falls gradually again as insulin signals the body to metabolize the glucose. In someone with diabetes, blood glucose rises and remains high after consumption of the liquid.

A doctor can decide, based on these tests and a physical exam, whether someone has diabetes. If a blood test is borderline abnormal, the doctor may want to monitor the person's blood glucose regularly. If a person is overweight, he or she probably will be advised to lose weight. The doctor also may monitor the patient's heart, since diabetes increases the risk of heart disease.

Treating Diabetes

The goals of diabetes treatment are to keep blood glucose within normal range and to prevent long-term complications. Why control blood glucose? In the first place, diabetes can cause short-term effects: some are unpleasant and some are dangerous. These include thirst, frequent urination, weakness, lack of ability to concentrate, loss of coordination, and blurred vision. Loss of consciousness is possible with very high or low blood sugar levels, but is more of a danger in insulin-dependent than in noninsulin-dependent diabetes.

In the second place, the long-term complications of diabetes may result from many years of high blood glucose. Research is under way to find out if this is true and to learn if careful control can help prevent complications. Meanwhile, most doctors feel that if people with diabetes keep their blood glucose levels under control, they will reduce the risk of complications.

In 1986, a National Institutes of Health panel of experts recommended that the best treatment for noninsulin-dependent diabetes is a diet that helps the person maintain normal weight. In people who are overweight, losing weight is the one treatment that is clearly effective in controlling diabetes.

In some people, exercise can help keep weight and diabetes under control. However, when diet and exercise alone can't control diabetes, two other kinds of treatment are available: oral diabetes medications and insulin. The treatment a doctor suggests depends on the person's age, lifestyle, and the severity of the diabetes.

Diabetes Diet

The proper diet is critical to diabetes treatment. It can help someone with diabetes:

- Achieve and maintain desirable weight. Many people with diabetes can control their blood glucose by losing weight and keeping it off.
- Maintain normal blood glucose levels.
- Prevent heart and blood vessel diseases, conditions that tend to occur in people with diabetes.

A doctor will usually prescribe diet as part of diabetes treatment. A dietitian or nutritionist can recommend a diet that is healthy, but also interesting and easy to follow. No one has to be limited to a preprinted, standard diet. Someone with diabetes can get assistance in the following ways:

- A doctor can recommend a local nutritionist or dietitian.
- The local American Diabetes Association, American Heart Association, and American Dietetic Association can provide names of qualified dietitians or nutritionists and information about diet planning.
- Local diabetes centers at large medical clinics, hospitals, or medical universities usually have dietitians and nutritionists on staff.

The guidelines for diabetes diet planning include the following:

- Many experts, including the American Diabetes Association, recommend that 50 to 60 percent of daily calories come from carbohydrates, 12 to 20 percent from protein, and no more than 30 percent from fat.
- Spacing meals throughout the day, instead of eating heavy meals once or twice a day, can help a person avoid extremely high or low blood glucose levels.
- With few exceptions, the best way to lose weight is gradually: one or two pounds a week. Strict diets *must never* be undertaken without the supervision of a doctor.

- People with diabetes have twice the risk of developing heart disease as those without diabetes, and high blood cholesterol levels raise the risk of heart disease. Losing weight and reducing intake of saturated fats and cholesterol, in favor of unsaturated and monounsaturated fats, can help lower blood cholesterol.

  For example, meats and dairy products are major sources of saturated fats, which should be avoided; most vegetable oils are high in unsaturated fats, which are fine in limited amounts; and olive oil is a good source of monounsaturated fat, the healthiest type of fat. Liver and other organ meats and egg yolks are particularly high in cholesterol. A doctor or nutritionist can advise someone on this aspect of diet.

- Studies show that foods with fiber, such as fruits, vegetables, peas, beans, and whole-grain breads and cereals may help lower blood glucose. However, it seems that a person must eat much more fiber than the average American now consumes to get this benefit. A doctor or nutritionist can advise someone about adding fiber to a diet.

- Exchange lists are useful in planning a diabetes diet. They place foods with similar nutrients and calories into groups. With the help of a nutritionist, the person plans the number of servings from each exchange list that he or she should eat throughout the day. Diets that use exchange lists offer more choices than preprinted diets. More information on exchange lists is available from nutritionists and from the American Diabetes Association.

Continuing research may lead to new approaches to diabetes diets. Because one goal of a diabetes diet is to maintain normal blood glucose levels, it would be helpful to have reliable information on the effects of foods on blood glucose. For example, foods that are rich in carbohydrates, like breads, cereals, fruits, and vegetables break down into glucose during digestion, causing blood glucose to rise. However, scientists don't know how each of these carbohydrates affect blood glucose levels. Research is also under way to learn whether foods with sugar raise blood glucose higher than foods with starch. Experts do know that cooked foods raise blood glucose higher than raw, unpeeled foods. A person with diabetes can ask a doctor or nutritionist about using this kind of information in diet planning.

Alcoholic Beverages

Most people with diabetes can drink alcohol safely if they drink in moderation (one or two drinks occasionally), because in higher quantities alcohol can cause health problems:

- Alcohol has calories without the vitamins, minerals, and other nutrients that are essential for maintaining good health. A doctor can discuss whether it's safe for an individual with diabetes to drink. People who are trying to lose weight need to account for the calories in alcohol in diet planning. A dietitian also can provide information about the sugar and alcohol content of various alcoholic drinks.
- Alcohol on an empty stomach can cause low blood glucose or hypoglycemia. Hypoglycemia is a particular risk in people who use oral medications or insulin for diabetes. It can cause shaking, dizziness, and collapse. People who don't know someone has diabetes may mistake these symptoms for drunkenness and neglect to seek medical help.
- Oral diabetes medications—tolbutamide and chlorpropamide—can cause dizziness, flushing, and nausea when combined with alcohol. A doctor can advise patients on the safety of drinking when taking these and other diabetes medications.
- Frequent, heavy drinking can cause liver damage over time. Because the liver stores and releases glucose, blood glucose levels may be more difficult to control in a person with liver damage from alcohol.
- Frequent heavy drinking also can raise the levels of fats in blood, increasing the risk of heart disease.

Exercise

Exercise has many benefits, and for someone with diabetes regular exercise combined with a good diet can help control diabetes. Exercise not only burns calories, which can help with weight reduction, but it also can improve the body's response to the hormone insulin. As a result, following a regular exercise program can make oral diabetes medications and insulin more effective and can help control blood glucose levels.

Exercise also reduces some risk factors for heart disease. For example, exercise can lower fat and cholesterol levels in blood, which increase heart disease risk. It also can lower blood pressure and increase production of a cholesterol, called HDL, that protects against heart disease.

However, infrequent, strenuous exercise can strain muscles and the circulatory system and can increase the risk of a heart attack during exercise. A doctor can decide how much exercise is safe for an individual. The doctor will consider how well controlled a person's diabetes is, the condition of the heart and circulatory system, and whether complications require that the person avoid certain types of activity.

Walking is great exercise, especially for an inactive person, and it's easy to do. A person can start off walking for 15 or 20 minutes, three or four times a week, and gradually increase the speed or distance of the walks. The purpose of a good exercise program is to find an enjoyable activity and do it regularly. Doing strenuous exercise for six months and then stopping isn't as effective. People taking oral drugs or insulin need to remember that strenuous exercise can cause dangerously low blood glucose and they should carry a food or drink high in sugar for medical emergencies. Signs of hypoglycemia include hunger, nervousness, shakiness, weakness, sweating, headache, and blurred vision. As a precaution, a person with diabetes should wear an identification bracelet or necklace to alert a stranger that the wearer has diabetes and may need special medical help in an emergency.

A doctor may advise someone with high blood pressure or other complications to avoid exercises that raise blood pressure. For example, lifting heavy objects and exercises that strain the upper body raise blood pressure.

People with diabetes who have lost sensitivity in their feet also can enjoy exercise. They should choose shoes carefully and check their feet regularly for breaks in skin that could lead to infection. Swimming or bicycling can be easier on the feet than running.

Oral Medications

Oral diabetes medicines, or oral hypoglycemics, can lower blood glucose in people who have diabetes, but are able to make some insulin. They are an option if diet and exercise don't work. Oral diabetes medications are not insulin and are not a substitute for diet and exercise. Although experts don't understand exactly how each oral medicine works, they know that they increase insulin production and affect how insulin lowers blood glucose. These medications are most effective in people who developed diabetes after age 40, have had diabetes less than 5 years, are normal weight, and have never received insulin or have taken only 40 units or less of insulin a day. Pregnant and nursing women shouldn't take oral medications because their effect on the fetus and newborn is unknown, and because insulin provides better control of diabetes during pregnancy.

There is also some question about whether oral diabetes medications increase the risk of a heart attack. Experts disagree on this point and many people with noninsulin-dependent diabetes use oral medicines safely and effectively. The Food and Drug Administration (FDA), the agency of the Federal Government that approves medications for use in this country, requires that oral diabetes medicines carry a warning concerning the increased risk of heart attack. Whether someone uses a medication depends on its benefits and risks, something a doctor can help the patient decide.

Six FDA-approved oral diabetes medications are now on the market. Their generic names are tolbutamide, chlorpropamide, tolazamide, acetohexamide, glyburide, and glipizide. The generic name refers to the chemical that gives each medicine its particular effect. Some of these medications are made by more than one pharmaceutical company and have more than one brand name. All six are different types of one class of medication, called sulfonylureas, but each affects metabolism differently. A doctor will choose a patient's medication based on the person's general health, the amount his or her blood glucose needs to be lowered, the person's eating habits, and the medicine's side effects.

The purpose of oral medications is to lower blood glucose. Therefore, the person taking them must eat regular meals and engage in only light to moderate exercise, to prevent blood glucose from dipping too low. Medications taken for other health problems, including illness, also can lower blood sugar and may react with the diabetes medicine. Therefore, a doctor needs to know all the medications a person is taking to prevent a harmful interaction. Lowering blood sugar too much can cause hypoglycemia with symptoms such as headache, weakness, shakiness, and if the condition is severe enough, collapse.

Oral diabetes medications usually don't cause side effects. However, a few people do experience nausea, skin rashes, headache, either water retention or diuresis (increased urination), and sensitivity to direct sunlight. These effects should gradually subside, but a person should see a doctor if they persist. For reasons that aren't always clear, sometimes oral diabetes medications don't help the person for whom they're prescribed. Investigations are under way to learn why this happens.

Insulin

Like oral diabetes medications, insulin is an alternative for some people with noninsulin-dependent diabetes who can't control their blood glucose levels with diet and exercise. In special situations, such as surgery and pregnancy, insulin is a temporary but important means of controlling blood glucose. A section of this booklet called "special situations" discusses insulin use during pregnancy and surgery.

Sometimes it's unclear whether insulin or oral medications are more effective in controlling blood glucose; therefore, a doctor will consider a person's weight, age, and the severity of the diabetes before prescribing a medicine. Experts do know that weight control is essential for insulin to be effective. A doctor is likely to prescribe insulin if diet, exercise, or oral medications don't work, or if someone has a bad reaction to oral medicines. A person also may have to take insulin if his or her blood glucose fluctuates a great deal and is difficult to control. A doctor will instruct a person with diabetes on how to purchase, mix, and inject insulin. Various types of insulin are available that differ in purity, concentration, and how quickly they work. They also are made differently. In the past, all commercially available insulin came from the pancreas glands of cows and pigs. Today, human insulin is available in two forms: one uses genetic engineering and the other involves chemically changing pork insulin into human insulin. The best sources of information on insulin are the company that makes it and a doctor.

Checking Blood Glucose Levels

When a person's body is operating normally, it automatically checks the level of glucose in blood. If the level is too high or too low, the body will adjust the sugar level to return it to normal. This system operates in much the same way that cruise control adjusts the speed of a car. With diabetes, the body doesn't do the job of controlling blood glucose automatically. To make up for this, someone with diabetes has to check blood sugar regularly and adjust treatment accordingly.

A doctor can measure blood glucose during an office visit. However, levels change from hour to hour and someone who visits the doctor only every few weeks won't know what his or her blood glucose is daily. Do-it-yourself tests enable people with diabetes to check their blood sugar daily.

The easiest test someone can do at home is a urine test. When the level of glucose in blood rises above normal, the kidneys eliminate the excess glucose in urine. Glucose in urine, therefore, reflects an excess of glucose in blood.

Urine testing is easy. Tablets or paper strips are dipped in urine. The color change that occurs indicates whether blood glucose is too high. However, urine testing is not completely accurate because the reading reflects the level of blood glucose a few hours earlier. In addition, not everyone's kidneys are the same. Even when the amount of glucose in two people's urine is the same, their sugar levels may be different. Certain drugs and vitamin C also can affect the accuracy of urine tests.

It's more accurate to measure blood glucose directly. Kits are available that allow people with diabetes to test their blood glucose at home. The test involves pricking a finger to draw a drop of blood. A spring-operated "lancet" does this automatically. The drop of blood is placed on a strip of specially coated plastic or into a small machine that "reads" how much glucose is in the blood. A doctor may suggest that someone test his or her blood glucose several times a day. Self blood glucose monitoring can show how the body responds to meals, exercise, stress, and diabetes treatment.

Another test that measures the effectiveness of treatment is a "glycosylated hemoglobin" test. It measures the glucose that has become attached to hemoglobin, the molecule in red blood cells that gives blood its red color. Over time, hemoglobin absorbs glucose, according to its concentration in blood. Once glucose is absorbed by hemoglobin it remains there until the blood cells die and new ones replace them. With the "glycosylated hemoglobin" test, a doctor can tell whether blood glucose has been very high over the last few months.

Diabetes Complications

A key goal of diabetes treatment is to prevent complications because, over time, diabetes can damage the heart, blood vessels, eyes, kidneys, and nerves, although the person may not know damage is taking place. It's important to diagnose and treat diabetes early, because it can cause damage even before it makes someone feel ill.

How diabetes causes long-term problems is unclear. However, changes in the small blood vessels and nerves are common. These changes may be the first step toward many problems that diabetes causes. Scientists can't predict who among people with diabetes will develop complications, but complications are most likely to occur in someone who has had diabetes for many years. However, because a person can have diabetes without knowing it, a complication may be the first sign.

Heart Disease

Heart disease is the most common life-threatening disease linked to diabetes, and experts say diabetes doubles a person's risk of developing heart disease. In heart disease, deposits of fat and cholesterol build-up in the arteries that supply the heart with blood. If this build-up blocks blood from getting to the heart, a potentially fatal heart attack can occur.

Other risk factors include hypertension or high blood pressure, obesity, high amounts of fats and cholesterol in blood, and cigarette smoking. Eliminating these risk factors, along with treating diabetes, can reduce the risk of heart disease. The American Heart Association has literature that explains what heart disease is and how to prevent it. The association's address is in the resources section of this booklet.

Kidney Disease

People with diabetes are also more likely to develop kidney disease than other people. The kidneys filter waste products from the blood and excrete them in the form of urine, maintaining proper fluid balance in the body. While people can live without one kidney, those without both must have special treatment, called dialysis. Most people with diabetes will never develop kidney disease, but proper diabetes treatment can further reduce the risk. High blood pressure also can add to the risk of kidney disease. Therefore, regular blood pressure checks and early treatment of the disorder can help prevent kidney disease.

Urinary tract infections are also a cause of kidney problems. Diabetes can affect the nerves that control the bladder, making it difficult for a person to empty his or her bladder completely. Bacteria can form in the unemptied bladder and the tubes leading from it, eventually causing infection. The symptoms of a urinary tract infection include frequent, painful urination, blood in the urine, and pain in the lower abdomen and back. Without prompt examination and treatment by a doctor, the infection can reach the kidneys, causing pain, fever, and possibly kidney damage. A doctor may prescribe antibiotics to treat the infection and may suggest that the person drink large amounts of water.

Kidney problems are one cause of water retention, or edema, a condition in which fluid collects in the body, causing swelling, often in the legs and hands. A doctor can decide if swelling or water retention relates to kidney function.

A nephrologist, a doctor specially trained to diagnose and treat kidney problems, can identify the cause of problems and recommend ways to reduce the risk of kidney disease.

Eye Problems

Diabetes can affect the eyes in several ways. Frequently, the effects are temporary and can be corrected with better diabetes control. However, long-term diabetes can cause changes in the eyes that threaten vision. Stable blood glucose levels and yearly eye examinations can help reduce the risk of serious eye damage.

Blurred vision is one effect diabetes can have on the eyes. The reason may be that changing levels of glucose in blood also can affect the balance of fluid in the lens of the eye, which works like a flexible camera lens to focus images. If the lens absorbs more water than normal and swells, its focusing power changes. Diabetes also may affect the function of nerves that control eyesight, causing blurred vision.

Cataract and glaucoma are eye diseases that occur more frequently in people with diabetes. Cataract is a clouding of the normally clear lens of the eye. Glaucoma is a condition in which pressure within the eye can damage the optic nerve that transmits visual images to the brain. Early diagnosis and treatment of cataract and glaucoma can reduce the severity of these disorders.

Diabetic Retinopathy

Retinopathy, a disease of the retina, the light sensing tissue at the back of the eye, is a common concern among people with diabetes. Diabetic retinopathy damages the tiny vessels that supply the retina with blood. The blood vessels may swell and leak fluid. When retinopathy is more severe, new blood vessels may grow from the back of the eye and bleed into the clear gel that fills the eye, the vitreous.

While most people with diabetes may never develop serious eye problems, people who have had diabetes for 25 years are more likely to develop retinopathy. Experts think high blood pressure may contribute to diabetic retinopathy, and that smoking can cause the condition to worsen. If someone experiences blurred vision that lasts longer than a day or so, sudden loss of vision in either eye, or black spots, lines, or flashing lights in the field of vision, a doctor should be alerted right away.

Treatment for diabetic retinopathy can help prevent loss of vision and can sometimes restore vision lost because of the disease. A yearly eye examination with dilated pupils makes it possible for an ophthalmologist, an eye doctor, to notice changes before the illness becomes harder to treat. Scientists are testing new means of treating diabetic retinopathy. For more information on eye complications of diabetes and the treatment of these conditions, see the resource list at the end of this booklet.

Legs and Feet

Leg and foot problems can arise in people with diabetes due to changes in blood vessels and nerves in these areas. Peripheral vascular disease is a condition in which blood vessels become narrowed by fatty deposits, reducing blood supply to the legs and feet. Diabetes also can dull the sensitivity of nerves. Someone with this condition, called peripheral neuropathy, might not notice a sore spot caused by tight shoes or pressure from walking. If ignored, the sore can become infected and because blood circulation is poor, the area may take longer to heal.

Proper foot care and regular visits to a doctor can prevent foot and leg sores and ensure that any that do appear don't become infected and painful. Helpful measures include inspecting the feet daily for cuts or sore spots. Blisters and sore spots are not as likely when shoes fit well and socks or stockings aren't tight. A doctor also may suggest washing feet daily, with warm, not hot water; filing thick calluses; and using lotions that keep the feet from getting too dry. Shoe inserts or special shoes can be used to prevent pressure on the foot.

Diabetic neuropathy, or nerve disease, dulls the nerves and can be extremely painful. A person with neuropathy also may be depressed. Scientists aren't sure whether the depression is an effect of neuropathy, or if it's simply a response to pain. Treatment, aimed at relieving pain and depression, may include aspirin and other pain-killing drugs.

Any sore on the foot or leg, whether or not it's painful, requires a doctor's immediate attention. Treatment can help sores heal and prevent new ones from developing. Problems with the feet and legs can cause life-threatening problems that require amputation—surgical removal of limbs—if not treated early.

Other Effects of Diabetic Neuropathy

Nerves provide muscle tone and feeling and help control functions like digestion and blood pressure. Diabetes can cause changes in these nerves and the functions they control. These changes are most frequent in people who have had other complications of diabetes, like problems with their feet. Someone who has had diabetes for some years and has other complications, may find that spells of indigestion or diarrhea are common. A doctor may prescribe drugs to relieve these symptoms. Diabetes also can affect the nerves that control penile erection in men, which can cause impotence that shows up gradually, without any loss of desire for sex. A doctor can find out whether impotence is the result of physical changes, such as diabetes, or emotional changes, and suggest treatment or counseling.

Skin and Oral Infection

People with diabetes are more likely to develop infections, like boils and ulcers, than the average person. Women with diabetes may develop vaginal infections more often than other women. Checking for infections, treating them early, and following a doctor's advice can help ensure that infections are mild and infrequent.

Infections also can affect the teeth and gums, making people with diabetes more susceptible to periodontal disease, an inflammation of tissue surrounding and supporting the teeth. An important cause of periodontal disease is bacterial growth on the teeth and gums. Treating diabetes and following a dentist's advice on dental care can help prevent periodontal disease.

Emergencies

Very high blood glucose levels cause symptoms that are hard to ignore: frequent urination and excessive thirst. However, in someone who is elderly or in poor health these symptoms may go unnoticed. Without treatment, a person with high blood glucose or hyperglycemia can lose fluids, become weak, confused, and even unconscious. Breathing will be shallow and the pulse rapid. The person's lips and tongue will be dry, and his or her hands and feet will be cool. A doctor should be called immediately.

The opposite of high blood glucose, very low blood glucose or hypoglycemia, is also dangerous. Hypoglycemia can occur when someone hasn't eaten enough to balance the effects of insulin or oral medicine. Prolonged, strenuous exercise in someone taking oral diabetes drugs or insulin also can cause hypoglycemia, as can alcohol.

Someone whose blood glucose has become too low may feel nervous, shaky, and weak. The person may sweat, feel hungry, and have a headache. Severe hypoglycemia can cause loss of consciousness. A person with hypoglycemia who begins to feel weak and shaky should eat or drink something with sugar in it immediately, like orange juice. If the person is unconscious, he or she should be taken to a hospital emergency room right away. An identification bracelet or necklace that states that the wearer has diabetes will let friends know that these symptoms are a warning of illness that requires urgent medical help.

Special Situations

Surgery

Surgery is stressful, both physically and mentally. It can raise blood glucose levels even in someone who is careful about control. To make sure that surgery and recovery are successful for someone with diabetes, a doctor will test blood glucose and keep it under careful control, usually with insulin. Careful control makes it possible for someone with diabetes to have surgery with little or no more risk than someone without diabetes.

To plan a safe and successful surgery, the surgeon and attending physicians must know that the person they're treating has diabetes. While tests done before surgery can detect diabetes, the patient should inform the doctor of his or her condition. A surgical team also will evaluate the possible effect of complications of diabetes, such as heart or kidney problems.

Pregnancy

Bearing a child places extra demands on a woman's body. Diabetes makes it more difficult for her body to adjust to these demands and it can cause problems for both mother and baby. Some woman may develop a form of diabetes during pregnancy called gestational diabetes. Gestational diabetes develops most frequently in the middle and later months of pregnancy, after the time of greatest risk for birth defects. Although this kind of diabetes often disappears after the baby's birth, treatment is necessary during pregnancy to make sure the diabetes doesn't harm the mother or fetus.

A woman who knows she has diabetes should keep her condition under control before she becomes pregnant, so that her diabetes won't increase the risk of birth defects. A woman whose diabetes isn't well controlled may have an unusually large baby. Diabetes also increases the risk of premature birth and problems in the baby, such as breathing difficulties, low blood sugar and occasionally, death.

Blood glucose monitoring and treatment with insulin can ensure that a baby born to a mother with diabetes will be healthy. Oral diabetes drugs aren't given during pregnancy because the effects of these drugs on the unborn baby aren't known. By following the advice of a doctor trained to treat gestational diabetes, the mother can make sure her blood glucose is normal and her baby is well nourished.

Approximately half of women with gestational diabetes will no longer have abnormal blood glucose tests shortly after giving birth. However, many women with gestational diabetes will develop noninsulin-dependent diabetes later in their lives. Regular check-ups can ensure that if a woman does develop diabetes later, it will be diagnosed and treated early.

Is *Diabetes Hereditary?*

Scientists estimate that the child of a parent with noninsulin-dependent diabetes has approximately a 10 to 15 percent chance of developing noninsulin-dependent diabetes. If both parents have diabetes, the child's risk of having the disease increases. The child's health habits throughout his or her life will affect the risk of developing diabetes. Obesity, for example, may increase the risk of diabetes or cause it to occur earlier in life.

Noninsulin-dependent diabetes in a parent has no effect on the chances that his or her child will have insulin-dependent diabetes, the more severe form of diabetes.

Stress and Illness

One way the body responds to stress is to increase the level of blood glucose. In a person with diabetes, stress may increase the need for treatment to lower blood glucose levels. Illnesses such as colds and flu are forms of physical stress that a doctor can treat. The doctor will advise the person to drink plenty of fluids. When blood glucose is high, the body gets rid of glucose through urine, and this fluid needs to be replaced.

If nausea makes eating or taking oral diabetes drugs a problem, a doctor should be consulted. Not eating can increase the risk of low blood glucose, while stopping oral medications or insulin during illness can lead to very high blood glucose. A doctor may prescribe insulin temporarily for someone with diabetes who can't take medicine by mouth.

Great thirst, rapid weight loss, high fever, or very high urine or blood glucose are signs that blood sugar is out of control. If a person has these symptoms, a doctor should be called immediately.

Like illness, stress that results from losses or conflicts at home or on the job can affect diabetes control. Urine and blood glucose checks can be clues to the effects of stress. If someone finds that stress is making diabetes control difficult, a doctor can advise treatment and suggest sources of help.

Dealing with Diabetes

Good diabetes care requires a daily effort to follow a diet, stay active, and take medicine when necessary. Talking to people who have diabetes or who treat diabetes may be helpful for someone who needs emotional support. The list of organizations at the back of this booklet can help patients find discussion groups or counselors familiar with diabetes. It's very important for people with diabetes to understand how to stay healthy, follow a proper diet, exercise, and be aware of changes in their bodies. People with diabetes can live long, healthy lives if they take care of themselves.

Finding Help

A person with diabetes is responsible for his or her daily care and a doctor is the best source of information on that care. A doctor in family practice or internal medicine can diagnose and treat diabetes, and may refer the patient to a doctor who specializes in treating diabetes. "Endocrinologists" and "diabetologists" are doctors with advanced training and experience in diabetes treatment. The local chapters of the American Diabetes Association or the Juvenile Diabetes Foundation have lists of doctors who specialize in diabetes. Another alternative is to contact a university-based medical center. These centers may have special diabetes clinics or may be able to suggest diabetes doctors who practice in the community.

Printed Information

While information in books and magazines can't replace a doctor's personal advice, it can provide a clear explanation of diabetes and describe advancements in diabetes treatment. The American Diabetes Association and Juvenile Diabetes Foundation have brochures about diabetes and diabetes treatment. These publications are for people without a medical background. The addresses of these organizations are in the resources section at the back of this booklet.

Brochures and books about diabetes also are available from public libraries and bookstores. Local chapters of the American Diabetes Association, hospitals, and medical centers frequently sponsor educational programs on diabetes and diabetes treatment. Information about diabetes programs is also available from a doctor's office, a local hospital or health department, or a local diabetes organization.

Resources on Diabetes

Agency for Health Care Policy and Research (AHCPR)
Medical Treatment Effectiveness Program
2101 East Jefferson Avenue
Rockville, MD 20852
(301) 227-8364—Division of Information and Publications

The Agency supports grant and contract research on the relationship between the use of medical services and procedures and patient outcomes.

American Association of Diabetes Educators (AADE)
444 N. Michigan Avenue, Suite 1240
Chicago, IL 60611
(312) 644-2233 or 1-800-338-3633

The AADE is a multidisciplinary organization, with state and regional chapters, for health professionals involved in diabetes education. It sponsors continuing education programs on both beginning and advanced levels and a certification program for diabetes educators, and provides grants, scholarships, and awards for educational research and teaching activities. The AADE publishes a monthly journal, curriculum guides, consensus statements, self-study programs, and other resources for diabetes educators.

American Diabetes Association
National Service Center
1660 Duke Street
P.O. Box 25757
Alexandria, VA 22313
(703) 549-1500 or 1-800-232-3472

A private, voluntary organization that fosters public awareness of diabetes and supports and promotes diabetes research. It publishes information on many aspects of diabetes, and local affiliates sponsor community programs. Local affiliates can be found in the telephone directory or through the national office.

American Dietetic Association
430 North Michigan Avenue
Chicago, IL 60611
(312) 822–0330

A professional organization that can help someone find a nutritionist in the community.

American Heart Association
7320 Greenville Avenue
Dallas, TX 75231
1–800-242–1793

A private, voluntary organization that has literature on heart disease and how to prevent it. Contact the local affiliate of the American Heart Association listed in telephone directories.

Centers for Disease Control (CDC)
National Center for Chronic Disease Prevention and Health Promotion
1600 Clifton Road
The Rodes Building MS K-13
Atlanta, GA 30333
Technical Information Services Branch (404) 488–5080

The CDC is an agency of the Federal Government that has information on the surveillance and prevention of diabetes for health care professionals and people with diabetes.

Juvenile Diabetes Foundation International
432 Park Avenue, South
New York, NY 10016
(212) 889–7575 or 1–800-223–1138

A private, voluntary organization with an interest in type I or insulin-dependent diabetes. Local affiliates are found across the country. It also has information on noninsulin-dependent diabetes.

National Diabetes Information Clearinghouse
Box NDIC
Bethesda, MD 20892
(301) 468–2162

The National Diabetes Information Clearinghouse has a variety of publications for distribution to the public and to health professionals. The clearinghouse is a program of the National Institute of Diabetes and Digestive and Kidney Diseases, a component of the National Institutes of Health, leading the Federal Government's research on diabetes.

National Eye Health Education Program
National Eye Institute
National Institutes of Health
Box 20/20
Bethesda, MD 20892
(301) 496–5248

Information about how diabetes affects the eyes is available from the National Eye Institute, a component of the Federal Government's National Institutes of Health.

National Heart, Lung, and Blood Institute
Building 31, Room 4A21
National Institutes of Health
Bethesda, MD 20892
(301) 496–4236

Information on heart disease is available from this component of the Federal Government's National Institutes of Health.

Chapter 10

Understanding Gestational Diabetes: A Practical Guide to a Healthy Pregnancy

(For the purpose of this text the words sugar and glucose are used synonymously.)

Approximately 3 to 5 percent of all pregnant women in the United States are diagnosed as having gestational diabetes. These women and their families have many questions about this disorder. Some of the most frequently asked questions are: What is gestational diabetes and how did I get it? How does it differ from other kinds of diabetes? Will it hurt my baby? Will my baby have diabetes? What can I do to control gestational diabetes? Will I need a special diet? Will gestational diabetes change the way or the time my baby is delivered? Will I have diabetes in the future?

This text will address these and many other questions about diet, exercise, measurement of blood sugar levels, and general medical and obstetric care of women with gestational diabetes. It must be emphasized that these are general guidelines and only your health care professional(s) can tailor a program specific to your needs. You should feel free to discuss any concerns you have with your doctor or other health care provider, as no one knows more about you and the condition of your pregnancy.

What is gestational diabetes and what causes it?

Diabetes (actual name is diabetes mellitus) of any kind is a disorder that prevents the body from using food properly. Normally, the body gets its major source of energy from glucose, a simple sugar that comes from foods

---

NIH Pub. No. 93–2788.

high in simple carbohydrates (e.g., table sugar or other sweeteners such as honey, molasses, jams, and jellies, soft drinks, and cookies), or from the breakdown of complex carbohydrates such as starches (e.g., bread, potatoes, and pasta). After sugars and starches are digested in the stomach, they enter the blood stream in the form of glucose. The glucose in the blood stream becomes a potential source of energy for the entire body, similar to the way in which gasoline in a service station pump is a potential source of energy for your car. But, just as someone must pump the gas into the car, the body requires some assistance to get glucose from the blood stream to the muscles and other tissues of the body. In the body, that assistance comes from a hormone called insulin. Insulin is manufactured by the pancreas, a gland that lies behind the stomach. Without insulin, glucose cannot get into the cells of the body where it is used as fuel. Instead, glucose accumulates in the blood to high levels and is excreted or "spilled" into the urine through the kidneys.

When the pancreas of a child or young adult produces little or no insulin we call this condition juvenile-onset diabetes or Type I diabetes (insulin-dependent). This is not the type of diabetes you have. Unlike women with Type I diabetes, women with gestational diabetes have plenty of insulin. In fact, they usually have more insulin in their blood than women who are not pregnant. However, the effect of their insulin is partially blocked by a variety of other hormones made in the placenta, a condition often called insulin resistance.

The placenta performs the task of supplying the growing fetus with nutrients and water from the mother's circulation. It also produces a variety of hormones vital to the preservation of the pregnancy. Ironically, several of these hormones such as estrogen, cortisol, and human placental lactogen (HPL) have a blocking effect on insulin, a "contra-insulin" effect. This contra-insulin effect usually begins about midway (20 to 24 weeks) through pregnancy. The larger the placenta grows, the more these hormones are produced, and the greater the insulin resistance becomes. In most women the pancreas is able to make additional insulin to overcome the insulin resistance. When the pancreas makes all the insulin it can and there still isn't enough to overcome the effect of the placenta's hormones, gestational diabetes results. If we could somehow remove all the placenta's hormones from the mother's blood, the condition would be remedied. This, in fact, usually happens following delivery.

How does gestational diabetes differ from other types of diabetes?

There are several different types of diabetes. Gestational diabetes begins during pregnancy and disappears following delivery. Another type is referred to as juvenile-onset diabetes (in children) or Type I (in young adults). These individuals usually develop their disease before age 20. People with Type I diabetes must take insulin by injection every day. Approximately 10 percent of all people with diabetes have Type I (also called insulin-dependent diabetes).

Type II diabetes or noninsulin-dependent diabetes (formerly called adult-onset diabetes) is also characterized by high blood sugar levels, but these patients are often obese and usually lack the classic symptoms (fatigue, thirst, frequent urination, and sudden weight loss) associated with Type I diabetes. Many of these individuals can control their blood sugar levels by following a careful diet and exercise program, by losing excess weight, or by taking oral medication. Some, but not all, need insulin. People with Type II diabetes account for roughly 90 percent of all diabetics.

Who is at risk for developing gestational diabetes and how is it detected?

Any woman might develop gestational diabetes during pregnancy. Some of the factors associated with women who have an increased risk are obesity; a family history of diabetes; having given birth previously to a very large infant, a stillbirth, or a child with a birth defect; or having too much amniotic fluid (polyhydramnios). Also, women who are older than 25 are at greater risk than younger individuals. Although a history of sugar in the urine is often included in the list of risk factors, this is not a reliable indicator of who will develop diabetes during pregnancy. Some pregnant women with perfectly normal blood sugar levels will occasionally have sugar detected in their urine.

The Council on Diabetes in Pregnancy of the American Diabetes Association strongly recommends that all pregnant women be screened for gestational diabetes. Several methods of screening exist. The most common is the 50-gram glucose screening test. No special preparation is necessary for this test, and there is no need to fast before the test. The test is performed by giving 50 grams of a glucose drink and then measuring the blood sugar level 1-hour later. A woman with a blood sugar level of less than 140 milligrams per deciliter (mg/dl) at 1-hour is presumed not to have gestational diabetes and requires no further testing. If the blood sugar level is greater than 140 mg/dl the test is considered abnormal or "positive." Not all women with a positive screening test have diabetes. Consequently, a 3-hour glucose tolerance test must be performed to establish the diagnosis of gestational diabetes.

If your physician determines that you should take the complete 3-hour glucose tolerance test, you will be asked to follow some special instructions in preparation for the test. For 3 days before the test, eat a diet that contains at least 150 grams of carbohydrates each day. This can be accomplished by

Table 10.1 3-Hour Glucose Tolerance Test for Gestational Diabetes

	Diagnostic Criteria Blood Glucose Level	Normal Mean Values* Blood Glucose Level
Fasting	105 mg/dl	80 mg/dl
1 hour	190 mg/dl	120 mg/dl
2 hour	165 mg/dl	105 mg/dl
3 hour	145 mg/dl	90 mg/dl

From 752 Unselected Pregnancies

including one cup of pasta, two servings of fruit, four slices of bread, and three glasses of milk every day. For 10 to 14 hours before the test you should not eat and not drink anything but water. The test is usually done in the morning in your physician's office or in a laboratory. First, a blood sample will be drawn to measure your fasting blood sugar level. Then you will be asked to drink a full bottle of a glucose drink (100 grams). This glucose drink is extremely sweet and occasionally makes some people feel nauseated. Finally, blood samples will be drawn every hour for 3 hours after the glucose drink has been consumed. The normal values for this test are shown in [Table 10–1].

If two or more of your blood sugar levels are higher than the diagnostic criteria, you have gestational diabetes. This testing is usually performed at the end of the second trimester or the beginning of the third trimester (between the 24th and 28th weeks of pregnancy) when insulin resistance usually begins. If you had gestational diabetes in a previous pregnancy or there is some reason why your physician is unusually concerned about your risk of developing gestational diabetes, you may be asked to take the 50-gram glucose screening test as early as the first trimester (before the 13th week). Remember, merely having sugar in your urine or even having an abnormal blood sugar on the 50-gram glucose screening test does not necessarily mean you have gestational diabetes. The 3-hour glucose tolerance test must be abnormal before the diagnosis is made.

How does gestational diabetes affect pregnancy and will it hurt my baby?

The complications of gestational diabetes are manageable and preventable. The key to prevention is careful control of blood sugar levels just as soon as the diagnosis of gestational diabetes is made.

You should be reassured that there are certain things gestational diabetes does not usually cause. Unlike Type I diabetes, gestational diabetes generally does not cause birth defects. For the most part, birth defects originate sometime during the first trimester (before the 13th week) of pregnancy. The insulin resistance from the contra-insulin hormones produced by the placenta does not usually occur until approximately the 24th week. Therefore, women with gestational diabetes generally have normal blood sugar levels during the critical first trimester.

One of the major problems a woman with gestational diabetes faces is a condition the baby may develop called "macrosomia." Macrosomia means "large body" and refers to a baby that is considerably larger than normal. All of the nutrients the fetus receives come directly from the mother's blood. If the maternal blood has too much glucose, the pancreas of the fetus senses the high glucose levels and produces more insulin in an attempt to use the glucose. The fetus converts the extra glucose to fat. Even when the mother has gestational diabetes, the fetus is able to produce all the insulin it needs. The combination of high blood glucose levels from the mother and high insulin levels in the fetus results in large deposits of fat which causes the fetus to grow excessively large, a condition known as macrosomia. Occasionally, the baby grows too large to be delivered through the vagina and a cesarean delivery becomes necessary. The obstetrician can often determine if the fetus is macrosomic by doing a physical examination. However, in many cases a special test called an ultrasound is used to measure the size of the fetus. This and other special tests will be discussed later.

In addition to macrosomia, gestational diabetes increases the risk of hypoglycemia (low blood sugar) in the baby immediately after delivery. This problem occurs if the mother's blood sugar levels have been consistently high causing the fetus to have a high level of insulin in its circulation. After delivery the baby continues to have a high insulin level, but it no longer has the high level of sugar from its mother, resulting in the newborn's blood sugar level becoming very low. Your baby's blood sugar level will be checked in the newborn nursery and if the level is too low, it may be necessary to give the baby glucose intravenously. Infants of mothers with gestational diabetes are also vulnerable to several other chemical imbalances such as low serum calcium and low serum magnesium levels.

All of these are manageable and preventable problems. The key to prevention is careful control of blood sugar levels in the mother just as soon as the diagnosis of gestational diabetes is made. By maintaining normal blood sugar levels, it is less likely that a fetus will develop macrosomia, hypoglycemia, or other chemical abnormalities.

What can be done to reduce problems associated with gestational diabetes?

In addition to your obstetrician, there are other health professionals who specialize in the management of diabetes during pregnancy including internists or diabetologists, registered dietitians, qualified nutritionists, and diabetes educators. Your doctor may recommend that you see one or more of these specialists during your pregnancy. In addition, a neonatologist (a doctor who specializes in the care of newborn infants) should also be called in to manage any complications the baby might develop after delivery.

One of the essential components in the care of a woman with gestational diabetes is a diet specifically tailored to provide adequate nutrition to meet the needs of the mother and the growing fetus. At the same time the diet has to be planned in such a way as to keep blood glucose levels in the normal range (60 to 120 mg/dl). Specific details about diet during pregnancy are discussed later.

An obstetrician, diabetes educator, or other health care practitioner can teach you how to measure your own blood glucose levels at home to see if levels remain in an acceptable range on the prescribed diet. The ability of patients to determine their own blood sugar levels with easy-to-use equipment represents a major milestone in the management of diabetes, especially during pregnancy. The technique called "self blood glucose monitoring" (discussed in detail later) allows you to check your blood sugar levels at home or at work without costly and time-consuming visits to your doctor. The values of your blood sugar levels also determine if you need to begin insulin therapy sometime during pregnancy. Short of frequent trips to a laboratory, this is the only way to see if blood glucose levels remain under good control.

What is self blood glucose monitoring?

Once you are diagnosed as having gestational diabetes, you and your health care providers will want to know more about your day-to-day blood sugar levels. It is important to know how your exercise habits and eating patterns affect your blood sugars. Also, as your pregnancy progresses, the placenta will release more of the hormones that work against insulin. Testing your blood sugar level at important times during the day will help determine if proper diet and weight gain have kept blood sugar levels normal or if extra insulin is needed to help keep the fetus protected.

Self blood glucose monitoring is done by using a special device to obtain a drop of your blood and test it for your blood sugar level. Your doctor or other health care provider will explain the procedure to you. Make sure that you are shown how to do the testing before attempting it on your own. Some items you may use to monitor your blood sugar levels are:

Lancet—a disposable, sharp needle-like sticker for pricking the finger to obtain a drop of blood.

Lancet device—a spring-loaded finger sticking device.

Test strip—a chemically treated strip to which a drop of blood is applied.

Color chart—a chart used to compare against the color on the test strip for blood sugar level.

Glucose meter—a device which "reads" the test strip and gives you a digital number value.

Your health care provider can advise you where to obtain the self-monitoring equipment in your area. You may want to inquire if any places rent or loan glucose meters, since it is likely you won't be needing it after your baby is born.

How often and when should I test?

You may need to test your blood several times a day. Generally, these times are fasting (first thing in the morning before you eat) and 2 hours after each meal. Occasionally, you may be asked to test more frequently during the day or at night. As each person is an individual, your health care provider can advise the schedule best for you.

How should I record my test results?

Most manufacturers of glucose testing products provide a record diary, although some health care providers may have their own version. A Self Blood Glucose Monitoring Diary is included at the end of this [document. See form 10–1].

You should record any test result immediately because it's easy to forget what the reading was during the course of a busy day. You should always have this diary with you when you visit your doctor or other health care provider or when you contact them by phone. These results are very important in making decisions about your health care.

Are there any other tests I should know about?

In addition to blood testing, you may be asked to check your urine for ketones. Ketones are by-products of the breakdown of fat and may be found in the blood and urine as a result of inadequate insulin or from inadequate calories in your diet. Although it is not known whether or not small amounts of ketones can harm the fetus, when large amounts of ketones are present they are accompanied by a blood condition, acidosis, which is known to harm the fetus. To be on the safe side, you should watch for them in your urine and report any positive results to your doctor.

How do I test for ketones?

To test the urine for ketones, you can use a test strip similar to the one used for testing your blood. This test strip has a special chemically treated pad to detect ketones in the urine. Testing is done by passing the test strip through the stream of urine or dipping the strip in and out of urine in a container. As your pregnancy progresses, you might find it easier to use the container method. All test strips are disposable and can be used only once. This applies to blood sugar test strips also. You cannot use your blood sugar test strips for urine testing, and you cannot use your urine ketone test strips for blood sugar testing.

When do I test for ketones?

Overnight is the longest fasting period, so you should test your urine first thing in the morning every day and any time your blood sugar level goes over 240 mg/dl on the blood glucose test. It is also important to test if you become ill and are eating less food than normal. Your health care provider can advise what's best for you.

Is it ever necessary to take insulin?

Yes, despite careful attention to diet some women's blood sugars do not stay within an acceptable range. A pregnant woman free of gestational diabetes rarely has a blood glucose level that exceeds 100 mg/dl in the morning before breakfast (fasting) or 2 hours after a meal. The optimum goal for a gestational diabetic is blood sugar levels that are the same as those of a woman without diabetes.

There is no absolute blood sugar level that necessitates beginning insulin injections. However, many physicians begin insulin if the fasting sugar exceeds 105 mg/dl or if the level 2 hours after a meal exceeds 120 mg/dl on two separate occasions. Blood sugar levels measured by you at home will help your doctor know when it is necessary to begin insulin. The ability to perform self blood glucose monitoring has made it possible to begin insulin therapy at the earliest sign of high sugar levels, thereby preventing the fetus from being exposed to high levels of glucose from the mother's blood.

Will my baby be healthy?

The ultimate concern of any expectant mother is, "Will my baby be all right?" There is an array of simple, safe tests used to assess the condition of the fetus before birth and these can be particularly valuable during a pregnancy complicated by gestational diabetes. Tests that may be given during your pregnancy include:

Ultrasound. Ultrasound uses short pulses of high-frequency, low-intensity sound waves to create images. Unlike x rays, there is no radiation exposure to the fetus. First used during World War II to detect enemy submarines below the surface of the water, ultrasound has since been used safely in obstetrics. Occasionally, the date of your last menstrual period is not sufficient to determine a due date. Ultrasound can provide an accurate gestational age and due date that may be very important if it is necessary to induce labor early or perform a cesarean delivery. Ultrasound can also be used to determine the position of the placenta if it is necessary to perform an amniocentesis (another test discussed later).

Fetal movement records. Recording fetal movement is a test you can do by yourself to help determine the condition of the baby. Fetal activity is generally a reassuring sign of well-being. Women are often asked to count fetal movements regularly during the last trimester of pregnancy. You may be asked to set aside specific times to lie down on your back or side and count the number of times the baby moves or kicks. Three or more movements in a 2-hour period is considered normal. Contact your obstetrician if you feel fewer than three movements to determine if other tests are needed.

Fetal monitoring. Modern instruments make it possible to monitor the baby's heart rate before delivery. Currently, there are two types of fetal monitors—internal and external. The internal monitor consists of a small wire electrode attached directly to the scalp of the fetus after the membranes have ruptured. The external monitor uses transducers secured to the mother's abdomen by an elastic belt. One transducer records the baby's heart rate by a sensitive microphone called a doppler. The other transducer measures the firmness of the abdomen during a contraction of the uterus. It is a crude measure of the strength and frequency of contractions. Fetal monitoring is the basis for the non-stress test and the oxytocin challenge test described below.

Non-stress test. The "non-stress" test refers to the fact that no medication is given to the mother to cause movement of the fetus or contraction of the uterus. It is often used to confirm the well-being of the fetus based on the principle that a healthy fetus will demonstrate an acceleration in its heart rate following movement. Fetal activity may be spontaneous or induced by external manipulation such as rubbing the mother's abdomen or making a loud noise above the abdomen with a special device. When movement of the fetus is noted, a recording of the fetal heart rate is made. If the heart rate goes up, the test is normal. If the heart rate does not accelerate, the fetus may merely be "sleeping"; if, after stimulation, the fetus still does not react, it may be necessary to perform a "stress test" (oxytocin challenge test).

Stress test (oxytocin challenge test). Labor represents a stress to the fetus. Every time the uterus contracts, the fetus is momentarily deprived of its usual blood supply and oxygen. This is not a problem for most babies. However, some babies are not healthy enough to handle the stress and demonstrate an abnormal heart rate pattern. This test is often done if the non-stress test is abnormal. It involves giving the hormone oxytocin (secreted by every mother when normal labor begins) to the mother to stimulate uterine contractions. The contractions are a challenge to the baby, similar to the challenge of normal labor. If the baby's heart rate slows down rather than speeds up after a contraction, the baby may be in jeopardy. The stress test is considered more accurate than the non-stress test. Nevertheless, it is not 100 percent fool-proof and your obstetrician may want to repeat it on another occasion to ensure its accuracy. Most women describe this test as mildly uncomfortable but not painful.

Amniocentesis. Amniocentesis is a method of removing a small amount of fluid from the amniotic sac for analysis. Either the fluid itself or the cells shed by the fetus into the fluid can be studied. In mid-pregnancy the cells in amniotic fluid can be analyzed for genetic abnormalities such as Down syndrome. Many women over the age of 35 have amniocentesis for just this reason. Another important use for amniocentesis late in pregnancy is to study the fluid itself to determine if the lungs of the fetus are mature and able to withstand early delivery. This information can be very important in deciding the best time for a woman with Type I diabetes to deliver. It is not done as frequently to women with gestational diabetes.

Amniocentesis can be performed in an obstetrician's office or on an outpatient basis in a hospital. For genetic testing, amniocentesis is usually performed around the 16th week when the placenta and fetus can be located easily with ultrasound and a needle can be inserted safely into the amniotic sac. The overall complication rate for amniocentesis is less than 1 percent. The risk is even lower during the third trimester when the amniotic sac is larger and easily identifiable.

Does gestational diabetes affect labor and delivery?

Most women with gestational diabetes can complete pregnancy and begin labor naturally. Any pregnant woman has a slight chance (about 5 percent) of developing preeclampsia (toxemia), a sudden onset of high blood pressure associated with protein in the urine, occurring late in pregnancy. If preeclampsia develops, your obstetrician may recommend an early delivery. When an early delivery is anticipated, an amniocentesis is usually performed to assess the maturity of the baby's lungs.

Gestational diabetes, by itself, is not an indication to perform a cesarean delivery, but sometimes there are other reasons your doctor may elect to do a cesarean. For example, the baby may be too large (macrosomic) to deliver vaginally, or the baby may be in distress and unable to withstand vaginal delivery. You should discuss the various possibilities for delivery with your obstetrician so there are no surprises.

Careful control of blood sugar levels remains important even during labor. If a mother's blood sugar level becomes elevated during labor, the baby's blood sugar level will also become elevated. High blood sugars in the mother produce high insulin levels in the baby. Immediately after delivery high insulin levels in the baby can drive its blood sugar level very low since it will no longer have the high sugar concentration from its mother's blood.

Women whose gestational diabetes does not require that they take insulin during their pregnancy, will not need to take insulin during their labor or delivery. On the other hand, a woman who does require insulin during pregnancy may be given insulin by injection on the morning labor begins, or in some instances, it may be given intravenously throughout labor. For most women with gestational diabetes there is no need for insulin after the baby is born and blood sugar level returns to normal immediately. The reason for this sudden return to normal lies in the fact that when the placenta is removed the hormones it was producing (which caused the insulin resistance) are also removed. Thus, the mother's insulin is permitted to work normally without resistance. Your doctor may want to check your blood sugar level the next morning, but it will most likely be normal.

Should I expect my baby to have any problems?

One of the most frequently asked questions is, "Will my baby have diabetes?" Almost universally the answer is no. However, the baby is at risk for developing Type II diabetes later in life, and of having other problems related to gestational diabetes, such as hypoglycemia (low blood sugar) mentioned earlier. If your blood sugars were not elevated during the 24 hours before delivery, there is a good chance that hypoglycemia will not be a problem for your baby. Nevertheless, a neonatologist (a doctor who specializes in the care of newborn infants) or other doctor should check your baby's blood sugar level and give extra glucose if necessary.

Another problem that may develop in the infant of a mother with gestational diabetes is jaundice. Jaundice occurs when extra red blood cells in the baby's circulation are destroyed, releasing a substance called bilirubin. Bilirubin is a pigment that causes a yellow discoloration of the skin (jaundice). A minor degree of jaundice is common in many newborns. However, the presence of large amounts of bilirubin in the baby's system can be harmful and requires placing the baby under special lights which help get rid of the pigment. In extreme cases, blood transfusions may be necessary.

Will I develop diabetes in the future?

For most women gestational diabetes disappears immediately after delivery. However, you should have your blood sugars checked after your baby is born to make sure your levels have returned to normal. Women who had gestational diabetes during one pregnancy are at greater risk of developing it in a subsequent pregnancy. It is important that you have appropriate screening tests for gestational diabetes during future pregnancies as early as the first trimester.

Pregnancy is a kind of "stress test" that often predicts future diabetic problems. In one large study more than one-half of all women who had gestational diabetes developed overt Type II diabetes within 15 years of pregnancy. Because of the risk of developing Type II diabetes in the future, you should have your blood sugar level checked when you see your doctor for your routine check-ups. There is a good chance you will be able to reduce the risk of developing diabetes later in life by maintaining an ideal body weight and exercising regularly.

Why is a special diet recommended?

A nutritionally balanced diet is always essential to maintaining a healthy mother and successful pregnancy. The foods you choose become the nutrient building blocks for the growth of the fetus. For a woman with gestational diabetes, proper diet alone often keeps blood sugar levels in the normal range and is generally the first step to follow before resorting to insulin injections. Careful attention should be paid to the total calories eaten daily, to avoid foods which increase blood sugar levels, and to emphasize the use of foods which help the body maintain a normal blood sugar. A registered dietitian is the best person to help you with meal planning to meet your individual needs. Your physician can help you find a dietitian if this service is not a part of his or her office or clinic. Your local chapter of the American Dietetic Association or the American Diabetes Association can also help you locate a registered dietitian.

How much weight should I gain?

Of all questions asked by pregnant women, this is the most common. The answer is particularly important for women with gestational diabetes. The weight that you gain is a rough indication of how much nutrition is available to the fetus for growth. An inadequate weight gain may result in a small baby who lacks protective calorie reserves at birth. This baby may have more illness during the first year of life. An excessive weight gain during preg-

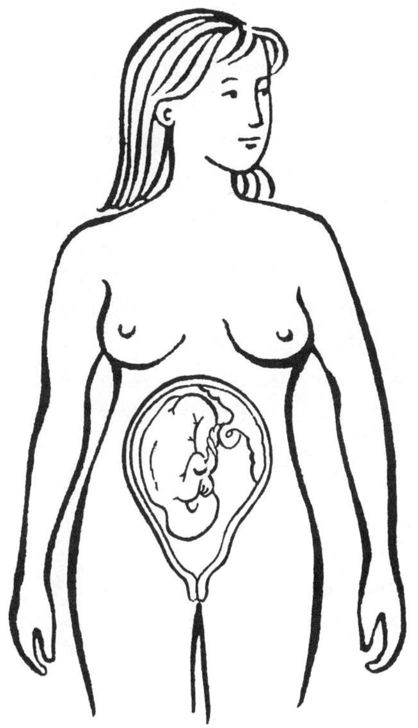

WEIGHT IN POUNDS	
7.5-8.5	FETUS
7.5	STORES OF FAT & PROTEIN
4.0	BLOOD
2.7	TISSUE FLUIDS
2.0	UTERUS
1.8	AMNIOTIC FLUID
1.5	PLACENTA & UMBILICAL CORD
1.0	BREASTS
28-29.0 POUNDS	

Figure 10.1 Distribution of Weight Gain During Pregnancy

nancy, however, has an insulin-resistant effect, just like the hormones produced by the placenta, and will make your blood sugar level higher.

The "optimal" weight to gain depends on the weight that you are before becoming pregnant. Your pre-pregnancy weight is also a rough indication of how well-nourished you are before becoming pregnant. If you are at a desirable weight for your body size before you become pregnant, a weight gain of 24 to 27 pounds is recommended. If you are approximately 20 pounds or more above your desirable weight before pregnancy, a weight gain of 24 pounds is recommended. Many overweight women, however, have healthy babies and gain only 20 pounds. If you become pregnant when you are underweight, you need to gain more weight during the pregnancy to give your baby the extra nutrition he or she needs for the first year. You should gain 28 to 36 pounds, depending on how underweight you are before becoming pregnant. Your nutrition advisor or health care provider can recommend an appropriate weight gain. How your weight gain is distributed is illustrated in [Figure 10–1].

Total recommended weight gain is often not as helpful as a weekly rate of gain. Most women gain 3 to 5 pounds during the first trimester (first 3 months) of pregnancy. During the second and third trimesters, a good rate of weight gain is about three-quarters of a pound to one pound per week. Gaining too much weight (2 or more pounds per week) results in putting on too much body fat. This extra body fat produces an insulin-resistant effect which requires the body to produce more insulin to keep blood sugar levels normal. An inability to produce more insulin, as in gestational diabetes, causes your blood sugar levels to rise above acceptable levels. If weight gain has been excessive, often limiting weight gain to approximately three-quarters of a pound per week (3 pounds per month) can return blood sugar levels to normal. Fetal growth and development depend on proper nourishment and will be placed at risk by drastically reducing calories. However, you can limit weight gain by cutting back on excessive calories and by eating a nutritionally-sound diet that meets your needs and the needs of your baby. Remember that dieting and severely cutting back on weight gain may increase the risk of delivering prematurely. If blood sugar levels continue to go up and you are not gaining excessive weight or eating improperly, the safest therapy for the well-being of the fetus is insulin.

Occasionally, your weight may go up rapidly in the last trimester (after 28 weeks) and you may notice an increase in water retention, such as swelling in the feet, fingers, and face. If there is any question as to whether the rapid weight gain is due to eating too many calories or too much water retention, keeping records of how much food you eat and your exercise patterns at this time will be very helpful. A Food and Exercise Record Sheet is included at the end of this [text. See Form 10–2]. By examining your Food and Exercise Record Sheet, your nutrition advisor can help you determine which is causing the rapid weight gain. In addition, by examining your legs and body for signs of fluid retention, your physician can help you to determine the cause of your weight gain. If your weight gain is due to water retention, cutting back drastically on calories may actually cause more fluid retention. Bed rest and resting on your side will help you to lose the build-up of fluid. Limit your intake of salt (sodium chloride) and very salty foods, as they tend to contribute to water retention.

Marked fluid retention when combined with an increase in blood pressure and possibly protein in the urine are the symptoms of preeclampsia. This is a disorder of pregnancy that can be harmful to both the mother and baby. Inform your obstetrician of any rapid weight gain, especially if you are eating moderately and gaining more than 2 pounds per week. Should you develop preeclampsia, be especially careful to eat a well-balanced diet with adequate calories.

After being diagnosed as having gestational diabetes, many women notice a slower weight gain as they start cutting the various sources of sugar out of their diet. This seems to be harmless and lasts only 1 or 2 weeks. It may be that sweets were contributing a substantial amount of calories to the diet.

How should I eat during my pregnancy?

As with any pregnancy, it is important to eat the proper foods to meet the nutritional needs of the mother and fetus. An additional goal for women with gestational diabetes is to maintain a proper diet to keep blood sugars as normal as possible.

The daily need for calories increases by 300 calories during the second and third trimesters of pregnancy. If non-pregnant calorie intake was 1800 calories per day and weight gain was maintained, a calorie intake of 2100 calories per day is usual from 14 weeks until delivery. This is the equivalent of an additional 8 ounce glass of 2% milk and one-half of a sandwich (1 slice of bread, approximately 1 ounce of meat, and 1 teaspoon of margarine, mayonnaise, etc.) per day. The need for protein also increases during pregnancy. Make sure your diet includes foods high in protein, but not high in fat. Most vitamins and minerals are also needed in larger amounts during pregnancy. This can be attained by increasing dairy products, especially those low in fat, and making sure you include whole grain cereals and breads, as well as fruits and vegetables in your diet each day. To make sure you get enough folate (a B vitamin critical during pregnancy) and iron, your obstetrician will probably recommend a prenatal vitamin. Prenatal vitamins do not replace a good diet; they merely help you to get the nutrients you need. To absorb the most iron from your prenatal vitamin, take it at night before going to bed, or in the morning on an empty stomach.

The Daily Food Guide [Table 10–2] serves as a guideline for food sources that provide important vitamins and minerals, as well as carbohydrates, protein, and fiber during pregnancy. The recommended minimal servings per day appear in parentheses after each food group listed. This guide emphasizes foods that are low in fat and in sugar (discussed later).

The food guide is divided into six groups: milk and milk products; meat, poultry, fish, and meat substitutes; breads, cereals, and other starches; fruits; vegetables; and fats. Each group provides its own combination of vitamins, minerals, and other nutrients which play an important part in nutrition during pregnancy. Omitting the foods from one group will leave your diet inadequate in other nutrients. Plan your meals using a variety of foods within each food group, in the amounts recommended, and you'll be most likely to get all the vitamins, minerals, and other nutrients the fetus needs for growth and development.

Table 10.2 Daily Food Guide

Milk and Milk Products *(4 Servings Per Day)*	1 cup milk, skim or low-fat 1/3 cup powdered non-fat milk 1 cup reconstituted powdered non-fat milk 1½ oz. low-fat cheese* (no more than 6 grams of fat per ounce) 1 cup low-fat yogurt**	(high protein calcium, vitamin D)
Meat, Poultry, Fish, and Meat Substitutes *(5-6 Servings Per Day)*	1 oz. cooked poultry, fish, or lean meat (beef, lamb, pork) 1 tbsp. peanut butter 1 egg 1/4 cup low-fat cottage cheese 1/2 cup cooked dried beans or lentils	(high protein, B vitamins, iron)
Breads, Cereals, and Other Starches *(5-6 Servings Per Day)*	1 slice whole grain bread 5 crackers 1 muffin, biscuit, pancake, or waffle 3/4 cup dry cereal, unsweetened 1/2 cup pasta (macaroni, spaghetti), rice, mashed potatoes, or cooked cereal 1/3 cup sweet potatoes or yams 1/2 cup cooked dried beans or lentils 1/2 bagel, 1/2 english muffin, or 1/2 flour tortilla 1 small baked potato 2 taco shells	(high complex carbohydrates) (emphasize whole grains, or use fortified or enriched) (a good source of protein, B-vitamins, fiber and minerals)

Table 10.2 (Continued)

Fruit *(2 servings per day)*	1/2 cup fresh fruit, 1/2 banana, or 1 medium-sized fruit (apple, orange) 1/2 cup, orange, grapefruit, or other juice fortified with vitamin C 1/2 medium-sized grapefruit 1 cup strawberries 1/2 cup fresh apricots, nectarines, purple plums, cantaloup, or 4 halves dried apricots (vitamin A source)	(fresh fruit provides fiber) (include one vitamin C source daily)
Vegetables*** *(2 servings per day)*	1/2 cup cooked or 1 cup raw: broccoli, spinach, carrots, (vitamin A source) 1/3 cup mixed vegetables	(include good vitamin A sources at least every other day)
Fats	1 tsp. butter or margarine 1 tsp. oil or mayonnaise 1 tbsp. regular salad dressing 2 tbsp. low-calorie salad dressing 1/4 cup nuts or seeds	

**1 oz. low-fat cheese can also be used as 1 serving from the Meat, Poultry, Fish, and Meat Substitutes group if sufficient calcium is already being provided from 4 servings.*

***This refers to plain yogurt. Commercially fruited yogurt contains a lot of added sugar.*

****Starchy vegetables such as corn, peas, and potatoes are included in Breads, Cereals, and Other Starches list.*

Other Nutritional and Non-Nutritional Considerations:

Alcohol. There is no known safe level of alcohol to allow during pregnancy. Daily heavy alcohol intake causes severe defects in development of the body and brain of the fetus, called Fetal Alcohol Syndrome. Even moderate drinking is associated with delayed fetal growth, spontaneous abortions, and lowered birth weight in babies. The Surgeon General's office warns: "Women who are pregnant or even considering pregnancy should avoid alcohol completely and should be aware of the alcohol content of food and drugs."

Salt. Salt restriction is no longer routinely advised during pregnancy. Recent research shows that during pregnancy the body needs salt to help provide the proper fluid balance. Your health care provider may recommend that you use salt in moderation.

Caffeine. Studies conflict on the potential danger of caffeine to the fetus. Caffeine is found primarily in coffee, tea, and some sodas [Table 10–3]. Moderation is recommended. Talk to your doctor or other health professional about the maximum amount of caffeine recommended.

Megavitamins. Megavitamins are defined as 10 times the Recommended Dietary Allowance (dietary allowances established by the National Academy of Sciences—National Research Council) of vitamins and minerals and are not recommended for pregnant women. Although it is possible to get all of the necessary nutrients from food alone, your doctor may prescribe some prenatal vitamins and minerals. If taken regularly, along with a balanced diet, you will be getting all the vitamins and minerals needed during your pregnancy.

Smoking. Research has shown without question that smoking during pregnancy increases the risk of fetal death and preterm delivery, impairs fetal growth, and can lead to low birth weight. It is best to stop smoking entirely and permanently, or at the very least, to cut back drastically on the number of cigarettes you smoke.

What foods patterns help keep blood sugar levels normal?

The following outlines food patterns which help to keep blood sugar levels within an acceptable range.

Avoid sugar and foods high in sugar. Most women with gestational diabetes, just like those without diabetes, have a desire for something sweet in their diet. In pregnant women, sugar is rapidly absorbed into the blood and requires a larger release of insulin to maintain normal blood sugar levels. Without the larger release of insulin, blood sugar levels will increase excessively when you eat sugar-containing foods.

Table 10.3 Caffeine Comparisons

Food	Serving	Amount of Caffeine
Regular coffee	8 oz.	80-200 mg.
Instant coffee	8 oz.	60-100 mg.
Decaffeinated coffee	8 oz.	3-5 mg.
Tea	8 oz.	60-65 mg.
Carbonated drinks, e.g., colas	12 oz.	30-65 mg.
Hot chocolate	8 oz.	13 mg.

There are many forms of sugar such as table sugar, honey, brown sugar, corn syrup, maple syrup, turbinado sugar, high fructose corn syrup, and molasses. Generally, food that ends in "ose" is a sugar (e.g., sucrose, dextrose, and glucose).

Foods that usually contain high amounts of sugar include pies, cakes, cookies, ice cream, candy, soft drinks, fruit drinks, fruit packed in syrup, commercially fruited yogurt, jams, jelly, doughnuts, and sweet rolls. Many of these foods are high in fat as well.

Be sure to check the list of ingredients on food products. Ingredients are listed in order of amount. If an ingredient is first on the list, it is present in the highest amount. If some type of sugar is listed first, second, or third on the list of ingredients, the product should be avoided. If sugar is further down, fourth, fifth, or sixth, it probably will not cause your blood sugar levels to go up excessively.

Fruit juices should only be taken with a meal and limited to 6 ounces. Tomato juice is a good choice because it is low in sugar. Six ounces of most other juice (apple, grapefruit, orange) with no sugar added still contain approximately 4 to 5 teaspoons of sugar. However, these do not contain much of the fiber of a piece of fruit which normally would act to slow the absorption of sugar into the blood. If you drink juice frequently to quench your thirst during the day, a high blood sugar level may result. Use only whole fruit for snacks.

To help with the occasional sweet tooth that we all have, artificial sweeteners may be used in foods. Aspartame has been extensively tested for safety. Use during pregnancy has been approved by the Food and Drug Administration and by the American Medical Association's Review Board. However, aspartame has not been tested for long-term safety and has not been on the market very long. It may be best to avoid its use until more tests have been done.

Saccharin is not advised during pregnancy. Likewise, use of mannitol, xylitol, sorbitol, or other artificial sweeteners is not recommended until further research is done.

Fructose is a special type of sugar that is slowly absorbed into the system. A small amount of fructose can be used if your blood sugar levels are within normal range. However, fructose still has 4 calories per gram, as much as table sugar. High fructose corn syrup is part fructose and part corn syrup, making it very similar to table sugar in composition. It will raise blood sugar levels and should definitely be avoided.

Emphasize the use of complex carbohydrates. These include vegetables, cereal, grains, beans, peas, and other starchy foods. A well-balanced diet with plenty of fiber provided by vegetables, dried beans, cereals, and other starchy foods decreases the amount of insulin your body needs to keep blood sugars within a normal range. Anything that decreases the need for insulin is beneficial. The American Diabetes Association recommends that at least one-half of your calories come from complex carbohydrates. Starchy foods include pasta, rice, grains, cereals, crackers, bread, potatoes, dried beans, peas, and legumes. Also, contrary to popular belief, carbohydrates are not highly fattening when eaten in moderate amounts and without the rich sauces and toppings often added.

Emphasize foods high in dietary fiber. Fiber is the edible portion of foods of plant origin that is not digested (e.g., skins, membranes, seeds, bran). Foods with a high fiber content include whole grain cereals and breads, fruits, vegetables, and legumes (dried peas and beans). Fiber aids digestion and helps prevent constipation. The fiber found in fruits, vegetables, and legumes also helps keep your blood sugar level from becoming too high without requiring extra insulin.

Keep your diet low in fat. Some fat is needed to help with the absorption of certain vitamins and to provide the essential fatty acids necessary for fetal growth. A diet which is high in fat causes the insulin to react in a less efficient manner, necessitating more insulin to keep blood sugar levels within normal range. Foods high in saturated fats such as fatty meats, butter, bacon, cream (light, coffee, sour cream, etc.), and whole milk cheeses are likely to be high in total fat. Most foods with saturated fat are also high in cholesterol because they are fats from animal origin. However, foods such as crackers made with coconut, palm, or palm kernel oil can be high in saturated fats as well. Read labels carefully. Unsaturated fats are found in foods such as fish, margarine and vegetable oils. Keep your use of salad dressings to a minimum and whenever possible use those prepared with olive oil. To help keep the diet lower in fat, avoid adding extra fats such as rich sauces and creamy desserts, and bake or broil foods instead of frying them. Replacing fatty foods with those high in complex carbohydrates is also helpful.

Include a bedtime snack that is a good source of protein and complex carbohydrates. Women with gestational diabetes have a tendency toward lower than normal blood sugar levels during the night. This causes the body to increase its utilization of fats as a fuel source. As fat is used, ketones (discussed later) are produced as a by-product of the breakdown of fats, and in large amounts, may be harmful to the fetus. This can be prevented by having a bedtime snack that provides protein and complex carbohydrates such as starchy foods. Starch will stabilize your blood sugar level in the early night, while protein acts as a long-acting stabilizer. Examples of a bedtime snack are:

1 oz. American-processed cheese + 5 crackers

1/2 chicken sandwich on whole wheat bread

3 cups unbuttered popcorn + 1/4 cup nuts

If you need to take insulin, a bedtime snack is critical and you should not omit it. When taken by injection, insulin acts to lower blood sugar level, even during the night when meals are not eaten. A bedtime snack is protective against low blood sugars while sleeping or upon arising. If a bedtime snack causes heartburn, sleep with your head raised on pillows, and be careful that you are not eating too large a bedtime snack.

How do I plan meals?

A registered dietitian or qualified nutritionist can help you plan a meal pattern that is right for you. Most women with gestational diabetes need three meals and a bedtime snack each day. It is unwise for anyone who is pregnant to go long periods of time (greater than 5 hours) without eating, as this will produce ketones. Extra snacks are necessary if your schedule results in a long time between meals. Blood sugars will be easier to keep in the normal range if meal times and amounts (total calories) are evenly spaced. It's more likely that a higher blood sugar will result if the majority of calories are eaten at dinner, than if they are distributed more evenly throughout the day. If insulin injections prove necessary, the time at which meals are eaten and the amounts eaten should be approximately the same from day to day. Do not skip meals and snacks, as this often results in hypoglycemia (low blood sugar), which may be harmful to the fetus and makes you feel irritable, shaky, or may result in a headache.

What can be done to slow weight gain during pregnancy?

Gaining too much weight during pregnancy will make blood sugar levels higher than normal for women with gestational diabetes. Yet, for many pregnant women it is very difficult to gain weight slowly and still get all of the recommended nutrients. Luckily, fat, which is high in calories (9 calories per gram), is needed in only small amounts during pregnancy. Carbohydrates and protein, in contrast to fat, provide only 4 calories per gram. To cut calories without depriving the fetus of any necessary nutritional factors, it is best to avoid fats and fatty foods.

- Avoid high-fat meats. Choose lean cuts of beef, pork, and lamb. Emphasize more fish and poultry (without the skin).
- Avoid frying meat, fish, or poultry in added oil, shortening, or lard. Bake, broil, or roast instead.
- Avoid foods fried in oil such as chips, french fries, and doughnuts. Substitute pretzels, unbuttered popcorn, or breadsticks instead.

Table 10.4 Sample Menu—2000 Calories

This diet is planned for women whose normal non-pregnant weight should be 130-135 lbs. For women who weigh less than 130 before pregnancy, the diet should contain fewer calories. Women who are overweight are at higher risk for gestational diabetes. Your health care provider can discuss this and help you make necessary changes.

BREAKFAST

1/2 grapefruit
3/4 cup oatmeal, cooked
1 tsp. raisins
1 cup 2% milk
1 whole wheat English muffin
1 tsp. margarine

LUNCH

Salad with:
  1 cup romaine lettuce
  1/2 cup kidney beans, cooked
  1/2 fresh tomato
1 oz. part skim mozzarella cheese
2 tbsp. low-calorie Italian dressing
1 bran muffin
1/2 cup cantaloupe chunks

AFTERNOON SNACK

2 rice cakes
6 oz. low-fat yogurt, plain
1/2 cup blueberries

DINNER

3/4 cup vegetable soup with
  1/4 cup cooked barley
3 oz. chicken, without skin
1 baked potato
1/2 cup cooked broccoli
1 piece whole wheat bread
1 tbsp. margarine
1 fresh peach

BEDTIME SNACK

1 apple
2 cups popcorn, plain
1/4 cup peanuts

- Avoid using cream sauces and butter sauces, as well as salt pork for seasoning on vegetables. Season with herbs instead.
- Avoid using the fat drippings from meat or poultry for gravy. Use broth or bouillon instead and thicken with cornstarch.
- Avoid using mayonnaise or oil for salads. Use vinegar, lemon juice, or low-calorie salad dressings instead.

To help reduce calories choose low-fat dairy products. During pregnancy you need 1200 mg calcium daily to build the fetal skeleton without drawing from maternal calcium stores. [Tabale 10–5] points out foods in which the calcium content is almost the same, yet the calories are not due to the difference in fat content.

The difference between 600 calories and 340 calories is only 260 calories and may seem insignificant. Yet, if your diet is cut by 260 calories daily for 1 week, your weight gain slows down by approximately 1/2 pound per week.

In other words, instead of gaining 1+ pounds per week you will only gain 1 pound per week.

If cheese is a part of your daily diet, use low-fat cheeses such as low-fat cottage cheese, Neufchatel, mozzarella, farmers, and pot cheese. Avoid using cream cheese, as it has little protein and most of its calories come from fat.

Even though pregnancy can be a very hectic time, with little time for meal preparation, eat less and less often at "fast food" restaurants. Studies have shown that some foods from fast food restaurants average 40 to 60 percent of their calories from fat, and are quite high in calories (*Fast Food Facts: Nutritive and Exchange Values for Fast Food Restaurants,* Marion J. Franz, International Diabetes Center, Minneapolis, Minnesota, 1987. 54 pp.). For example, chicken and fish that are coated with batter and deep-fried in fat may contain more fat and calories than a hamburger or roast beef sandwich.

Go lightly when using butter and margarine. Adding only an extra three pats of butter or margarine (same calories) daily could add an extra pound of weight gain next month. It may be better to emphasize the use of foods rich in complex carbohydrates that don't use butter, margarine, or cream sauce to make them palatable. Many people find rice, noodles, and spaghetti tasty without a lot of butter. Use a variety of spices and herbs (such as curry, garlic, and parsley) to flavor rice and tomato sauce to flavor pasta without additional fats.

It is also a good idea to eat small amounts frequently, thereby keeping the edge off your appetite. This will assist your "self-control" in avoiding large portions of food that you should not have. Avoid skipping meals or trying to cut back drastically on breakfast or lunch. It will leave you too hungry for the next meal to exercise any control. Your doctor or dietitian can help you determine how you can cut extra calories.

You may find it helpful to keep food records of what you eat, as most of us tend to forget or not realize the extent of our snacking. Recording everything you eat or drink tends to be a sobering and instructive experience. A Food and Exercise Record Sheet is included at the end of this [text. See Form 10–2].

Be careful to maintain a weight gain of at least 1/2 pound per week, over several weeks, if you are in the second trimester (14 weeks or more of gestation). Cutting back more than this may increase the risk of having a low-birth-weight infant.

Is breast-feeding recommended?

Breast-feeding is strongly encouraged. For most women this represents the easiest way back to pre-pregnancy weight after delivery. The body draws

Table 10.5 Calorie Comparisons

Food	Calories
4-8 oz. glasses whole milk	600
4-8 oz. glasses 2% milk	480
4-8 oz. glasses skim milk	340
2-8 oz. glasses whole milk plus 3 oz. American processed cheese	600
2-8 oz. glasses 2% milk plus 3 oz. American processed cheese	540
2-8 oz. glasses skim milk plus 3 oz. American processed cheese	470

on the calories stored during the first part of pregnancy to use in milk production. Approximately 800 calories per day are used during the first 3 months of milk production, and even more during the next 3 months. By 6 weeks after delivery, women who breast-feed usually have lost 4 pounds more than women who bottle-feed. This can be a very important factor, as it is strongly recommended that women with gestational diabetes return to their desirable body weight 4 to 5 months postpartum. As previously mentioned, maintaining a weight appropriate for your height and frame may reduce the risk of developing diabetes later in life.

In addition, breast-feeding has many advantages for your baby. Protection from infection and allergies are transferred to the baby through breast milk. This milk is also easier to digest than formula, and its minerals are better absorbed than those in formula.

Should I exercise?

A daily exercise program is an important part of a healthy pregnancy. Daily exercise helps you feel better and reduces stress. In addition, being physically fit protects against back pain, and maintains muscle tone, strength, and endurance. For women with gestational diabetes, exercise is especially important.

- Regular exercise increases the efficiency or potency of your body's own insulin. This may allow you to keep your blood sugar levels in the normal range while using less insulin.
- Moderate exercise also helps blunt your appetite, helping you to keep your weight gain down to normal levels. Maintaining the correct weight gain is very important in preventing high blood sugar levels.

Talk with your doctor about what exercise program is right for you. Your doctor can advise you about limitations, warning signs, and any special considerations. Generally, you can continue any exercise program or sport you participated in prior to pregnancy. Use caution, however, and avoid sports or exercises where you might fall, or that involve jolting. Pre-pregnancy bicycling, jogging, and cross-country skiing are good exercises to continue during pregnancy. If you plan to start an exercise program during pregnancy, talk to your doctor before beginning and start slowly. Vigorous walking is good for women who need to start exercising and have not been active before pregnancy.

Exercising frequently, 4 to 5 days per week, is necessary to get the "blood sugar lowering" advantages of an exercise program. Don't omit a warm-up period of 5 to 10 minutes and a cool-down period of 5 to 10 minutes. Always stop exercising if you feel pain, dizziness, shortness of breath, faintness, palpitations, back or pelvic pain, or experience vaginal bleeding. Also, avoid vigorous exercise in hot, humid weather or if you have a fever. It is important to prevent dehydration during exercise, especially during pregnancy. The American College of Obstetricians and Gynecologists (ACOG) recommends drinking fluids prior to and after exercise, and if necessary, during the activity to prevent dehydration.

An ACOG report (*Home Exercise Program: Exercise During Pregnancy and the Postnatal Period.* American College of Obstetricians and Gynecologists. May 1985. 6 pp.) issued in 1985, warned that target heart rates for pregnant and postpartum women should be set approximately 25 to 30 percent lower than rates for non-pregnant women. It may be that exercising too vigorously will direct blood flow away from the uterus and fetus. ACOG recommends that pregnant women measure their heart rate during activity and that maternal heart rate not exceed 140 beats per minute.

If you need to be on insulin during your pregnancy, take a few precautions. Because both insulin and exercise lower blood sugar levels, the combination can result in hypoglycemia or low blood sugar. You need to be aware that this is a potential problem, and you should be familiar with the symptoms of hypoglycemia (confusion, extreme hunger, blurry vision, shakiness, sweating). When exercising, take along sugar in the form of hard, sugar-sweetened candies just in case your blood sugar becomes too low. When on insulin, you should always carry some form of sugar for potential episodes of hypoglycemia.

It may be necessary for you to eat small snacks between meals if the exercise results in low blood sugar levels.

- One serving of fruit will keep blood sugars normal for most short-term activities (approximately 30 minutes).

- One serving of fruit plus a serving of starch will be enough for activities that last longer (60 minutes or more).

If you exercise right after a meal, eat the snack after the exercise. If the exercise is 2 hours or more after a meal, eat the snack before the exercise.

What happens if diet and exercise fail to control my blood sugars?

If your blood sugars tend to go over the acceptable levels (105 mg/dl or below for fasting, 120 mg/dl or below 2 hours after a meal) you may need to take insulin injections. Insulin is a protein and would be digested like any other protein in food if it were given orally. The needles used to inject insulin are extremely fine, so there is little discomfort. If insulin injections are necessary, you will be taught how to fill the syringe and how to do the injections yourself.

Your physician will calculate the amount of insulin needed to keep blood sugar levels within the normal range. It is very likely that the amount or dosage of insulin needed to keep your levels of blood sugar normal will increase as your pregnancy advances. This does not mean your gestational diabetes is getting worse. As any healthy pregnancy progresses, the placenta will grow and produce progressively higher levels of contra-insulin hormones. As a result you will likely need to inject more insulin to overcome their effect. Some women may even require two injections each day. This does not imply anything about the severity of the problem or the outcome of the pregnancy. The goal is to maintain normal blood sugar levels with whatever dosage of insulin is needed.

Can my blood sugar level go too low, and if so, what do I do?

Occasionally, your blood sugar level may get too low if you are taking insulin. This can happen if you delay a meal or exercise more than usual, especially at the time your insulin is working at its peak. This low blood sugar is called "hypoglycemia" or an "insulin reaction." This is a medical emergency and should be promptly treated, never ignored.

The symptoms of insulin reaction vary from sweating, shakiness, or dizziness to feeling faint, disoriented, or a tingling sensation. Remember, if you take insulin injections, you need to keep some form of sugar-sweetened candy in your purse, at home, at work, and in your car. In case of an episode of hypoglycemia, you will be prepared to treat it immediately. Be sure to eat something more substantial afterward. Also, report any insulin reactions or high blood sugar levels to your doctor right away in case an adjustment in your treatment needs to be made.

As you can see from reading this text, extra care, work, and commitment on the part of you and your spouse or partner are required to provide the special medical care necessary. Don't worry if you occasionally go off your diet or miss a planned exercise program. Your doctor and other health care professionals will work along with you to make sure you receive the specialized care that has resulted in dramatically improved pregnancy outcome.

An ounce of prevention is worth a pound of cure! Eat as directed. Exercise as directed. Monitor as directed. Do these things and you are doing your part toward a happy, healthy pregnancy.

Glossary

Gestational diabetes—A form of diabetes which begins during pregnancy and usually disappears following delivery.

Health care providers—Health care professionals who specialize in the management of certain conditions. In the case of gestational diabetes, the health care providers may include an obstetrician, an internist, a diabetologist, a registered dietitian, a qualified nutritionist, a diabetes educator, and a neonatologist.

Hormone—A chemical substance produced within the body which has a "regulatory" effect on the activity of a certain tissue in the body. Estrogen, cortisol, and human placental lactogen are hormones produced by the placenta which cause changes in the mother's body to prepare her for the pregnancy and birth. These hormones also have a contra-insulin effect.

Insulin-resistance—A partial blocking of the effect of insulin. This interference can be caused by hormones produced by the placenta or by excessive weight gain.

Legumes—Beans, peas, and lentils which supply fiber and nutrients and are high in vegetable protein.

Macrosomia—A term meaning "large body". This refers to a baby that is considerably larger than normal. This condition occurs when the mother's blood sugar levels have been higher than normal during the pregnancy. This is a preventable complication of gestational diabetes.

Nutrients—Proteins, carbohydrates, fats, vitamins, and minerals. These are provided by food and are necessary for growth and the maintenance of life.

Placenta—A special tissue that joins the mother and fetus. It provides hormones necessary for a successful pregnancy, and supplies the fetus with water and nutrients (food) from the mother's blood.

Recommended Dietary Allowances—Recommendations for daily intake of specific nutrients for groups of healthy individuals. There is a specific recommendation for pregnant and for lactating women: These recommendations are set by the Food and Nutrition Board of the National Research Council of the National Academy of Science.

Trimester—A period of 3 months. Pregnancy is divided into three trimesters. The first trimester is 0–13 weeks gestation. The second trimester is 14–26 weeks gestation. The third trimester is 27 weeks gestation until birth.

[For additional terms, see the *Diabetes Dictionary* which is reproduced in Chapter 1.]

Self Blood Glucose Monitoring Diary

DATE	Before eating **am**	2 hr. after **breakfast**	2 hr. after **lunch**	2 hr. after **dinner**	Amount of **insulin**	NOTES

Form 10-1.

Food and Exercise Record Sheet

The following chart is intended to help you and your health care providers keep track of your food and exercise habits and enable you to plan a regimen tailored to your particular needs.

1) Write down everything you eat or drink.

2) Write down items added to foods (e.g., sugar, butter).

3) Write down how your food was prepared (e.g., broiled, fried, baked).

4) Write down the amount you eat in household measures (e.g., 1/2 cup or 2 tbsp.).

5) Write down any exercising you have done, type of exercise, and time spent.

DAY	TIME	FOOD AND TYPE OF PREPARATION	AMOUNT	EXERCISE

Form 10-2.

Chapter 11

Diabetes Goals for the Nation

Complication-Specific Goals

The complications of diabetes increase with age and disease duration. They develop slowly, vary in severity, and are rarely reversible. For most complications of diabetes, similar methods can be used to address patient and professional education, health care financing, access to health care, minority problems, and the needs of high-risk groups. These overall strategies are described below in "Interdisciplinary Diabetes Interventions." Certain complications, however, will require additional, more specific strategies and methods to achieve the goals for effective prevention and treatment. . . .

The first annual report of the DTC will include detailed identification of the available methods for achieving reductions in these complications and strategies for implementing the interdisciplinary interventions. Other Federal agencies that are responsible for health care delivery programs will describe their progress in meeting complication-specific and interdisciplinary goals and objectives in their own annual reports.

Diabetes and Pregnancy

Offspring of women with diabetes are at increased risk of macrosomia, hypoglycemia, respiratory distress syndrome, and congenital malformations. Current statistics, although limited, suggest that the mortality rates of infants

---

Excerpts from: *The National Long-Range Plan to Combat Diabetes.* NIH Pub. No. 88–1587.

of mothers with diabetes is approximately 7 percent. In diabetes centers that have experience in intensive treatment, however, mortality rates are closer to 2 percent. It is becoming clear that pregnancy counseling and management are critical and that normal glycemia at the time of conception will decrease the rate of fetal anomalies, which currently account for 40 percent of neonatal deaths. There is a need both for educational efforts and disease surveillance in the health care community to clearly establish the problems and the effects of interventions.

In spite of the increased knowledge about the importance of gestational diabetes, universal screening of pregnant women for the presence of diabetes mellitus does not occur. Followup and treatment in accordance with current guidelines for patient care is not uniform. . . .

Diabetic Eye Disease

Ocular complications of diabetes are the leading cause of new cases of legal blindness in people ages 20 to 74 in the United States. Retinopathy is the single largest cause of this blindness. Some factors that increase the risk of blindness, such as longer duration of diabetes or younger age at diagnosis of diabetes, cannot be changed; however, other associated factors can be eliminated or reduced. Better control of elevated blood glucose and blood pressure levels in persons with diabetes may decrease the risk of blindness. Laser photocoagulation treatment for proliferative retinopathy or macular edema can reduce the progression to severe vision loss by as much as 60 percent. Therefore, all persons with IDDM of longer than 5 years' duration and past puberty and all persons with NIDDM should have annual examinations by skilled practitioners for early diagnosis and management of ophthalmic changes.

Surveys suggest that improvements in eye care of persons with diabetes are necessary to reduce their risk of blindness. Therefore, the roles of various vision care providers should be clarified to identify optimal care within different community settings. Individuals with diabetes and their health care providers must be aware that thorough and competent eye examinations and followup are crucial. Primary care physicians should arrange for referrals for examination on a routine basis. In populations where adequate eye care for examination and treatment is not available, improvements in the availability of such care must be made. . . .

Prevention of Foot Complications and Lower Extremity Amputations

The risk for lower extremity amputation (LEA) is 15 times greater in individuals with diabetes than in individuals without it. Estimates suggest that persons with diabetes undergo over one-half of the approximately

125,000 LEA's performed annually in the United States. The causes of LEA are complex, encompassing combinations of vascular and neurologic pathology with metabolic factors, lower extremity ulcers, infections, and trauma.

Despite a number of patient care programs that suggest reductions in amputations would be possible with intensive prevention-oriented foot care, available preventive and therapeutic strategies are not used fully in public or private health care delivery settings. Although there has been improvement in reducing perioperative mortality associated with LEA's, much less progress has been made in preventing amputations, improving postoperative LEA survival, and enhancing patient function and quality of life. Moreover, the extent of the problem may be understated because of the absence of a surveillance system to monitor care practices and all hospital discharge data. . . .

Cardiovascular Disease Control and Hypertension

The most common cause of death among persons who have diabetes in the United States is coronary heart disease. Not only is heart disease more common in people with IDDM or NIDDM than in other members of the population, it also occurs at a younger age, is more often fatal, and is as common in women with diabetes as it is in men. The risk factors for coronary heart disease (e.g., high blood pressure, platelet and lipid abnormalities) are more commonly observed in persons with diabetes than in the general population. It has been estimated that treating and eliminating these risk factors could reduce the risk of heart attacks in individuals with diabetes by 60 percent.

The combination of diabetes and hypertension may hasten the progression of nephropathy, retinopathy, and vascular disease, resulting in such complications as coronary artery disease (which could lead to heart attacks and heart failure), peripheral vascular disease (which could lead to amputations), and cerebrovascular disease (which could lead to strokes).

While the NDAB supports the DHHS's objectives for the Nation for reduction of cardiovascular and cerebrovascular diseases for all individuals, specific emphasis on smoking cessation and control of hypertension, obesity, and blood cholesterol levels in individuals with diabetes is needed. . . .

Kidney Disease

Kidney disease is a frequent and serious complication of diabetes. Approximately 30 percent of all new patients in the United States being treated for end-stage renal disease (ESRD) have diabetes. This percentage is increasing at a rate of approximately 2 percent annually; therefore, within the next decade, diabetes-related kidney disease will account for more than one-half of all enrollees in the End-Stage Renal Disease Program. Although the importance of control of elevated blood pressure to slow the rate of progression of renal disease is recognized, the roles of other factors such as tight blood glucose control, special protein-restricted diets, and certain antihypertensive drugs require additional research.

Patients with diabetes fare poorly once ESRD begins. The mortality of diabetes patients with ESRD on dialysis is two to five times higher than the mortality of dialysis patients without diabetes. Although dialysis and renal aspects are carefully monitored in patients with ESRD, preventing or delaying other complications is often underemphasized. Because ESRD patients are at high risk for morbidity and mortality, a special comprehensive approach is needed for their care. . . .

Periodontal Disease

Individuals with diabetes are at increased risk for periodontal disease. Periodontal infections advance rapidly and lead not only to loss of teeth but also to compromised metabolic control. A study of Pima Indians has documented a twofold to tenfold increase in the prevalence of tooth loss in people with diabetes, depending on the age group, compared with those people of comparable age without diabetes.

Periodontal infection responds to appropriate dental treatment. Early detection and prompt treatment can prevent infection and tooth loss. Primary care providers, dental professionals, and patients are not uniformly aware of this association. Efforts to disseminate information about periodontal disease and diabetes to primary care practitioners are under way. . . .

Neuropathy

Diabetic neuropathy is one of the most frequent long-term complications of diabetes, and until recently, it was also one of the most poorly understood. New knowledge about the metabolism of peripheral nerves has contributed to a better understanding of the abnormalities found in diabetic neuropathy, including a link between hyperglycemia and abnormal nerve conduction. Proper diagnosis and treatment of cardiovascular and gastrointestinal problems and impotence related to neuropathy is important for both the patient and the health care provider. However, short of primary prevention of neuropathy via tight metabolic control or an as yet unknown method, immediate intervention is possible only in the area of the treatment and prevention of the devastating consequences of neurotrophic ulcer disease of the lower extremities. The role of peripheral neuropathy in amputations is recognized and also is addressed in the goal for the reduction of lower extremity amputations. . . .

Diabetic Ketoacidosis, Hyperosmolar Coma, and Hypoglycemia

Diabetic ketoacidosis (DKA) and hyperosmolar coma place the person with diabetes at high risk for morbidity and mortality. The pathogenic mechanisms and prevalence of cerebral edema—a malignant complication of DKA—are poorly understood. DKA is preventable assuming early diagnosis of diabetes, better understanding of self-care during acute illness or stress, identification of effective ways to ensure continuity of adherence to a rational therapeutic program, and meaningful psychological support and attention to the psychosocial problems in patients, particularly those with repetitive DKA. Many pathophysiologic mechanisms have been clarified over the past 10 years, yet the basic causes and ideal management of nonketotic hyperosmolar coma remain to be elucidated. Further, no progress has been made to help those patients who, for whatever reason, manifest either repetitive DKA or hyperosmolar coma. . . .

Psychosocial Issues

Serious and lifelong complications of diabetes include the emotional and social stresses that accompany the physical problems of the disease. Patients must become their own physicians on a daily basis as they attempt to act for the pancreas. Self-care tasks divert time and money as well as energy from normal activities. They further impose limitations on families and peers in work and recreation. Both health providers and patients experience frustration when diabetes and life events come into conflict.

Although it is not possible to measure psychological stress in the same way, for example, that glycosylated hemoglobin is measured, stress itself interferes with the already disturbed humoral regulatory processes. Identifying and accepting psychosocial issues are crucial to self-management of this disease because behavior can be a major factor in developing diabetes complications. . . .

Multidisciplinary Interventions

Given the multiple dimensions of diabetes and the variety of possible complications along the pathologic and psychologic continuum, five major areas have an impact on the care of individuals with diabetes: patient education, professional education, the ability of third-party payers to cover the costs of patient education and prescribed diabetes therapies, access to diabetes care, and special diabetes problems of minority populations. Each of these five specialty areas is important in the prevention and control of diabetes. The strategies presented will be adaptable to all complications and should be considered as methods to achieve complication-specific goals.

Patient Education

Patient education is considered to be an integral part of patient care. Education for diabetes self-management, in conjunction with a treatment plan, has been associated with reductions in hospitalizations and with the prevention or alleviation of some of the complications of diabetes. However, there are several barriers to providing adequate patient education to persons with diabetes. These barriers include the following: Significant information on the advances in clinical care has not reached health professionals who teach patients with diabetes; the time of health professionals who care for these patients is limited, and education often is not considered a priority; inpatient education is restricted because of reduced hospital stays, and often, the stress of hospitalization makes it a poor time for learning; most people with diabetes are not hospitalized at the time they need education, yet ambulatory patient education is generally not covered by third-party payers; access to existing outpatient education programs is limited, particularly in rural or geographically inaccessible areas; materials and educational approaches are lacking for people with cultural differences, learning disabilities, and low literacy levels; there is a lack of interaction among the many components of the health care system used by the person with diabetes, and as a result, there is little continuity and documentation of patient education; and, finally, there is little support for research into educational strategies that promote motivation and behavioral change. Efforts to eliminate these barriers are now being implemented by several organizations. . . .

Professional Education

Despite the technical and clinical advances in diabetes patient care over the past 10 years, a number of professionals have not changed their care practices to reflect these advances. Many physicians receive little training on the management of the uncomplicated patient with diabetes and the early management of complications. Professional education is conducted by a variety of agencies and organizations and differs depending on the providing agency, the professional subspecialty, and discipline. Therefore, many professionals remain unaware of beneficial and cost-effective patient care methods to prevent or delay complications of diabetes and to ameliorate their effects. . . .

Health Care Financing

Persons with diabetes have direct medical costs that are three times greater than the costs for persons without diabetes. Unless covered by a group health insurance plan, individuals with diabetes can have problems obtaining and affording health insurance. In 1985, Federal, state, and local funds underwrote more than 40 percent of medical costs, private insurance paid slightly more than 30 percent, and individuals themselves paid slightly less than 30 percent. Because people with diabetes have greater difficulty obtaining third-party coverage, significant cost burdens may be associated with the health care of individuals with diabetes.

Progress is being made in health care financing in three areas: (1) pooled risk health insurance plans for state residents unable to get health insurance because of poor health, (2) third-party coverage for diabetes outpatient education programs, and (3) third-party coverage of selected technologies, services, and medical devices.

In a growing number of states, Blue Cross/Blue Shield, Medicare, Medicaid, or insurance coverage is available for diabetes outpatient education programs. The criteria for reimbursement generally specify that patients must be referred by a physician, the program must meet national standards, the program must be offered by a certified provider, and the education program must be tailored to meet individual needs. Coverage of self blood glucose meters and supplies varies from state to state and among major payers. . . .

Access to Diabetes Health Care

In spite of the many research and translation advances, many patients diagnosed with diabetes may receive little or no diabetes health care because of lack of access to quality health care and the inability to utilize the health care system. This lack of health care is not unique to those with diabetes. It may result from large geographic distances between patients and providers, absence (or limited numbers) of skilled providers, the individual's inability to make choices within the health care system, or the cost of receiving preventive and other health care. . . .

Special Problems of Diabetes in Minority Populations

The prevalence of diabetes among black, Native American, Hispanic, and Asian and Pacific Island populations greatly exceeds that in the white population. Mortality data for blacks and American Indians suggest that their age-adjusted diabetes-related mortality rates are twice those experienced in white populations. Although there may be some risk factors in the development of diabetes (NIDDM) that are more prevalent in these populations (e.g., obesity), the disparity in morbidity and mortality from diabetes between minority and nonminority populations is unacceptable. . . .

Guidelines for Patient Care

Technology used to treat individuals with diabetes has expanded greatly over the past 10 years as a result of research advances. The goal of developing and implementing guidelines for the care of persons with diabetes is to establish criteria for diabetes health care. This will ensure state-of-the-art, individualized patient care aimed at maintaining health in the diabetes patient without complications and at preventing, delaying, or ameliorating complications of diabetes in others. Straightforward brief treatment guidelines based on medical consensus will motivate many health care providers to intervene effectively and more often.

In 1982, the NDAB, working with representatives of the NIH and CDC and with health care providers, developed initial guidelines, entitled *The Prevention and Treatment of Five Complications of Diabetes: A Guide for Primary Care Practitioners*. This document, based on consensus in the medical community, provided an impetus for many health care providers to incorporate this information into their everyday practice. As hoped, it also led to several complementary efforts to develop brief guides for other diabetes issues. [A copy of the revised document, *The Prevention and Treatment of Complications of Diabetes*, is reproduced in Chapter 35.]

PART TWO

DIABETES MANAGEMENT

Chapter 12

Who's the Doctor Around Here?

Most doctors go to Medical School because they want to help make people who are ill get well. Treating diabetes turns this arrangement on its head. There is no cure for diabetes. Also, more than ninety-five percent of the daily treatment of diabetes is provided by the patient. When you have diabetes, you may be asked to do blood tests, take pills or inject insulin, examine your feet, treat low blood sugar reactions, follow sick day guidelines, and do other diabetes care practices. The kind of diabetes care that you have to provide for yourself is what doctors went to medical school to learn to provide for their patients. This situation sometimes makes patients and their doctors uncomfortable.

In order for diabetes care to be successful, both you and the doctor must recognize that this disease demands new roles for both of you. Because diabetes is cared for largely by the patient, your role is more like the role of the doctor. The doctor's role is more like that of a consulting specialist. Patients who are unwilling to accept responsibility for treating their own diabetes or doctors who are unwilling to allow their patients to accept this responsibility will find diabetes care frustrating. Doctors may be frustrated that they cannot cure diabetes or even provide the majority of the daily diabetes treatment. Diabetes can be equally frustrating for patients because you may not want the responsibility for treating diabetes. As you carry out the many steps involved in diabetes care you may think, "If I wanted to be a doctor I would have gone to medical school. I never bargained for this." You're right, no one bargains to get diabetes.

Developed by the Michigan Diabetes Research and Training Center.
Used by permission.

It may be very useful to discuss with your doctor the fact that your roles are very different than the traditional doctor/patient roles. If you feel anxious or even resentful of the fact that the responsibility of daily diabetes care falls on your shoulders, you should share these feelings with your doctor. Diabetes care can be a satisfying experience for you and your doctor. However, it requires both of you to change your ideas about the usual doctor and patient relationship. In this new relationship, patients should be thought of as their own doctors. Your doctor can be viewed as your "diabetes coach" who helps you carry out your daily self-care plan.

Diabetes care can be a rewarding experience for both the patient and the doctor when they both accept the fact that the patient is responsible for the daily treatment. More than most other diseases, diabetes care requires good communication and a great deal of trust between you and your doctor. Ask your doctor to refer you to a diabetes education program to help prepare you to be your own "diabetes doctor."

ASK YOUR DOCTOR THE FOLLOWING QUESTION:

1. ***Is there a diabetes education program that I could attend to help me take care of my diabetes?***

Chapter 13

What You Don't Know About Diabetes Can Hurt You

If you have diabetes you have to treat it every day. Your doctor and other health care professionals will help you develop a daily treatment plan but you must carry it out. That means you need to learn about diabetes because with diabetes, what you don't know can hurt you. Here are just three of the many reasons why you should learn as much as you can about caring for your diabetes.

First, safety. Many people with diabetes (especially people taking insulin) must make daily and sometimes emergency self-care decisions. For example, if you take insulin you must know how to give it safely. You should learn how to identify, treat, and prevent both low blood sugar and high blood sugar. You also need to know about monitoring your blood sugar and what to do when you have a cold or the flu and much more. Whether you take insulin or not, you need to learn about diet, exercise, foot care, and sometimes diabetes pills. The problems caused by poor diabetes self-care may take a long time to appear, but when they do they can be tragic.

Second, motivation. Sometimes people avoid learning about diabetes because not knowing makes it easier to believe that their diabetes is not serious. Diabetes should always be thought of as a serious matter. Learning about diabetes not only gives you knowledge and skills but can help you to feel more like caring for your diabetes as well. Learning how serious diabetes can be, and all the things you and your health care team can do to keep you well, may help you prevent major problems with your diabetes later on.

Developed by the Michigan Diabetes Research and Training Center.
Used by permission.

Third, team care. Taking care of your diabetes is a team effort. In addition to yourself, your health care team may include your family, doctors, nurses, dietitians, pharmacists, psychologists, ophthalmologists, social workers, foot and exercise specialists, and others. All of the professionals on your health care team have the knowledge and skills needed to help treat diabetes. However, you are the key member of the team; it's your diabetes. In order for you to be a good team member you need to learn about diabetes care as well.

How can you tell if you know enough about your diabetes? Ask your doctor or diabetes educator to review your diabetes knowledge and skills with you. They can help you correct any weak areas. Remember, learning about diabetes can help you to control your diabetes rather than being controlled by it.

ASK YOUR DOCTOR, NURSE, OR DIETITIAN THE FOLLOWING QUESTIONS:

1. ***Is there a diabetes patient education program in this area that I can attend?***
2. ***Would you please check my diabetes knowledge to make sure I know how to take care of my diabetes correctly?***

Chapter 14

Putting Together an all Star Diabetes Care Team

You may have heard that caring for diabetes takes a team effort. Why this is true and who should be on your diabetes care team may not be clear to you. Caring for diabetes takes a team made up of different experts. Your doctor is an expert on the medical treatment of diabetes but you also need help with your meal plan from a dietitian, and education about diabetes self-care from a nurse. In addition, your eyes should be examined by an eye doctor every year. Depending on your needs you may want to see a podiatrist for help with your feet and a psychologist or social worker when your diabetes care causes you emotional or financial problems. Your pharmacist and dentist are important members of your health care team and you may want to see an expert on exercise.

These experts can help you develop the best diabetes care plan possible. However, the most important expert on your diabetes care team is ***you***. This is because diabetes care affects almost every part of your life and ***you*** are the expert about your own life. For example, you know the most about your family, your work, and your social life. But most importantly, ***you*** are the one that has to carry out most of your daily diabetes care and ***you*** are the one who will see the results of that diabetes care. The members of your health care team should listen to you. If they do not listen to you and fit your ideas into your diabetes self-care plan, the plan may not work. When you are looking for health care professionals to be part of your diabetes care team, find people who are willing to begin with your point of view.

Developed by the Michigan Diabetes Research and Training Center.
Used by permission.

When putting together your team, look for health care professionals who are experts and are interested in diabetes care. Many type of doctors can treat diabetes. For example, internists, family practice physicians, general practitioners, and endocrinologists can all care for patients with diabetes. When choosing a doctor it is useful to talk with that doctor about how much interest and experience he or she has in caring for diabetes. Some doctors are very interested in diabetes care, others less so. Nurses, dietitians, and other health care professionals who specialize in diabetes education will often have the letters C.D.E. after their names. C.D.E. stands for Certified Diabetes Educator. It means that these diabetes educators have passed a national exam showing that they are experts in diabetes. Psychologists should have a Ph.D. and a social worker should have a Masters Degree (M.S. or M.S.W.). A podiatrist should have a Doctor of Podiatric Medicine (D.P.M.) and have completed a residency in podiatry.

You can ask your local chapter of the American Diabetes Association, local hospital, health department, or other people in your area with diabetes about who are the diabetes experts in your area. It is in your best interest to spend the time and effort you need to put together an all star team for your diabetes care.

ASK YOUR PHYSICIAN, NURSE, DIETITIAN, OR OTHER DIABETES TEAM MEMBER THE FOLLOWING QUESTIONS:

1. ***Would you be willing to tell me about your expertise and interest in treating diabetes?***
2. ***Do you belong to a professional diabetes organization such as the American Diabetes Association or the American Association of Diabetes Educators?***
3. ***Do you have any special degrees, residencies, or certifications related to diabetes care?***
4. ***What do you think the patient's role on the diabetes care team should be?***

Chapter 15

Take Charge of Your Diabetes

Preface

Take Charge of Your Diabetes: A Guide for Patients was written to help you take care of your health—today, tomorrow, and in the coming years. You'll learn about certain problems that sometimes occur with diabetes. Then you'll learn how you and your health care providers can work as a team to prevent or treat these problems.

Ask your health care providers to look at this guide with you. Let them know that this goes along with a guide recently published for them, *The Prevention and Treatment of Complications of Diabetes: A Guide for Practitioners.*

At the [end of the text] you'll find record sheets to help you keep track of important facts about your health. Have your health care providers regularly review these records. Working together, you can take charge of your diabetes!

William H. Herman, M.D.
University of Michigan Medical Center
Ann Arbor, Michigan

Thanks

This guide was prepared by the Department of Health and Human Services, Public Health Service, Centers for Disease Control, National Cen-

U.S. Department of Health & Human Services, CDC, 1991.

ter for Chronic Disease Prevention and Health Promotion, Division of Diabetes Translation.

William H. Herman, M.D., was the general editor. Alacia Lyons was the Project Coordinator. Dawn Satterfield and Rick Hull helped prepare the final version of this guide.

The American Association of Diabetes Educators lent expert guidance and support in the development and evaluation of this guide.

Introduction

Diabetes touches almost every part of your life. It's a serious disease, but you can work to control it. You can take charge of your own good health—not only for today, but for the coming years.

Today and every day, you need to balance your food, activity, and medicine. Testing your own blood sugars (glucoses) helps you see how this balance is working out. You can then make choices that help you feel well day-to-day.

You can also work to guard against some of the problems that diabetes can cause. As time goes on, diabetes can hurt your eyes, your kidneys, and your nerves. It can lead to problems with the blood flow in your body. Even your teeth and gums can be affected. And diabetes in pregnancy can cause special problems.

Many of these problems don't have to happen. You can do a lot to prevent them.

You'll read in this guide about day-to-day and long-term problems of diabetes. Learning about these can help you cope with your fears. You can then work to keep these problems from happening. And if they do happen, you can learn to deal with them in a positive way. For example, you can learn how to use your blood sugar readings to prevent or treat blood sugars that are too low or too high. You can learn the warning signs of other problems. And you can remind your health care team when it's time to do certain tasks.

Write down the names and telephone numbers of your health care providers—your primary doctor, eye doctor, foot doctor, dentist, dietitian, diabetes educator, counselor, and others. Also write down any questions you'd like to ask and any important points you want to remember from your talks with these experts.

In this guide, you'll learn how to be an active member of your health care team. You'll read how important it is to keep a record of certain facts about your health. [Following the text of this document], you'll find forms for writing down these facts. [You may photocopy these forms, re-create similar forms, or obtain a personal copy of this document by contacting the ***Division of Diabetes Translation, Centers for Disease Control and Prevention***

(CDC). The address is located in the *Directory of Diabetes Organizations* in the Appendix of this volume.] These records will help you and the rest of your health care team keep track of your health.

Take your time reading this guide. There's a lot of material, but you don't have to read it all at once. You may want to look first at the parts that deal with your own special concerns.

Feelings About Having Diabetes

Living with diabetes isn't easy. It's normal to have bad feelings about it. Tell your health care provider how you feel. Point out any problems you have with your diabetes care plan. Your diabetes educator or other health care provider may be able to help you think of ways to deal with these problems.

Talk about the stresses you feel at home, school, and work. How do you cope with these pressures? If your feelings are getting in the way of taking care of yourself, you need to ask for help.

On [Form 15–1], you'll find a form to write down the date you discuss these feelings with your health care provider. This date is one of the important health facts you'll be keeping track of in your guide.

It helps to talk with other people who have problems like your own. Ask your health care provider about support groups for people with diabetes and their families and friends. Many people like to attend these meetings regularly.

One-on-one and family counseling sessions may also help. Be sure to see a counselor who knows about diabetes and its treatment. You can ask your health care provider to help you find a counselor.

Knowing Your Blood Sugars

Testing your own blood sugars (self-monitoring blood glucose) tells you how they are doing minute-to-minute and day-to-day. Keep records of your blood sugars in a logbook or on a record sheet. If you don't have one of these, ask your health care provider how to get one.

Blood sugar testing can help you understand how food and activity affect your blood sugars. Testing can help you make day-to-day choices about food, activity, and diabetes medicine. Testing can also tell you when your blood sugar is too low or too high so that you can treat these problems.

A glycohemoglobin test or hemoglobin Al test is a blood test that helps sum up your diabetes control for the past month or two. This test measures how much sugar has been sticking to your red blood cells.

If most of your recent blood sugars have been normal (70 to 120 mg/dL), the glycohemoglobin test will be normal or near normal (usually about 6%

to 8%). If you've had many blood sugars above normal, the extra sugar sticking to your red blood cells will make your glycohemoglobin test read higher. You should have a glycohemoglobin blood test 4 times a year. Ask your health care provider for the results and record them on [Form 15–2]. This test will help you and your diabetes care team keep track of your average blood sugar control.

Ask your health care provider what the normal range of values is in the laboratory that does your test. Set a target goal with your diabetes care team. If your test is high, you'll know you need to work closer with your diabetes care team. You and your team can then adjust your balance of food, activity, and diabetes medicine. When your glycohemoglobin test result is near your target goal, you'll know you've balanced things well.

Problems With High Blood Sugars

Eating too much food, being less active than usual, or taking too little diabetes medicine are some common reasons for high blood sugars. Your blood sugars can also go up when you're sick or under stress.

Some common signs of high blood sugars are feeling tired, having blurred vision, and losing weight without trying. Other signs include having a dry mouth, being thirsty, and urinating (passing water) a lot. If your blood sugars are very high, you may have stomach pain, feel sick to your stomach, or even throw up.

If you have any signs that your blood sugar is high, test your blood. In your logbook or on your record sheet, write down your blood sugar and the time you did the test. If your blood sugar is high, think about what could have caused it to go up. If you think you know of something, write this down beside your blood sugar reading.

Show your blood sugar records to your health care provider. Ask how you can change your food, activity, and medicine to avoid or treat high blood sugars. Ask when you should call for help. On [Form 15–3], record the date you discuss these points. Your blood sugars are more likely to go up when you're sick—for example, when you have the flu or an infection. You'll need to take special care of yourself during these times. The guide that follows can help you do this.

How to Take Care of Yourself When You're Sick

Medicine

Be sure to keep taking your diabetes pills or insulin. Don't stop taking them even if you can't eat. Your health care provider may even advise you to take more insulin or pills during sickness.

Table 15.1

What to Eat or Drink When You're Sick
(each item equals one bread or fruit exchange)

Food Item	Amount
Fruit juice	1/3 to 1/2 cup
Fruit-flavored drink	1/2 cup
Soda pop (not diet)	1/2 cup
* Jell-O™ (not sugar-free)	1/2 cup
* Popsicle™ (not sugar-free)	1/2 twin
Sherbert	1/4 cup
Hot cereal	1/2 cup (cooked)
Milk	1 cup
Thin soup (examples: vegetable, chicken noodle)	1 cup
Thick soup (examples: cream of mushroom, tomato)	1/2 cup
Ice cream (vanilla)	1/2 cup
Pudding (sugar-free)	1/2 cup
Pudding (regular)	1/4 cup
Macaroni, noodles, rice, mashed potatoes	1/2 cup (cooked)

*Use of trade names is for identification only and does not imply endorsement by the U.S. Department of Health and Human Services.

Food

Try to eat the same amount of fruits and breads as usual. If you can, eat your regular diet. If you're having trouble doing this, eat enough soft foods or drink enough liquids to take the place of the fruits and breads you usually eat. Use the list in [Table 15–1] to make these exchanges.

Liquids

Drink extra liquids. Try to drink at least 1/2 to 3/4 cup every half-hour to hour, even if you have to do this in small sips. These liquids should *not* have calories. Water, diet soda pop, or tea without sugar are good choices.

Testing

Test your blood sugar at least every 4 hours. If your blood sugar is 240 mg/dL or higher, test your urine for ketones.

Weigh yourself every day.

Check your temperature every morning and evening.

Every 4 to 6 hours, check how you're breathing and decide how alert you feel. Having trouble breathing, feeling more sleepy than usual, or not thinking clearly can be danger signs.

Record Keeping

Use the *Records for Sick Days* on [Form 15–4]. Ask a family member or friend to help if you need it.

Calling

Ask your health care provider when you should call. During your sick times, you may need to call every day for advice.

You should call your health care provider or go to an emergency room if any of the following happens:

- You feel too sick to eat normally and can't keep food or liquids down for more than 6 hours.
- You have severe diarrhea.
- You lose 5 pounds or more.
- Your temperature is over 101°F.
- Your blood sugar level is lower than 60 mg/dL or remains over 300 mg/dL.

- You have moderate or large ketones in your urine.
- You're having trouble breathing.
- You feel sleepy or can't think clearly.

Problems With Low Blood Sugars

In general, blood sugars lower than 70 mg/dL are too low. If you take a diabetes pill or insulin, you can have a low blood sugar. Low blood sugars are usually caused by eating less or later than usual, being more active than usual, or taking too much diabetes medicine. Drinking beer, wine, or liquor may also cause low blood sugars or make them worse.

Low blood sugars happen more often to persons who are trying to keep their blood sugars near normal. This is no reason to stop trying to control your diabetes. It just means you have to watch carefully for low blood sugars.

Some possible signs of a low blood sugar are feeling nervous, shaky, or sweaty. Sometimes people just feel tired.

The signs are usually mild at first. But a low blood sugar can quickly drop much lower if you don't treat it. When your blood sugar is very low, you may get confused, pass out, or have seizures.

If you're having any signs that your blood sugar is low, test it right away. If your sugar is low, recheck it and treat it. In your blood sugar logbook or record sheet, write down the numbers and the times when the low sugars happen. Think about what may be causing them. If you think you know the reason, write it beside the low sugars.

Show your logbook or record sheet to your health care provider. Be sure to tell your provider if you're having one or more low blood sugars a week. On [Form 15–3], record the date you talk about this.

If you get confused, pass out, or have a seizure, you need emergency help. Remember, it may not be safe to drive when you're having a lot of low blood sugars.

After you've been treated, call your health care provider as soon as you can. Talk about changing your diet, activity, or diabetes medicine.

You and your family, your friends, and the people you work with need to know how to treat low blood sugars. Study the guidelines that begin [in the next section]. Talk to your health care provider about these guidelines.

How to Prevent and Treat Low Blood Sugars

Be Prepared

Always wear something (like an identification bracelet) that says you have diabetes. Carry a card in your wallet that says you have diabetes and tells if you use medicine to treat it.

Table 15.2

Foods and Liquids for Low Blood Sugars
(each item equals about 10 to 15 grams of sugar)

Food Item	Amount
Glucose tablets	2 to 3
Glucose gel	1 tube
Sugar packets	2 to 3
Fruit juice	1/2 cup (4 oz.)
Soda pop (not diet)	1/2 cup (4 oz.)
Hard candy	3 to 5 pieces
Sugar or honey	3 teaspoons

Always carry some type of sugar with you so you'll be ready to treat a low blood sugar anywhere.

Don't Wait

When you feel your blood sugar is low or when it tests less than 60 to 70 mg/dL, you should eat 10 to 15 grams of sugar *right away.* See the list [in Table 15–2] for examples of foods and liquids with this amount of sugar.

Keep Checking

Check your blood sugar again in 15 minutes. Eat another 10 to 15 grams of sugar every 15 minutes until your blood sugar is above 70 mg/dL or your signs have gone away.

Sugar (10 to 15 grams) will keep your blood sugar up for only about 30 minutes. So if your next planned meal or snack is more than 30 minutes away, you should also eat a small snack.

Play It Safe

If you feel a low blood sugar coming on but can't test right then, play it safe—go ahead and treat it. Waiting is *not* safe.

If you ignore a low blood sugar or don't know that your sugar is low, it can get worse quickly. You may be in danger of passing out.

Let Others Know

Tell family members, close friends, teachers, and people at work that you have diabetes. Tell them how to know when you have a low blood sugar. Show them what to do if you can't treat yourself. Someone will need to give you fruit juice, soda pop (not diet), or sugar.

If you can't swallow, someone will need to give you a shot of glucagon and call for help. Glucagon is a prescription medicine that raises the sugar and is injected like insulin. If you take insulin, you should have a glucagon kit handy. Teach family members, roommates, and friends when and how to use it.

Pregnancy

Women with diabetes can have healthy babies, but it takes planning and hard work.

Pregnancy can make high and low blood sugars happen more often. It can worsen diabetic eye disease and diabetic kidney disease. High blood sugars during pregnancy are dangerous for the baby, too.

Keeping blood sugars near normal before and during pregnancy can help protect the baby and the mother. That's why it's so important that women with diabetes plan their pregnancies ahead of time.

If you want to have a baby, tell your health care provider. Work with your diabetes care team to get your blood sugars in the normal or near-normal range before you become pregnant. Your blood sugar records and your glycohemoglobin test results will show when this has happened.

You may need to change your meal plan and your usual activity, and you may need to take more frequent insulin shots. Testing your blood sugars several times a day will help you see how well you're balancing things. Get a complete check of your eyes and kidneys before you try to become pregnant.

Don't smoke, drink alcohol, or use drugs—doing these things can harm you and your baby.

If you don't want to become pregnant, talk with your health care provider about birth control. On [Form 15–1], keep track of this important part of your care.

Dental Disease

Because of high blood sugars, people with diabetes are more likely to have problems with their teeth and gums. One of these problems, called gingivitis, can cause sore, swollen, and red gums that bleed when you brush your teeth. Another problem, called periodontitis, happens when your gums shrink or pull away from your teeth. Dental infections, like all infections, can make your blood sugar go up.

If you don't have a dentist, find one or ask your health care provider for the name of a dentist in your area. You should have your teeth cleaned and checked at your dentist's office at least every 6 months.

Daily teeth and gum care at home is important to prevent infections. The guide that begins [in the next section] offers some tips on good dental care.

How to Take Care of Your Teeth

Brushing

Brush your teeth at least twice a day to prevent gum disease and tooth loss. Be sure to brush before you go to sleep. Use a soft toothbrush and toothpaste with fluoride. To help keep bacteria from growing on your toothbrush, rinse it after each brushing and store it with the bristles at the top. Get a new toothbrush at least every 3 months.

Flossing

Besides brushing, you need to clean between your teeth to help remove plaque, a film that forms on teeth and can cause tooth problems. Your dentist or dental hygienist will help you choose a good method to remove plaque, such as dental floss, bridge cleaners, or water spray. If you're not sure of the right way to brush or floss, ask your dentist or dental hygienist for help.

Professional Dental Care

See your dentist at least twice a year. Make an appointment right away if you have any of the following signs of dental disease: bad breath, a bad taste in your mouth, bleeding or sore gums, red or swollen gums, sore or loose teeth, or difficulty chewing.

Give your dentist the name and telephone number of your diabetes health care provider. Each time you make an appointment, remind your dentist that you have diabetes.

Plan dental appointments so they don't change your insulin and meal schedule. Just after breakfast may be a good time for your appointment. Don't skip a meal or diabetes medicine before your appointment.

Eye Problems

Diabetic eye disease is a serious problem that can lead to loss of sight. It may be developing even when your sight is good. If you're having trouble reading, if your vision is blurred, or if you're seeing rings around lights, dark spots, or flashing lights, you may have eye problems.

Finding and treating eye problems early can help save sight. Laser surgery may help people who have advanced diabetic eye disease. An operation called vitrectomy may help others who have lost their sight from bleeding in the back of eye.

Regular, complete eye exams, even when you're seeing fine, are important to protect your sight. Before the exam, a doctor or nurse will put drops in your eyes to dilute the pupils. If you haven't already had this exam, you should have one *now* if any of the following apply to you:

- You've had insulin-dependent diabetes (type I diabetes) for 5 or more years.
- You have non-insulin-dependent diabetes (type II diabetes).
- You're going through puberty.
- You're pregnant.
- You're planning to become pregnant.

After your first exam, you should have your eyes dilated and examined once a year. Keep track of these exams on [Form 15–5].

If you have any sight problems, tell your health care provider. If you have diabetic eye disease, see an eye doctor who is an expert in diabetic eye care. Even if you've lost your sight from diabetic eye disease, you should still have regular eye care.

If your sight is poor, an eye doctor who is an expert in low vision may be able to give you glasses or other devices that can help you use your limited vision more fully. You may want to ask your health care provider about support groups and job training for people with low vision.

If you don't have an eye doctor, ask your health care provider for the name of one. If you can't afford an eye exam, ask about a payment plan or a free exam. If you're 65 or older, Medicare may pay for diabetic eye exams (but not glasses). You can ask your eye doctor to accept the Medicare fee as full payment.

Kidney Problems

The kidneys keep the right amount of water in the body and help filter out harmful wastes. These wastes then pass from the body in the urine.

Diabetes can cause kidney disease, which can lead to kidney failure. High blood pressure makes diabetic kidney disease worse. Eating too much meat, cheese, and milk and having high blood sugar may also worsen diabetic kidney disease.

Albumin or protein in the urine is an early sign of diabetic kidney disease. You should have your urine checked for albumin or protein every year.

You should also have a yearly blood test to measure your kidney function. If the tests show albumin or protein in the urine or if your kidney function isn't normal, you'll need to be checked more often.

On [Form 15–5], write down the dates and the results of these tests. Ask your health care provider to explain what the results mean. If you have diabetic kidney disease, you must have your blood pressure checked at least 4 times a year. High blood pressure (higher than 140/90) should be treated with diet and, if needed, pills.

You may want to check your blood pressure at home to be sure it stays lower than 140/90. You may also want to talk to your health care provider about cutting back on the meats in your meal plan.

Bladder and kidney infections can worsen diabetic kidney disease. If you see cloudy or bloody urine, feel pain or burning when you urinate, go to the bathroom a lot, or have to go in a hurry, call your health care provider right away. You may have a bladder infection. Back pain, chills, and fever are other danger signs that tell you to call right away. These signs may mean you have a kidney infection.

Your health care provider will test your urine. If you have a bladder or kidney infection, you'll be given an antibiotic. After you take all the medicine, you'll need to have your urine checked again to be sure the infection is gone.

If you have kidney disease, ask your health care provider about the possible bad effects that X-ray dyes and some medicines can have on your kidneys.

Problems With Blood Flow

Heart and blood flow problems are the main causes of sickness and death among people with diabetes. You're more likely to have heart and blood flow problems if you smoke cigarettes, have high blood pressure, or have too much cholesterol or other fats in your blood.

You should have several tests done regularly to check on your risk of having heart and blood problems. These tests can help you and your health care provider know if you need to change your treatment. On [Form 15–5], keep a record of these tests.

At least once a year, your health care provider will ask you about tobacco use. If you smoke, it's very important that you quit. In fact, quitting smoking is one of the best choices you can make for your health. Ask your health care provider about nicotine gum and stop-smoking programs.

Get your blood pressure checked at each visit. Record these numbers on [Form 15–2]. If your blood pressure is higher than 140/90 at two visits, you may want to buy a blood pressure cuff and check your own blood pressure at home.

If you have high blood pressure, you should begin a low-salt diet and drink little or no alcohol. If you're overweight, you should lose weight. Ask your health care provider about an activity program.

If your blood pressure is still high after 3 months, you'll probably need medicine to help control it. If you have side effects from the medicine, ask your health care provider to change it. Many medicines are available to treat high blood pressure.

Have your cholesterol checked once a year. Record the results on [Form 15–5]. Your total cholesterol should be lower than 200 mg/dL.

If your cholesterol is higher than 200 mg/dl on two or more checks, you can do several things to lower it. You can work with your diabetes care team to improve your sugar control, you can lose weight (if you're overweight), and you can cut down on fat and cholesterol in your meal plan. Meet with a dietitian to learn about foods that are low in fat and cholesterol. Ask your health care provider about an activity program.

If your cholesterol is still high after 6 months of treatment, you'll probably need a medicine to help control your cholesterol.

If you feel dizzy, have sudden loss of sight, slur your speech, or feel numb or weak in one arm or leg, you may be having serious problems. Your blood flow may not be getting to your brain as well as it should. Danger signs of blood flow problems to the heart include chest pain or pressure, shortness of breath, swollen ankles, or irregular heartbeats. If you have any of these signs, go to an emergency room or call your health care provider right away.

Blood flow problems to your legs can cause pain or cramping in your buttocks, thighs, or calves that happens during activity and goes away with rest. Report these signs to your health care provider.

Nerve Damage

Diabetic nerve damage is a common problem. Some warnings of nerve damage are pain, burning, tingling, or loss of feeling in the feet and hands. Having nerve damage can lead to other serious problems.

Nerve damage can happen slowly. You may not even be aware you're losing feeling in your feet. So at least once a year, your health care provider should test how well you can sense temperature, pinprick, vibration, and position in your feet. If you have signs of nerve damage, your health care provider may want to do more tests. Testing can help your health care provider know what is wrong and how to treat it.

Ask your health care provider to examine your feet at each visit. Keep track of these exams on [Form 15–2].

If you've lost feeling in your feet, you'll need to take special care of them. Examine your feet every day. Wear shoes that fit well.

You'll read more about foot care [in the following section].

Diabetic nerve damage can affect more than just your feet or hands. It can also cause you to sweat abnormally, make it hard for you to tell when your blood sugar is low, and make you feel light-headed when you stand up.

Nerve damage can also cause stomach and bowel problems, make it hard to urinate, cause dribbling with urination, and lead to bladder and kidney infections. Trouble with sexual function is a common problem for many people with diabetic nerve damage. If you have any of these problems, tell your health care provider. Many of these problems can be treated.

Foot Problems

Nerve damage, blood flow problems, and infections can cause serious foot problems, including amputations.

Nerve damage can cause you to lose feeling in your feet. Sometimes, nerve damage can deform or misshape your feet. Foot deformities can cause abnormal pressure points that can turn into blisters, sores, or ulcers. Poor blood flow can make these injuries slow to heal.

Ask your health care provider to look at your feet at each visit. As a reminder, take off your shoes and socks at every visit. On [Form 15–2], record your foot exams.

Have your sense of feeling and your pulses checked at least once a year. If you have nerve damage, deformed or misshaped feet, or a blood flow problem, your feet need special care. Ask your health care provider to show you how to care for your feet. Also ask if special shoes would help you.

Some guidelines for foot care [are listed below]. Safeguards like these have prevented many amputations.

How to Take Care of Your Feet

Inspecting Your Feet

You may have serious foot problems yet feel no pain. Look at your feet every day to see if you have scratches, cracks, cuts, or blisters. Always check between your toes and on the bottoms of your feet. If you can't bend over to see the bottoms of your feet, use an unbreakable mirror. If you can't see well, ask a family member to help you. Call your health care provider at once if you have a sore on your foot. Sores can worsen quickly.

Bathing

Wash your feet every day. Dry them with care, especially between the toes. Don't soak your feet—it can dry out your skin, and dry skin can lead to infections. If you have dry skin, rub a thin coat of oil, lotion, or cream on the tops and bottoms of your feet—but not between your toes. Moisture between the toes will let germs grow that could cause an infection.

Toenails

Trim your toenails after you've washed and dried your feet—the nails will be softer and safer to trim. Cut your toenails straight across and smooth them with an emery board. Don't cut into the corners.

If you can't see well, or if your nails are thick or yellowed, get them trimmed by a podiatrist (foot doctor) or another health care provider. Ask your health care provider for the name of a foot expert. If you see redness around the nails, see your health care provider at once.

Corns and Calluses

Don't cut corns and calluses. Ask your health care provider how to gently use a pumice stone to rub them. Don't use razor blades, corn plasters, or liquid corn or callus removers—they can damage your skin.

Keeping Your Feet Safe

Hot water or hot surfaces are a danger to your feet. Before bathing, test the water with a bath thermometer (90 to 95°F is safe) or with your elbow.

Wear shoes and socks when you walk on hot surfaces such as beaches or the pavement around swimming pools. In summer, be sure to use a sunscreen on the tops of your feet.

You also need to protect your feet from the cold. In winter, wear socks and footwear such as fleece-lined boots to protect your feet. If your feet are cold at night, wear socks. Don't use hot water bottles or heating pads—they can burn your feet.

Don't use strong antiseptic solutions or adhesive tape on your feet.

Shoes and Socks

Wear shoes and socks at all times. Don't walk barefoot—not even indoors.

Wear shoes that fit well and protect your feet. Don't wear plastic shoes or sandals with thongs between the toes. Ask your health care provider what types of shoes are good choices for you.

New shoes should be comfortable at the time you buy them—don't expect them to stretch out. Slowly break in new shoes by wearing them only one or two hours a day.

Always wear socks or stockings with your shoes. Choose socks made of cotton or wool—they help keep your feet dry.

Before you put on your shoes each time, look and feel inside them. Check for any loose objects, nail points, torn linings, and rough areas—these can cause injuries. If your shoe isn't smooth inside, wear other shoes.

Blood Flow

If you smoke, quit.

If you have high blood pressure or high cholesterol, work with your health care provider to lower it.

Professional Care

See your health care provider regularly. Be sure to get your feet examined each time. Tell your foot doctor that you have diabetes.

Form 15-1

At Least Once a Year

Discuss These Major Points With Your Health Care Provider

(Record the dates in the boxes below.)

Major Points	Dates of Discussions							
Feelings About Diabetes								
High Blood Sugars (knowing and treating)								
Low Blood Sugars (knowing and treating)								
Diabetes and Pregnancy								
Dental Care								
Foot Care								

Form 15-2

Each Visit

Have Your Health Care Provider Do These **Tests**
(Record the dates and results in the boxes below.)

Tests	Dates and Results							
Blood Sugar Test	____mg/dL	____mg/dL	____mg/dL	____mg/dL	____mg/dL	____mg/dL	____mg/dL	____mg/dL
Glycohemoglobin Test	____%	____%	____%	____%	____%	____%	____%	____%
Weight	____lb	____lb	____lb	____lb	____lb	____lb	____lb	____lb
Blood Pressure Test	___/___ mm Hg	___/___ mm Hg	___/___ mm Hg	___/___ mm Hg	___/___ mm Hg	___/___ mm Hg	___/___ mm Hg	___/___ mm Hg
Foot Check								

Form 15-3

At Least Once a Year

Have Your Health Care Provider Do These **Tests**

(Record the dates and results in the boxes below.)

Tests	Dates and Results							
Kidney Tests								
creatinine	_____ mg/dL	_____ mg/dL	_____ mg/dL	_____ mg/dL	_____ mg/dL	_____ mg/dL	_____ mg/dL	_____ mg/dL
protein or albumin	_____ mg	_____ mg	_____ mg	_____ mg	_____ mg	_____ mg	_____ mg	_____ mg
Blood Flow Tests								
cholesterol	_____ mg/dL	_____ mg/dL	_____ mg/dL	_____ mg/dL	_____ mg/dL	_____ mg/dL	_____ mg/dL	_____ mg/dL
EKG								
tobacco use								
Eye Exam								
Foot Exam (blood flow and nerves)								

Form 15-4

Records for Sick Days

How often	Question	Answer	
Every day	How much do you weigh today?	_____pounds	
Every evening	How much did you drink today?	_____glasses	
Every morning and every evening	What is your temperature?	______ A.M. ______ P.M.	
Every 4 hours or before every meal	How much diabetes medicine did you take?	Time	Dose
		_____	_____
		_____	_____
		_____	_____
		_____	_____
		_____	_____
		_____	_____
Every 4 hours or before every meal	What is your blood sugar?	Time	Blood sugar
		_____	__________
		_____	__________
		_____	__________
		_____	__________
		_____	__________
		_____	__________
Every 4 hours or each time you pass urine	What are your urine ketones?	Time	Ketones
		_____	__________
		_____	__________
		_____	__________
		_____	__________
		_____	__________
		_____	__________

Form 15-4 (continued)

Every 4 to 6 hours	How are you breathing?	Time	Condition
		_____	__________
		_____	__________
		_____	__________
		_____	__________
		_____	__________
		_____	__________

Reminders for Sick Days

Call your health care provider if any of the following happens to you:

- You feel too sick to eat normally and are unable to keep down food for more than 6 hours.
- You're having severe diarrhea.
- You lose 5 pounds or more.
- Your temperature is over 101 °F.
- Your blood sugar is lower than 60 mg/dL or remains over 300 mg/dL.
- You have moderate or large ketones in your urine.
- You're having trouble breathing.
- You feel sleepy or can't think clearly.

If you feel sleepy or can't think clearly, have someone call your health care provider or take you to an emergency room.

Form 15-5

Each Visit

Discuss These Major Points With Your Health Care Provider

(Record the dates in the boxes below.)

Major Points	**Dates of Discussions**							
Meal Plan								
Activity								
Self Blood Sugar Testing								
High and Low Blood Sugar Problems								
Medicines								
Birth Control and Family Planning								

Chapter 16

Dental Tips for Diabetics

Controlling your blood glucose is the most important step you can take to prevent tooth and gum problems. People with diabetes, especially those whose blood glucose levels are poorly controlled, are more likely to get gum infections than nondiabetics. A severe gum infection can also make it more difficult to control your diabetes. Once such an infection starts in a person with diabetes, it takes longer to heal. If the infection lasts for a long time, the diabetic person may lose teeth.

Much of what you eat requires good teeth for chewing, so it is extremely important to try to preserve your teeth. Because the bone surrounding the teeth may sometimes be damaged by infection, dentures may not always fit properly and may not be perfect substitutes for your natural teeth.

Taking good care of your gums and teeth is another important measure. Use a soft-bristle brush between the gums and the teeth in a vibrating motion. Place the rubber tip on the toothbrush between the teeth and move it in a circle.

If you notice that your gums bleed while you are eating or brushing your teeth, see a dentist to determine if you have a beginning infection. You should also notify your dentist if you notice other abnormal changes in your mouth, such as patches of whitish-colored skin.

Have a dental checkup every 6 months. Be sure to tell your dentist that you have diabetes and ask him or her to demonstrate procedures that will help you maintain healthy teeth and gums.

Prepared by: Office of Communications, National Institute of Dental Research, National Institutes of Health.

Chapter 17

Testing Your Blood Sugar Can Keep Your Diabetes on Course

In the early days of flying, pilots seldom flew at night because they could not see how high or low they were flying. Today, most planes have modern instruments that allow them to be flown safely after dark. If you have diabetes, you are trying to keep your diabetes on course. Like a pilot, you need accurate information. Luckily, there are modern blood testing instruments to help you as well. When you test the level of sugar (glucose) in your blood you can help keep your diabetes control from flying too high or too low.

Today most doctors urge their patients with diabetes to keep their blood sugars as close to normal as possible. This may prevent the short-term problems of diabetes such as dangerously high levels of blood sugar and the long-term complications of diabetes such as eye disease and kidney failure. To control your blood sugar you need to make many decisions. Some of them are made by you and your health care team together. Some are made by you alone. The information provided when you test your blood sugar allows you and your health care team to make wise choices.

For example, a record of blood sugar levels allows you and your doctor to see how medicines, physical activity, diet, colds and flu, stress and other things affect your blood sugar each day. With the help of your doctor and diabetes educators you can learn to adjust your own insulin, level of physical activity, and diet whenever needed. If you are not already testing your blood sugar, ask your doctor if doing so would help you care for your diabetes.

Developed by the Michigan Diabetes Research and Training Center.
Used by permission.

Testing your blood sugar level has become much simpler and less costly in recent years. There are two major ways to test blood sugar. Both ways involve taking a small drop of blood from your finger and putting it on the end of a plastic strip. The strip changes color depending on how much sugar is present in your blood. With the first method, you compare the color on the strip to a color chart to get a rough estimate of your blood sugar level. With the second method, you insert the strip into a meter which reads the strip. The second method gives you a more exact measure of your blood sugar. Both methods are much more accurate than urine testing. Your doctor or diabetes educator can help you decide which method would be best for you. Members of your health care team are like experts in the control tower who provide you with needed help. But, in terms of daily diabetes care, you are the pilot. Testing your blood sugar yourself can keep you flying safely.

ASK YOUR DOCTOR OR NURSE THE FOLLOWING QUESTIONS:

1. ***What blood testing method would be best for me?***
2. ***How often should I test my blood?***
3. ***How can I use the results of my blood tests to improve my diabetes care?***

Chapter 18

Hemoglobin A1—What's in a Name?

The hemoglobin A1 blood test—quite a name isn't it? But it is a name you should remember. This blood test, also called glycosylated (gly-kos-a-lated) hemoglobin, is an important tool to help you and your health care team control your diabetes. This test shows the ***average*** level of sugar (glucose) in your blood over the last six (6) to eight (8) weeks. This test is done in a laboratory and can be ordered by your doctor. The results give you and your doctor a "picture" of your diabetes control for the last couple of months. This is very useful information to help decide how well your treatment plan is working.

Hemoglobin is part of your red blood cells. The sugar in your blood attaches itself to the hemoglobin in your blood to form hemoglobin Al. The more sugar in your blood, the more hemoglobin Al you will have. Unlike an individual blood sugar test, your hemoglobin Al level reflects all the ups and downs of your blood sugar over the past six (6) to eight (8) weeks. In other words, the hemoglobin A1 is an average blood sugar level for you for the last two (2) months, whereas a single blood sugar (glucose) test only tells the state of your diabetes control at one point in time.

With the information in the hemoglobin Al test, you and your health care team can decide whether to make changes in your medication (insulin or pills), diet, and exercise plan. Then, by having your hemoglobin Al tested three (3) to four (4) months later, you can see if the changes you made have improved your blood sugar control. You can then make more changes in

---

Developed by the Michigan Diabetes Research and Training Center.
Used by permission.

your self-care plan, if needed, and then test your hemoglobin Al again to see how well you are doing.

The process of changing your treatment plan and testing your hemoglobin A1 should continue until your blood sugar levels are close to normal. Even when your diabetes is well controlled, you should continue to have your hemoglobin A1 tested three (3) or four (4) times a year. This is because both you and your diabetes are constantly changing. By testing your hemoglobin A1 regularly, you will be able to change your treatment plan whenever it becomes necessary.

The hemoglobin A1 (glycosylated hemoglobin) test is a very helpful tool in controlling diabetes—it is in your best interest to use it.

ASK YOUR DOCTOR THE FOLLOWING QUESTIONS:

1. ***Would you please test my hemoglobin A1 (glycosylated hemoglobin)?***
2. ***Would you please explain the results of my hemoglobin A1 test?***
3. ***Are there things that I should be doing to improve my hemoglobin Al level (diabetes control)?***

Chapter 19

Insulin—The Shot Heard 'Round the World

If you take insulin for your diabetes, you may think that taking shots is a burden. But if you had insulin-dependent diabetes before 1921, you would have died from it. When insulin was discovered, it saved the lives of tens of thousands of people with diabetes. Some of those people were only days or hours from death. To them, each shot of insulin was a life-saving miracle. Whether you think of insulin shots as a burden or miracle is largely a matter of your point of view.

The food that you eat causes your blood sugar to go up. Insulin helps this sugar move from your blood into your cells where it is needed for energy. After the sugar is in your cells, your blood sugar level goes back down to where it was before you ate. Before you got diabetes, your pancreas (a small organ near your stomach) squirted insulin into your blood stream every time you ate. Now you have to give your body the insulin it needs to fit with the food that you eat.

Some people who have diabetes take just one insulin shot each day. For most people who need insulin, this won't keep the blood sugar level near normal throughout the day. If you are taking one shot of insulin a day and your blood sugar levels are not yet in the normal range, you may need to take more than one shot. Many people take insulin both in the morning and at night. Some also take a shot before lunch. You and your doctor can work out an insulin plan that will work for you.

Also, it is usually wise to take at least two types of insulin. Short-acting

---

Developed by the Michigan Diabetes Research and Training Center.
Used by permission.

(regular) insulin works best in a few hours while intermediate (NPH, Lente) insulins work more slowly to lower your blood sugar. Taking two types of insulin helps your blood sugar levels to be more steady throughout the day. Both types of insulin can be put into the same syringe so that you don't have to take an extra shot.

Finally, it is a good idea to learn how to adjust your insulin dose based on your blood sugar level, diet, and physical activity. This gives you more control over your diabetes and your lifestyle. This is your diabetes—the decision to try for good blood sugar control is yours as well.

ASK YOUR DOCTOR THE FOLLOWING QUESTION:

1. ***Could taking more shots of insulin improve my diabetes control?***

Chapter 20

Can I Reuse My Insulin Syringe?

For years, patients were told to use their insulin syringes only once and then discard them to reduce the risk of getting an infection. However, recent research indicates that the risk of getting an infection from reusing a syringe is really very small. According to a 1989 statement from the American Diabetes Association, "for many patients it appears both safe and practical for the syringe to be reused if the patient so desires."

The advantages to reusing a syringe generally outweigh the disadvantages. The main disadvantage to reusing a syringe is the very slight risk of getting an infection. Even this slight risk can be reduced by following the guidelines for syringe reuse listed below. Another disadvantage is that the needle may become dull after several uses. Also, the lines that show the unit markings may wear off after a while, making it hard to draw up the right dose.

The most obvious advantage in reusing syringes is to save money. If a syringe that costs 20 cents each is used once a day, the total cost for a year is $73. If you take two injections a day and use a new syringe for each injection the cost is $146 a year, and if you take three injections a day and use a new syringe every time the cost is $219 a year. However, if you make each syringe last one week, you pay only about $10 a year. This means that, depending on how many injections of insulin you take, you could save from $63 to $209 a year by making each syringe last one week. Another reason for reusing plastic syringes is the problem of environmental waste. Plastic syringes do not biodegrade, and since no one else should ever use your

---

Developed by the Michigan Diabetes Research and Training Center. Used by permission.

syringe, they can not be recycled either. Every syringe that is thrown away becomes garbage. So every time a syringe is reused there is a little less pollution in the world and a little more money in your pocket.

Guidelines for Reuse of Syringes:

If you decide to reuse your syringes, we suggest that you follow these American Diabetes Association (ADA) guidelines:

- Store the syringe to be reused (dry) at room temperature.
- Recap the needle to store it.
- If the needle touches anything except your skin at the injection site and the top of the insulin bottle, throw it away.
- Do not clean the needle with alcohol. (This wipes off the coating that makes it less painful to stick yourself.)
- Do not reuse a needle that is bent or dull.
- Never use anyone else's syringe and never let anyone else use yours.

How long can you use a syringe?

It is not uncommon for people to use a syringe for up to a month.

How should I dispose of my used syringes?

- Put into a milk carton, 2 liter pop bottle, or coffee can.
- Tape the lid down when the container is full.
- Throw away according to local policy. (Call your local health department if you are not sure about local laws regarding syringe disposal.)

ASK YOUR DOCTOR OR NURSE THE FOLLOWING QUESTION:

1. ***Is there any reason why I should not reuse my insulin syringes?***

Chapter 21

Handle With Care: How to Throw Out Used Insulin Syringes and Lancets at Home

A Note to Adults

This booklet is for young people with insulin-dependent diabetes and for you.

People living in the United States use more than ***one billion*** (1,000,000,000) syringes, needles and lancets ***each year*** to take care of their diabetes. This booklet shows you the safe way to handle *and* throw out used insulin syringes and lancets at home.

It's simple. The easy directions on the following pages show you how to protect your family and waste handlers from injury—and help ***keep the environment clean and safe!***

While you are reading this booklet, keep in mind that your state, county or town may have ***special rules*** about how to dispose of syringes and lancets. Ask your doctor or diabetes educator how to find out about any rules in your area.

Did You Know?

People with insulin-dependent diabetes know how important syringes and lancets are for controlling their diabetes and staying healthy.

EPA Pub. No. 530-SW-90-089.

Most people with insulin-dependent diabetes use syringes and lancets every day. But what do you do with them when you're done?

Like anything else we throw out, lancets and syringes need to be disposed of properly. Otherwise they can end up in places they don't belong, like beaches. And because they have very sharp, pointy ends, they can hurt people by accident, like the person who collects your garbage, someone in your family, or even you!

But there's a simple way you can help protect people AND the environment. It's quick and easy!

Just follow these ***TWO*** steps.

Step #1: Put a Lid on It!

After you've given yourself an insulin shot, put your syringe *directly* into a strong ***plastic*** or ***metal container*** with a tight cap or lid.

This is the best thing to do! DON'T try to bend, break, or put the cap back on your needle . . . you might hurt yourself!

After you use a lancet put it into the same container too.

MAKE IT EASY! Keep your container in the same room you usually have your insulin shot or test your blood sugar.

Container Do's

The best container is one made of strong plastic with a tight screw-on cap, such as:

- a plastic bleach jug
- a liquid detergent bottle
- a plastic milk jug, or
- any other opaque or colored plastic bottle

These containers are all good because they are very strong (so that needles can't poke through) and because they have a small opening on top that can be closed tightly (to prevent any spills).

You can use a coffee can, too. But when it gets full, close the lid tightly and seal it with strong tape.

Container Don'ts

- Don't use glass containers (they can break)
- Don't use any container that will be *returned to the store or recycled* (syringes and lancets can't be recycled!)

Step #2: Pitch In!

When the container is full and tightly sealed, throw it out in the trash.

Congratulations!

Now you know how to handle and throw out used insulin syringes and lancets safely.

Pass It On!

Do you know others with insulin-dependent diabetes? Tell them what you've learned about handling and safe disposal of used syringes and lancets. By spreading the word, you can help others keep the environment clean and safe!

This Booklet Is Sponsored By:

American Association of Diabetes Educators
American Diabetes Association
American Medical Association
Association for Practitioners in Infection Control, Inc.
Childhood & Adolescent Diabetes Center
Children's National Medical Center
Juvenile Diabetes Foundation
National Association for Home Care
National Diabetes Information Clearinghouse

This booklet was prepared by the Environmental Law Institute pursuant to a grant from the United States Environmental Protection Agency, Office of Solid Waste.

For additional copies of this booklet, please call the RCRA Hotline Monday through Friday, 8:30 a.m. to 7:30 p.m. EST.

The national toll-free number is (800) 424–9346: for the hearing impaired it is TDD (800) 553–7672. In Washington, DC, the number is (202) 382–3000 or TDD (202) 475–9652.

Chapter 22

Research in Diabetes: Insulin Pumps

One of the more recent methods of therapy available for diabetes management is the portable insulin infusion pump (the "pump"). At the present time, the insulin pump is a device which is worn outside the body. This means that surgery is not required in order to use the pump. A needle (like the needle of an insulin syringe) is inserted under the skin in an area where it won't rub against clothing and where it can be taped securely in place. The needle is connected to plastic tubing which leads to the pump. The needles and tubing are called an infusion set. The pump works by pushing down on a syringe to provide insulin to the body. Every two or three days, the needle and tubing are thrown away and a new infusion set is reinserted under the skin.

Pumps vary in size, with some as small as a deck of cards, or even a credit card. The pump is usually worn on a belt and provides a constant trickle of short-acting insulin through the tubing and needle into the body. In this way, the pump provides an almost continuous flow of insulin under the skin. This continuous flow is called the basal rate. It can be adjusted depending on insulin requirements during different parts of the day. For example, before each meal a button on the pump can be pushed to provide a rapid push of insulin, similar to giving an injection. This is called an insulin bolus. Because the needle stays under the skin at all times, the extra insulin needed for meals is given as an insulin bolus instead of an extra insulin injection.

Insulin pumps are used by some people who have Type I, or insulin-

---

Developed by the Michigan Diabetes Research and Training Center.
Used by permission.

dependent diabetes, especially those people with hard-to-control diabetes—those who have trouble keeping their blood sugars in the normal range. Some people who use this method of therapy find that they feel better and their blood sugar levels are within the normal range more consistently.

Use of the insulin pump may be very beneficial, but it does not "manage" diabetes for the person using it. Pump users must still perform all the other tasks of diabetes care such as following a meal plan, monitoring blood glucose and ketones, and keeping accurate records. There are many things to consider before deciding whether or not to switch to pump therapy, but for some people, it may be the right answer for better management of diabetes.

QUESTIONS TO ASK YOUR DOCTOR:

1. ***Would using an insulin pump help to control my diabetes better?***
2. ***Is there some information I can read to learn more about insulin pumps?***

Chapter 23

Nerve Damage From Diabetes (Neuropathy)

Over time, diabetes can cause changes in many parts of your body. These are called the long-term complications of diabetes. These changes can cause eye and kidney problems and heart and blood vessel disease.

Another complication of diabetes is diabetic neuropathy or nerve damage from diabetes. In fact, this is the most common complication of diabetes. The nerves in the feet and legs are the ones most often damaged. (Your nerves are the long, thin strings that connect your brain to all parts of your body.) Sometimes the nerves in the hands and arms are also affected. No one really knows why this happens, but it may be partly due to the effects of high blood sugar.

Having neuropathy does not mean that you will feel or act nervous. Neuropathy has to do with your sense of touch. When nerves are damaged by diabetes, they become either ***less*** sensitive (you feel less than before), or ***more*** sensitive (you feel more than before). The way that you will feel depends on which nerves are affected and how they are affected.

Less sensitive nerves do not send feelings of pain, heat, or cold to the brain as easily. Some people notice numbness or heaviness (similar to when your foot "goes to sleep"). Other people don't notice any symptoms. Feeling pain is one way that the body protects itself. If you aren't able to feel pain, you can hurt yourself very easily. For example, you could burn your foot with your bathwater if you can't feel that it is too hot. You might walk around with a tack in your shoe and not know that you are hurting your foot.

Developed by the Michigan Diabetes Research and Training Center.
Used by permission.

Before your feet lost their sensitivity, they would let you know when something was wrong. Now you need to do what the nerves in your feet used to do for you. Take extra care with your feet and legs. Wear shoes that fit well to avoid blisters. Look at your feet (top and bottom) each time you take a shower to see if there are any cuts, red areas, signs of infections or other changes.

If your nerves become more sensitive, you may feel burning, numbness, tingling of feet, pain from the weight of clothing or sheets, or shooting pain in the legs and feet. These signs usually do not happen all at once. They may seem to come and go. You need to tell your doctor about these feelings, even though they may not seem very important at the time.

Pain from neuropathy can be severe. It can also be hard to treat. Pills with narcotics in them are not the best choice for this type of pain. You need to take pills that are better for the long-term. Good blood sugar control often helps the pain. Keeping your blood sugar in the target range has been shown to prevent and may also ease the pain.

Other ways of helping the pain include:

- Relaxation exercises
- Transcutaneous Nerve Stimulation (TENS) unit. A TENS unit is a box you wear which provides an electric shock to the painful nerves.
- Pain clinics. Your health care team can give you more information on a pain clinic in your area.

Neuropathy can also damage the nerves that control your stomach, your bladder, and how you digest food. Signs of this damage include diarrhea, nausea, vomiting, and urine staying in your bladder.

In the past, there was often very little that could be done to ease the pain of neuropathy. But, this is an area of a great deal of research. New medicines are being tested for neuropathy. Ask your health care team about a diabetes specialist, a diabetes center, or a neurologist if you need more help with your neuropathy. In the meantime, good blood sugar control can do a lot to ease the pain of neuropathy.

ASK YOUR DOCTOR OR NURSE THE FOLLOWING QUESTIONS:

1. ***Has my diabetes affected my nerves?***
2. ***What should I do if my diabetes has affected my nerves?***
3. ***Should I see a specialist or go to a Diabetes Center for treatment of my nerve damage (neuropathy)?***

Chapter 24

Diabetes and High Blood Pressure— A Challenging Combination

Often diabetes and high blood pressure (hypertension) go hand in hand. It is thought that 40 to 50 percent of people with diabetes have high blood pressure as well. High blood pressure, like diabetes, is a lifelong disease. It can be treated but not cured. If you have both diabetes and high blood pressure, it will be especially important to work closely with your doctor and other health care professionals to control both.

Blood pressure is the amount of force your blood exerts against the walls of your blood vessels. Blood pressure is usually measured as two numbers, such as 120/80 (normal blood pressure). The first and larger number (systolic pressure) is the blood pressure during a contraction (beat) of the heart. The second and smaller number (diastolic pressure) is the blood pressure when the heart is at rest (between beats). Your blood pressure can change many times during the day depending on physical activity, emotional state, and other reasons. Therefore a number of blood pressure readings are needed before a diagnosis of high blood pressure (hypertension) can be made. Blood pressure readings usually above 130/85 mean you have high blood pressure, if you are below age 65. For those over age 65, 160/90 is the normal limit.

Sometimes blood pressure that is too high will cause dizziness, headaches, or nosebleeds. Most often however, high blood pressure causes no outward signs of trouble. Because of this, high blood pressure is often referred to as a "silent" disease. It can be missed in people who do not have their blood pressure checked regularly. Because usually there are no symp-

---

Developed by the Michigan Diabetes Research and Training Center.
Used by permission.

toms, people who have high blood pressure sometimes stop taking their medicine because they feel okay. This is a serious mistake. High blood pressure that is not treated can lead to a heart attack, stroke or kidney failure.

If you have diabetes and high blood pressure, it is very important to take care of them both. High blood pressure can cause the complications of diabetes to be worse. High blood pressure can speed up the process of hardening of the arteries and kidney disease. This leads to an increased risk of heart attack, stroke, and kidney failure. High blood pressure further weakens damaged blood vessels in the eyes, and can make blood flow problems in the feet and legs worse. Taking good care of your diabetes and high blood pressure can decrease, delay, and sometimes prevent these problems.

The care of high blood pressure is somewhat like the care of diabetes. In fact, sometimes the same treatment works for both of them. Many people with diabetes and high blood pressure are overweight. Weight loss and regular exercise will help control both diabetes and high blood pressure. People with high blood pressure should also cut down on salt and faithfully take any medicine prescribed. By working with your health care team and following your treatment, you can meet the challenge of caring for diabetes and high blood pressure.

ASK YOUR DOCTOR OR NURSE THE FOLLOWING QUESTIONS:

1. ***What is my blood pressure?***
2. ***What should it be?***
3. ***What should I do to keep my blood pressure from going too high?***

Chapter 25

Is Your Blood Too Fat?

For years, doctors have thought that too much fat (cholesterol) in the blood helped cause heart disease. Now they know for sure. Recent studies have proven that high levels of cholesterol in the blood increase the risk for heart disease. If your cholesterol is high, for ***every*** 1% you reduce it, you will reduce your chance for heart disease by 2%.

There are other risk factors for heart disease. Some of the risk factors are things that you cannot change. For example, men have a higher risk than women. Also, someone who has heart disease in the family has a higher risk than someone without heart disease in the family. Neither of these can be changed. Diabetes is also a risk factor, but it is a risk factor you can do something about. You can lower your cholesterol and reduce your chances of getting heart disease by controlling your diabetes. High blood sugar levels can raise your triglyceride levels, which is part of your total cholesterol.

The first step is to find out your cholesterol level. A normal cholesterol is 200 or less and people with diabetes should keep their cholesterol in the normal range. The next time you visit your doctor, ask to have your blood tested. Then talk about your cholesterol level with your doctor. If your cholesterol level is too high, your doctor can refer you to a dietitian who can help you plan a diet that will fit with your life.

One of the best ways to lower your cholesterol is to eat less fat and less saturated or hard fat. One way to eat less fat is to find low-fat substitutes for the high-fat foods you eat. For example, if you drink whole milk you can

---

Developed by the Michigan Diabetes Research and Training Center.
Used by permission.

switch to 2% or 1/2% milk. Eat meats low in fat and trim fat before cooking. Also, avoid fried foods and use canola or olive oil for salads and cooking. Eat frozen yogurt instead of ice cream. You can make a lot of changes in your diet that will help lower your cholesterol. If you make these changes one at a time, you can work them into your eating habits without a big upset.

A low-fat diet can also help you lose weight and control your diabetes. Keeping your blood sugar near the normal range and eating less fat can go a long way toward helping you lower your cholesterol and reduce your chances for heart disease.

ASK YOUR DOCTOR THE FOLLOWING QUESTIONS:

1. ***What is my cholesterol?***
2. ***Will you send me to a dietitian who can help me plan a low-fat diet?***
3. ***What else can I do to lower my cholesterol?***

Chapter 26

You Are What You Eat

Good nutrition is the most basic part of your plan to control your diabetes. Usually the foods on your diabetes meal plan are the same foods that are healthy for *everyone* in your family! Special foods are not needed. It's a good idea to avoid foods that are high in sugar and fat. They are not good for anyone—whether they have diabetes or not. The goal is to eat a balanced diet and try not to overeat.

You can meet your basic nutrition needs by eating foods from the different food groups every day. These foods are:

1. Starches and breads include cereal, rice, and noodles. Eat whole grain, fortified or enriched starches, breads, and cereals.
2. Fruits and vegetables that are fresh, frozen, or canned without sugar. Have fruit or juice rich in vitamin C, such as oranges, grapefruit, cantaloupe, or strawberries, every day.
3. Plain vegetables that are fresh, frozen or canned. Include a dark green or orange vegetable such as broccoli, carrots, spinach, or winter squash at least every other day.
4. Milk and milk products such as low-fat or skim milk and plain low-fat yogurt.
5. Meats such as chicken, turkey, and lean cuts of beef and pork. You can also eat other protein foods such as tuna, salmon, and other fish, cottage cheese, peanut butter, cooked dried beans or peas, tofu, egg whites.

Developed by the Michigan Diabetes Research and Training Center.
Used by permission.

If you plan each meal to include food from each of the food groups you will be eating a balanced diet. Eating a variety of healthy foods is good for your diabetes, good for your body, and good for your family. It will help prevent heart and blood vessel disease and may lessen your chances of getting some kinds of cancer. If you want more information, a registered dietitian in your community can help you plan meals that are healthy and fit your lifestyle.

ASK YOUR DOCTOR OR NURSE THE FOLLOWING QUESTIONS:

1. ***Where is there a dietitian I can visit to help me plan my diet?***
2. ***What changes in my diet would help me control my diabetes better?***
3. ***Is my diet good for my whole family?***

ASK YOUR DIETITIAN THE FOLLOWING QUESTIONS:

1. ***What changes in my diet would help me control my diabetes better?***
2. ***Is my diet good for my whole family?***

Chapter 27

Ordering Fast Food Wisely

About a third of the average American's food budget is spent on eating out. Unfortunately, it's not always easy to eat a nutritious, balanced, and non-fattening meal away from home. Fast-food restaurants are probably the biggest challenge. You can still have a healthy, relatively low-calorie meal that can fit into your diabetes meal plan, if you know how to order.

Fast foods are generally very low in fiber and complex carbohydrates, but are high in fat, salt and sugar. Because fat has twice as many calories as an equal amount of carbohydrate or protein, most fast foods are very "calorie dense." It doesn't take very much food to add up to too many calories. Fast-food dinners such as fried chicken or a fish sandwich and fries get about half their calories from fat. Such a meal could easily top the 1000 mark—and exceed half the total suggested daily calories for most adults!

The easiest answer to the fast-food dilemma is to keep such foods to a minimum. But fast foods are here to stay and, admittedly, they're tasty, inexpensive and fast. Here are some suggestions for how to deal with them:

- When you eat a fast-food meal, try to balance this with healthier foods for the remaining meals of the day. Choose fresh vegetables and fruit, whole grain breads, and low-fat dairy products at your other meals.
- Don't assume that anything you get from a salad bar is low in calories and fat. A plate of prepared salads such as potato and macaroni salads

---

Developed by the Michigan Diabetes Research and Training Center.
Used by permission.

or cole slaw, covered with bacon bits, croutons, cheeses, and heavy dressings could exceed the calorie and fat content of a burger, fries, and shake!

- Many fast-food restaurants now offer broiled chicken, which is much lower in fat and calories than batter-fried. But whether you order broiled or fried chicken, remove the skin, which is where most of the fat lies. In addition, when ordering something fried, choose larger pieces rather than tidbits, which have more greasy batter.
- Shakes and colas are high in sugar and have little or no nutritive value. Skim milk, fruit juice, or even a glass of ice water are healthier alternatives.
- Go easy on the condiments or order your sandwich plain. Per serving, Big Mac sauce contains 126 calories; tartar sauce, 140 calories; mayonnaise, 153 calories; and most barbecue sauces, 60 calories.
- Many fast-food breakfasts are little more than grease on a bun. A croissant may contain as much as four and a half pats of butter or fat. If you're in a hurry, you're much better off having a quick breakfast at home of fresh fruit and cold cereal.
- Fast-food portions are intended for large appetites. In fact, fast-food advertisers emphasize "BIG," "JUMBO," and "SUPER" portions. Order smaller versions when you can. Choose fast-food restaurants with salad bars and have a salad of fresh fruit and vegetables on the side if you want more food.
- Get information on the calorie/nutrient values of fast foods so you know just what you're eating. Almost every fast-food restaurant has this information available.

ASK YOUR DIETITIAN THE FOLLOWING QUESTION:

1. ***Can you help me learn how to make healthy food choices when I go to a fast-food restaurant?***

Chapter 28

Why Exercise?

For those with diabetes, exercise is an important part of treatment. Along with diet and medication, exercise aids in keeping your blood glucose in good control. Regular exercise lowers blood glucose for two reasons. First, more energy (in the form of blood sugar) is used when the body is active. Second, exercise helps the body use insulin more efficiently and this lowers blood sugar. Exercise is also beneficial because it helps the heart to function well. Exercise can also result in an improved sense of well-being since it is a way to relieve tension and helps relaxation and sleep. Finally, along with a healthy diet, exercise can help control weight. This may be especially important for people with Type II diabetes if they are overweight.

Before beginning an exercise program, it is important to check with your doctor, particularly if you have been inactive. Your physician may recommend special tests to see what effect exercise has on your heart. This will help in planning an exercise program which suits your individual needs and physical condition. If you are in good health, it is likely that your physician will recommend rhythmic, repetitive activities which use large muscles and stimulate the circulatory system so that the heart, lungs, and other organs and muscles work together more efficiently. Anyone starting such a program should not go "all-out" from the start. It is important to begin easily, gradually adding more demanding activities after becoming accustomed to a certain level of exercise. Doing this will help avoid the problem of severe muscle soreness and the feeling that exercise is "too much," which may cause

---

Developed by the Michigan Diabetes Research and Training Center.
Used by permission.

you to give up. As with almost any regular activity, there may be times when you are not motivated to continue, which is natural. It may help to find activities that are fun for you. Examples of such activities may include walking, bicycling, swimming, and active sports or games. Exercising with family members or friends may also be more fun and help you to maintain a regular schedule.

For people with diabetes, the activity level (exercise) must be balanced with diet and medication. In addition, a person who takes insulin may need a snack before exercising or may need to decrease the insulin dose on an exercise day to avoid low blood sugar. Checking your blood glucose level before and after exercising will also help you to see the effect exercise has on blood sugar levels. The more constant the amount of exercise day to day, the more constant will be the control of your diabetes.

When you decide to make exercise a regular part of your daily life, you are making a good decision about taking care of yourself and your diabetes. Exercise can be fun, and healthy.

QUESTIONS TO ASK YOUR DOCTOR, NURSE, OR DIETITIAN:

1. ***Is there a type of exercise that would improve my diabetes control and fit with my age and overall health?***
2. ***Is there a program or group that I could join to exercise?***

Chapter 29

Taking Care of Yourself by Walking

You ***can*** control your blood sugar. One way is to walk. This booklet will help you plan a good walking program.

Why Walk?

Walking helps you.

It uses up blood sugar. Walking uses up some of your blood sugar for energy. The more you walk, the more you can lower your blood sugar.

It uses up fat. Walking can help you lose fat. Your body uses fat for energy during long walks.

You feel better. Best of all, walking makes you feel better. You feel more calm during the day. You have more strength. You handle daily stresses better.

How Much?

3 times a week for 30 minutes. Walk steadily, for 30 minutes or longer, each time. Walk often, 3 times a week or more.

Have fun! Walk with family or friends. Enjoy talking. Take scenic routes.

Walking during work is not enough. Most people walk more than 30 minutes during a day. They walk 3 minutes here, 4 minutes there.

IHS 1987. Produced by the Portland Area Diabetes Program in cooperation with the Northwest Portland Area Indian Health Board and the Indian Health Service Diabetes Program, Headquarters West, Albuquerque, New Mexico.

But, to get help from walking, you need to walk steadily, for 30 minutes at a time. And you must walk often, 3 times a week or more.

Protect Your Feet!

Prevent damage to your feet. Try to avoid all foot problems. Treat even small problems right away.

- Look at your feet after every walk.
- Look for red areas, blisters, or sores.

Good shoes. Wear good shoes that fit, cushion, and support your feet. Good shoes do not cause blisters.

Break in new shoes slowly. Wear them for short periods of time.

Wear a clean pair of socks to help cushion and protect your feet.

If you have any foot problems, see a doctor or nurse.

Have Fun!

Have a walking partner, or two or lots!

Tell your friends about your walking. They may join you!

Talk with friends while you walk.

Make it a habit. Walk the same time each day.

Walk for at least 30 minutes.

Have a weekly schedule. Walk at least three times each week.

Start Slow

Go Easy! Start with slow short walks. Make your first walks short—10 minutes—with a slow pace.

If you cannot talk while you walk, you are walking too fast.

Increase slowly. Increase your time in stages, by 5 minutes every 2 weeks. Work your way up, to a total of 30 minutes.

Increase your walking pace in stages, after you can walk for 30 minutes.

Stretching. Do arm and leg stretches before and after long walks. Stretching helps prevent aches and muscle cramps.

Start by stretching easy.

Other exercise is good for you, too.

Such as:

- aerobics
- riding a bike

- hiking the hills
- dancing
- walking in shallow water
- canoeing
- swimming, and
- walking to the store or work.

Do any of them 3 times a week for 30 minutes.
Start by stretching easy.

Chapter 30

Coping With Stress

Stress is part of life and we all have things happen to us now and then that we define as stressful. Each person defines what is stressful to him or her. Some stress in our lives is good. It makes our lives more interesting and gives purpose and meaning. Things that we believe are harmful or causing a great deal of change may be too stressful. Too much stress at one time can also cause an overload.

The body responds to stress by making certain hormones. These can cause the heart to beat faster, the blood pressure to go up, and faster breathing. If this energy is not used to either fight or run away you may feel tense, tired, or have a headache.

Stress can also affect your diabetes. The hormones your body makes when it feels stress can cause the blood sugar to go up. However, some people find that their blood sugar goes down during stressful times. Thus stress can make your diabetes harder to control. It can lead to blood sugars that are too high, too low, or changing often. Some people find that they do not handle stress as well when they have diabetes. They spend so much energy taking care of their diabetes that they don't feel like they cope with other problems as well as they used to do.

Before you can cope with stress, you first need to be aware of when you feel under stress. There are some signs that your body needs a rest. These are headaches, tight muscles in your neck or jaw, a change in eating or sleeping patterns, feeling angry or tense most of the time, loss of interest in

---

Developed by the Michigan Diabetes Research and Training Center.
Used by permission.

sex, and not feeling sure of yourself. Some people find it helps to keep track of how they feel under stress, what causes the stress, and how they handle it. This information can be added to your blood sugar record or food diary. Putting these facts together can give you a picture of how your diabetes control and eating habits are affected by stress.

Everyone handles stress in their own way. Some ways of coping give you more problems even though they may help at the time. Eating too much, smoking, alcohol, drugs or not taking care of a problem are not positive ways to cope with stress. Positive ways to cope with stress help you to feel in control, informed, and supported by other people. It is helpful to have several positive ways to cope with different kinds of stress.

Here are some tips that can help you to deal with stress each day.

- Talk about your stressors with others.
- Know your limits and don't try to do more than you can.
- Realize that it is okay to cry.
- Realize that it is good to laugh each day.
- Exercise or become more active.
- Take care of yourself and your health.
- Plan your day and set goals you can meet.
- Take breaks during stressful hours.
- Don't try to do everything yourself.
- Practice your religion.
- Do fewer things and do them better.
- Avoid stressful situations when possible. If you can't, plan ahead how you will handle the stress.
- Use the energy in other ways. Hobbies, exercise, shopping, or spending time with others can reduce stress.
- Join a support group.

Feeling under stress happens to everyone. It is important to learn to cope with stress. Your diabetes control, your overall health and the way you feel about yourself will all be better if you do.

QUESTIONS TO ASK YOUR DOCTOR, NURSE, OR DIETITIAN:

1. ***How can I learn more about stress and diabetes?***
2. ***Are there any programs or groups that can help me manage my stress?***

Chapter 31

Don't Let Your Life Go Up In Smoke

You may be wondering why a newsletter about diabetes has an issue on smoking. The reason is, if you have diabetes you have ***another*** reason not to smoke. If you don't smoke, don't start. If you do smoke, this is a good time to think about quitting. You know some of the reasons not to smoke. For example, smoking is the #1 cause of lung cancer and lung cancer causes over 100,000 deaths each year. Illnesses related to smoking cause more than 325,000 deaths each year. In fact, a smoker's risk for early death is 70% higher than for a nonsmoker. Almost everyone who smokes will damage their health and shorten their life.

But why is smoking a special problem for people with diabetes? The reason is because both smoking and diabetes are risk factors which greatly increase your chances of getting heart disease. Smoking does a lot of things to your heart—all of them bad. Smokers have a 50–100% greater chance of having a heart attack than nonsmokers do. Also, when people who smoke have heart attacks, they are more severe than when nonsmokers have them. For example, smoking makes high blood pressure worse. It also increases the chances of getting angina (a severe chest pain caused by not enough blood getting to the heart). Smoking also restricts blood flow to your hands and feet.

You may already know many of these facts. You may want to quit smoking but believe that you just can't do it. Maybe you have tried quitting in the past and failed. Each year in this country, 80,000 people stop smoking.

Developed by the Michigan Diabetes Research and Training Center.
Used by permission.

Most of these people have failed many times before. Keep trying. Ask yourself—"Do I want to live?" "Do I want to stay as healthy as I can?" "Am I willing to learn not to smoke?" If the answer is yes, many programs in your community can help you learn not to smoke. Find out about them—join one. This may be one of the hardest things you'll ever do but it is worth it!

ASK YOUR DOCTOR OR NURSE THE FOLLOWING QUESTIONS:

1. ***How does smoking affect my chances of getting diabetes complications?***
2. ***Will you refer me to a program to help me learn not to smoke?***

Chapter 32

A Journey of a Thousand Miles is Taken Step-by-Step

Caring for your diabetes means making changes—sometimes lots of them. You're asked to change things about the way you eat and your activity level. You may also have to take pills or learn how to take shots, test your blood, and recognize the symptoms of low and high blood sugar. It's not always easy to make changes in your life, but there are ways to help you. If you are ready, you may be able to make big changes in your diet and level of activity all at once. But many people who try to make big changes do not succeed. Trying to change too much at one time is one reason why crash diets seldom work. For many people, a good way to make a big change is to break it down into small steps. If you have tried to change your diet before and it did not work, the step-by-step approach may be for you. Make a list of small changes you can make in your diet. Each of the small steps can be taken one at a time. In this way a big change can be made bit-by-bit.

You will probably have much more success in making a big change in the way you eat if you make it slowly. If you tried to stop eating all the foods that are high in sugar and fat, it might be too big a change for you to make. You might feel upset and hungry much of the time and, if you did, there is a good chance that you would go back to your old way of eating. However, you could cut down on sugar and fat a bit at a time. For example, if you drink whole milk, which is high in fat, you could change to low-fat milk. A good way to make the change is to switch to 2% milk for a while. When you are used to that, you can switch to 1/2% milk or skim milk. It's easier to make the change a little at a time.

Developed by the Michigan Diabetes Research and Training Center.
Used by permission.

You can substitute many low-fat and low-sugar foods for foods that you may now be eating. Replace high-fat and sweet foods one at a time. For example, if you use mayonnaise, switch to a light or diet mayonnaise. After you are used to the diet mayonnaise, switch from your regular butter or margarine to a diet margarine. Wait another week and then make another change and then another. If one change doesn't work for you, try a different one.

Over time, you will change your entire way of eating. As your body becomes used to the new way of eating, you will come to like and enjoy more of the new foods. We all learned to like the foods we eat now—we can learn to like new foods too.

So if you want to eat a more healthy diet, think about changing what you eat one step at a time. It isn't easy to change your food habits, but by making one change a week you will find yourself eating foods that are low in fat, sugar, and calories. As time goes on you will notice that you have lost weight and lowered your blood sugar level. Remember, always talk about any changes you plan to make in your diet with your health care team.

ASK YOUR DOCTOR OR NURSE THE FOLLOWING QUESTION:

1. ***Where is there a dietitian I can see to help me plan a low-sugar and low-fat diet?***

ASK YOUR DIETITIAN THE FOLLOWING QUESTIONS:

1. ***Can you help me make a list of food changes and substitutions that will help me control my diabetes?***
2. ***Which of the food changes on my list will do me the most good?***

Chapter 33

Diabetes Translation

Impediments to Better Care

Despite the progress of the past decade, a significant disparity continues to exist between advances of science and their reflection in the care provided to most patients. Effective and widespread application of research findings in diabetes does not occur automatically because a variety of gaps and barriers are inherent in the health care system. First, practitioners and their patients are not always aware of current medical and self-care advances. Second, both practitioners and patients frequently are confronted with health care reimbursement practices that impede the application of effective therapies. Finally, patients are expected to develop an exceptional degree of "consumer sophistication" to gain access to necessary medical care within complex and confusing health care systems. Overcoming these obstacles to optimal patient care requires a systematic coordinated effort.

The National Commission on Diabetes recognized that Federal support and leadership would be needed to facilitate the translation of research into clinical practice. Translation may be defined as the implementation of the results of scientific research and the evaluation of that implementation. This process of translation is not one action but rather a series of coordinated steps involving Government agencies, professional and voluntary groups, third-party payers, patients, and others, which ultimately benefit the individual with diabetes.

Excerpts from: *The National Long-Range Plan to Combat Diabetes.* NIH Pub. No. 88-1587.

The initial long-range plan therefore provided for the establishment and support of specific Federal translation activities. Among these were the DRTC's, diabetes control programs supported by the CDC and IHS, and the National Diabetes Information Clearinghouse. Each of these activities has increased our capacity to improve diabetes care. The CDC and IHS programs have demonstrated in selected populations that the application of currently available prevention and treatment information can lead to significant reductions in mortality, morbidity, and associated economic costs. However, these programs do not have the resources or the mandate to effect widespread implementation of the research advances and clinical opportunities [reviewed in Chapters 11, 49, and 50]. Therefore, the new long-range plan recommends support for a new initiative and for existing Federal programs so that we may build upon the success of the past decade to systematically bridge the gap between research and patient.

Diabetes Translation Center: A New Strategy for Coordinating the Federal Translation Program

The major recommendation of the long-range plan as it relates to translation is the establishment of the DTC within the CDC. The DTC will have two major goals:

- To plan, conduct, coordinate, and evaluate Federal efforts to translate diabetes research into patient care.
- To serve as the focal point for coordination between Federal programs and the private sector. . . .

Activities of the Diabetes Translation Center

- Coordinate the Collection, Surveillance, Analysis, Evaluation, and Dissemination of Diabetes Data Related to the Translation of Research Results to Patient Care . . .
- Coordinate the Development of Clinical Management Consensus for Diabetes Mellitus and Its Complications . . .
- Design and Evaluate Translation Strategies . . .
- Develop Diabetes Health Care Indicators . . .
- Provide Support for Statewide Programs . . .
- Develop Mechanisms for Financing Cost-Effective Health Care . . .

- Conduct Professional Education and Training Programs for Community Diabetes Control . . .
- Promulgate the Results of Research and Translation . . .

Recommendations for Current Federal Translation Programs

Many Federal agencies conduct programs that directly or indirectly influence the delivery of health care through professional education, patient and public education, reimbursement of health care expenses, data collection and analysis, and related activities. A few agencies also provide health care services directly to specific populations. Some of these programs already have developed initiatives that focus on or include diabetes and its complications. Each of the following programs warrants increased support for diabetes-related activities.

Model Diabetes Care Program of the Indian Health Service

Whether expressed in terms of prevalence, morbidity, premature mortality, or economic impact, diabetes among American Indians is significantly more severe than in other U.S. population groups. Diabetes occurred quite infrequently in American Indians 50 years ago, but the diagnosis of diabetes became progressively more common by the 1960's. Today, diabetes in some tribes has achieved epidemic proportions. A startling 50 percent of Pima Indians over the age of 35 have diabetes, and prevalence rates greater than 20 percent among adults have been reported in several tribes in Arizona, Florida, Nevada, New Mexico, New York, North Carolina, and Oklahoma.

The serious complications of diabetes, especially renal failure, amputations, and blindness, are increasing in frequency among American Indians. The costs of managing diabetes and its complications also are increasing rapidly. Because the IHS, an agency of the HRSA, is responsible for the health care of American Indians, these rising health care costs of diabetes are borne directly by the Federal Government. The following are only two examples:

- The treatment for renal failure—kidney dialysis or transplantation—is particularly expensive. The annual cost of treating the current patient population of American Indians with chronic renal failure exceeds $10 million.
- American Indians with diabetes account for approximately 75 percent of all amputations within the IHS health care system. The annual

hospital-related costs alone of these amputations exceed $3 million, exclusive of the costs of rehabilitation and disability.

Prevention and treatment strategies are available to reduce the rate and severity of these and other complications of diabetes. The National Commission on Diabetes recommended, and Congress authorized and funded, the Model Diabetes Health Care Program to develop and evaluate effective and culturally acceptable methods to reduce the severity of the disease and to reduce the expense to the IHS of related medical services. The program emphasizes the effective application of clinical advances to prevent or reduce the severity of several diabetes complications. Because of the success of the model program, many of these treatment advances are now being incorporated throughout the IHS. Plans for the next decade include further development of culturally acceptable methods to reduce the severity of diabetes and widespread incorporation of comprehensive diabetes control activities throughout the IHS. . . .

Other Programs of the Health Resources and Services Administration

Many individuals with diabetes, particularly in medically underserved and rural areas, are served by HRSA health care delivery programs. These include the IHS (described earlier), the Maternal and Child Health Program, Crippled Children Services, Migrant Health and Community Health Centers, and the Federal Employee Occupational Health Program. In addition, the HRSA is responsible for health manpower programs vital to the implementation of the translation goal of this long-range plan. . . .

National Center for Health Services Research

The National Center for Health Services Research (NCHSR) seeks to create new knowledge and better understanding of the processes by which health services are made available and how they may be provided more efficiently and effectively. Because diabetes translation involves many complex health services, problems in health care delivery frequently influence care and patient outcomes. Few individuals are conducting research in this important area. Potential diabetes research topics include access, acceptability, organization, technology, utilization, quality, and financing of health services and systems; supply, distribution, quality, utilization, organization, and cost of health manpower; role of market forces in the health care delivery system and their part in restraining cost increases and improving the availability and quality of care; and safety, efficacy, effectiveness, cost, and economic and social impact of various health care technologies. . . .

National Center for Health Statistics

The NCHS conducts national studies to provide data on the medical, economic, and social impact of diabetes. This information is an important resource for the DTC, the NDDG, and other diabetes organizations concerned with research, health care services, and formulation of public policy related to diabetes. For example, the National Health Interview Survey and the National Health and Nutrition Examination Survey provide valuable prevalence data and information about the use of health care resources for diabetes. The National Ambulatory Medical Care Survey samples physicians in office-based practices and provides information about morbidity among the outpatient population with diabetes, while the National Hospital Discharge Survey samples the records of all inpatients who have been discharged from U.S. hospitals. The National Nursing Home Survey provides information about long-term care facilities. . . .

Health Care Financing Administration

The Health Care Financing Administration is responsible for the Federal Medicare and Medicaid programs. The success of many diabetes translation recommendations contained in this report [portions of which are also reproduced in Chapters 11, 49, and 50] is dependent upon the implementation of reimbursement practices that support effective health care practices. . . .

Veterans Administration

The VA is unique among Federal agencies in that it is involved in the research, education, and patient care aspects of diabetes. The VA is the largest health care agency in the world, with 172 medical centers, 57 independent satellite outpatient clinics, and 117 nursing home care units. The VA has the legislative mandate to care for the Nation's 28 million veterans, many of whom have diabetes. The annual health care budget for the VA is $9.5 billion. Survey data indicate that approximately 11 percent of VA hospital inpatients have diabetes as one of their medical problems. Because the VA has long-term responsibility for the care of a fixed population of entitled patients, preventive care for diabetes is an important aspect of the VA's health care goals.

The VA also is an important component of physician training programs. Over two-thirds of all physicians in the United States have had at least part of their training at a VA medical center. The total trainee budget for the VA in fiscal year 1986 was $247,834,000, with an additional $8,534,000 for continuing education of VA medical center staff. The size of this program places the VA in a unique position to train physicians and other health care professionals in the latest techniques for the diagnosis and treatment of diabetes and its complications.

Whereas the research budget of the VA is modest when compared with the budget of the NIH, VA investigators have long been in the forefront of many research accomplishments described in other portions of this plan [which are reproduced in Chapters 40 and 50], and one VA scientist recently was awarded the Nobel prize for research conducted in a VA research laboratory. Many VA investigators are conducting diabetes-related research projects. . . .

Department of Defense

The DOD provides health care programs for the uniformed services and for authorized beneficiaries. A variety of hospital and outpatient professional services for diabetes patient care are routinely available. These include physician and nursing care, dietary instruction, physical therapy, podiatric care, pharmacy support, and social services. Each branch of the military service also supports biomedical research on a variety of subjects related to the health care needs of its members. In addition, training programs in diabetes-related topics are conducted for physicians, paramedical and other health science personnel, and research investigators. . . .

Department of Agriculture

The Department of Agriculture conducts major research programs in nutrition, some of which are applicable to diabetes mellitus. In addition, the Cooperative Extension Service supports nutrition education programs, which are an important resource for diabetes control programs. . . .

National Institute of Diabetes and Digestive and Kidney Diseases

The NIDDK is primarily responsible for biomedical research. However, many NIDDK activities are important resources for the translation of research to patient care. One such program, the National Diabetes Information Clearinghouse (NDIC), is particularly important to the translation component of the long-range plan.

NDIC serves health professionals, the public, and patients by identifying, collecting, and disseminating current information about diabetes and its complications. The NDIC works closely with professional and voluntary organizations to facilitate these activities.

PART THREE

COMPLICATIONS OF DIABETES

Chapter 34

Diabetes Control and Complications Trial: Results of a 10-year Study

Support for the Diabetes Control and Complications Trial (DCCT) from Major Diabetes Voluntary Organizations

We wish to extend our gratitude for the efforts of the National Institute of Diabetes and Digestive and Kidney Diseases and all those involved in the Diabetes Control and Complications Trial (DCCT). The DCCT is a model clinical trial—one of the very best designed and executed large-scale clinical trials in history. The clinical investigators, trial coordinators and the entire team, including the patient participants, deserve our highest accolades both for their expertise and their unwavering commitment to the study.

The Diabetes Control and Complications Trial would not have been possible without an exceptional partnership—among government, voluntary organizations and industry. The cooperation among all parties and the corporate support for the Trial demonstrates a model relationship for future health care initiatives.

The DCCT and its findings create opportunities for the millions of people with diabetes to receive better treatment to help them lead healthier lives and reduce or prevent the very serious complications of diabetes. We are delighted to be able to play a role in disseminating the results of the Trial over the coming months and years to health care professionals and people with diabetes.

Continued research will help us in our quest to improve diabetes care—

Taken from a report issued by the National Institute of Diabetes & Digestive & Kidney Diseases, June 2, 1993.

and someday reach our ultimate goal, to find a cure for this disease. The importance of continued support for diabetes research from both the public and private sectors is demonstrated by the Diabetes Control and Complications Trial. This study represents the rewards of the very best kind of collaborative research effort.

THE DIABETES CONTROL AND COMPLICATIONS TRIAL: A 10-Year Study of Intensive Treatment of Insulin-Dependent Diabetes Mellitus (IDDM).

What Is the DCCT?

In 1983, the National Institute of Diabetes and Digestive and Kidney Diseases (NIDDK) launched the DCCT, a 10-year controlled, randomized clinical trial to assess the safety and determine the benefits of intensive blood sugar control. The most comprehensive diabetes study ever conducted, it compared the effects of two different treatment regimens on the development of long-term diabetes complications including eye, kidney and nerve disease.

Patients in the conventional treatment group followed a regimen used by most people with IDDM:

- insulin injections once or twice a day
- daily blood glucose tests
- clinical visits every three months

Those in the intensive treatment group learned to adjust their insulin doses to keep blood sugar levels as close to normal as possible. Their treatment included:

- three or more insulin injections a day or use of an insulin pump
- blood sugar tests four or more times a day
- a diet and exercise plan
- an initial hospital stay to implement treatment
- weekly to monthly clinical visits

What Were the Results of the DCCT?

The DCCT showed that intensive treatment that keeps blood glucose levels as close to normal as possible slows the onset and progression of long-term diabetes complications including eye, kidney and nerve disease.

Effects of intensive treatment on retinopathy

- Slowed progression of retinopathy (diabetic eye disease) by more than 50 percent. This reduction occurred both in people without eye damage and with eye damage at time of entry into the study.
- Slowed progression to severe retinopathy and requirement for laser surgery by approximately 50 percent.

Diabetes is the most common cause of blindness in adults in the United States.

Effects of intensive treatment on nephropathy

- Decreased development of nephropathy (diabetic kidney disease) by nearly 50 percent in people who had no signs of kidney disease at time of entry into the study.
- Slowed progression of more severe kidney damage (clinical grade proteinuria) by more than 50 percent.

Diabetes is the most common cause of end-stage renal disease in the United States. The disease costs the Federal Government an estimated $7.26 billion per year to treat.

Effects of intensive treatment on neuropathy (diabetic nerve damage)

- Reduced clinically significant neuropathy by 60 percent.

Neuropathy leads to lower extremity amputation in more than 25,000 patients each year in the United States.

Were There Side Effects from Intensive Treatment?

Intensively treated patients experienced a three-fold increase in the risk of hypoglycemia (low blood sugar reactions). Modest weight gain also occurred. While the benefits of intensive treatment outweigh the risks for most patients with diabetes, intensive treatment should be undertaken with added caution by patients with other diseases that increase the risk of hypoglycemia, and by those who cannot recognize or recover normally from hypoglycemia.

Who Volunteered?

Twenty-nine medical centers in the U.S. and Canada enrolled 1,441 volunteers. Half were male and half were female, and their average age at entry was 27. To participate in the trial, volunteers had to:

- be 13 to 39 years old
- have had IDDM for at least 1 year but no more than 15 years
- have no, or only early, signs of diabetic complications
- be taking no more than two insulin injections a day

The summary manuscript of the main results from the DCCT will be published in the *New England Journal of Medicine* in early fall. Other articles related to the DCCT will be forthcoming in various journals throughout the next few years. For reprints of the journal article, please write to the National Diabetes Information Clearinghouse, Box NDIC/DCCT, 9000 Rockville Pike, Bethesda, Maryland 20892.

Diabetes Complications Studied by the DCCT

Widely recognized as one of the leading causes of death and disability in the U.S., diabetes costs this country more than $40 billion annually. Medical complications from diabetes affect virtually every part of the body, causing blindness, heart disease, stroke, kidney failure, nerve damage, and amputations. The DCCT studied three major types of complications: microvascular, involving changes in small blood vessels; macrovascular, related to changes in large blood vessels; and neuropathy, related to disease of the peripheral and autonomic nervous system.

Microvascular Complications

Diabetic Retinopathy. The major threat to vision from diabetes is diabetic retinopathy. Retinopathy means disease of the retina, the light-sensing tissue at the back of the eye. After a person has had diabetes for 5 to 10 years, changes occur in the tiny vessels that supply the retina with blood. These vessels may leak fluid and small amounts of blood. This form of the disease, called nonproliferative or background retinopathy, usually does not cause symptoms. However, if the part of the retina responsible for most vision, called the macula, becomes swollen, a condition called macular edema will lead to loss of vision. When retinopathy is more advanced, new blood vessels may grow on the surface of the eye, a disease called proliferative retinopathy. These new vessels are fragile, and can rupture easily, releasing blood into the center of the eye and causing sudden loss of vision. The healing process can cause scarring and retinal detachment, which can lead to blindness.

Scientists have found that when laser treatment is used to correct macular edema or certain stages of proliferative retinopathy, it can prevent many cases of blindness caused by diabetes. But despite the effectiveness of laser therapy, diabetes remains the most common cause of new cases of blindness in people under age 65. A yearly eye examination with dilated pupils enables an ophthalmologist to diagnose retinal changes early and provide effective treatment.

All DCCT participants were monitored carefully for diabetic retinopathy. Special stereoscopic photographs of the retina were taken every 6 months and evaluated for degree of retinopathy.

Diabetic Nephropathy. Diabetic nephropathy, or kidney disease caused by diabetes, is the most common cause of kidney failure in the U.S. The single greatest health risk to adults with insulin-dependent diabetes, nephropathy usually occurs in people who have had diabetes 15 years or longer. The kidneys are a complex network of small blood vessels that filter impurities from blood for excretion in urine. Diabetes can damage these small blood vessels so the kidneys cannot perform their waste-filtering work. As nephropathy progresses, the kidneys become unable to eliminate waste. Once waste products build up in the bloodstream to the point of causing illness, patients must undergo a kidney transplant or rely on dialysis to cleanse the blood regularly.

The DCCT included several measures of kidney function. Regular urine collections and special tests were performed to assess kidney function and efficiency in filtering and removing waste products from the blood.

Macrovascular Complications

Diabetes is associated with acceleration of atherosclerosis, or damage to major arteries. Symptoms of macrovascular disease depend on which blood vessels are affected. Disease of the vessels supplying the heart muscle may cause angina, heart attacks or heart failure. If the vessels to the brain are affected, stroke may result. Impaired circulation in the feet and legs, often in concert with nerve damage, can impair the ability to walk, slow healing of infections and ultimately, lead to amputation.

Heart Disease. People with diabetes are 2 to 5 times more likely to suffer heart attacks and experience other circulatory problems than people without the disease. The reason for this increase in vascular disease is unknown, but many scientists believe it may be related to high blood sugar levels. While further studies are needed to confirm this theory, most experts believe people with diabetes should maintain low cholesterol levels and keep high blood pressure under control. High blood pressure accelerates the development of kidney disease and increases the risk of heart disease and stroke.

DCCT volunteers were not expected to have many macrovascular problems because they were on average 27 years old when the study began. Most people, even those with diabetes, do not begin to suffer circulatory problems until they are middle aged or older. Procedures used to monitor circulatory problems in DCCT patients included regular physical examinations and cardiograms. In addition, investigators monitored risk factors for cardiovascular disease, including hypertension, cholesterol, and other lipids on a regular basis.

Neuropathy Complications. Nerve damage from diabetes, called diabetic peripheral neuropathy, can dull sensation in the feet, legs, and fingertips. When this occurs, bruises or sores on the legs and feet may go unnoticed until deep ulcers or infections develop. Reduced blood flow, caused by diabetes' effects on blood vessels, can slow healing. The combination of neuropathy and poor circulation places people with diabetes at increased risk for amputation when ulcers develop. Diabetes is a leading cause of amputation, second only to trauma-related injuries.

Patients may not be aware they have peripheral neuropathy because it develops gradually and may only cause mild numbness at first. Regular foot examinations by a health care professional and proper foot care are the best way to diagnose neuropathy early and prevent amputations.

Diabetes also affects the autonomic part of the nervous system, which controls blood pressure, heart rate, and digestive and sexual function. Diabetes can cause abnormal blood pressure fluctuations, impotence in men, and other nervous system problems.

Participants in the DCCT had regular examinations to detect the development of peripheral and autonomic neuropathy. Researchers conducted special examinations of nerve function in the hands and feet at prescribed intervals.

News Statement: Phillip Gorden, M.D.
Diabetes Control and Complications Trial
June 13, 1993, Las Vegas, Nevada

Good Morning:

The Diabetes Control and Complications Trial was initiated in 1983 to answer the most important diabetes research question of the past 60 years. Can intensive treatment that keeps blood sugar levels as close to normal as possible decrease the long-term complications of diabetes? The answer, we now know, is yes.

Intensive treatment very significantly slows the progression of eye, nerve, and kidney complications of diabetes. With intensive treatment, patients can expect to lead lives that are healthy and free of these devastating complications for a much longer time.

I want to summarize for you the effects of intensive treatment seen in the diabetes control and complications trial:

Progression of eye damage was reduced by 62 percent. This reduction occurred in people without eye damage and people with eye damage at the time of entry into the study.

Progression of eye damage to a severe degree, requiring referral to an ophthalmologist for close follow-up and possible laser surgery, was reduced by 46 percent.

The need for treatment of sight-threatening eye damage, which is done with laser surgery, was reduced by 49 percent.

These findings are of extreme clinical importance because diabetes is the most common cause of blindness in adults in the United States.

The intensive treatment program also had a very significant effect on nerve damage. Clinically significant neuropathy was reduced by 60 percent.

This result is important, because diabetic nerve damage leads to

lower extremity amputation in more than 25,000 patients each year in the United States.

A significant effect was also seen on kidney damage. Evidence of early kidney damage was decreased by 46 percent in those who were normal at the time of entry. Evidence of more severe kidney damage, (clinical grade proteinuria) was significantly reduced by 56 percent.

These findings are important because diabetes is the most common cause of kidney failure in the United States.

I will give you some details about how these results were obtained. The study enrolled 1,441 volunteers at 29 clinics in the United States and Canada. The same number of men and women were enrolled. The average age was 27. The participants were between the ages of 13 and 39. They were studied for an average of 6.5 years. Patients who entered the clinical trial in 1983 were studied for almost 10 years.

The Diabetes Control and Complications Trial compared two different treatment programs. One group followed the regimen recommended for most people with insulin-dependent diabetes. They took one or two insulin shots each day, did daily blood or urine tests, and followed a standard diabetes diet.

The other group was treated very intensively with the goal of maintaining their blood sugar levels as close to normal as possible. They took insulin shots three or four times a day or used an external insulin pump, and they adjusted the insulin doses based on frequent blood sugar tests done by finger prick. Their insulin was also adjusted according to diet and exercise.

A number of tests were done to determine the effects of near normalization of blood sugar on the development and progression of diabetes complications. These tests included state-of-the-art tests for eye, nerve, and kidney disease. Risk factors for heart disease such as cholesterol and blood pressure were also evaluated. Tests were also done to see if intensive treatment had harmful side effects.

We learned during the study that intensive treatment results in a threefold increase in the risk of low-blood sugar reactions. Modest weight gain also occurred. We feel that the benefits of this form of treatment outweighs these risks for most patients with diabetes.

Patients below the age of 13, those with other diseases that make hypoglycemia risky, and those who cannot recognize or recover normally from hypoglycemia are poor candidates for intensive treatment.

Now, Dr. Oscar Crofford, professor of medicine at Vanderbilt University in Nashville, Tenn., who served as our Study Chairman, will discuss clinical implications of these results.

News Conference Statement by DCCT Study Chairman

Oscar B. Crofford, M.D., Professor of Medicine, Vanderbilt University, Nashville, Tennessee

EMBARGOED until 11:00 AM, PDT June 13, 1993

The Diabetes Control and Complications Trial provides compelling evidence that if people with insulin dependent diabetes are changed to a program of intensive treatment, major benefits can be expected. If intensive treatment is started early, before complications develop, the onset of severe complications can be delayed substantially and perhaps prevented. If intensive treatment is started in people who have already begun to develop complications, progression of complications can be slowed and perhaps halted. The avoidance of the eye, kidney, and nerve complications of diabetes will lead to fewer hospital admissions, fewer tests, less surgery, lower health care costs, and an improved quality of life.

It is important to understand that intensive diabetes treatment is not just "more insulin." The goal of intensive diabetes treatment is to maintain the blood sugar level as close to normal as possible. It involves frequent self-monitoring of blood sugar, careful attention to diet and exercise, and complicated insulin delivery systems or routines. It requires a skilled and experienced treatment team and a patient who is highly motivated and well skilled in self-management techniques. Hypoglycemia, meaning that the blood sugar has dropped below a safe level, is a definite risk even when intensive treatment is applied under ideal circumstances.

The large number of patient volunteers and the long follow-up period have enabled us to assess the balance between the benefits and the risks that are associated with intensive diabetes treatment. In most patients, the benefits of avoiding severe complications heavily outweigh the risks.

At the present time, there are not enough diabetes treatment teams with the skills and resources to provide intensive diabetes treatment for all the people who can benefit. Family doctors, diabetes specialists, health planners, health educators, and health payors must work together to meet the immediate needs. Research teams must accelerate the development of better methods to keep the blood sugar in the near-normal range. But until a "cure" for diabetes is discovered, intensive diabetes treatment is the best way to avoid the complications of diabetes.

DIRECTORY OF DCCT CENTERS AND KEY STAFF

CALIFORNIA

University of California, San Diego in La Jolla
Principal Investigator:
Orville G. Kolterman, M.D., Adjunct Professor of Medicine

Trial Coordinator:
Gayle Lorenzi, R.N., C.D.E.

Public Affairs Officer:
Denine Denlinger (619) 534–4977

CONNECTICUT

Yale University School of Medicine, New Haven
Principal Investigator:
William V. Tamborlane, M.D., Professor of Pediatrics

Trial Coordinator:
JoAnn Ahern, R.N., M.S.N, C.D.E.

Public Affairs Officer:
Helaine Patterson (203) 785–5824

FLORIDA

University of South Florida College of Medicine, Tampa
Principal Investigator:
John I. Malone, M.D., Professor, Department of Pediatrics

Trial Coordinator:
Nancy Grove, R.N., B.A., B.S., M.A.

Public Affairs Officer:
Michael Hoad (813) 974–3300

ILLINOIS

Northwestern University, Chicago
Principal Investigator:
Mark E. Molitch, M.D., Professor of Medicine

Trial Coordinator:
Barbara Schaefer, B.S.N., M.S.

Public Affairs Officer:
Elizabeth Crown (312) 503–8928

IOWA

University of Iowa, Iowa City
Principal Investigator:
Rodney Zeitler, M.D., M.S.
Assistant Professor, Dept. of Internal Medicine
William Sivitz, M.D.
Associate Professor, Dept. of Internal Medicine

Trial Coordinator:
Meg Bayless, B.S.N., R.N., C.D.E.

Public Affairs Officer:
Mary Abboud-Kamps (319) 335–8037

MARYLAND

University of Maryland, Baltimore
Principal Investigator:
A. Avinoam Kowarski, M.D.
Professor of Pediatrics
Philip A. Levin, M.D.
Associate Professor of Medicine and Pediatrics

Trial Coordinator:
Debra K. Ostrowski, B.S.N.

Public Affairs Officer:
Ellen Beth Levitt (410) 328–8919

MASSACHUSETTS

Joslin Diabetes Center, Boston
Principal Investigator:
Alan M. Jacobson, M.D.
Chief, Mental Health Unit, Joslin Diabetes Center
Associate Professor of Psychiatry, Harvard Medical School

Trial Coordinator:
Susan Crowell, B.S.N., R.N., C.D.E.

Public Affairs Officer:
Tom McCullough (617) 732–2415

Massachusetts General Hospital, Boston
Principal Investigator:
David M. Nathan, M.D.
Associate Professor of Medicine, Harvard Medical School

Trial Coordinator:
Mary Larkin, R.N.

Public Affairs Officer:
Martin Bander (617) 726–2206

MICHIGAN

Henry Ford Hospital, Detroit
Principal Investigator:
Fred W. Whitehouse, M.D.
Head, Division of Endocrinology and Metabolism

Trial Coordinator:
Davida F. Kruger, M.S.N., R.N., C., C.D.E.

Public Affairs Officer:
Rick Swanson (313) 876–8700

University of Michigan, Ann Arbor
Principal Investigator:
Douglas A. Greene, M.D., Professor of Internal Medicine
Director, Michigan Diabetes Research and Training Center

Trial Coordinator:
Catherine L. Martin, B.S.N., C.D.E.

Public Affairs Officer:
Toni Shears (313) 764–6375

MINNESOTA

Mayo Foundation, Rochester
Principal Investigator:
F. John Service, M.D., Ph.D., F.A.C.P., F.R.C.P(C).
Professor of Medicine, Mayo Medical School

Trial Coordinator:
A. LeVuo Schmidt, R.N., C.D.E.

Public Affairs Officer:
Michael O'Hara (507) 284–9522

International Diabetes Center, Minneapolis
Principal Investigator:
Donnell D. Etzwiler, M.D.
President and Chief Medical Officer
International Diabetes Center
Clinical Professor of Family Practice and Community Medicine
University of Minnesota

Trial Coordinator:
Patricia L. Callahan, R.N., B.S., C.D.E.

Public Affairs Officer:
Amy Pak (612) 927–3740

University of Minnesota, Minneapolis
Principal Investigator:
John P. Bantle, M.D., Associate Professor

Trial Coordinator:
Michael V. Mech, R.N., B.S.N., C.D.E.

Public Affairs Officer:
Mary Stanik (612) 624–5100

MISSOURI

University of Missouri, Columbia
Principal Investigator:
David E. Goldstein, M.D. Professor of Child Health, Internal Medicine and Pathology

Trial Coordinator:
Melba R. Hall, R.N. M.S.

Public Affairs Officer:
Jo Ann Wait (university hospital) (314) 882–1081
Delores Shearon (School of Medicine) (314) 882–5660

Washington University at St. Louis
Principal Investigator:
Julio V. Santiago, M.D., Professor of Pediatrics and Medicine
Director, Diabetes Research and Training Center

Trial Coordinator:
Lucy A. Levandoski, B.S., PA-C.

Public Affairs Officer:
Joni Westerhouse (university) (314) 362–8257
Daryle Bollinger (St. Louis Children's Hospital) (314) 454–5432

NEW MEXICO

University of New Mexico School of Medicine, Albuquerque
Principal Investigator:
David S. Schade, M.D., Professor of Medicine

Trial Coordinator:
Carolyn O'Hearn Johannes, R.N., B.S.N.

Public Affairs Officer:
Carolyn R. Tinker (505) 277–3322

NEW YORK

Albert Einstein College of Medicine, Bronx
Principal Investigator:
Harry Shamoon, M.D., Professor of Medicine

Trial Coordinator:
Helena Duffy, R.N., B.S.N., C.D.E.

Public Affairs Officer:
Art Oceans (718) 430–3101

Cornell University Medical College, New York
Principal Investigator:
Robert G. Campbell, M.D.
Director, General Clinical Research Center

Trial Coordinator:
Mary Ellen Lackaye, B.S.N., C.D.E.

Public Affairs Officer:
Diana Goldin, New York Hospital (212) 746–1401

OHIO

Case Western Reserve University, Cleveland
Principal Investigator:
Saul Genuth, M.D., Professor of Medicine

Trial Coordinator:
Betty Brown, R.N., B.S.N.

Public Affairs Officer:
Beth Schmittle, Mt. Sinai Medical Center (216) 421–4035

PENNSYLVANIA

University of Pennsylvania, Philadelphia
Principal Investigator:
Lester Baker, M.D. Professor of Pediatrics

Trial Coordinator:
Patricia Ilves-Corressel, R.N., C.D.E.

Public Affairs Officer:
Sarah Jarvis, Children's Hospital of Philadelphia (215) 590–4092
Harriet Levy, (university) (215) 349–5658

University of Pittsburgh, Pittsburgh
Principal Investigator:
Allan L. Drash, M.D., Professor of Pediatrics

Trial Coordinator:
Jacqueline Wesche, R.N., B.S.N., C.D.E.

Public Affairs Officer:
Jane Duffield (412) 624–2607

SOUTH CAROLINA

Medical University of South Carolina, Charleston
Principal Investigator:
John A. Colwell, M.D., Ph.D., Professor of Medicine

Trial Coordinator:
Denise Turner-Wood, R.N., M.S.N., C.D.E.

Public Affairs Officer:
Scott Regan (803) 792–3621

TENNESSEE

University of Tennessee, Memphis
Principal Investigator:
Abbas E. Kitabchi, Ph.D., M.D.
Professor of Medicine and Biochemistry

Trial Coordinator:
Laura Taylor, R.N., B.S.N., C.D.E.

Public Affairs Officer:
Gilbert I. Hayes (901) 528–5544

Vanderbilt University Medical Center, Nashville
Principal Investigator:
Rodney Lorenz, M.D., Associate Professor of Pediatrics

Trial Coordinator:
Janie Lipps, M.S.N., R.N., C.S., F.N.P.

Public Affairs Officer:
William N. Hance (615) 322–4747

TEXAS

University of Texas, Dallas
Principal Investigator:
Philip Raskin, M.D., C.D.E., Professor of Internal Medicine

Trial Coordinator:
Suzanne Strowig, M.S.N., R.N., C.D.E.

Public Affairs Officer:
Ann Harrell (214) 688–3404

WASHINGTON

University of Washington, Seattle
Principal Investigator:
Jerry P. Palmer, M.D., Professor of Medicine

Trial Coordinator:
Janice C. Ginsberg, R.N., B.S.N., C.D.E.

Public Affairs Officer:
Kathleen Klein (206) 543–3620

CANADA

University of British Columbia, Vancouver
Principal Investigator:
A. D. Morrison, M.D., Associate Professor of Medicine

Trial Coordinator:
Alison Jalbert, R.N.

Public Affairs Officer:
Michelle Perreault (604) 875–4838

University of Toronto, Ontario
Principal Investigator:
Bernard Zinman, M.D.C.M., F.R.C.P., F.A.C.P.
Professor of Medicine

Trial Coordinator:
Annette Barnie, R.N.

Public Affairs Officer:
Jody McPherson (416) 586–5065

University of Western Ontario, London
Principal Investigator:
John Dupre, F.R.C.P.(C), F.R.C.P.(London), F.A.C.P.
Professor of Medicine and Physiology

Trial Coordinator:
Pamela Colby, B.Sc.(F.Sc), R.P.Dt.

Public Affairs Officer:
Leigh-Anne Stradeski (519) 663–3113

Chapter 35

The Prevention and Treatment of Complications of Diabetes Mellitus

Preface

This publication is designed to help the primary care practitioner in the day-to-day management of patients with diabetes. The recommendations relate to the prevention, detection, and treatment of the major complications of diabetes. The emphasis is on early application of currently available measures that, if systematically applied, may reduce the incidence or severity of these complications. Because of the need for brevity and practicality, we have neither discussed areas of controversy nor provided in-depth discussions of pathophysiology and the scientific rationale for treatment.

An office guide is included as an appendix. The office guide is a brief synopsis of the recommendations contained in the body of the text and is designed so that it may be photocopied and placed in the patient's medical record.

A companion publication entitled *Take Charge of Your Diabetes: A Guide for Patients* is available [and is reproduced in Chapter 15 of this volume]. It is written in nontechnical language and emphasizes the same preventive measures and treatments. The sequence of the chapters corresponds with the sequence in this document.

William H. Herman, M.D.
University of Michigan Medical Center
Ann Arbor, Michigan

NIH Pub. No. 93-3464.

Psychosocial Problems

Background

Description. Like other chronic illnesses, diabetes mellitus poses a wide range of problems for patients and their family members. These problems include pain, hospitalization, changes in lifestyle and vocation, physical disabilities, and threatened survival. Direct psychological consequences can arise from any one of these factors, making it harder for patients to treat their diabetes and live productive, enjoyable lives.

Populations at risk. Diabetes itself does not cause changes in personality or psychiatric illness, but particular subgroups of the diabetic population appear to be at risk for developing psychosocial problems. Young people with insulin-dependent diabetes mellitus (IDDM) may have a higher prevalence of eating disorders, such as anorexia nervosa and bulimia, and adults with longstanding diabetes and major medical complications have a higher prevalence of symptoms of depression and anxiety. Elderly persons who have non-insulin-dependent diabetes mellitus (NIDDM) and other symptomatic medical conditions may also have a higher risk of developing psychological problems.

Patients with IDDM diagnosed before age 5 and older patients with NIDDM may have associated alterations in cognitive or intellectual functioning. The pathophysiology of these cognitive changes is not well understood. In the young patients, these cognitive changes may be linked to recurring episodes of severe hypoglycemia. In the older patients, both microvascular and artherosclerotic disease are possible factors.

Barriers to self-care. Research has indicated that psychological and social factors can profoundly influence a patient's success at adhering to a prescribed regimen of self-care. Patients may fail to care for themselves if they have certain attitudes or beliefs, including the following:

- Anticipating an early cure.
- Believing that their self-care regimen is too difficult.
- Believing that treatment is unlikely to improve or control their health problems.

Several other psychosocial factors can influence how well patients care for themselves:

- Stressful events in the patient's life.
- Development of a new complication.
- The availability and quality of social support for the patient.

- Psychiatric problems unrelated to the patient's diabetes.
- The health care provider's approach to medical care.

Prevention

To help anticipate or identify psychosocial problems that could interfere with a patient's self-care regimen, the practitioner should strive to establish an ongoing, therapeutic alliance with the patient. The stronger the alliance, the more likely the patient is to share inner concerns and psychosocial issues. This leads to improved detection and permits more rapid institution of treatment.

This therapeutic alliance will take shape over time, through discussions identifying the patient's expectations of, and feelings about, treatment. Although the patient should not be forced to set particular goals, the practitioner may be able to broaden or refine existing objectives to include improving the patient's adjustment to having diabetes.

Over time, this alliance may lead to better glycemic control by helping the patient address such self-care barriers as low motivation, preconceived judgments about treatment, and fears about diabetes

Detection

The practitioner should be sensitive to possible psychosocial issues when diabetes is first diagnosed and when complications, however minor, first develop.

Some psychosocial barriers stem from personal, family, and cultural beliefs that may conflict with suggested treatment. A patient may resist following a prescribed diet, for instance, because of certain cultural beliefs about weight. Such beliefs should be given their due respect; patients respond best to advice that does not seem to prejudge their beliefs.

Certain medical conditions can be reliable indicators of psychosocial barriers. Recurrent hypoglycemia, frequent episodes of diabetic ketoacidosis, and very high glycosylated hemoglobin levels should each be recognized as a possible sign of personal or family problems. Although brittle, or unstable, diabetes can sometimes have a metabolic basis, interrupted or erratic self-care is by far a more common cause—and psychosocial problems may underlie this cause.

To help uncover problem areas, the practitioner may want to conduct discussions along the following lines:

- Ask patients to describe how they feel about the following issues of self-care: the importance of glycemic control; the feasibility of adhering to a prescribed diet; the importance of self-monitoring of blood glucose; the patient's susceptibility to developing complications; the efficacy of treating complications; the reasonableness of the practitioner's recommendations and expectations.

- Ask patients to describe any stressful events or situations, such as changes in job, school, place of residence, and immediate family (for example, death or divorce). Ask whether any other events could be creating barriers to a self-care program.
- Determine whether patients have adequate social and family support. Specifically, ask patients to whom they can turn for help in caring for themselves.
- Ask about problems concerning mood, anxiety, and sense of well-being.
- Ask young women who might be at risk for eating disorders whether they have skipped insulin doses, dieted excessively, eaten in binges, or vomited.
- Ask specific questions about topics that patients may hesitate to talk about, such as sexual problems.
- Determine how effectively patients use available information about diabetes. Ask whether they find it difficult to retain or add to such knowledge.

Thc practitioner may then be able to counsel patients and provide useful solutions.

Treatment

Try to actively engage the patient in determining as well as pursuing a course of treatment. Ask the patient both specific and open-ended questions. Open-ended questions may elicit information that can help detect problems as well as tailor the course of treatment. Such discussions may identify individual strengths and problem-solving strategies that have helped the patient successfully face previous challenges.

The practitioner will need to identify, for possible referral, mental health professionals who are knowledgeable about diabetes and who can serve as collaborators in treating the patient. If these individuals are not familiar with diabetes, they can be given materials (such as this guide) that provide basic information.

Refer the following persons:

- Parents of children or adolescents in whom diabetes has recently been diagnosed. A single psychosocial evaluation of the family unit may be important to the overall educational process of raising a child who has diabetes.

- Patients who in one year have had two or more episodes of severe hypoglycemia or diabetic ketoacidosis without obvious causes.
- Patients whom you—the health care professional—find frustrating. The mental health professional may prove a valuable consultant for treating these patients.

Remember that diabetes is a chronic illness. Even if treatment activities fail to bring change within a short time, remaining involved with the patient and the patient's family and providing an accepting atmosphere may lead to fincreased motivation for change.

Encourage patients and their families to attend group sessions. Medical and psychosocial information can be given at these sessions, which can also provide a forum for discussion of personal concerns. These sessions can be led by health care professionals, including physicians, nurses, and dietitians, and may meet several times a year. Local diabetes organizations may sponsor or know of such groups.

Patient Education Principles

- Inform patients about the typical personal concerns that come with diabetes, about the problems faced in accepting the disease and adapting to it, and about the impact diabetes has on emotional and social functioning.
- Involve families in treatment and education sessions.
- Encourage parents to help their young children and adolescents who are having problems controlling their diabetes.
- Encourage parents to give adolescents increasing responsibility for their diabetes—but not to force them to take these steps.
- Encourage families to provide help for their older relatives, who may find insulin difficult or frightening to use or who may have trouble changing lifelong dietary habits.
- Encourage families to ensure that school nurses and teachers are educated about the needs of children with diabetes and that nursing homes provide proper treatment to elderly patients with diabetes.

References

Bradley C. Psychological aspects of diabetes. In: Alberti KGMM, Krall LP, eds. *The Diabetes Annual/*1. New York: Elsevier, 1985.

Feste C. *The Physician Within.* Minneapolis: Diabetes Center, 1987.
Jacobson AM, Hauser ST. Behavioral and psychological aspects of diabetes. In: Ellenberg M, Rifkin H, eds. *Diabetes Mellitus: Theory and Practice.* 3rd ed. Vol. 2. New Hyde Park. New York: Medical Examination, 1983.

Acute Glycemic Complications

Introduction

In diabetes mellitus, severe hyperglycemia may result from absolute or relative insulin deficiency. In some patients, the condition may culminate in diabetic ketoacidosis or hyperglycemic hyperosmolar nonketotic coma. Profound hypoglycemia may result from a relative excess of insulin. Symptoms associated with acute hyperglycemia generally develop more slowly (over hours or days) than do symptoms associated with an acute fall in the level of blood glucose (over minutes).

Diabetic Ketoacidosis

Background

Definition. Diabetic ketoacidosis (DKA) develops when absolute insulin deficiency and excess contra-insulin hormones increase hepatic glucose production, decrease peripheral glucose utilization, and stimulate release of fatty acids from fat cells and production of ketones by the liver. These changes cause hyperglycemia, osmotic diuresis, volume depletion, and acidosis.

Occurrence. The annual incidence of DKA ranges from three to eight episodes per 1,000 persons with diabetes. It is much more common among persons with insulin-dependent diabetes mellitus (IDDM) than among those with non-insulin-dependent diabetes mellitus (NIDDM).

DKA may be the initial manifestation of previously unrecognized IDDM. More often, DKA develops in persons known to have diabetes. Patients with IDDM who fail to take insulin or who do not receive extra insulin during flulike illness pneumonia, or myocardial infarction may develop DKA. Patients with NIDDM who experience severe stress may secrete more contra-insulin hormones; these further compromise limited insulin secretion, which may in turn lead to DKA.

Morbidity and mortality. Before insulin was available, patients with diabetes often died of DKA; now, the mortality rate associated with DKA is less than 5%. However, persons who develop DKA experience pain and suffering, lose time from school or work, have increased hospitalization rates, and have high medical costs. Serious medical sequelae include cerebral edema (in young people), aspiration pneumonia, and adult respiratory distress syndrome.

Prevention

Why DKA occurs. Ultimately, DKA results from lack of insulin. Early recognition of metabolic disarray, by monitoring glucose and ketones and by properly using exogenous insulin and fluids, can prevent further decompensation. Thus, DKA should be considered preventable. Said differently, when DKA occurs, a breakdown in care has occurred that should have been prevented.

Three general circumstances may allow DKA to develop:

- Low index of suspicion.
- Inappropriate cessation of insulin therapy.
- Mismanagement of intercurrent illness, often due to inadequate education.

Index of suspicion. Many people may not know the signs and symptoms of diabetes. At times, even when a person seeks medical help, a health care provider may fail to recognize the warning signs of hyperglycemia—particularly when the patient is very young (an infant), is very old (such as an octogenarian), or has unusual symptoms (such as mental deterioration without nausea or vomiting).

Therefore, to prevent DKA or to minimize its extent, the health care provider must have a high index of suspicion for DKA. In emergency rooms, clinics, and physicians' offices, routine use of a glucose/ketone urine dipstick may allow for early identification of decompensating diabetes.

Inappropriate cessation of insulin therapy. Under circumstances such as those described below, insulin therapy may be inappropriately discontinued.

- Adolescents with diabetes may not adhere to a prescribed program, and their parents may not provide appropriate supervision.
- Patients with major emotional or psychosocial problems may fail to adhere to their usual medical program.

Intercurrent illness. Both patients and health care providers may incorrectly assume that when no food or fluid is consumed, no insulin should be taken. However, when ill or stressed, the patient with diabetes should promptly test the glucose level in blood and/or urine and test the urine for ketones. The patient should follow a sick-day protocol and consult with the health care provider. Both patients and providers must understand the proper management of diabetes during intercurrent illness. (See "Guidelines for Sick Days" below.)

The guidelines and record for sick days below are adapted from *Take Charge of Your Diabetes: A Guide for Patients*. Review these guidelines and discuss them with patients before illness occurs. Explain how to keep a record, and stress the importance of self-monitoring.

Guidelines for Sick Days

Keep a daily record of your sick days by following the guidelines below. If you feel too sick to follow any of these guidelines, ask a family member or a friend to help you. By following these instructions and by keeping a diary, you can work with your health care provider to feel better.

Health care provider's name:

Health care provider's telephone number:

1. If you feel too sick to eat normally, call your health care provider right away. Describe in detail how you feel.

2. Keep taking insulin when you feel sick. Don't stop taking insulin even if you can't eat. Your health care provider may change your insulin dose or may tell you to drink liquids that have sugar in them.

3. Weigh yourself every day and write down your weight.

4. Take your temperature every morning and evening. Write down the readings. (For small children or for someone who is breathing through the mouth, use a rectal thermometer.) If your temperature is above normal (99°F), drink extra liquids.

5. If you weigh 80 pounds or more, try to drink at least 12 eight-ounce glasses of liquid per day. Write down how much you drink. If you throw up, call your health care provider right away. You may need to go to the hospital or have special medical treatment.

6. Every 4 hours or before every meal, measure the glucose level in your blood. Write down the results. If the level is less than 60 mg/dL or consistently higher than 240 mg/dL, call your health care provider. Every 4 hours or each time you pass urine, test your urine for ketones and write down the results.

7. If you start to have trouble breathing, call your health care provider (or have someone do it for you) or go to a nearby emergency room.

8. Every 4 to 6 hours, write down whether you feel awake or sleepy. If you feel very sleepy or can't concentrate, have someone call your health care provider right away.

9. If your health care provider asks you to, call every day to describe your daily record. Your health care provider may adjust your daily insulin dosage.

Analysis and referral. For the patient who has experienced DKA, the health care provider should do the following:

- Determine why DKA occurred.
- Assess the patient's self-care practices.
- Modify individual guidelines (as appropriate).
- Implement preventive measures to prevent subsequent episodes.

When recurrent episodes of DKA occur, the practitioner should determine the medical and psychosocial components of the episodes. Patients with difficult-to-manage IDDM should be referred to a diabetologist. Patients with underlying psychosocial problems should be referred to a mental health professional.

Detection

Symptoms. Suspect diabetes and DKA in any person at any age who has symptoms compatible with hyperglycemia and ketosis, including:

- Altered mental status.
- Fatigue.
- Weight loss.
- Blurred vision.
- Thirst.
- Excessive urination.
- Enuresis.
- Abdominal pain.
- Nausea or vomiting.

Results of a simple glucose/ketone urine dipstick may give guiding information about the presence of diabetes or DKA. If glucose or ketones are present in the urine, the blood glucose level must be measured.

Monitoring. All patients with IDDM should be taught to prevent DKA. Encourage patients to monitor their blood glucose level and advise them to monitor the urine for ketones when the blood glucose level is 240 mg/dL or more and/or acute illness develops.

Insist that patients contact you promptly when the blood glucose level remains at 240 mg/dL or more, ketonuria develops, or acute illness persists.

Periodically assess how proficient patients are with self-monitoring and reassess their understanding of self-care during acute illness. (See "Guidelines for Sick Days" above.)

Treatment

Identify the causes of DKA by taking a thorough history, performing a physical examination, and requesting appropriate laboratory tests. In adult patients, an electrocardiogram should be performed to rule out a silent acute myocardial infarction. Treatment should be initiated while this information is being collected.

If DKA is mild and the patient is quickly responding to therapy, replacement of fluids, electrolytes, and insulin may occur in the emergency room. If DKA is more severe, hospitalize the patient at once to ensure adequate treatment and monitoring of the clinical state until recovery ensues. An intensive care unit is the preferred site for the treatment of severe DKA.

Health care providers whose experience with DKA is episodic and infrequent should not hesitate to arrange for the patient's prompt referral to a specialist experienced in the care of patients with DKA. A detailed summary of the treatment of DKA is available in the American Diabetes Association's *Physician's Guide to Insulin-Dependent (Type I) Diabetes.*

Note: See "Patient Education Principles" at the end of this section.

Hyperglycemic Hyperosmolar Nonketotic Coma

Background

Definition. Hyperglycemic hyperosmolar nonketotic coma (HHNKC) is characterized by severe hyperglycemia (glucose level typically greater than 600 to 800 mg/dL), dehydration, and altered mental status—in the absence of ketosis. In HHNKC, hyperglycemia causes glycosuria. Osmotic diuresis results in volume contraction and a reduction in both the glomerular filtration rate and glucose excretion. Worsening hyperglycemia causes further extracellular hypertonicity and intracellular dehydration.

Central nervous system dysfunction in persons with HHNKC is probably due to hyperosmolarity. The absence of ketosis has not been entirely explained but may be due to the secretion of insulin in amounts sufficient to suppress ketogenesis.

Occurrence. HHNKC occurs most often among persons over 60 years of age. Most persons with HHNKC have a history of NIDDM, but in a sizable minority, NIDDM is undiagnosed or untreated. When persons who are chronically ill, debilitated, or institutionalized have mild renal insufficiency and lack normal thirst mechanisms or access to water, they are at risk of developing HHNKC. Acute illnesses (stroke, myocardial infarction, or pneumonia), drugs (diuretics or glucocorticoids), surgery, and, occasionally, large glucose loads (through enteral or parenteral nutrition or peritoneal dialysis) may precipitate HHNKC.

Severity. The mortality rate for HHNKC has been reported to be as high as 50%, primarily because of the age of the population most at risk and the acute precipitating causes.

Prevention

Be alert to the elderly patient who:

- Has a history of NIDDM.
- Has an altered level of consciousness.
- Takes diuretics or glucocorticoids.
- Lacks free access to drinking water.
- Has a poor support system at home or lives in a nursing home.
- Is receiving enteral or parenteral nutrition.

For persons with several of these characteristics, periodically monitor the glucose level in the urine or blood. (Monitoring blood glucose is preferred.) If the fasting blood glucose level is above 200 mg/dL, monitor the glucose level more frequently and initiate or adjust hypoglycemic medications as necessary.

Early diagnosis of diabetes or early identification of worsening hyperglycemia will permit appropriate therapy that will prevent the development of HHNKC.

Detection

The patient with HHNKC has severe hyperglycemia and azotemia without ketoacidosis. The intravascular volume is contracted, and the patient shows signs and symptoms of hypovolemia and severe dehydration. Both diffuse and focal central nervous system deficits may occur. These may include hallucinations, aphasia, nystagmus, hemianopsia, hemiplegia, hemisensory deficits, and focal or grand mat seizures. Coma may ensue.

Treatment

Therapy is primarily directed at replacement of fluid and electrolytes while supportive care is given. Insulin therapy is designed to slowly—over 24 to 48 hours—return the blood glucose level to a near normal range.

When therapy is successful, the patient may be significantly sensitive to further insulin. Ultimately, the patient may achieve metabolic control through diet and/or oral agents.

Note: See "Patient Education Principles" at the end of this section.

Hypoglycemia

Background

Occurrence. Any person with diabetes who takes an oral hypoglycemic agent or insulin may experience low blood glucose. Severe hypoglycemia occurs more often in patients who are following an intensified insulin therapy protocol (with the target glucose level near the normal range), whose diet and activity vary widely, who have a long duration of diabetes, and/or who have autonomic neuropathy. Patients with a history of severe hypoglycemia are at increased risk for future episodes. Often the cause is multifactorial. A delay or decrease in food intake, vigorous physical activity, and alcohol consumption all may contribute.

Prevention

Patient education and self-monitoring of blood glucose are the best approaches to preventing hypoglycemia.

By emphasizing the relation between hypoglycemia and delayed or decreased food intake or increased physical activity, you may help patients anticipate and avoid the condition. If patients regularly and correctly monitor their blood glucose level, impending hypoglycemia may be avoided. Patients who know how to treat hypoglycemia can reduce its impact and severity.

To minimize the risk of hypoglycemia, cooperation is required between the patient, family members, other persons close to the patient (including friends, teachers, and colleagues), and health care providers. Stress the importance of such persons knowing the signs and symptoms of hypoglycemia and how to treat it.

Detection

Clinical hypoglycemia (blood glucose level below approximately 60 mg/dL) is associated with adrenergic symptoms (apprehension, tremors, sweating, or palpitations) and neuroglycopenic symptoms (fatigue, headache, confusion, coma, or seizure). Usually, the symptoms of low blood glucose are mild, related to catecholamine release, and easily treated by the patient.

Severe hypoglycemia occurs when the patient ignores, inappropriately treats, lacks, or does not recognize the early warning signs or when glucose counterregulation fails to return the blood glucose level to normal.

Treatment

Guidelines for treating hypoglycemia are as follows:

Person	Action
Patient	Eat 10 to 15 grams of rapidly absorbable carbohydrate (3 to 5 pieces of hard candy, 2 to 3 packets of sugar, or 4 ounces of fruit juice) to abort the episode. Repeat in 15 minutes, as necessary.
Friend or family member	If the patient is unable to treat himself or herself, administer oral carbohydrate. If the patient is unable to swallow, administer glucagon subcutaneously or intramuscularly. For children younger than 3 years of age, give 0.5 mg glucagon; for children 3 years of age and older and for adults, give 1.0 mg.
Practitioner	If the patient shows signs and symptoms of severe hypoglycemia, administer glucagon or inject 25 grams of sterile 50% glucose intravenously. Analyze the cause of the episode. Often, a modest reduction in the insulin dosage should be advised. Reeducate the patient about preventing hypoglycemia by discussing the timing of meals and physical activity, the use of alcohol, and the frequency of self-monitoring of blood glucose. Those patients who develop hypoglycemia while taking oral hypoglycemic agents should be closely monitored for at least 48 to 72 hours to prevent a possible recurrence.

Teaching Patients to Avoid Acute Glycemic Complications

Thorough and repetitive patient education is essential to preventing the development of acute glycemic complications. In particular, teach patients how to care for themselves when they are ill and how to monitor themselves.

Patient Education Principles

For patients with diabetic ketoacidosis

- Be sure your patients with diabetes know the following: If they are at risk for DKA; When they are most susceptible to DKA; What they can do to prevent DKA; When they should contact you.

For patients with hyperglycemic hyperosmolar nonketotic coma

- Remind persons responsible for the elderly the infirm, or the chronically ill to look for the signs and symptoms of diabetes when their patients do not thrive. Recommend that a blood glucose screening test be performed at the bedside.

For patients with hypoglycemia

- Ensure that patients who use oral hypoglycemic agents or insulin understand the signs and symptoms, causes, and treatment of hypoglycemia.
- Instruct patients who use oral hypoglycemic agents or insulin to wear a bracelet or necklace that identifies them as having diabetes and to carry sugar or some other source of simple carbohydrate that can be used to promptly treat hypoglycemia.
- Advise persons with diabetes to tell close friends, teachers, or colleagues about their diabetes, how to recognize hypoglycemia, and what to do if an emergency occurs.
- Ensure that patients particularly prone to hypoglycemia who are treated with insulin have glucagon available and that family members and friends know how to administer it.
- Instruct patients with diminished awareness of the signs and symptoms of hypoglycemia to monitor their blood glucose levels at frequent intervals so that unexpected episodes can be recognized early and more severe hypoglycemia forestalled.
- Consider changing the level of diabetes control in the following patients: Those who do not or cannot recognize the early warning signs of hypoglycemia; Those who do not understand the educational

details of avoiding or treating hypoglycemia; Those whose lifestyle makes them vulnerable to life-threatening episodes of hypoglycemia.

References

Bergenstal RM. Diabetic ketoacidosis. *Postgraduate Medicine*. 1985;77:151–161.

Butts DE. Fluid and electrolyte disorders associated with diabetic ketoacidosis and hyperglycemic hyperosmolar nonketotic coma. *Nursing Clinics of North America*. 1987;22:827–836.

Carroll P, Matz R. Uncontrolled diabetes in adults. *Diabetes Care*. 1983;6:579–585.

Casparie AF, Elzing LD. Severe hypoglycemia in diabetic patients. *Diabetes Care*. 1985;8:141–145.

Consensus statement of self-monitoring of blood glucose. *Diabetes Care*. 1987;10: 95–99

The DCCT Research Group. Diabetes Control and Complications Trial (DCCT): results of feasibility study. *Diabetes Care*. 1987;10:1–19.

Foster DW, McGarry JD. The metabolic derangements and treatment of diabetic ketoacidosis. *New England Journal of Medicine*. 1983;309:159–169.

Keller U. Diabetic ketoacidosis: current views on pathogenesis and treatment. *Diabetologia*. 1986;29:71–77.

Kitabchi AE, Matteri R. Murphy MB. Optimal insulin delivery in diabetic ketoacidosis and hyperglycemic, hyperosmolar nonketotic coma. *Diabetes Care*. 1982;5(suppl 1):78–87.

Physician's Guide to Insulin-Dependent (Type I) Diabetes: Diagnosis and Treatment. Alexandria, Virginia: American Diabetes Association, 1988.

Physician's Guide to Non-Insulin-Dependent (Type 11) Diabetes: Diagnosis and Treatment. 2nd ed. Alexandria, Virginia: American Diabetes Association, 1988.

Sperling MA. Diabetic ketoacidosis. *Pediatric Clinics of North America*. 1984;31: 591–610.

Adverse Outcomes of Pregnancy

Introduction

When a woman who is known to have diabetes becomes pregnant, she is said to have pregestational diabetes. When a woman develops diabetes during pregnancy or is first recognized as having this condition during pregnancy, she is said to have gestational diabetes. Each year, approximately 10,000 infants are born to women with pregestational diabetes, and 60,000 to 90,000 infants are born to women with gestational diabetes.

The factor most important to the outcome of pregnancy is how well the mother's glucose level is controlled before and during pregnancy. When women with diabetes receive optimal care, the perinatal mortality rate for their offspring approaches the corresponding rate for the general population. However, when pregnant women with diabetes do not receive expert treatment, the perinatal mortality rate for their offspring more than doubles.

Pregestational and Gestational Diabetes

Background

Metabolic changes. Normal pregnancy is characterized by increasing insulin resistance, which is probably due to human placental lactogen, a growth-hormone-like protein secreted by the placenta. Although pregnant women develop compensatory hyperinsulinemia, postprandial glucose levels increase significantly throughout pregnancy. During late pregnancy, fasting glucose levels fall because of increased glucose consumption by the placenta and the fetus.

Human placental lactogen reaches its peak late in pregnancy; during the third trimester, insulin requirements rise. Gestational diabetes most often appears during this period of maximum insulin resistance, and ketoacidosis may be seen—particularly in patients with insulin-dependent diabetes mellitus who do not increase their insulin dose appropriately.

Effect on the fetus. Because glucose crosses the placenta by facilitated diffusion, maternal hyperglycemia produces fetal hyperglycemia. Fetal hyperinsulinemia occurs in response to this abnormal metabolic environment. Hyperinsulinemia, combined with hyperglycemia, leads to excessive fetal growth. It may also contribute to intrauterine fetal death, delayed fetal pulmonary maturation, and neonatal hypoglycemia.

The incidence of major congenital malformations is increased approximately fourfold among infants of women with pregestational diabetes. Approximately 9% of pregnancies complicated by pregestational diabetes result in the birth of infants with central nervous system, cardiac, renal, skeletal, and other malformations. Major malformations may occur in 20% to 25% of infants born to women with very poor glycemia control during organogenesis, as evidenced by markedly elevated glycosylated hemoglobin levels during the first trimester.

Other factors that may increase the risk for fetal anomalies include early age at onset of maternal diabetes and microvascular disease in the mother. The earlier the age at onset of pregestational diabetes, the worse the prognosis is for successful pregnancy.

Effect on the mother. Pregnancy may be associated with exacerbation of diabetic eye disease, especially in women with unrecognized or untreated proliferative diabetic retinopathy. Diabetic women with nephropathy and hypertension are at greater risk for preeclampsia and fetal growth retardation than are women without nephropathy. Death has been reported among pregnant women with diabetes and coronary artery disease.

Caring for the Patient With Pregestational Diabetes

Prevention

The outcome of pregnancy complicated by pregestational diabetes is improved when care begins before conception. Each visit with a woman of childbearing age who has diabetes should be considered a preconceptional visit. Discuss family planning and ask the patient her thoughts about a future pregnancy.

Results of a glycosylated hemoglobin test provide overall assessment of glycemic control. Pregnancy should be deferred until excellent glycemic control is achieved, as indicated by a normal or near normal glycosylated hemoglobin level. Counsel patients about nutrition and teach them how to monitor their blood glucose levels and how to adjust their insulin treatment.

For patients who are planning to become pregnant, establish baseline data that can be used to assess maternal and perinatal risk, including the following:

- History of diabetic ketoacidosis and severe hypoglycemia.
- Blood pressure measurement.
- Eye examination.
- Quantitative assessment of renal function and urinary protein or albumin excretion.
- Electrocardiogram (if indicated).

Patients whose pregnancy is complicated by diabetes often experience significant emotional and financial stresses. Assess the patient's emotional or psychosocial support and financial resources through discussion with the patient, her partner, and her family.

Emphasize the dangers of smoking and of consuming alcohol when pregnant.

Treatment

Health care team. An experienced health care team is required to care for a patient with pregestational diabetes. The team should include the following persons:

- An obstetrician or a specialist in maternal-fetal medicine.
- An internist or diabetologist.
- A pediatrician or neonatologist.
- A diabetes educator.
- A dietitian.
- A social worker.

Every effort should be made to refer patients to medical centers that can provide comprehensive support. If such referral is not possible, members of the health care team should frequently consult with each other by telephone.

Glucose level. Excellent control of maternal diabetes is a critical objective both before and during pregnancy. During normal pregnancy, mean maternal plasma glucose levels rarely exceed 120 mg/dL and range from fasting levels of 60 mg/dL to 2-hour postprandial levels of 120 mg/dL. Use these values as the therapeutic objective for patients whose pregnancies are complicated by pregestational diabetes.

Diet. During the latter half of pregnancy, the patient with pregestational diabetes needs to eat approximately 35 kilocalories per kilogram of her ideal prepregnancy body weight each day, or approximately 2200 to 2400 calories per day. A weight gain of 24 to 28 pounds is recommended for most patients; however, for obese patients with noninsulin-dependent diabetes mellitus, the preferred daily dietary intake is 25 kilocalories per kilogram of ideal prepregnancy body weight, or approximately 1600 to 1800 calories per day.

The calories should be derived as follows: approximately 50% from complex carbohydrates, 30% from fats, and 20% from proteins. Patients will require three meals and up to three snacks each day. A bedtime snack is particularly important to decrease the risk of nocturnal hypoglycemia.

Monitoring. Patients with insulin-treated diabetes should monitor their blood glucose levels at least four times a day either before or 2 hours after each meal and at bedtime. Before breakfast, patients should test for ketones in their urine. Ask patients to record results in a log book and to note any changes in diet and exercise and any problems with hypoglycemia.

Measure the glycosylated hemoglobin level at least once each trimester to assess overall glycemic control.

Insulin therapy. Patients treated with oral hypoglycemic agents should be switched to insulin before they become pregnant. Human insulin should generally be used. Patients with insulin-treated diabetes require an individualized insulin regimen based on their exercise plan and blood glucose levels.

Most patients will require at least two injections a day of a mixture of intermediate-acting (NPH or lente) and short-acting (regular) insulin. Selected patients may be treated with multiple daily injections (that is, regular insulin before each meal and an injection of intermediate- or long-acting (ultralente) insulin at bedtime). For some patients, continuous subcutaneous insulin infusion is an option, but it appears to offer no significant advantage over multiple daily injections. Patients who prefer the flexibility offered by the pump may be started on such therapy, and those who have used a pump before pregnancy may continue to do so.

Fetal assessment. Maintain a program of fetal assessment throughout pregnancy. Measure the maternal serum alpha-fetoprotein level at 16 weeks of gestation to screen for neural tube defects and other fetal anomalies. Perform a detailed ultrasonographic examination at 16 to 18 weeks of gestation. If indicated, assess the fetal cardiac structure by echocardiography at 20 weeks of gestation. When performed by experienced professionals, such tests allow detection of most major fetal malformations. If an anomaly is found skilled counseling must be provided for the patient.

During the third trimester, assessment of fetal growth and well-being becomes most important. Fetal growth may be evaluated by serial ultrasonographic examination every 4 to 6 weeks. Fetal well-being may be determined by a variety of techniques, including the following:

- Maternal monitoring of fetal activity.
- Antepartum heart rate testing by using the nonstress or contraction stress test.
- Biophysical profile that includes an ultrasonographic evaluation of fetal activity, fetal breathing movements, fetal tone, and amniotic fluid volume.

Although these tests may be initiated at 28 weeks of gestation, they are most often begun at 32 weeks and performed once or twice a week until delivery.

Delivery. If the patient maintains excellent glucose control, if her blood pressure is normal, and if antepartum fetal testing shows no evidence of fetal compromise, delivery may occur at term. If delivery is planned before term, assess fetal pulmonary maturation by measuring the ratio of amniotic fluid lecithin to sphingomyelin (L/S) and the level of acidic phospholipid phosphatidyglycerol. If ultrasound suggests excessive fetal size, delivery by cesarean section may be elected.

Delivery must take place where expert maternal and neonatal care are available. Breast-feeding should be encouraged.

Postpartum care. In the immediate postpartum period, reassess the patient's meal plan and adjust her treatment program. Maternal insulin requirements fall significantly, usually to—or even below—prepregnancy levels.

During the patient's postpartum follow-up visit, encourage her to diet, if necessary, to achieve her ideal body weight. Contraception should be discussed. Low-dose oral contraceptives or a progestin-only pill may be offered to patients who have no evidence of hypertension or vascular disease. For patients with hypertension or vascular disease, a barrier method of contraception, such as a diaphragm, is preferred. If the patient has completed her family or if she has serious vascular disease, sterilization should be discussed.

Caring for the Patient With Gestational Diabetes

Detection

Screening. All pregnant women should be screened for gestational diabetes. If only those patients with recognized historical or clinical risk factors are screened, a significant number of cases of gestational diabetes will be missed.

Timing. Screen for gestational diabetes at approximately 24 to 28 weeks of gestation. Screening may be indicated before 24 weeks if the patient has a history of any of the following:

- Polydipsia or polyuria.
- Recurrent vaginal and/or urinary tract infections.
- Glycosuria of 1+ or greater on two or more occasions or 2+ or greater on one occasion.
- Hydramnios.
- Having given birth to an infant who was large for gestational age.
- Gestational diabetes

Method for screening. Patients need not be fasting when the screening test is performed. Use a 50-gram oral glucose load and measure the patient's glucose level after one hour. If the venous plasma glucose is 140 mg/dL or higher, schedule a 100-gram oral glucose tolerance test (see next paragraph).

Method for diagnosis. In pregnancy, the oral glucose tolerance test should be performed as follows:

- Perform the test in the morning, after at least 3 days of unrestricted diet (more than 150 grams of carbohydrate per day) and unrestricted physical activity and after an overnight fast of at least 8 hours but not more than 14 hours.
- Ask the patient to remain seated. If she smokes, ask her not to do so during the test.
- Administer a 100-gram oral glucose load.
- Measure venous plasma glucose when the patient is fasting and at 1, 2, and 3 hours after administering the glucose load.

- Diagnose gestational diabetes when two or more of the following concentrations are met or exceeded.

Time of Test	Glucose Concentration
Fasting	105 mg/dL
After glucose	
1 hour	190 mg/dL
2 hours	165 mg/dL
3 hours	145 mg/dL

- If the initial glucose tolerance test is normal but the patient is thought to be at high risk for gestational diabetes, or if one concentration is met or exceeded, consider repeating the glucose tolerance test at 32 weeks of gestation.

Although blood glucose measurements using glucose-oxidase-impregnated test strips are useful for monitoring treatment, they are not sufficiently precise for diagnostic purposes. Glycosuria and glycosylated hemoglobin tests are also not sensitive enough to be used to diagnose gestational diabetes.

Treatment

Most women with gestational diabetes can be cared for as outpatients. The patient should be seen at 1- to 2-week intervals to assess glucose control, weight gain, and blood pressure. The patient may need to be hospitalized if she does not maintain acceptable glucose control or if she develops hypertension or an infectious complication such as pyelonephritis.

Diet. Dietary therapy is the mainstay of treatment for patients with gestational diabetes. The daily dietary plan should contain approximately 2000 to 2400 calories distributed among three meals and a bedtime snack.

Monitoring. Ideally, the efficacy of the diet is assessed by daily self-monitoring of blood glucose. Weekly measurements of fasting and postprandial glucose levels are also an acceptable method of monitoring.

Pharmacologic therapy. If the fasting plasma glucose level exceeds 105 mg/dL and/or the 2-hour postprandial value exceeds 120 mg/dL, treatment with human insulin should be initiated. Patients who require insulin should be instructed in glucose self-monitoring.

Oral hypoglycemic agents should not be used during pregnancy.

Fetal assessment. Patients with insulin-treated gestational diabetes require a program of fetal surveillance identical to that recommended for patients with pregestational diabetes (see the earlier discussion). Begin fetal surveillance by 34 weeks of gestation for patients with non-insulin-treated gestational diabetes who develop preeclampsia or have a history of intrauterine death. Begin fetal surveillance at 40 weeks of gestation for patients with uncomplicated non-insulin-treated gestational diabetes who have not delivered.

Postpartum care. All patients with gestational diabetes should undergo a 75-gram oral glucose tolerance test at 6 to 8 weeks postpartum to determine whether abnormal carbohydrate metabolism has persisted.

The glucose tolerance test should be performed as follows:

- Perform the test in the morning, after at least 3 days of unrestricted diet (more than 150 grams of carbohydrate per day) and unrestricted physical activity and after an overnight fast of between 8 and 14 hours.
- Ask the patient to remain seated. If she smokes, ask her not to do so during the test.
- Administer a 75-gram oral glucose load.
- Measure the venous plasma glucose when the patient is fasting and 30, 60, 90, and 120 minutes after administering the glucose load.

Diagnose abnormal glucose tolerance according to the following criteria:

	Glucose Concentration		
Time of Test	Normal Glucose Tolerance	Impaired Glucose Tolerance	Diabetes Mellitus
Fasting	<115 mg/dL *and*	<140 mg/dL *and*	>140 mg/dL *or*
After glucose (30, 60, and 90 minutes)	<200 mg/dL mg/dl *and*	1 value >200 mg/dL *and*	1 value >200 mg/dL *and*
120 minutes	<140 mg/dL	>140 mg/dL but <200 mg/dL	>200 mg/dL

Encourage patients to achieve their ideal body weight to decrease their likelihood of developing non-insulin-dependent diabetes mellitus. Patients with a history of gestational diabetes should be annually evaluated for onset of diabetes.

For contraception, patients may use low-dose oral contraceptive pills, progestin-only pills, or barrier methods.

Patient Education Principles

For patients with pregestational diabetes

- Emphasize the importance of prepregnancy care.
- Work with the patient, her partner, her family, and other health care providers to improve the patient's nutrition, exercise program, and glucose control.
- Recommend that conception be delayed until the patient's blood glucose control is excellent and the glycosylated hemoglobin level is normal or near normal.
- Explain the risks of birth defects and adverse perinatal outcomes and the need for fetal surveillance.
- Recommend that the patient's vascular condition be thoroughly evaluated before she becomes pregnant. Explain that pregnancy may exacerbate advanced diabetic retinopathy but generally does not permanently worsen diabetic nephropathy.
- Explain that, overall, pregnancy does not shorten the life expectancy of a woman with diabetes but does increase her risk for hypoglycemia and ketoacidosis and for associated mortality.
- Inform patients with coronary atherosclerosis that their risks for morbidity or mortality may be greater during pregnancy.
- Discuss the emotional and financial demands of pregnancy with the patient, her partner, and her family.
- Inform patients about lifestyle elements—such as drinking alcoholic beverages and smoking—that increase the risk for a poor outcome of pregnancy. Emphasize that patients will need to modify such behaviors before becoming pregnant.

For patients with gestational diabetes

- Work with the patient, her partner, her family, and other health care providers to improve the patient's nutrition, exercise program, and glucose control.
- Explain the risks of adverse perinatal outcomes and the need for fetal surveillance.

- Inform patients that they are at increased risk both for developing gestational diabetes during future pregnancies and for developing overt diabetes later in life.
- Encourage physical activity and postpartum weight loss to decrease the likelihood of developing diabetes later in life.
- Recommend an evaluation at 6 to 8 weeks postpartum, and annually thereafter, for detecting the development of diabetes.

For patients with a history of gestational diabetes

- Recommend screening for overt diabetes before subsequent pregnancies.
- Recommend early screening for the onset of carbohydrate intolerance during subsequent pregnancies.

References

Freinkel N, Dooley SL, Metzger BE. Care of the pregnant woman with insulin-dependent diabetes mellitus. *New England Journal of Medicine.* 1985;313:96–101.

Freinkel N, Gabbe SG, Hadden DR, et al. Summary and recommendations of the Second International Workshop-Conference on Gestational Diabetes Mellitus. *Diabetes.* 1985;34(suppl 2): 123–126.

Fuhrmann K, Reiher H. Semmler K, Fischer F. Fischer M, Glockner E. Prevention of congenital malformations in infants of insulin-dependent diabetic mothers. *Diabetes Care.* 1983;6:219–223.

Gabbe SG. Management of diabetes mellitus in pregnancy. *American Journal of Obstetrics and Gynecology.* 1985;153:824–828.

Greene MF, Hare JW, Cloherty JP, et al. First-trimester hemoglobin A_1 and risk for major malformation and spontaneous abortion in diabetic pregnancy. *Teratology.* 1989;39:225–231.

Landon MB, Gabbe SG. Glucose monitoring and insulin administration in the pregnant diabetic patient. *Clinical Obstetrics and Gynecology.* 1985;28:496–506.

Mills JL, Knopp RH, Simpson JL, et al. Lack of relation of increased malformation rates in infants of diabetic mothers to glycemic control during organogenesis. *New England Journal of Medicine.* 1988;318:671–676.

Mills JL, Simpson JL, Driscoll SG, et al. Incidence of spontaneous abortion among normal women and insulin-dependent diabetic women whose pregnancies were identified within 21 days of conception. *New England Journal of Medicine.* 1988;319:1617–1623.

Schwartz R. The infant of the diabetic mother. In: Davidson JK, ed. *Clinical Diabetes Mellitus.* New York: Thieme, 1986.

Steel JM. Prepregnancy counseling and contraception in the insulin-dependent diabetic patient. *Clinical Obstetrics and Gynecology.* 1985;28:553–566.

Periodontal Disease

Background

Definition. The term periodontal disease describes a group of localized infections that affect the tissue surrounding and supporting the teeth.

The two most common forms of periodontal disease are gingivitis and periodontitis. Gingivitis, an early and reversible condition, is an inflammation of the soft tissues surrounding the teeth. Persons with gingivitis have tender, edematous, red gums that may bleed upon gentle pressure, such as from toothbrushing.

Periodontitis is a progressive inflammatory condition that destroys periodontal ligament fibers and alveolar bone and can eventually cause tooth loss. Although gingivitis usually precedes periodontitis, not all gingivitis progresses to periodontitis.

For all persons, the keys to preventing periodontal disease are good oral hygiene and regular dental care. A third element crucial to persons with diabetes is good glycemic control; poorly controlled diabetes can invite or promote periodontal disease.

Occurrence. Periodontal disease is widely prevalent. Forty to 50% of U.S. adults report gingival bleeding, and over 80% of adults have objective evidence of previous periodontal disease. The prevalence and severity of periodontal disease increase markedly with age. Eight percent of adults younger than age 65 and 34% of adults 65 and older have evidence of advanced periodontal destruction.

Among children and adolescents with poorly controlled insulin-dependent diabetes mellitus and among adults with poorly controlled non-insulin-dependent diabetes mellitus, the prevalence of periodontal disease is considerably greater than it is among their nondiabetic peers. The severity of periodontal disease is also usually greater among persons with diabetes.

Pathophysiology. Periodontal disease is initiated by the toxic metabolic products of bacteria in dental plaque. Other associated factors include smoking, vitamin C deficiency, dental restorations, and prostheses.

Periodontal disease appears to be aggravated by increased levels of blood glucose and by other conditions associated with poor glycemic control. Altered microbial flora, impaired immunity, vascular changes, and abnormal collagen metabolism may contribute to the development and severity of periodontal disease among persons with diabetes.

Prevention

Effective self-care is essential to periodontal health. To ensure that patients with diabetes are aware of the importance of maintaining good glycemic control as well as an effective regimen of oral hygiene, the health care provider should do the following:

- Inform patients of their increased risk of developing periodontal disease.
- Inform patients of the association between poor glycemic control and periodontal disease.
- Explain that severe periodontal disease and other oral infections may adversely affect glycemic control.
- Motivate patients to care for their teeth and gums: explain how dental plaque contributes to periodontal disease; inform patients that they can partly remove plaque by brushing and flossing their teeth at least twice a day; explain that teeth lost to periodontal disease may be difficult to replace. Dentures often fit poorly over gums damaged by periodontitis; the resulting discomfort may limit a patient's dietary choices and may thus impede diabetes management.

To ensure that patients receive the regular professional dental care critical to preventing periodontal disease, the health care provider should do the following:

- Instruct patients to see a dentist at least every 6 months. Patients with periodontal disease will need to schedule more frequent appointments.
- Provide a list of recommended dentists or local dental clinics if the patient does not have a dentist.
- Urge patients to inform their dentist that they have diabetes. If possible, ask for the dentist's name and telephone number; you may need to alert this person to the special problems of treating a person with diabetes.

Efficient brushing and flossing removes the more superficial supragingival dental plaque. Subgingival plaque, as well as calculus (hard deposits of plaque, also called tartar), will require professional removal. For some patients, the dentist may prescribe antiplaque rinses, such as chlorhexidene.

To evaluate personal oral hygiene, the dentist or dental hygienist should ask patients to demonstrate how they remove plaque. Patients can then be shown, if necessary, how to more effectively care for their teeth.

Detection

To determine whether a patient is at increased risk for developing periodontal disease, the health care provider should ask about the patient's oral hygiene habits. Does the patient brush and floss twice daily? Does the patient use any other devices for cleaning teeth? When did the patient last see a dentist? Is the patient experiencing any of the following: bad taste in the mouth, bad breath, sore gums, swollen or red gums, bleeding gums, difficulty chewing, loose teeth, or oral pain?

The health care provider should inspect the patient's mouth for the following signs of dental disease:

- Puffy, red gums.
- A buildup of plaque.
- Obviously decayed teeth.
- The characteristic bad breath of periodontitis.

Patients showing these possible indicators of periodontal disease should be referred to a dentist.

Severe periodontal disease can be present without obvious inflammation. A complete dental examination, including periodontal probing of gum pockets, is necessary to determine the presence and severity of periodontal infection.

Treatment

The health care provider can treat periodontal disease by helping the patient achieve good glycemic control. Further measures fall to the dental health professional, who initially treats periodontal disease by removing plaque from infected areas of the patient's mouth. If infection or destruction has progressed too far, the dentist may prescribe antibiotic treatment, perform restorative procedures, perform surgery, or extract teeth.

The health care provider should work with the dentist in planning treatment and scheduling dental appointments. The health care provider should also be consulted before the patient is pretreated with an antibiotic or is hospitalized.

Patient Education Principles

- Help patients maintain good control of their blood glucose levels.
- Instruct patients to do the following to remove plaque: brush their teeth with a soft toothbrush and a fluoridated toothpaste at least twice a day, especially before going to sleep; rinse their toothbrush thoroughly after each brushing, store it vertically (with the bristles at the top), and replace it at least every 3 months. (Toothbrushes can harbor bacteria.); use dental floss, bridge cleaners, water sprayers, or other cleaning aids recommended by their dentist;

- Emphasize the importance of seeking regular preventive dental care at least every 6 months (or according to the dentist's recommended schedule).
- Encourage patients to ask their dentist for further instructions or advice on caring for their teeth.
- Instruct patients to see a dentist if they have bad breath, an unpleasant taste in the mouth, bleeding gums, sore gums or teeth, red or swollen gums, difficulty chewing, or loose teeth.
- Urge patients to inform their dentist that they have diabetes and to remind their dentist of this when they make appointments. Patients should also give their dentist their health care provider's name and telephone number.
- Stress the importance of scheduling dental appointments that do not interfere with the patient's insulin and meal schedule. The best time for an appointment may be a few hours after breakfast. Tell patients not to skip a meal or insulin before an appointment.

References

Epidemiology and Oral Disease Prevention Program, National Institute of Dental Research. *Oral Health of United States Adults—the National Survey of Oral Health in US Employed Adults and Seniors: 1985–1986.* Bethesda, Maryland: US Department of Health and Human Services, Public Health Service, 1987. Publication NIH 87–2868.

Manouchehr-Pour M, Bissada NF. Periodontal disease in juvenile and adult diabetic patients: a review of the literature. *Journal of the American Dental Association.* 1983;107:766–770.

Murrah VA. Diabetes mellitus and associated oral manifestations: a review. *Journal of Oral Pathology.* 1985;14:271–281.

National Institute of Dental Research. *Detection and Prevention of Periodontal Disease in Diabetes.* Bethesda, Maryland: US Department of Health and Human Services, Public Health Service, 1986. Publication NIH 86–1148.

Williams RC. Periodontal disease. *New England Journal of Medicine.* 1990;322: 373–382.

Eye Disease

Background

Diabetes mellitus is a major cause of blindness in the United States and is the leading cause of new blindness in working-aged Americans. Diabetic retinopathy alone accounts for at least 12% of new cases of blindness each year in the United States. People with diabetes are 25 times more at risk for blindness than the general population. The estimated annual incidence of new cases of proliferative diabetic retinopathy and diabetic macular edema are 65,000 and 75,000, respectively. Approximately 700,000 Americans have proliferative diabetic retinopathy—the most sight-threatening form of retinopathy—and 500,000 have diabetic macular edema. Over a lifetime, 70% of people with insulin-dependent diabetes mellitus (IDDM) will develop proliferative diabetic retinopathy, and 40% will develop macular edema. Both complications, if untreated, frequently lead to serious visual loss and disability.

Diabetic retinopathy is often asymptomatic in its most treatable stages. Unfortunately, only about half of persons with diabetes receive adequate eye care. Early detection of diabetic retinopathy is critical.

The results of National Eye Institute-supported multicenter clinical trials of laser surgery and vitrectomy surgery have demonstrated that the risk of blindness from diabetes can be reduced.

- Timely laser surgery can reduce the risk of visual loss from high-risk proliferative diabetic retinopathy by approximately 60%.
- Timely laser surgery can reduce the risk of moderate visual loss from clinically significant diabetic macular edema by 50%.
- Vitrectomy can restore useful vision in some diabetic patients whose retinopathy is too advanced for laser surgery.

Diabetic retinopathy and macular edema. The process by which diabetes results in retinopathy and macular edema is not fully understood. It is known that diabetes causes the retinal capillaries to become functionally less competent. Five clinical pathological processes can be recognized in diabetic retinopathy:

- Formation of microaneurysms (outpouchings of the capillary walls).
- Increased vascular permeability of retinal capillaries.
- Closure of retinal capillaries and arterioles.
- Proliferation of new vessels and fibrous tissues.
- Contraction of fibrous tissue and hemorrhage and/or retinal detachment due to traction.

Nonproliferative and proliferative diabetic retinopathy and macular edema have several clinical manifestations. Diabetic macular edema can be associated with any stage of diabetic retinopathy.

* * *

Clinical Manifestations of Eye Diseases

Nonproliferative Diabetic Retinopathy

- *Nonproliferative Diabetic Retinopathy*

- Retinal microaneurysms.
- Occasional blot hemorrhages.
- Hard exudates.
- One or two soft exudates.

- *Preproliferative Diabetic Retinopathy*

- Presence of venous beading.
- Significant areas of large retinal blot hemorrhages.
- Multiple cotton wool spots (nerve fiber infarcts).
- Multiple intraretinal microvascular abnormalities.

Proliferative Diabetic Retinopathy

- New vessels on the disc (NVD).
- New vessels elsewhere on the retina (NVE).
- Preretinal or vitreous hemorrhage.
- Fibrous tissue proliferation.

High-Risk Proliferative Diabetic Retinopathy

- NVD with or without preretinal or vitreous hemorrhage.
- NVE with preretinal or vitreous hemorrhage.

Diabetic Macular Edema

- Any thickening of retina < 2 disc diameters from center of macula.
- Any hard exudate < 2 disc diameters from center of macula with associated thickening of the retina.

- Any nonperfused retina inside the temporal vessel arcades.
- Any combination of the above.

* * *

Cataracts. Cataracts are 1.6 times more common in people with diabetes than in those without diabetes. Furthermore, cataracts occur at a younger age and progress more rapidly in people with diabetes. Young people with IDDM occasionally develop snowflake or metabolic cataracts. These may lessen or resolve with improved glycemic control. Fortunately, cataract extraction with or without lens implantation is 90% to 95% successful in restoring useful vision, but the surgery is not without potential complications that are more frequent in patients with diabetes.

Open-angle glaucoma. Open-angle glaucoma is 1.4 times more common in the diabetic population. The prevalence of glaucoma increases with the patient's age and with the length of time the patient has had diabetes. Medical therapy for open-angle glaucoma is generally effective. Argon laser trabeculoplasty may normalize intraocular pressure in over 80% of patients in whom medical therapy has proven ineffective.

Neovascular glaucoma. Neovascular glaucoma is a more severe type of glaucoma that most commonly occurs among patients with severe proliferative diabetic retinopathy and retinal detachments. It occasionally follows vitrectomy or cataract surgery. Early recognition and emergency panretinal laser surgery may prevent full development of this devastating type of glaucoma. Diagnosis and evaluation require slit-lamp examination of the iris and gonioscopic evaluation of the filtration angle.

Prevention of Diabetic Retinopathy

Epidemiological studies have suggested that diabetic retinopathy and diabetic macular edema are associated with poorer glycemic control and higher blood pressure levels. Health care providers should work with their patients to achieve good blood glucose and blood pressure control. While the National Institute of Health-sponsored Diabetes Control and Complications Trial is investigating whether very strict control of blood glucose levels is effective in preventing development of retinopathy and slowing its progression, it is prudent to maintain good control of blood glucose levels without causing significant hypoglycemia.

Because coexisting medical problems—including hypertension and renal disease—may affect the development and progression of diabetic retinopathy, blood pressure should be routinely measured. If hypertension exists even at borderline levels, it should be monitored and treated as needed. Aspirin treatment (650 mg per day) neither alters the progression of diabetic retinopathy nor increases the risk of vitreous hemorrhage. Therefore, diabetic retinopathy is not a contraindication for the medical use of aspirin.

Because diabetic retinopathy and diabetic macular edema cannot be prevented, routine early evaluation, timely laser surgery, and careful follow-up are critical.

Detection and Monitoring of Diabetic Retinopathy

Laser surgery, as defined by the National Eye Institute-sponsored Diabetic Retinopathy Study and Early Treatment Diabetic Retinopathy Study, can ameliorate the devastating effects of diabetic retinal disease, particularly when laser surgery is initiated at the most treatable stages. Emphasis, therefore, must be placed on early detection of diabetic retinopathy and timely referral to ophthalmologists experienced in the management of diabetic eye disease. Because mild, moderate, and even severe retinopathy may be present without any symptoms, the responsibility to screen or examine the patient with diabetes for retinopathy is significant.

The following examination schedule is designed to ensure the early detection and monitoring of diabetic eye disease:

- All patients with IDDM of more than five years' duration and all patients with non-insulin-dependent diabetes mellitus should have yearly eye examinations including a history of visual symptoms, measurement of visual acuity, measurement of intraocular pressure, and dilation of the pupils with thorough vitreous and retinal examination including stereoscopic examination of the macula.
- Retinopathy may progress more rapidly during puberty. Children in this developmental stage should have yearly eye examinations, regardless of how long they have had diabetes.
- Any woman who is planning pregnancy should be examined before pregnancy by a practitioner experienced in the diagnosis and classification of diabetic retinopathy. Any woman with known diabetes who becomes pregnant should be examined for retinopathy early in the first trimester. Retinopathy may progress very rapidly during pregnancy; close cooperation among the health care team is critical.

The practitioner may elect to perform the examination, but because proper stereoscopic examination requires dilation of the pupils and specialized techniques, such as binocular indirect ophthalmoscopy, referral to ophthalmologists or optometrists appropriately trained and skilled in the diagnosis and classification of diabetic eye disease is preferred.

After the initial eye examination, persons with diabetes should receive complete examinations once a year, unless more frequent examinations are indicated by the presence of abnormalities.

The patient should be under the care of a retinal specialist or ophthalmologist experienced in the treatment of diabetic retinopathy when any of the following conditions are identified:

- Proliferative retinopathy.
- Macular edema.
- Preproliferative retinopathy (severe or very severe nonproliferative retinopathy).
- Nonproliferative retinopathy in children during puberty or women during pregnancy.

People with any degree of retinal disease—including those who have lost vision from retinopathy—should continue to receive regular eye care. Vitrectomy surgery may restore usable vision for some individuals who have lost sight from vitreous hemorrhage or fibrous tissue proliferation with traction detachment. Postsurgical treatment requires proper refraction, low vision evaluation, optical aids, and other techniques and devices to enable the person to use even severely limited vision. Referral to optometrists or ophthalmologists specializing in low vision may be appropriate. Support groups for the visually challenged and organizations providing vocational rehabilitation are available in most areas. All practitioners should be familiar with appropriate rehabilitative referral sources for their patients with visual impairment.

Treatment and Referral

Patients with high-risk proliferative diabetic retinopathy should receive immediate laser photocoagulation surgery. Some patients with diabetic macular edema are candidates for immediate macular laser surgery. If careful follow-up can be maintained, it is safe to defer treatment in those with severe nonproliferative diabetic retinopathy and non-high-risk proliferative retinopathy until it approaches or reaches the high-risk stage. Alternatively, in patients with bilateral non-high-risk proliferative retinopathy, one eye may be considered for laser surgery prior to the high-risk stage.

Certain patients with vitreous hemorrhage or recent traction retinal detachment may be candidates for vitrectomy. Laser surgery and vitrectomy surgery should be performed by a retinal specialist or other ophthalmologist experienced in laser surgery and the management of diabetic eye disease.

Patients with functionally decreased visual acuity should be referred for low vision evaluation and appropriate visual, vocational, and psychosocial rehabilitation .

Patient Education Principles

- Inform patients that sight-threatening eye disease is a common complication of diabetes and may be present even with good vision. Remind them to report all ocular symptoms, since essentially any symptoms may be diabetic in origin. Blurred vision while reading may indicate macular edema. The presence of floaters may indicate hemorrhage, and flashing lights may indicate retinal detachment. Inform patients that early detection and appropriate treatment of diabetic eye disease greatly reduces the risk of visual loss.
- Inform patients about the possible relationship between glycemic control and the subsequent development of ocular complications.
- Tell patients about the association between hypertension and diabetic retinopathy. Stress the importance of the diagnosis and continuing treatment of hypertension. Urge patients to work closely with their health care team.
- Help patients understand the natural course and treatment of diabetic retinopathy and the importance of yearly eye examinations.
- Tell patients with diabetic retinopathy about the availability and benefits of early and timely laser photocoagulation therapy in reducing the risk of visual loss.
- Inform patients about their higher risks of cataract formation, open-angle glaucoma, and neovascular glaucoma.
- Tell all patients with any visual impairment (including blindness) about the availability of visual, vocational, and psychosocial rehabilitation programs.

References

Aiello LM, Rand LI, Sebestyen JG, et al. The eyes and diabetes. In: Marble A, Krall LP, Bradley RS, Christlieb AR, Soeldner JS, eds. *Joslin's Diabetes Mellitus.* 12th ed. Philadelphia: Lea & Febiger, 1985.

Diabetic Retinopathy Study Research Group. Photocoagulation treatment of proliferative diabetic retinopathy: clinical application of Diabetic Retinopathy Study (DRS) findings, DRS report no. 8. *Ophthalmology.* 1981;88:583–600.

Early Treatment Diabetic Retinopathy Study Research Group. Photocoagulation for diabetic macular edema: Early Treatment Diabetic Retinopathy Study report no. 1. *Archives of Ophthalmology.* 1985;103:1796–1806.

Klein BEK, Moss SE, Klein R. Effect of pregnancy on progression of diabetic retinopathy. *Diabetes Care.* 1990;13:34–40.

Klein R. The epidemiology of diabetic retinopathy: findings from the Wisconsin Epidemiologic Study of Diabetic Retinopathy. *International Ophthalmology Clinics.* 1987;27:230–238.

Klein R, Klein BEK, Moss SE, et al. The Wisconsin Epidemiologic Study of Diabetic Retinopathy. II. Prevalence and risk of diabetic retinopathy when age at diagnosis is less than 30 years. *Archives of Ophthalmology.* 1984;102:520–526.

Klein R, Klein BEK, Moss SE, et al. The Wisconsin Epidemiologic Study of Diabetic Retinopathy. III. Prevalence and risk of diabetic retinopathy when age at diagnosis is 30 or more years. *Archives of Ophthalmology.* 1984;102:527–532.

Klein R, Moss SE, Klein BEK, et al. The Wisconsin Epidemiologic Study of Diabetic Retinopathy. XI. The incidence of macular edema. *Ophthalmology.* 1989;96:1501–1510.

Preferred Practice Pattern—Diabetic Retinopathy. San Francisco: American Academy of Ophthalmology, 1989.

Kidney Disease

Background

Description. Diabetic nephropathy represents a distinct clinical syndrome characterized by albuminuria, hypertension, and progressive renal insufficiency. Diabetic nephropathy can lead to end-stage renal disease (ESRD), a serious condition in which a patient's survival depends on either dialysis or kidney transplantation.

Occurrence. Among persons who have had insulin-dependent diabetes mellitus (IDDM) for 20 years, the incidence of ESRD approaches 40%. Among whites, the incidence of ESRD is lower among those with non-insulin-dependent diabetes mellitus (NIDDM) than among those with IDDM. Because NIDDM is much more common than IDDM, the number of whites with NIDDM who develop renal failure each year is about the same as for those with IDDM. In certain populations-including blacks, Hispanics, and Native Americans—persons with NIDDM have a higher incidence of ESRD.

About a third of new cases of ESRD in the United States are attributed to diabetes. These persons account for about a third of the $2.8 billion per year that is spent for the care of patients with ESRD

Pathophysiology-IDDM. The natural history of renal involvement in persons with IDDM has been well characterized. When diabetes is first diagnosed, the histological appearance of the kidney is normal. Within three years, however, the typical changes of diabetic glomerulosclerosis appear: thickening of the glomerular basement membrane and mesangial expansion.

Renal blood flow and the glomerular filtration rate (GFR) are characteristically elevated, correlating with an increase in kidney size and weight. Mild albuminuria may be present if glycemia is not well regulated. Because of renal hyperfiltration, serum creatinine and urea nitrogen concentrations are usually slightly reduced.

After 10 to 15 years, the first laboratory evidence of renal damage may appear with the presence of persistent microalbuminuria (30 to 300 mg per 24 hours). In IDDM, the prevalence of hypertension increases markedly in patients with microalbuminuria, and hypertension clearly contributes to the progression of renal disease.

Clinical diabetic nephropathy is said to be present when a patient who has had diabetes for more than five years and has evidence of diabetic retinopathy develops clinically apparent albuminuria (>300 mg per 24 hours) and has no evidence of any other cause of kidney disease. When these criteria are fulfilled, a clinical diagnosis of diabetic nephropathy can generally be made without performing a renal biopsy.

About four years after the onset of clinical diabetic nephropathy, the serum creatinine level rises to 2 mg/dL or greater. Within an additional three years, about one-half of patients will have developed ESRD.

Pathophysiology-NIDDM. The natural history of renal involvement in persons with NIDDM is not well established. Although microalbuminuria has been shown to be associated with the development of clinical diabetic nephropathy, the precise level of microalbuminuria that reliably predicts this condition has yet to be determined. Some individuals with low levels of albuminuria do not develop renal failure. In these persons, albuminuria may be due to the presence of other complicating renal diseases, such as obstructive uropathy, hypertension, or arteriolosclerosis, or may reflect an age-related increase in urinary albumin excretion.

Prevention

At present, strategies for preventing diabetic nephropathy must be viewed as limited in their effectiveness, since the exact pathogenic factors responsible for this condition are unknown.

In patients with albuminuria, blood pressure regulation is of critical importance in slowing the progression to renal failure. Other strategies that may slow the progression of renal disease include limiting the patient's protein intake, maintaining good glycemic control, promptly treating urinary tract infections, and avoiding potentially nephrotoxic drugs and radiographic dyes.

Detection

At the time of initial diagnosis, all diabetic patients should have a urinalysis performed. If bacteria or white blood cells are seen, a culture should be obtained.

Each year, obtain a sensitive quantitative measure of urinary albumin or protein excretion. In general, the protein excretion rate is about one-third greater than that for albumin. Thus, a protein excretion rate of approximately 400 mg per 24 hours would correspond to an albumin excretion rate of 300 mg per 24 hours.

Measure renal function (serum creatinine and/or creatinine clearance) each year.

Before establishing a diagnosis of diabetic nephropathy, exclude other possible causes of renal disease particularly, obstructive uropathy and infection. If diabetic retinopathy is not present, suspect a nondiabetic cause of renal disease.

Hypertension is a common development with the onset of diabetic nephropathy or shortly thereafter. If the patient's initial blood pressure is higher than 140/90 mm Hg, at least three additional readings should be obtained over the next month.

Treatment

At present, no known interventions have been shown to reverse clinical diabetic nephropathy. However, practitioners can take several actions to monitor and perhaps slow the progress of this complication:

- Aggressively monitor and treat high blood pressure (>140/90 mm Hg) or significant increments in blood pressure (20/10 mm Hg or greater on careful follow-up) in patients with renal disease.
- Encourage all nonpregnant adults with diabetes, especially those with renal involvement, to limit their daily protein intake to 0.8 g/kg of body weight, as recommended by the American Diabetes Association.
- Strive to achieve good glycemic control, without undue side effects from hypoglycemia, in all diabetic patients, especially those with microalbuminuria.
- Recommend consultation with a diabetologist and/or a nephrologist if patients have microalbuminuria (30 to 300 mg per 24 hours), clinically overt albuminuria (>300 mg per 24 hours), nephrotic syndrome, elevated serum creatinine (>2 mg/dL), or diminished GFR (<50 mL per minute).

- Instruct patients with microalbuminuria or diabetic nephropathy to receive yearly eye examinations.
- Assess cardiovascular risk factors—particularly hypercholesterolemia and cigarette smoking—and provide appropriate treatment, especially for patients with NIDDM.
- Seek and treat other causes of renal disease, particularly obstructive uropathy and infection. Promptly treat any urinary tract infections. Repeat a urine culture after treatment to ensure resolution.

Patients who have developed ESRD will require kidney transplantation, hemodialysis, or peritoneal dialysis to prolong their lives. Because diabetic complications—especially retinopathy and neuropathy—progress more rapidly with the onset of renal failure, dialysis is usually instituted earlier (when the concentration of serum creatinine reaches about 6 mg/dL) for people with diabetes than for those without diabetes. Kidney transplantation is preferable to dialysis when a living relative of the patient is available as a donor; the patient's chances of survival are otherwise about equal among these three courses of treatment. The ultimate choice will require the input of the patient, the patient's family, the primary health care provider, and a nephrologist.

Patient Education Principles

- Inform patients about the potential renal complications of diabetes.
- Inform patients about the association between hypertension and accelerated renal disease. Discuss the need for regular blood pressure measurements and encourage patients to measure their own blood pressure at home. Stress the importance of treating hypertension.
- Explain the potential role that excessive protein in the diet may play in the pathogenesis and progression of diabetic nephropathy.
- Explain the possible relationship between poor glycemic control and the development of diabetic renal disease.
- Emphasize the importance of achieving and maintaining ideal body weight and of undertaking a regular physical exercise program as strategies for preventing hypertension and improving glycemic control.
- Review with patients the symptoms of urinary tract infection. Instruct patients to contact their health care provider if such symptoms occur.
- Review with patients which drugs are potentially nephrotoxic. Explain the danger of radiographic dye studies.

- Review the natural history of clinical diabetic nephropathy with patients who have this condition. Discuss the therapeutic options—dialysis versus transplantation—for ESRD.

References

American Diabetes Association. Nutritional recommendations and principles for individuals with diabetes mellitus: 1986. *Diabetes Care.* 1987;10:126–132.

Consensus statement. Proceedings from the International Symposium on Preventing the Kidney Disease of Diabetes Mellitus: public health perspectives. *American Journal of Kidney Diseases.* 1989; 13:2–6.

DeFronzo RA. Diabetes and the kidney: an update. In: Olefsky JM, Sherwin RS, eds. *Diabetes Mellitus: Management and Complications.* New York: Churchill Livingstone, 1985.

Kaplan NM, Rosenstock J, Raskin P. A differing view of treatment of hypertension in patients with diabetes mellitus. *Archives of Internal Medicine.* 1987;147:1160–1162.

Mogensen CE, Schmitz A, Christensen CK. Comparative renal pathophysiology relevant to IDDM and NIDDM patients. *Diabetes/Metabolism Reviews.* 1988: 4:453–483.

Viberti GC, Walker JD. Diabetic nephropathy: etiology and prevention. *Diabetes/ Metabolism Reviews.* 1988;4:147–162.

The Working Group on Hypertension in Diabetes. Statement on hypertension in diabetes mellitus. *Archives of Internal Medicine.* 1987:147:830–842.

Cardiovascular Disease

Background

Occurrence. Cardiovascular disease is the leading cause of morbidity and mortality among persons with diabetes. In the United States in 1986, approximately 80,000 deaths from cardiovascular disease were associated with diabetes.

The annual risk for death from cardiovascular disease is two to three times greater for persons with diabetes than for persons without diabetes. For persons with diabetes, the risk for cerebrovascular disease and for coronary artery disease is two to three times greater, and the risk for peripheral vascular disease is five times greater. Among persons without diabetes, women have a lower rate of cardiovascular disease than men do; among persons with diabetes, women are not preferentially spared.

Risk factors. In persons with diabetes, smoking is a powerful risk factor for cardiovascular disease, and the prevalence of smoking appears to be higher in young people (less than 21 years old) with diabetes than in young people without diabetes.

Hypertension, also a strong risk factor for cardiovascular disease, occurs two to three times more often in persons with diabetes than in persons without diabetes. The risk for cardiovascular disease increases linearly with increases in blood pressure.

Abnormalities in the concentration of lipids and lipoproteins in plasma have been reported to occur in almost 30% of persons with diabetes. The risk for cardiovascular disease is directly proportional to the concentration of low-density lipoprotein (LDL) cholesterol and inversely proportional to the concentration of high-density lipoprotein (HDL) cholesterol. Although hypertriglyceridemia is common among persons with non-insulin-dependent diabetes mellitus, whether the triglyceride level independently predicts cardiovascular disease is uncertain.

The precise relationship between hyperglycemia and atherosclerosis is also unknown. Among persons with diabetes, several concomitant conditions may affect the etiology of atherosclerosis: obesity, inactivity, hyperinsulinemia, abnormalities in platelet function, and defects in blood coagulation and flow.

Among persons with diabetes, part of the increased likelihood of cardiovascular disease appears to be a consequence of the increased frequency of risk factors. Yet diabetes itself is an independent risk factor for cardiovascular disease.

Prevention

Although the benefit of controlling smoking, hypertension, and hypercholesterolemia has not been well studied in diabetic populations, there is no reason to believe that persons with diabetes will not benefit from controlling these risk factors. However, the precise benefit that can be achieved is not known.

Smoking. Smoking cessation may be the most important modification in behavior that can be made to reduce the risk for cardiovascular disease. Stress to patients the importance of not smoking. Encourage those who smoke to quit, and remind those who do not smoke not to start.

Blood pressure. Blood pressure should be closely monitored in patients with diabetes. When blood pressure is increased over 140/90 mm Hg, nonpharmacologic therapy should be instituted. Medication may need to be initiated early, depending on the blood pressure level. When selecting drugs for treating hypertension, consider their potential adverse effects on other risk factors for cardiovascular disease.

Plasma lipids. The incidence of atherosclerotic heart disease and the morbidity associated with this condition can be decreased in nondiabetic populations by reducing the plasma cholesterol level. When the total cholesterol is more than 200 mg/dL and the LDL cholesterol is more than 130 mg/dL, nonpharmacologic therapy should be instituted.

Plasma glucose. The relationship between plasma glucose and the development of cardiovascular disease is less clear. However, poor glycemic control is often associated with hyperlipidemia. Improved glycemic control has been shown to lower the concentration of cholesterol and triglycerides in plasma and to raise the concentration of HDL cholesterol in persons with diabetes who are either hyperlipidemic or normolipidemic.

Weight, exercise, and aspirin therapy. Additional recommendations for preventing cardiovascular disease in diabetic patients include weight loss (for obese persons) and an increased level of physical activity. For patients who have had cardiovascular events, aspirin therapy may help to prevent mortality or additional morbidity from cardiovascular disease.

Detection

The following guidelines may help in the detection of cardiovascular disease.

At every office visit (at least four times a year)

- Measure the patient's blood pressure with a cuff appropriate for the patient's size.
- Ask patients whether they have had symptoms of the following conditions:

Condition	Symptoms such as
Cerebral vascular disease	Transient blindness, dysarthria, or unilateral weakness.
Coronary artery disease and congestive heart failure	Chest pain or pressure, dyspnea, orthopnea, paroxysmal nocturnal dyspnea, or edema. (Painless myocardial infarction is common among diabetic patients, and they may have angina or myocardial infarction with atypical symptoms.)
Peripheral vascular disease	Intermittent claudication or foot ulcers that do not heal.

At least once a year

- Ask patients about their use of tobacco.
- Auscultate for bruits over all large arteries and palpate all peripheral pulses.

Once a year

- Measure triglycerides (TG), total cholesterol (TC), and HDL cholesterol levels in the fasting state, and calculate the level of LDL cholesterol. For TG under 400 mg/dL,

$$LDL = TC - HDL - (TG \div 5)$$

  For children, consider measuring lipids every two years.

- Obtain a baseline electrocardiogram in all patients with diabetes and repeat the procedure yearly for those with clinically apparent cardiovascular disease.

Treatment

Smoking. Strongly advise patients who smoke to quit. Both the health hazards of smoking and the improved health that patients will enjoy when they stop smoking should be emphasized. Work with each patient to set a quit date, and follow up after that date. Nicotine gum may be used for physiological dependency. Behavioral treatment is recommended for psychological and social dependency. Health care providers should refer patients to smoking cessation programs in the community that are appropriate to patients' individual needs.

Hypertension. If the patient's blood pressure exceeds 140/90 mm Hg at two visits, begin nonpharmacologic therapy, including a low-sodium, alcohol-restricted diet designed for weight reduction. Regular exercise has also been shown to have a beneficial effect on blood pressure. Blood pressure should be maintained below 140/90 mm Hg. For individual patients, consider earlier pharmacologic intervention when indicated by clinical conditions (for example, diastolic blood pressure greater than 110 mm Hg) and the presence of other risk factors (such as albuminuria).

After three months of nonpharmacologic therapy, if the diastolic blood pressure remains above 90 mm Hg, begin pharmacologic treatment. Select drugs that do not worsen other risk factors for cardiovascular disease (including lipids) and that do not induce or worsen autonomic neuropathic complications of diabetes (including hypoglycemia unawareness, orthostatic hypotension, or impotence).

Hyperlipidemia. When the calculated LDL cholesterol level is greater than 130 mg/dL, consider the following guidelines for glycemic control, diet, and exercise.

Glycemic control. Glycemic control should be improved through diet, use of sulfonylureas, or insulin therapy. Weigh the benefits of improved glycemic control against the potential risk for hypoglycemia.

Dietary therapy. Dietary therapy should be instituted to reduce the weight of obese patients and to try to lower the LDL cholesterol level to below 130 mg/dL. Consider the following restrictions on diet:

- Calorie restriction for weight reduction if obesity is present.
- Total fat less than 30% of total calories.
- Saturated fats less than 10% of total calories. Complex carbohydrates and fiber (especially soluble fiber) can be substituted for the usual intake of saturated fats. Preliminary studies suggest that some diabetic patients with hypertriglyceridemia may benefit by restricting carbohydrate intake to 40% to 45% of total calories. In those patients, monounsaturated fats may be used to maintain caloric balance.
- Cholesterol less than 300 mg per day.

Exercise. Weigh the potential benefits of exercise against the risks and recommend an exercise program, if appropriate. Regular aerobic exercise has been shown to be a useful adjunct to weight loss and to have a beneficial effect on lipids, especially levels of triglycerides and HDL cholesterol. Exercise may also cause a modest drop in the LDL cholesterol level. Before patients begin an exercise program, determine whether they have hypoglycemia unawareness, postural hypotension, proliferative retinopathy, painless myocardial ischemia, or insensitive feet. An exercise stress test is recommended for all diabetic patients over 40 years old who are considering an exercise program.

Reevaluation. After six months of therapy, if a patient's LDL cholesterol level is above 160 mg/dL, consider drug therapy. Drugs used to treat patients with hypercholesterolemia include bile acid sequestrants (cholestyramine or colestipol), HMGCoA reductase inhibitors (lovastatin), fibrin acid derivatives (gemfibrozil or clofibrate), nicotinic acid, and probucol. Drugs used to treat patients with hypertriglyceridemia include fibrin acid derivatives (gemfibrozil or clofibrate) and nicotinic acid.

Existing cardiovascular disease. Clinically apparent cardiovascular disease poses considerable diagnostic and therapeutic challenges to the practitioner. Consider consulting with specialists (such as cardiologists, neurologists, and vascular surgeons) early in the course of such disease. The guidelines below address some of the cardiovascular diseases common among persons with diabetes.

Cerebral vascular disease. Patients with signs or symptoms of cerebral vascular disease should be referred for specialized diagnostic tests, including noninvasive Doppler flow studies and, if necessary, carotid arteriography. Caution should be used with dye studies in patients with preexisting renal disease and/or dehydration. Patients with symptomatic cerebral vascular disease may be treated with aspirin and anticoagulants. If symptoms persist despite pharmacological treatment and if correctable vascular lesions are present, surgery may be considered.

Coronary artery disease. Heart disease due to coronary atherosclerosis is the most common cause of morbidity and mortality in patients with diabetes. Patients with signs or symptoms of coronary artery disease should receive a complete evaluation, including exercise testing and, if necessary, coronary arteriography. Contrast-dye studies should be used with caution because of the possible coexistence of diabetic nephropathy. Nitrates, calcium channel blockers, and beta blockers may be prescribed for patients with angina. Consider coronary angioplasty or bypass surgery for patients with appropriate coronary lesions or intractable angina. Unless contraindicated, aspirin should be given after acute myocardial infarction. Because of their ability to prevent reinfarction in nondiabetic subjects, beta blockers may be used in patients with diabetes after myocardial infarction—with attention to possible hypoglycemia and/or hyperlipidemia.

Peripheral vascular disease. Generally, no effective medical treatment is available for patients with peripheral vascular disease, although some patients may benefit from pentoxifylline. Patients who have incapacitating symptoms of peripheral vascular disease (such as rest pain) or who have foot lesions that are poorly healing require careful evaluation. To detect surgically correctable peripheral vascular disease, first use clinical examination of the pulses and then consider noninvasive means (Doppler flow study). Contrast-dye studies should be used with caution because of the possible coexistence of diabetic nephropathy. Refer patients for surgery, as appropriate.

Patient Education Principles

- Inform patients with diabetes that their risk of developing cardiovascular disease is higher than that of persons without diabetes.
- Inform patients of the absolute necessity of not smoking.
- Emphasize to patients the importance of following dietary principles appropriate for their conditions (such as hypertension or hyperlipidemia).

- Inform patients that hypertension and hyperlipidemia must be treated vigorously.
- Tell patients to immediately report symptoms of cardiovascular disease (for example, transient ischemic attack, chest pain, and claudication) so that investigation and treatment can begin promptly.

References

American Diabetes Association. Nutritional recommendations and principles for individuals with diabetes mellitus: 1986. *Diabetes Care.* 1987;10:126–132.

Kannel WB, McGee DL. Diabetes and cardiovascular disease: the Framingham Study. *Journal of the American Medical Association.* 1979;241:2035–2038.

Kaplan NM, Rosenstock J, Raskin P. A differing view of treatment of hypertension in patients with diabetes mellitus. *Archives of Internal Medicine.* 1987;147:1160–1162.

Lipid Research Clinics Program. The Lipid Research Clinics Coronary Primary Prevention Trial results. II: the relationship of reduction in incidence of coronary heart disease to cholesterol lowering. *Journal of the American Medical Association.* 1984;251:365–374.

National Diabetes Data Group. *Diabetes in America.* Bethesda, Maryland: US Department of Health and Human Services, 1985. Publication NIH 85–1468.

1984 report of the Joint National Committee on Detection, Evaluation, and Treatment of High Blood Pressure. *Archives of Internal Medicine.* 1984;144:1045–1057.

Steering Committee of the Physicians' Health Study Research Group. Preliminary report: findings from the aspirin component of the ongoing physicians' health study. *New England Journal of Medicine.* 1988;318:262–264.

Working Group on Diabetes in Hypertension. Statement on hypertension in diabetes mellitus. *Archives of Internal Medicine.* 1987;147:830–842.

Neuropathy

Background

Persons with diabetes who develop neuropathy may have no symptoms or may experience pain, sensory loss, weakness, and autonomic dysfunction. Neuropathy may result in significant morbidity and may contribute to other major complications, such as lower extremity amputation.

There are three major types of diabetic neuropathy:

- Distal symmetrical polyneuropathy.
- Focal neuropathy.
- Autonomic neuropathy.

Distal symmetrical polyneuropathy. This most common of the diabetic neuropathies is characterized by insidious onset, symmetrical distribution, and progressive course. Although its cause is unclear, distal symmetrical polyneuropathy is believed to result from abnormal neural metabolism, generalized neural ischemia, or both. The onset and course of illness cannot be predicted for an individual patient, but increasing age, male sex, increasing height, longer duration of diabetes, poorer glucose control, hypertension, alcohol consumption, and smoking may be independent risk factors.

Estimates of the prevalence of distal symmetrical polyneuropathy differ greatly, but approximately 12% of patients have this condition when diabetes is diagnosed, and nearly 60% have it after 25 years.

Three overlapping clinical syndromes have been described:

- Acute painful neuropathy, an uncommon but extremely unpleasant complication of diabetes, often occurs without evidence of other significant neurologic impairment. It may occur early or late in the course of diabetes and may be associated with the institution of insulin treatment or with abrupt or considerable weight loss. Patients develop dysesthesia and paresthesia in the lower extremities. The severe, burning pain is often associated with cutaneous hyperesthesia and is worse at night. Objective evidence of neuropathy may be minimal. Symptoms generally resolve slowly, within months of achieving good glycemic control. Relapses are rare.
- Small fiber neuropathy may occur after only a few years of diabetes. Patients have varying degrees of pain and sensory loss; they usually feel a burning pain and may develop dysesthesia. Prominent features of small fiber neuropathy are distal loss of temperature sensation and of pinprick or pressure sensation. Vibratory sensation, position sense, muscle strength, and ankle reflexes are generally unimpaired. Neuropathic ulcers occasionally occur at sites of trauma.
- Large fiber neuropathy generally occurs in the setting of small fiber neuropathy. Patients have impaired distal vibration sensation and impaired distal position sense. Ankle reflexes are reduced or lost. In more severe instances, patients develop sensory ataxia and have a positive Romberg's test. Large fiber neuropathy is most strongly associated with the development of neuropathic foot ulcers and neuropathic arthropathy affecting the interphalangeal, metatarsophalangeal, and ankle joints.

Focal neuropathy. Focal neuropathy is an uncommon condition believed to occur after the acute occlusion of a blood vessel produces ischemia in a nerve or group of nerves. The characteristics of focal diabetic neuropathy are sudden onset, an asymmetrical nature, and a self-limited course. Near-total recovery generally occurs within two weeks to 18 months. Examples of focal diabetic neuropathies are cranial neuropathies, truncal neuropathies, mononeuropathies, radiculopathies, and plexopathies. Both sensory and motor components may be present.

Autonomic neuropathy. This troubling complication of diabetes encompasses multiple disturbances affecting the following systems: sudomotor (possible symptoms include heat exhaustion), pupillary (poor night vision), adrenomedullary (hypoglycemia unawareness), cardiovascular (orthostatic hypotension and painless myocardial ischemia), gastrointestinal (gastroparesis, constipation, diarrhea, and fecal incontinence), and urogenital (bladder dysfunction and sexual dysfunction).

The following complications can occur with autonomic neuropathy:

Condition	Description
Orthostatic hypotension	Suspect this condition when a patient reports having postural faintness, weakness, visual impairment, or syncope. In patients whose intravascular volume is not depleted, autonomic neuropathy may be diagnosed if the systolic blood pressure falls more than 30 mm Hg or if the diastolic blood pressure falls more than 10 mm Hg when the patient changes from a lying to a standing position.
Gastroparesis	May be associated with symptoms of anorexia, early satiety, bloating, abdominal pain, nausea, and vomiting. Signs may include weight loss and erratic glycemic control.
Constipation	A common manifestation that may be difficult to treat.
Diabetic diarrhea	May last from a few hours to several weeks. May be severe and watery, is generally worse at night, and is often preceded by abdominal cramps. During remissions, the patient may report constipation.

Fecal incontinence	Associated with a reduced threshold of conscious rectal sensation, low basal internal sphincter pressure, and reduced voluntary control of the external anal sphincter.
Diabetic bladder dysfunction	Associated with defective perception of bladder filling and decreased reflex bladder emptying. Patients may strain to initiate a stream, may be unable to completely void, may dribble when urinating, and may have recurrent urinary tract infections.
Sexual dysfunction	Men may experience impotence. Women may experience decreased vaginal lubrication and dyspareunia.

Prevention

Studies have not firmly established that glucose control is effective in preventing or treating diabetic neuropathy. It seems prudent, however, to promote good glycemic control until the benefits and risks of trying to achieve euglycemia are clarified by large clinical trials.

Practitioners should urge patients to avoid other risk factors associated with the development of peripheral polyneuropathy. These include consumption of alcohol, poor nutrition, exposure to chemical toxins, use of certain drugs, and physical injury to the nerves (such as entrapment and compression).

Detection

Interview. The practitioner should conduct an interview at each visit—at least four times a year—to determine whether the patient is experiencing the following:

- Peripheral pain, paresthesia, or numbness.
- Weakness.
- Hypoglycemia awareness.
- Orthostatic lightheadedness.
- Gastrointestinal symptoms, such as bloating, nausea, vomiting, constipation, diarrhea, and loss of bowel control.

- Urogenital symptoms, such as loss of bladder control and sexual dysfunction.

Physical examination. The practitioner should inspect the feet at each visit—at least four times a year. At least once a year, the practitioner should perform a physical examination to assess neurologic function. The practitioner should measure blood pressure and pulse rate—both when the patient is lying down and standing—and should assess the patient's muscle strength, deep tendon reflexes, and sense of touch. Four modalities of touch should be assessed.

Distal temperature sensation. Touch a cool piece of metal (such as a tuning fork) to the patient's foot; ask the patient to describe the object's temperature. Another method is to alternately touch the patient's foot with a test tube containing cool water and another containing warm water; ask the patient to distinguish between these objects.

Distal pinprick or pressure sensation. Have the patient close his or her eyes. Hold a pin lightly between your thumb and forefinger and touch it to the patient's foot. Ask the patient to say when a sensation is felt and whether the sensation is sharp or dull. Clarify a doubtful response by alternately touching the patient with the point and the head of the pin. As an alternative, pressure sensation can be assessed with a monofilament.

Distal vibratory sensation. Tap a 128 hz tuning fork and place the end of the handle on a bony surface of the patient, such as the distal first metatarsal head or the malleoli of the ankles. Ask the patient to say when the vibration ceases.

Position sense. Have the patient close his or her eyes. Grasp between your thumb and index finger the lateral and medial sides of the patient's toe. Ask the patient to describe the toe's position as you alternately flex and extend it.

Differential Diagnosis

The practitioner should exclude other potential causes of neuropathy before attributing a patient's neuropathy to diabetes.

Distal symmetrical polyneuropathy. The differential diagnosis includes the following:

- Medications.
- Exposure to toxins, including ethanol, organic solvents, and heavy metals.
- Uremia.
- Hypothyroidism.
- Pernicious anemia.

- Intoxication from vitamin B6.
- Syphilis.
- Gammopathy or myeloma.
- Malignancy.
- Collagen vascular disease.
- Porphyria.
- Hereditary neuropathy.

Focal neuropathy. The differential diagnosis includes the following:

Type	Differential Diagnosis
Cranial neuropathy	Increased intracranial pressure, aneurysm, tumor.
Truncal neuropathy	Cardiopulmonary disease, degenerative joint disease, disc disease, tumor, Paget's disease.
Mononeuropathy multiplex	Trauma, hemorrhage, tumor.

Autonomic neuropathy. The differential diagnosis includes the following:

Manifestation	Differential Diagnosis
Hypoglycemia unawareness	Medications, lack of knowledge about hypoglycemia.
Orthostatic hypotension	Medications, hypovolemia, panhypopituitarism, pheochromocytoma, Shy-Drager syndrome.
Gastroparesis	Medications, ketoacidosis, gastric or intestinal obstruction.
Constipation	Medications, dehydration, intestinal obstruction.

Diarrhea	Medications, dietary sorbitol or lactose, enteric pathogens, bacterial overgrowth, primary intestinal diseases, pancreatic exocrine insufficiency.
Impotence	Medications, hormonal abnormalities, vascular disease, psychogenic disease.

Treatment

Distal symmetrical polyneuropathy. Often the pain resolves. For patients with painful neuropathy, the practitioner should institute rigorous glucose control. If pain continues, consider using pharmacologic agents such as amitriptyline, imipramine, nortriptyline plus fluphenazine, carbamazepine, mexiletine, or capsaicin.

Inform patients with distal sensory or motor abnormalities about foot care. Tell patients who have lost sensation in their feet to wear special protective footwear and to avoid activities (such as jogging) that can traumatize the feet (see "Foot Problems").

If painful neuropathy persists or worsens, consider referring the patient to a diabetologist.

Focal neuropathy. After other causes are excluded (see previous section under differential diagnosis), management is palliative. Spontaneous resolution generally occurs within a period of months but may persist over years.

Autonomic neuropathy. Various treatments are available for autonomic neuropathy. If signs or symptoms of autonomic neuropathy are present, consider referring the patient to a diabetologist.

Hypoglycemia unawareness. If necessary, alter patients' targeted goals for glycemic control. Encourage patients to monitor their blood glucose regularly. Instruct patients to carry with them a source of simple sugar and to wear a necklace or bracelet that identifies them as having diabetes. Patients should also have glucagon available; their family and friends need to know how and when to use it.

Orthostatic hypotension. Patients may benefit from improved glycemic control (to reduce glycosuria), from volume and salt repletion, and from mechanical support with waist-high elastic stockings. Vasoconstrictors may be indicated.

Gastroparesis. Patients may benefit from correction of metabolic abnormalities (including hyperglycemia, ketosis, and hypokalemia), from dietary modification (eating small, liquid, low-fiber, low-fat meals), and from a prokinetic agent such as metoclopramide.

Constipation. Patients may benefit from correction of glycosuria, adequate hydration, a high-fiber diet, and psyllium.

Diarrhea. Patients may benefit from a bowel program that includes ingesting dietary fiber and making regular efforts to move the bowels. Another possible treatment is a short-term trial of an antidiarrheal agent (such as loperamide or diphenoxylate hydrochloride and atropine sulfate) or a broad-spectrum antibiotic with anaerobic coverage (such as tetracycline or metronidazole hydrochloride). Metoclopramide may occasionally be beneficial.

Fecal incontinence. Patients may be candidates for biofeedback training.

Diabetic bladder dysfunction. Patients may benefit from treatment to improve bladder emptying and to reduce the risk of urinary tract infection.

Impotence. Patients may benefit from noninvasive devices to assist erection, from a semirigid or inflatable penile prosthesis, or from papaverine injections.

Patient Education Principles

- Inform patients about the possible relationship between poor glycemic control and the subsequent development of diabetic neuropathy.
- Explain possible risk factors (such as consumption of alcohol and exposure to chemical toxins) and concomitant neural insults that may hasten the development or progression of diabetic neuropathy.
- Stress that because sensory or motor neuropathy may be asymptomatic, routine evaluation is necessary even for patients who have no symptoms of neuropathy.
- Explain that diabetic neuropathy can contribute to the development of other complications, including loss of limb.
- Inform patients who have lost sensation in their feet about the importance of caring for their feet, wearing proper shoes, and getting appropriate exercise.
- Discuss the signs and symptoms of autonomic neuropathy.
- Explain the benefits of treatment to patients with autonomic neuropathy.

References

Broadstone VL, Cyrus J, Pfeifer MA, Greene DA. Diabetic peripheral neuropathy, part I: sensorimotor neuropathy. *The Diabetes Educator.* 1987;13:30–35.

Cyrus J, Broadstone VL, Pfeifer MA, Greene DA. Diabetic peripheral neuropathy, part II: autonomic neuropathies. *The Diabetes Educator.* 1987;13:111–114.
Dyck PJ, Thomas PK, Asbury AK, Winegrad AI, Porte D Jr, eds. *Diabetic Neuropathy.* Philadelphia: W.B. Saunders, 1987.
Pfeifer MA, Greene DA. *Diabetic Neuropathy.* Kalamazoo, Michigan: The Upjohn Company, 1985. (Current Concepts booklet).
Physician's Guide to Insulin-Dependent (Type I) Diabetes: Diagnosis and Treatment. Alexandria, Virginia: American Diabetes Association, 1988.

Foot Problems

Background

Persons with diabetes are at significant risk for lower extremity amputations; such procedures are 15 times more common among persons with diabetes than among those without diabetes. Yet if patients whose feet are particularly at risk are aggressively sought out and treated, up to 50% of amputations can be prevented.

Pathophysiology. Peripheral neuropathy, peripheral vascular disease, and infection all may contribute to amputation in patients with diabetes. Peripheral neuropathy may contribute to loss of sensation in the feet and to the development of foot deformities. In insensitive feet, deformities can cause pressure points that are vulnerable to ulceration. Inadequate blood supply and infection can then lead to osteomyelitis and gangrene.

Many persons with diabetes who undergo a lower extremity amputation have an amputation of the contralateral leg within a few years. This occurs not only because of peripheral neuropathy and peripheral vascular disease but also because the remaining foot bears increased pressure and frequently develops ulceration and infection.

The in-hospital mortality rate for diabetic patients who receive an amputation is higher than the rate for nondiabetic patients. In general, morbidity and mortality are high among diabetic patients who have amputations. All diabetic patients who undergo amputation require close supervision for other medical problems, particularly coronary artery disease.

Occurrence. Persons with diabetes account for approximately 50,000 (or 50%) of all nontraumatic amputations performed in the United States each year. The risk is greater for patients over 40 years old who have had diabetes for more than 10 years.

Cost. Although there is some variation, the average hospital stay for an amputation is approximately 25 days, and the average in-hospital cost is $25,000.

Prevention

Saving the diabetic foot and preventing amputation requires the following:

- Identification of feet at risk.
- Prevention of foot ulcers.
- Treatment of foot ulcers.
- Prevention of recurrence of foot ulcers.

Achieving these goals requires patient and family education in the care of the foot, frequent foot inspection, and teamwork among medical disciplines.

Identification of feet at risk. The diabetic patient with distal symmetrical polyneuropathy and peripheral vascular disease has feet at risk for problems. At each visit, the health care provider should inquire for symptoms of peripheral neuropathy, including pain, burning, tingling, and numbness. Patients with insensitive feet may not be aware of ulcerations or lesions. Therefore, the shoes and stockings must be removed at every visit—at least four times a year—and the feet inspected for dryness, calluses, corns, and ulcers. The health care provider should also inspect between the toes and inspect for deformities. At least once a year, the health care provider should assess the patient's ability to sense temperature, pinprick or pressure, touch, and vibration and should test muscle strength and deep tendon reflexes (see "Neuropathy").

At every visit, the health care provider should also ask the patient about symptoms of intermittent claudication. In persons with diabetes and neuropathy, severe ischemia may exist without symptoms. At least once a year, the health care provider should palpate the following pulses: dorsalis pedis, posterior tibial, popliteal, and femoral.

Prevention of foot ulcers. Diabetic patients with feet at risk must learn foot hygiene and how to protect their feet. Changes in activity may be needed. Patients with foot deformities almost always require specially molded, extra-depth shoes. Deformed feet will not fit into ordinary shoes, although the patient, because of loss of sensation, may think they fit. The wearing of ordinary shoes on deformed feet may result in abrasions, ulcerations, and infection, which can lead to gangrene and amputation. If the patient's circulation is good, prophylactic correction of foot deformities should be considered.

Peripheral polyneuropathy may have a number of etiologies, such as drugs, alcohol, chemical toxins, and uremia. These must always be considered in the differential diagnosis of neuropathy in the patient with diabetes.

Factors that contribute to peripheral vascular disease should be avoided or treated. Smoking, the most significant risk factor for peripheral vascular disease, is associated with atherosclerosis, and even one cigarette can cause vasoconstriction that lasts for an hour or longer. Other risk factors for peripheral vascular disease should be treated, including hypertension, hypercholesterolemia, and perhaps hyperglycemia.

Rest pain and night pain are major indications for vascular surgery. Other indications are ulcers that will not heal, infections resistant to treatment, and incipient gangrene. In recent years, there has been an increase in the success of vascular surgical procedures. There are, however, risks to persons with diabetes who undergo vascular surgery, including the risk of angiography (see "Kidney Disease"). Conservative measures should thus always be considered before vascular surgery. Pentoxifylline may improve the circulation in patients with peripheral vascular disease; aspirin and dipyridamole have not been conclusively shown to be effective. Oral vasodilators are ineffective in improving blood flow, and sympathectomy is not helpful in these patients.

Treatment of foot ulcers. Carefully evaluate and vigorously debride foot ulcers to establish the depth of the ulcer. Use X-ray studies to help exclude the possibility of imbedded foreign objects or osteomyelitis. If osteomyelitis is suspected, use follow-up radiographs and appropriate scans to help establish the diagnosis. Where there is significant infection, use parenteral antibiotics. Since anaerobes frequently occur in the foot ulcers of diabetic patients, take both aerobic and anaerobic bacterial cultures to help select antibiotics.

Ulcers that occur in areas other than the usual plantar area, that cannot be explained by previous trauma or ill-fitting shoes, or that do not respond to aggressive treatment should be biopsied.

Ensure that patients do not put weight on the affected foot. Patients who do not feel pain will likely continue to walk; the resulting pressure on the foot will prevent healing. Total bed rest or the use of crutches may be required. Total-contact casts have been shown to help patients with foot ulcers ambulate while ulcers heal; the casts redistribute pressure so that the area of the ulcer bears much less weight than it would otherwise.

Good glycemic control also may help the patient's foot to heal. Topical use of hyperbaric oxygen, however, is not effective.

If foot ulcers do not respond to therapy, vascular surgery must be considered.

Prevention of recurrence of foot ulcers. Without special post-ulcer care, recurrence of the ulcer is almost certain. Such care may entail a change in job, a change in walking habits, and most importantly, special shoes. Extra-depth shoes with molded plastic insoles help redistribute weight and may prevent recurrent ulcers. In one study, ulcers recurred in only about 20% of patients who wore these special shoes, whereas ulcers recurred in 80% of patients who resumed wearing ordinary shoes.

If ulcers recur despite protective shoes, the most likely cause is a bony deformity. If the patient's circulation is good, orthopedic procedures to repair such deformities may help prevent recurrence of the ulcer.

Detection and Monitoring

All patients with diabetes should be given a complete foot examination at each visit (or at least four times a year).

The health care provider should ensure that these patients are instructed in proper foot care [see "How to Take Care of Your Feet" in *Take Charge of Your Diabetes*, which is reproduced in Chapter 15 of this volume]. A member of the health care team should instruct patients to do the following:

- Wash their feet daily.
- Inspect their feet daily.
- Use foot creams or lubricating oil.
- Cut their toenails correctly.
- Never cut calluses or corns.
- Avoid self-medication and extremes of temperature.
- Never walk barefooted.
- Wear appropriate shoes.
- Inspect the inside of the shoes daily.
- Seek medical care for all skin lesions.

If these patient instructions cannot be given during regular office visits, the health care provider should arrange to collaborate with another qualified specialist.

Treatment

Calluses. Assess the shoes of patients who have calluses. Teach patients to manage calluses with an emery board, callus file, or pumice stone—but strongly caution patients against trying to perform "home surgery" on calluses.

Deformities. If the foot is deformed, the patient will likely need consultation and should benefit from having specially molded shoes. Surgical correction should be considered for bunions, claw toes, or hammer toes—if the patient's circulation is good.

Neuropathic ulcers. When a neuropathic ulcer is present, consultation may be necessary, and the patient may need to be hospitalized where resources for proper treatment are available. Whenever a patient is hospitalized for any reason or is put at bed rest, heel protection should be used; the heels must be checked daily for evidence of pressure injury.

Additional considerations. Caring for the feet of persons with diabetes is complex. The expertise of professionals from many disciplines is often required. Health care providers may not be able to manage all aspects of foot care by themselves and may need to consult with other professionals:

- A diabetes nurse educator can teach about foot care.
- A pedorthist can provide special shoes for the patient with foot deformities.
- A podiatrist can help with the design and selection of special shoes and shoe inlays and can teach the patient how to manage calluses, corns, toenails, and minor foot deformities.
- A neurologist can help with the differential diagnosis of complicated peripheral neuropathies.
- A vascular surgeon can help improve peripheral blood flow in cases of peripheral vascular disease.
- An expert in infectious diseases can advise on the treatment of infected foot ulcers (with or without osteomyelitis).
- An orthopedist may be needed to treat major foot deformities or perform amputation.
- A social worker and a rehabilitation expert can help with the various socioeconomic problems, including loss of job, that may result from foot problems and particularly from amputation.

Patient Education Principles

- Instruct patients on the importance of regular foot care.
- Inform patients about the relationship between neuropathy, peripheral vascular disease, and foot ulcers.
- Urge patients to avoid risk factors associated with worsening of neuropathy (see "Neuropathy").
- Urge patients not to smoke—particularly if they have peripheral vascular disease.
- Inform patients about special shoes for preventing or treating foot problems.

- Refer patients to a certified pedorthist if they have foot deformities or otherwise need special shoes.
- Inform patients about the availability of podiatric services; encourage patients to use these services.

References

Bild DE, Selby JV, Sinnock P, Browner WS, Braveman P, Showstack JA. Lower-extremity amputation in people with diabetes: epidemiology and prevention. *Diabetes Care.* 1989;12:24–31.

Boulton AJM, Bowker JH, Gadia M, et al. Use of plaster casts in the management of diabetic neuropathic foot ulcers. *Diabetes Care.* 1986;9:149–152.

Edmonds ME, Blundell MP, Morris ME, Thomas EM, Cotton LT, Watkins PJ. Improved survival of the diabetic foot: the role of a specialised foot clinic. *Quarterly Journal of Medicine.* 1986;60:763–771.

Levin ME, O'Neal LW, eds. *The Diabetic Foot.* 4th ed. St. Louis: CV Mosby, 1988.

Chapter 36

Intensive Treatment of Diabetes Prevents Complications

Intensive management of insulin-dependent diabetes mellitus (IDDM) prevents the onset of complications and slows their progression in diabetic patients, according to the findings of the Diabetes Control and Complications Trial (DCCT), a comprehensive study that many have termed one of the most important milestones in the history of the disease. IDDM, a leading cause of death and disability, affects nearly 1.5 million Americans and incurs health care costs in excess of $40 billion each year.

In IDDM insulin-secreting beta cells in the pancreas are destroyed by the immune system for reasons that are still unknown. Insulin, a hormone that allows cells to absorb glucose and other substrates from the blood to use for energy and growth, is conventionally replaced in one or two injections. Although this therapy is life-saving and controls diabetes, it does not mimic the natural, minute-to-minute fluctuations in insulin levels that occur in response to food intake and energy expenditure. Instead, conventional insulin therapy is characterized by wide swings in blood glucose levels, which in turn may damage blood vessels and nerves.

The resulting disease complications include damage to blood vessels in the eye (retinopathy), which can cause blindness; injury of the kidney blood vessels (nephropathy), necessitating regular renal dialysis or even kidney transplantation; peripheral nerve damage (neuropathy) and injury to the peripheral blood vessels that may lead to amputation of the feet and legs; and cardiovascular problems including hypertension, heart attack, and stroke.

NCRR Reporter, January/February 1944.

Since the development of insulin therapy more than 60 years ago, the central question in diabetes management has been whether more intensive treatment would go beyond controlling the short-term symptoms of diabetes and actually prevent or slow the advancement of long-term complications. Intensive treatment requires frequent insulin dosing to more closely simulate normal plasma insulin profiles and stricter monitoring of blood sugar levels to ensure that they remain closer to the nondiabetic range. But aggressively lowering blood sugar levels can induce hypoglycemia, an abnormally low level of blood sugar that can cause loss of consciousness, seizures, coma, and even death. Nevertheless, if the long-term complications could be prevented or delayed, the benefits of intensive treatment might outweigh its risks.

The results of the DCCT answered this question so definitively that the study was halted early, so all subjects, as well as IDDM patients in the general population, could begin the clearly superior intensive therapy as soon as possible.

The 10-year study involved 1,441 patients with IDDM (also known as type I diabetes) who were followed at 29 American and Canadian research centers, including 19 General Clinical Research Centers (GCRC's) supported by the National Center for Research Resources. "The success of this study is due in large part to investigators' access to these high-quality research facilities. GCRC's provide a wonderful environment for conducting multicenter clinical trials," says Carolyn Siebert, director of the IDDM Clinical Trials Program at the National Institute of Diabetes and Digestive and Kidney Diseases (NIDDK). The NIDDK provided primary funding for the trial, which also received support from other NIH institutes and corporate sponsors.

Patients were randomly assigned to receive either conventional therapy or a more intensive treatment regimen aimed at achieving the tightest possible control of blood sugar levels. The conventional treatment involved one or two daily doses of insulin, regular monitoring of blood sugar levels, and a standard program of nutrition and exercise instruction. The intensive treatment required three or more insulin injections daily, or the use of an insulin pump that infused the hormone continuously. Insulin doses were adjusted frequently, corresponding to the subjects' food intake, level of exercise, and blood sugar levels as obtained by tests done at least four times per day.

The use of GCRC's was indispensable to this work, according to several investigators. Dr. Abbas E. Kitabchi, professor of medicine and chief of endocrinology at the University of Tennessee in Memphis and principal investigator of the trial at the GCRC there, says, "We used the GCRC extensively. Outpatient visits for this trial accounted for 3,400 patient days, and inpatient visits for more than 500 patient days."

After an average of 6.5 years of follow-up at all the participating DCCT centers, the intensive treatment had reduced the risk of retinopathy by 76 percent and slowed progression of already existing retinopathy by 54 percent. Similarly, intensive therapy reduced the level of the protein albumin in the urine—an indicator of nephropathy—by as much as 54 percent. And it decreased the development of neuropathy by 60 percent.

The intensive regimen's effect on complications such as heart disease and stroke could not be assessed adequately in this trial because of the relative youth of the subjects and the short duration of their disease. However, the DCCT data suggest a beneficial effect on these later developing, life-threatening complications as well, which the investigators hope to document with continued follow-up.

The most dangerous side effect of the intensive therapy is the increased risk of hypoglycemia. The incidence of severe hypoglycemia was three times higher in subjects receiving intensive treatment (62 episodes per 100 patient years) than in those receiving conventional treatment (19 episodes per 100 patient years), a risk the investigators deemed well worth the obvious benefits of the regimen. Despite this risk and the greater inconvenience of the intensive treatment, compliance throughout the years of the study was a remarkable 98 percent.

In addition to continuing the surveillance of these subjects to assess the treatment's effect on heart disease and stroke, DCCT investigators are turning their attention to two related areas of research.

Their first concern is to reduce the risks related to hypoglycemia, since that problem undoubtedly will become more common once patients in the general population begin the intensive therapy. Dr. William V. Tamborlane, chief of pediatric endocrinology at Yale University School of Medicine in New Haven, Connecticut, and program director of the pediatric GCRC at Yale, notes that scientists now will focus on developing noninvasive means of monitoring blood sugar levels. Patients can then more readily prevent hypoglycemia. In addition, the investigators will try to develop methods for augmenting the body's own ability to counteract hypoglycemia when it does occur.

According to Ms. Siebert, another large-scale, long-term study that will also call on the resources of several GCRC's is now in the final stages of planning. The subjects in this study will be IDDM patients' relatives who do not yet have the disease. The relatives will be assigned to a low-risk or a high-risk group based on immunologic and genetic tests that show their likelihood of developing IDDM.

Many DCCT investigators are concerned with the more immediate problem of enabling their study participants to continue intensive therapy now that the clinical trial is over, as well as making the therapy available to millions of others who have diabetes. "It's a real challenge now for us to find ways to get our patients who have inadequate health insurance or no insurance to continue intensive therapy. The supplies alone [mainly insulin and syringes] cost about $1,000 a year," says Dr. David S. Shade, professor of medicine at the University of New Mexico School of Medicine in Albuquerque and laboratory director at the GCRC there.

Add to that the cost of frequent outpatient visits, occasional inpatient visits, and the required treatment team that includes a nutritionist, psychologist or social worker, nurses, and a physician, and it becomes clear that expanding this treatment to the general population is a very costly proposition. "With 25 or 30 patients at our center, which has a very supportive and highly competent diabetes treatment team, intensive therapy was very doable. But it remains to be seen how this approach will be funneled into regular medical care," Dr. Tamborlane notes. "We hope that with the proof the DCCT has furnished, primary care physicians now will be motivated to provide the best possible care for diabetes patients, and to more effectively refer them to treatment centers that specialize in intensive therapy," he adds.

—*Mary Ann Moon*

Additional Reading

1. Diabetes Control and Complications Trial Research Group, The effect of intensive treatment of diabetes on the development and progression of long-term complications in insulin-dependent diabetes mellitus. *New England Journal of Medicine* 329:977–986, 1993.

2. Reichard, P., Nilsson, B.-Y., and Rosenqvist, U., The effect of long-term intensified insulin treatment on the development of microvascular complications of diabetes mellitus. *New England Journal of Medicine* 329: 304–309, 1993.

This research was supported by the General Clinical Research Centers Program of the National Center for Research Resources; the National Institute of Diabetes and Digestive and Kidney Diseases; the National Heart, Lung, and Blood Institute; and the National Eye Institute.

Chapter 37

Prevention Of Spontaneous Abortion In Diabetic Pregnancies

Good glycemic control decreases the rate of spontaneous abortion in diabetic pregnancies, according to researchers at the University of Cincinnati College of Medicine in Ohio. "Our studies have shown that the rate of spontaneous abortion in women with insulin-dependent diabetes mellitus (IDDM) is about 30 percent, or roughly twice that of the normal population," says principal investigator Dr. Menachem Miodovnik, associate professor in obstetrics and gynecology.

"Through a series of studies we have shown that very good glycemic control in early pregnancy can reduce the rate of spontaneous abortions and will probably reduce the number of birth defects as well," Dr. Miodovnik says.

The investigators monitored the glycemic status of the women by determining whether certain proteins found in the blood were glycosylated—had sugar molecules attached. "We looked at the concentration of glycohemoglobin A_1 (Hb A_1), a normal variant of hemoglobin that reflects the concentration of blood glucose during the preceding 4 to 8 weeks; at glycosylated serum albumin, which reflects glucose status during the previous 2 to 4 weeks; and at glycosylated serum total proteins, which reflect control in the previous 1 to 2 weeks," explains Dr. Miodovnik. "Looking at all of these proteins allows us to assess glucose status at conception, in early pregnancy, and close to the abortive event itself."

In a study of 68 IDDM women during 84 pregnancies the researchers found that the concentration of glycohemoglobin A_1 was significantly higher

---

Research Resources Reporter, November 1990.

in women who had spontaneous abortions than in women who had successful pregnancies. In contrast, the concentrations of total glycosylated serum proteins and glycosylated serum albumin did not differ between the two groups of women. "What this tells us is that it is the glycemic control in very early pregnancy or even preconception that is important in determining whether a spontaneous abortion will occur, since glycohemoglobin A_1 reflects glucose status in the previous 4 to 8 weeks," explains Dr. Miodovnik.

To evaluate whether careful glycemia control was capable of reducing the incidence of spontaneous abortion, Dr. Miodovnik and Dr. Francis Mimouni, associate professor of pediatrics, and their colleagues recruited 45 insulin-dependent diabetic women with two consecutive pregnancies. The women were recruited before the ninth week of pregnancy. Blood glucose measurements were made both before eating and 90 minutes after eating at each weekly visit to the clinic, and glycohemoglobin A_1 concentrations were measured at 9 weeks of pregnancy. Diabetes management included a split dosage regimen of insulin, including both a short and intermediate acting insulin, along with dietary regulation.

"Our results have given us four classes of patients," explains Dr. Miodovnik. "One class contains 20 women who had a successful pregnancy followed by another successful pregnancy, a second class contains 15 women who had an abortion followed by a successful pregnancy. The last two classes contain five women who had a successful pregnancy followed by an abortion and three women who had two abortions, respectively. We included only the first two classes in the statistical analysis, and we found that the abortion/successful pregnancy patients had a significant decrease in Hb A_1 and average postprandial blood glucose from the first to the second pregnancy, which resulted in a 50-percent reduction in the abortion rate."

Dr. Miodovnik believes this reduction in the spontaneous abortion rate owes much of its success to patient education and close management. "Today we use glucometers with memory chips to measure blood sugar as often as eight times a day, and for our patients who live some distance from the clinic we use modems to transmit the information. We also start educating them as early as possible, preferably before they become pregnant, on good diabetes management. In fact, now we have a program for teenagers and parents and try to get them in as early as we can," he explains.

The investigators believe that there might be an association between poor glycemic control and malformations in infants of diabetic women. "We have observed for quite a long time that babies of mothers with IDDM have a much higher rate of malformations than do offspring of normal mothers," says Dr. Mimouni. In 165 first pregnancies there were 13 infants with malformation (7.9 percent), including live-born infants and stillbirths. "Because all spontaneous abortions in that study occurred between 9 and 15 weeks of gestation—a time period believed to be associated with major malformations in the fetus—we suggest that such malformations are the cause of the higher spontaneous abortion rate in IDDM mothers, and that good glycemic control will reduce the rates of both malformations and abortions," he says. Neither maternal age nor duration of diabetes had a significant impact on the rate of spontaneous abortion.

According to Dr. Mimouni, "Cardiac problems occur most frequently. In addition, some very rare malformations occur much more frequently in these infants than in normal infants. One example is the caudal regression syndrome in which the sacrum (a bone situated between the two hip bones) can actually be completely missing. This defect may be accompanied by severe deformation of the lower limbs."

The malformations in the recent study were associated with elevated Hb A_1 concentrations at approximately 9 weeks of pregnancy and the presence of blood vessel disorders, or vasculopathies, in the retina or kidney of the mother. "We're not sure of the exact role played by maternal vascular disease in producing congenital malformations," says Dr. Mimouni. "The significance of elevated Hb A_1 may be the same as in animal studies that have shown a teratogenic (malformation-producing) effect of hyperglycemia, although other studies have shown hypoglycemia to be even more teratogenic."

Insulin that has crossed the placenta and magnesium deficiency in the diabetic women may be two additional causes of birth defects and spontaneous abortions. Dr. Mimouni notes that "it is well known that diabetic women are at risk of magnesium deficiency predominantly due to increased urinary magnesium losses. Because of the very important role magnesium plays in the function of enzymes and critical metabolic processes, magnesium deficiency could contribute to lethal fetal malformations and spontaneous abortions," he says.

Dr. Miodovnik is currently working on a study looking at "strict" versus "customary" glycemic control in pregnant IDDM women. Factors to be assessed include pregnancy outcome, complications of pregnancy, and the influence of hypoglycemic episodes on spontaneous abortion and malformation rates. Dr. Mimouni adds that the glucometers will allow separate analysis of the influence of hypoglycemic and hyperglycemic periods. Both physicians agree that identifying the exact mechanisms of malformation and spontaneous abortion in insulin-dependent diabetic women will help more of them achieve successful pregnancies and bear healthy children.

—M. Elisabeth Tracey

Additional Reading:

1. Menon, R. K., Cohen, R. M., Sperling, M. A., et al., Transplacental passage of insulin in pregnant women with insulin-dependent diabetes mellitus: Its role in fetal macrosomia. *New England Journal of Medicine* 323: 309–315, 1990.

2. Miodovnik, M., Mimouni, F., Siddiqi, T. A., et al., Spontaneous abortions in repeat diabetic pregnancies: A relationship with glycemic control. *Obstetrics and Gynecology* 75:75–78, 1990.

3. Miodovnik, M., Mimouni, F., Dignan, P. S. J., et al., Major malformations in infants of IDDM women. Vasculopathy and early first-trimester poor glycemic control. *Diabetes Care* 11:713–718, 1988.

4. Mimouni, F., Miodovnik, M., Tsang, R. C., et al., Decreased maternal serum magnesium concentration and adverse fetal outcome in insulin-dependent diabetic women. *Obstetrics and Gynecology* 70:85–88, 1987.

5. Miodovnik, M., Mimouni, F., Tsang, R. C., et al., Glycemic control and spontaneous abortion in insulin dependent diabetic women. *Obstetrics and Gynecology* 68:366–369, 1986.

6. Miodovnik, M., Lavin, J. P., Knowles, H. C., et al., Spontaneous abortion among insulin-dependent diabetic women. *American Journal of Obstetrics and Gynecology* 150:372–376, 1984.

This work was supported by the General Clinical Research Centers Program of the National Center for Research Resources and by the National Institute of Child Health and Human Development.

Chapter 38

Diabetic Neuropathy: The Nerve Damage of Diabetes

What is Diabetic Neuropathy?

Diabetic neuropathy is a nerve disorder caused by diabetes. People who have had diabetes for years may experience numbness and sometimes pain in their hands, feet, and legs. Nerve damage caused by diabetes can also lead to problems with indigestion, diarrhea or constipation, dizziness, bladder infections, and impotence. In some cases, damaged nerves can strike suddenly, causing pain, weakness, and weight loss. Depression may follow. While some treatments are available, a great deal of research still needs to be done to understand how diabetes affects the nerves and to find better treatments for this complication.

How Common is Diabetic Neuropathy?

Nerve problems can affect anybody with diabetes, but they are most common in people who have had diabetes more than 10 years. The majority of patients with neurological impairment due to diabetes do not have symptoms such as pain or numbness. However, some recent studies have reported that:

- 10 years after diagnosis, 30 percent of diabetes patients have symptoms or signs of diabetic neuropathy;
- 25 years after diagnosis, 40 percent of diabetes patients have symptoms or signs of neuropathy;

NIH Pub. No. 91-3185.

- 50 years after diagnosis, half of all diabetes patients have symptoms or signs of neuropathy.

Diabetic neuropathy appears to be more common in smokers, people over 40 years of age, and those who have had problems controlling the levels of glucose in their blood.

What Causes Diabetic Neuropathy?

Scientists do not know how diabetic neuropathy occurs, but it is likely that several factors come into play. High blood glucose causes chemical changes in nerves, impairing their ability to transmit nerve signals. High blood glucose also damages blood vessels that carry oxygen and nutrients to the nerves. Also, inherited factors probably unrelated to diabetes may make some people more susceptible to nerve disease than others.

The study of the chemical changes that happen to nerves exposed to high blood glucose is a very active area of research. A normal substance called aldose reductase converts glucose to a type of sugar alcohol called sorbitol. Scientists have found that when tissues have a high level of glucose, sorbitol builds up and apparently damages the membranes lining body tissues.

Scientists have noted that in animals and humans with diabetes, nerves have less than normal amounts of a substance called myoinositol. It is thought that myoinositol plays a role in how nerve cells use energy to maintain the correct balance of salts. This balance is important to cells' ability to conduct nerve impulses.

Studies have also shown that proteins age more quickly when exposed to high glucose. This has the effect of weakening certain connective proteins called collagens, which line and support nerve tissue. While these changes occur with normal aging, high blood glucose speeds up the damage.

It is likely that all three processes are chemically linked. Scientists are studying how these changes occur, how they are connected, how they cause nerve damage, and how the damage can be prevented and treated.

What are the Symptoms of Diabetic Neuropathy?

The symptoms of diabetic neuropathy vary a great deal. Some people notice no symptoms, while others are disabled by severe problems. Neuropathy may cause both pain and insensitivity to pain in the same person. Often, symptoms are slight at first, and since most nerve damage occurs over years, mild cases may go unnoticed for a long time. In some people, though, mainly those afflicted by mononeuorpathy, the onset of pain may be sudden and severe.

Peripheral Neuropathy (also called "somatic neuropathy" or "distal sensory polyneuropathy")

The most common type of neuropathy, peripheral neuropathy can affect any of the nerves that transmit sensation throughout the body. However, the nerves of the limbs, and especially the feet, seem affected most often. Peripheral neuropathy usually involves nerves on both sides of the body. Some of the most common symptoms of this kind of neuropathy are:

- numbness or insensitivity to pain or temperature;
- tingling, burning, or prickling;
- sharp pains or cramps; and
- extreme sensitivity to touch, even very light touch.

These symptoms are often worse at night.

After years of peripheral neuropathy, the damage to nerves may result in loss of reflexes and muscle weakness. These, in turn, may cause:

- loss of balance and coordination;
- inability to raise the foot;
- curling of the toes or other foot problems.

Often the foot becomes wider and shorter, the gait changes, and foot ulcers appear as pressure is put on parts of the foot that are less protected.

Loss of sensation may occur without the warning signs of pain, numbness or tingling. As the damaged nerve grows less sensitive to pain, it is easy to overlook foot problems when they first happen. Injuries can easily become infected because the poor circulation caused by diabetes impedes healing. If an injury is not treated in time, the infection may lead to gangrene, sometimes requiring amputation of the limb. However, problems caused by minor injuries can usually be controlled if they are caught in time.

Autonomic Neuropathy (also called "visceral neuropathy")

Autonomic neuropathy is usually found in people who already have peripheral neuropathy. Autonomic neuropathy affects the nerves that serve the heart and internal organs and produces changes in:

Urination and Sexual Response

Autonomic neuropathy most often affects the organs that control urination and reproduction. Nerve damage prevents the bladder from emptying completely, so bacteria grow more easily in the urinary tract (bladder or kidneys). When the nerves of the bladder are damaged, it may be difficult to control the bladder or to know when it is full.

The nerve damage and circulatory problems of diabetes can also lead to frequent vaginal infections and a gradual loss of sexual sensation or response in both men and women, although sex drive is unchanged. A man may be unable to have erections or may reach sexual climax without ejaculating normally.

Digestion

Autonomic neuropathy can also affect how food is digested. Nerve damage can cause the stomach to empty too slowly, a disorder called gastric stasis. When the condition is severe (gastroparesis), a person can have persistent nausea and vomiting, bloating, and loss of appetite. Blood glucose levels tend to fluctuate wildly.

If nerves in the esophagus are involved, swallowing may be difficult. Nerve damage to the bowels can cause constipation or frequent diarrhea, especially at night. Problems with the digestive system often lead to weight loss.

Cardiovascular System

Autonomic neuropathy least often affects the cardiovascular system, which controls the circulation of blood throughout the body. When it occurs, the nerve impulses from various parts of the body which signal the need for blood are not transmitted normally. As a result, blood pressure may drop sharply after sitting or standing, causing a person to feel dizzy or lightheaded, or even to faint (orthostatic hypotension).

Neuropathy that affects the cardiovascular system may also cause painless heart attacks and may raise the risk of a heart attack during general anesthesia. It can also hinder the body's normal response to low blood sugar or hypoglycemia.

Sweating and Salivation

Autonomic neuropathy can affect the nerves that control sweating and salivation. Sometimes, nerve damage interferes with the activity of the sweat glands, making it difficult to tolerate heat. Other times, it causes profuse sweating at night or while eating (gustatory sweating).

Mononeuropathy (including "multiplex neuropathy")

Occasionally, diabetic neuropathy appears suddenly and affects specific nerves, most often in the torso, leg, or head. When mononeuropathy occurs, it may cause:

- pain in the front of the thigh;
- severe pain in the lower back or pelvis;
- chest or abdominal pain sometimes mistaken for angina, heart attack, or appendicitis;
- aching behind the eye;
- inability to focus the eye:
- double vision;
- paralysis on one side of the face (Bell's palsy); or problems with hearing.

This kind of neuropathy is unpredictable and occurs most often in older people who have mild diabetes. Although mononeuropathy can be very painful, it tends to improve by itself after a period of weeks or months without causing long-term damage.

How do Doctors Diagnose Diabetic Neuropathy?

A doctor diagnoses neuropathy from symptoms and a physical exam. During the exam, the doctor may check muscle strength, reflexes, and sensitivity to position, vibration, temperature, and light touch. Sometimes special tests are used to help pinpoint the cause of symptoms and suggest treatment:

- ***Ultrasound*** employs sound waves too high to hear, which produce an image showing how well the bladder and other parts of the urinary tract are functioning.
- ***Nerve conduction*** studies check the flow of electrical current through a nerve. With this test, an image of the nerve impulse is projected on a screen as it transmits an electrical impulse. Impulses that seem slower or weaker than usual indicate possible damage to the nerve. This test allows the doctor to assess the condition of all of the nerves in the limb.
- ***Electromyography (EMG)*** is used to see how well muscles respond to electrical impulses transmitted by the nerves nearby. With an EMG, the electrical activity of the muscle is displayed on screen. A response that is slower or weaker than usual suggests damage to the muscle. This test is often done at the same time as nerve conduction studies.

- ***Nerve biopsy*** involves removing a sample of nerve tissue, which is examined for damage. This test is most often used in research settings.

If your doctor suspects autonomic neuropathy, you may also be referred to a specialist in digestive disorders (gastroenterologist) for additional tests.

How is Diabetic Neuropathy Usually Treated?

Treatment aims at relieving discomfort and preventing further tissue damage. The first step is to bring blood sugar under control by diet and oral drugs or insulin injections, if needed. Although symptoms can sometimes worsen as blood sugar is brought under control with intensive treatment, careful long-term monitoring of blood sugar helps reverse the pain or loss of sensation that neuropathy can cause. Good control of blood sugar with diet and, if necessary, drug therapy may also help prevent or delay the onset of further problems.

Another important part of treatment involves special care of the feet, which are especially prone to problems. (See section under foot care.)

Relieving Symptoms

A number of medications are used to relieve the symptoms of diabetic neuropathy:

- ***Pain, burning, tingling, or numbness.*** Your doctor may suggest an analgesic such as aspirin or acetaminophen; an anti-inflammatory drug containing ibuprofen; antidepressant medications such as amitriptyline, sometimes used with fluphenazine; or nerve medications such as carbamazepine or phenytoin sodium. Codeine is sometimes prescribed for short-term use to relieve severe pain.

Your doctor may also prescribe a therapy known as transcutaneous electronic nerve stimulation (TENS). In this treatment, small amounts of electricity block pain signals as they pass through a patient's skin. Other treatments include hypnosis, relaxation training, biofeedback, and acupuncture. Some people find that walking regularly or using elastic stockings helps relieve leg pain. Warm (not hot) baths, massage, or an analgesic ointment such as Ben Gay may also help.

- ***Indigestion, belching, nausea or vomiting.*** For patients with mild symptoms of slow stomach emptying, doctors suggest eating small, frequent meals and avoiding fats. Eating less fiber may also relieve symptoms. For patients with severe gastroparesis, the doctor may prescribe metoclopramide, which speeds digestion and relieves nausea. Other drugs that help regulate digestion or reduce stomach acid secretion may also be used. In each case, the potential benefits of these drugs need to be weighed against their side effects.

- ***Diarrhea or other bowel problems.*** Antibiotics or clonidine HCl, a drug used to treat high blood pressure, are some times prescribed. A wheat-free diet may also help bring relief since the gluten in flour sometimes causes diarrhea.
- ***Urinary tract infections.*** Your doctor may prescribe an antibiotic to clear up an infection and suggest drinking more fluids to prevent further infections. It is also a good idea to urinate at regular times (every 3 hours, for example) since you may not be able to tell when your bladder is full.
- ***Lightheadedness, dizziness, or fainting.*** Sitting or standing very slowly may help prevent these problems. Raising the head of your bed and wearing elastic stockings may also help. Increased salt in the diet and treatment with salt-retaining hormones such as fludrocortisone are other possible approaches. In research studies, drugs used to treat hypertension have increased blood pressure in some patients.
- ***Muscle weakness or loss of coordination.*** Physical therapy can often help strengthen muscles and improve coordination.

Sexual Problems

The nerve and circulatory problems of diabetes can disrupt normal sexual function. After ruling out a hormonal cause of impotence, your doctor can advise you about the different methods available to treat impotence caused by neuropathy. Short-term solutions involve using a mechanical vacuum device or injecting a drug called a vasodilator into the penis before sex. Both methods raise blood flow to the penis, making it easier to have and maintain an erection. Surgical procedures, in which an inflatable or semi-rigid device is implanted in the penis, offer a more permanent solution. For some people, counseling may help relieve the stress caused by neuropathy and restore sexual function.

In women who feel their sexual life is not satisfactory, the role of diabetes and the solutions are less clear. Illness, vaginal or urinary infections, and anxiety about pregnancy complicated by diabetes can, for example, interfere with a woman's ability to enjoy intimacy. Infections can be reduced by good blood glucose control. Counseling may also help a woman identify and cope with sexual concerns.

Foot Care

People with diabetes have to take special care of their feet. Since the nerves to the feet are the longest in the body, they are most often affected by neuropathy. At least 15 percent of all people with diabetes eventually have a foot ulcer, and 6 out of every 1,000 lose a limb to infection. However, doctors estimate that nearly three quarters of all amputations caused by neuropathy can be prevented with careful foot care.

Every day, you should check your feet and toes for any cuts, sores, bruises, bumps, or infections—using a mirror if necessary. Since diabetic neuropathy often causes numbness, you may be able to see injuries before you feel any discomfort. Also, poor circulation may cause infections to heal more slowly. To prevent foot problems from developing:

- Wash your feet daily, using warm water and a mild soap. (If you have neuropathy, you should test water temperature with your wrist.) Doctors do not advise soaking your feet for long periods since you may lose protective calluses. Dry your feet carefully with a soft towel, especially between toes.
- Cover your feet (except for the skin between the toes) with petroleum jelly, a lotion containing lanolin, or cold cream before putting on shoes and socks. The diabetic foot tends to sweat less than normal, leading to dry, cracked skin.
- Wear thick, soft socks, and avoid wearing slippery stockings, mended stockings, or stockings with seams.
- Wear shoes that fit your feet well and allow your toes to move. Break in new shoes gradually, wearing them for only an hour at a time. After years of neuropathy, as reflexes are lost, it is common for the feet to become wider and flatter. If you have problems finding shoes that fit well, ask your doctor to refer you to a specialist who can fit you with corrective shoes or inserts.
- Examine your shoes before putting them on to make sure they have no tears or sharp edges that might injure your feet.
- Cut your toenails straight across, but be careful not to leave any sharp corners that could cut the next toe.
- Use an emery board or a pumice stone to file away dead skin, but don't remove calluses, which act as protective padding. Don't try to cut off any growths yourself, and avoid using harsh chemicals such as wart remover on your feet.

- Don't take very hot baths and never go barefoot, even on the beach or by a pool.
- Wear socks if feet are cold at night—no heating pads or hot water bottles.
- Avoid sitting with your legs crossed. This can reduce the flow of blood to the feet.
- Ask your doctor to check your feet at every visit, and call your doctor if you notice that a sore isn't healing well.
- If you're not able to take care of your own feet, ask your doctor to recommend a podiatrist (specialist in the care and treatment of feet) who can help.

Some General Hints

- If you smoke, try to stop since smoking makes circulatory problems worse and increases the risk of neuropathy and heart disease.
- Ask your doctor to suggest an exercise routine that's right for you. Many people who exercise regularly find the pain of neuropathy is less severe. Aside from helping you reach and maintain your ideal weight, exercise also improves the body's use of insulin, helps improve circulation, and strengthens muscles. Check with your doctor before starting exercise that can be hard on your feet, such as running or aerobics.
- Cut back on the amount of alcohol you drink. Recent research has indicated that as few as four drinks per week can worsen neuropathy.

Are There Any Experimental Treatments for Diabetic Neuropathy?

Though still under study, new therapies may eventually prevent or reverse diabetic neuropathy. Extensive testing is required by the U.S. Food and Drug Administration to establish the safety and efficacy of drugs before they are approved for widespread use.

A new topical cream, capsaicin, is now in clinical trials and may prove to reduce the pain of neuropathy. Scientists believe that the ointment, a cayenne pepper extract, depletes the chemical that transmits pain signals to the brain.

Many doctors prescribe vitamin B1 because it appears to keep neuropathy from progressing, but there is no hard evidence of its benefits, and others feel it should not be prescribed. In addition, researchers are exploring treatment with another B vitamin called myoinositol. Early findings have shown that nerves in diabetic animals and humans have less than normal amounts of this substance. With supplements, myoinositol levels are increased in tissues of diabetic animals, but research is still needed to show any concrete, lasting benefits.

Another area of research concerns the drug aminoguanidine. In animals, aminoguanidine blocks cross-linking of proteins that occurs more quickly than normal in tissues exposed to high glucose. Very early clinical tests are under way to determine the effects of aminoguanidine in humans.

One approach that appeared promising involved the use of aldose reductase inhibitors. These are a class of drugs that block the formation of the sugar alcohol sorbitol, which is thought to damage nerves. Scientists hoped these drugs would prevent and might even repair nerve damage. But so far, clinical trials have shown these drugs to have major side effects while improving neuropathy in only a small number of patients.

Future Research

The National Institutes of Health (NIH) is an agency of the Public Health Service under the U.S. Department of Health and Human Services. Its mission is to improve human health through biomedical research. Several components of NIH—the National Institute of Diabetes and Digestive and Kidney Diseases, the National Institute of Neurological Disorders and Stroke, and the National Institute of Dental Research—conduct and support research on the nerve complications of diabetes. The knowledge gained from this research may one day offer a way to prevent or cure diabetic neuropathy and bring relief to millions of people.

Chapter 39

Facts About Diabetic Eye Disease

There are approximately 14 million Americans who have either Type I (juvenile onset) or Type II (adult onset) diabetes. All are at risk of developing sight-threatening eye diseases that are common complications of diabetes. Although early detection and timely treatment can substantially reduce the risk of severe visual loss or blindness from diabetic eye disease, many people at risk are not having their eyes examined regularly to detect these problems before they impair vision. Increased awareness of the sight-saving benefits of annual eye examinations through dilated pupils is essential to reduce the significant social and personal costs of diabetic eye disease.

What is Diabetic Eye Disease?

Diabetic eye disease refers to a group of sight-threatening eye problems that people with diabetes may develop as a complication of the disease. They include:

- *Diabetic retinopathy*. This disease damages blood vessels in the retina, the light-sensitive tissue at the back of the eye that translates light into electrical impulses that the brain interprets as vision.
- *Cataract*. A cataract is an opacity of the eye's crystalline lens that results in blurring of normal vision. People with diabetes are twice as likely to develop a cataract as someone who does not have the

---

National Eye Institute, National Eye Health Education Program, March 1993.

disease. In addition, cataracts tend to develop at an earlier age in people with diabetes, around late middle-age.

- *Glaucoma*—This disease occurs when increased fluid pressure in the eye leads to progressive optic nerve damage. People with diabetes are nearly twice as likely to develop glaucoma as other adults.

Cataract and glaucoma also affect many people who do not have diabetes.

What is the Most Common Diabetic Eye Disease?

Diabetic retinopathy. About half of the nation's estimated 14 million people with diabetes have at least early signs of diabetic retinopathy. Of this group, about 700,000 have serious retinal disease, with approximately 65,000 Americans progressing each year to proliferative retinopathy, the disease's most sight-threatening stage. Annually, as many as 24,000 people go blind from the disorder, making it a leading cause of blindness among working-age Americans.

Although anyone with diabetes can develop diabetic retinopathy, research shows two important risk factors: (1) type of diabetes, and (2) duration of disease. People with Type I diabetes are generally more likely to develop diabetic retinopathy than Type II patients. In fact, virtually all people who have had Type I diabetes for 15 years or more have some degree of diabetic retinopathy. Among people with Type II diabetes, duration of disease is also an important risk factor. Insulin-taking Type II patients who have had diabetes for five to 10 years have about a 2 percent incidence of proliferative retinopathy. This rate increases to more than 50 percent in insulin-taking Type II patients who have had diabetes for more than 20 years.

What is the Cost of Diabetic Retinopathy?

It is estimated that a year of blindness costs the U.S. government approximately $13,607 annually per person in Social Security benefits, lost income tax revenue, and health care expenditures. If Americans at risk for developing diabetic eye disease were regularly screened and treated to preserve their sight, the net annual savings to the government would be more than $100 million.

What Causes It?

Diabetic retinopathy is a complex disease. Although scientists understand much about the disease's natural history, they are still unclear about its specific pathological causes. There is, however, a consensus that diabetic retinopathy probably does not stem from a single retinal change. Rather, the disease may be triggered by a combination of biochemical, metabolic, and hematologic abnormalities.

In people with diabetes, three metabolic and hematologic changes are suspected of being involved in the early stages of diabetic retinopathy:

- Hyperglycemia: A chronic increase in normal blood-glucose levels may gradually alter cell metabolism in the retinal blood vessels.
- Blood platelet abnormalities: Diabetes-related biochemical changes may make circulating blood platelets abnormally sticky.
- Blood vessel narrowing: Hematologic changes may cause the retinal blood vessels to constrict.

These abnormalities may cause certain cells to die inside the retinal blood vessels. This leads to altered blood flow, increased blood vessel permeability, and the growth of certain blood vessel components. As a result, tiny outcroppings—called microaneurysms—may bulge from the weak blood vessel walls. The microaneurysms, which resemble tiny blisters on the blood vessels, may leak blood onto the central retina, or macula, causing an early, sight-impairing swelling of this area called macular edema.

The disease enters its proliferative stage when new blood vessels begin to grow into the retina and optic disc to increase blood flow to these tissues. New blood vessels may form because of hormonal signals, i.e., growth hormone, sent to the eye. These new blood vessels are fragile and often leak blood and protein into the vitreous—the transparent, gel that fills two-thirds of the inner eye—and retina, causing visual impairment.

As the disease progresses, the new blood vessels may also grow into the vitreous and cause it to detach gradually from the back of the eye. As the vitreous pulls away, it may detach the retina as well. As a result, severe visual loss or blindness will occur.

What are the Symptoms of Diabetic Retinopathy?

For many people with diabetic retinopathy, there are no early symptoms. There is no pain, no blurred vision, and no ocular inflammation. In fact, many people do not develop any visual impairment until the disease has advanced well into its proliferative stage. At this point, the vision that has been lost cannot be restored.

However, some people in the early and advanced stages of diabetic retinopathy may notice a change in their central and/or color vision. The loss of central vision results from macular edema, which can often be effectively treated.

How is Diabetic Eye Disease Detected?

Because diabetic eye disease often has no early symptoms, it is detected during a comprehensive eye examination through dilated pupils. Dilation consists of the eye care professional placing medicated drops into the eye to enlarge the pupil. By so doing, the practitioner can better examine the back of the eye for early signs of disease, such as microaneurysms, before noticeable vision loss occurs.

For example, if the eye care professional detects diabetic retinopathy early, he or she can then monitor the patient's condition and determine the best time to treat the problem, should it progress to that point. The National Eye Health Education Program—coordinated by the National Eye Institute, one of the federal National Institutes of Health—recommends that people with diabetes should undergo a comprehensive eye examination through dilated pupils at least once a year.

How is Diabetic Retinopathy Treated?

Laser surgery, also called photocoagulation, is now being used successfully to treat proliferative retinopathy. It is performed by aiming a narrow, high-energy beam of light through the pupil and onto the retina. The beam of light is used to make hundreds of small burns over the retinal surface that destroy the growing blood vessels.

Laser surgery is also used to treat macular edema. In this procedure, however, the laser is aimed directly onto leaking blood vessels in the macula. The beam of light then seals the blood vessels to stop their sight-impairing leakage.

Current treatment guidelines are so successful that even people with proliferative retinopathy have a 95 percent chance of maintaining their vision. Current treatment guidelines call for (1) regular eye examinations through dilated pupils, (2) timely laser surgery, and (3) when needed, vitrectomy, a surgical procedure that clears hemorrhaged blood from inside the eye that can cloud vision.

What Research is Being Conducted?

During the last 25 years, scientists have made great progress in managing and treating diabetic eye disease. Laser surgery, cataract surgery, and glaucoma medications and surgery have all been either developed or improved considerably during this period. But if this research progress is to continue, additional understanding is needed of the cellular and biochemical basis of each disease.

For example, NEI scientists have developed the first animal research model for advanced (proliferative) retinopathy. This model will allow researchers to study better the vascular changes associated with this disease. It will also allow them to initiate studies on new drugs that are designed to prevent and treat diabetic retinopathy.

Other NEI-funded scientists are studying several growth factors to determine whether they influence the development of weak new blood vessels that proliferate in advanced diabetic retinopathy. In other studies, NEI scientists have inoculated bacterial cells with the DNA sequence that codes for the enzyme aldose reductase, which has been demonstrated as being a major mechanism by which early retinal capillary cells breakdown in the formation of diabetic retinopathy. The inoculated cells are yielding abundant and active aldose reductase, which is valuable for use in the development of a safe and effective enzyme inhibitor.

A well-coordinated public health effort also requires accurate data on disease prevalence, progression, and associated factors. For this reason, the NEI is supporting a long-term epidemiologic study in southern Wisconsin on diabetic retinopathy.

As science moves forward in its study of diabetic eye disease, it is likely that new treatments will be a result of basic and clinical research. Improved treatment, coupled with heightened public awareness, should go far toward reducing diabetic eye disease as a future national health problem.

Chapter 40

Diabetic Retinopathy

Why is it Important to Know How Diabetes Affects the Eyes?

If you are among the 10 million people in the United States who have diabetes—or if someone close to you has this disease—you should know that diabetes can affect the eyes and cause visual impairment.

Fortunately, there are ways to prevent or lessen the eye damage caused by diabetes. That is why it is so important for people with this disease to have a professional eye examination as soon as their diabetes is diagnosed, and at least once a year thereafter.

Regular eye examinations are especially important for people who have had diabetes 5 years or longer, for those who have difficulty controlling the level of sugar in their blood, and for diabetic women who are pregnant. All of these people are at increased risk for diabetes-associated eye problems.

What is Diabetic Retinopathy?

Diabetic retinopathy is a potentially serious eye disease caused by diabetes. It affects the retina—the light-sensitive tissue at the back of the eye that transmits visual messages to the brain. Damage to this delicate tissue may result in visual impairment or blindness.

Diabetic retinopathy begins with a slight deterioration in the small blood vessels of the retina. Portions of the vessel walls balloon outward and fluid starts to leak from the vessels into the surrounding retinal tissue. Generally,

---

NIH Pub. No. 93-2171.

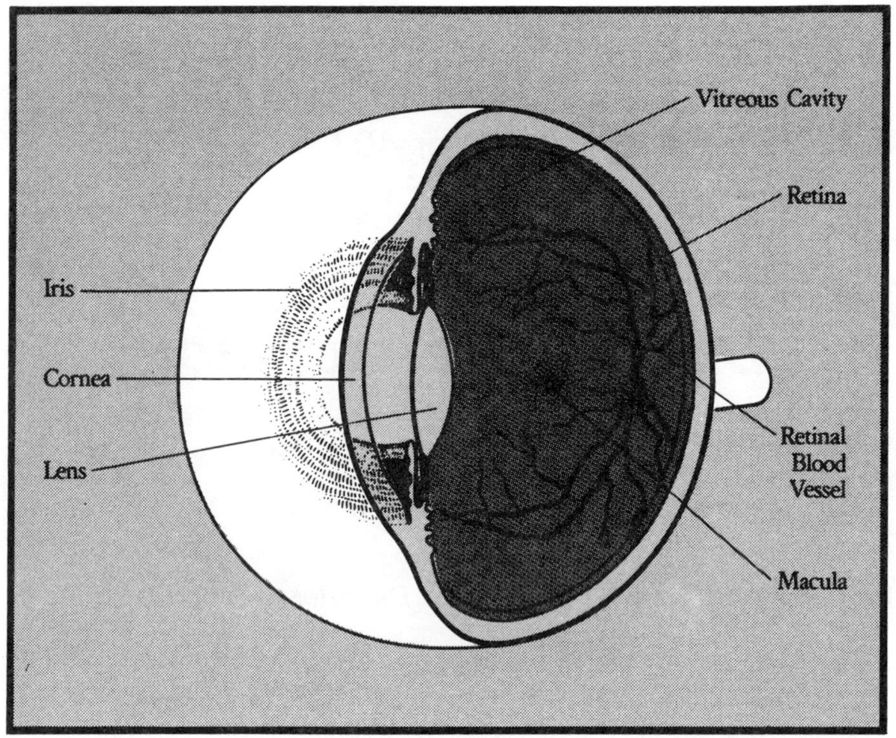

Figure 40-1.

these initial changes in the retina cause no visual symptoms. However, they can be detected by an eye specialist who is trained to recognize subtle signs of retinal disease.

In many people with diabetic retinopathy, the disease remains mild and never causes visual problems. But in some individuals, continued leakage from the retinal blood vessels leads to *macular edema*. This is a build-up of fluid in the macula—the part of the retina responsible for the sharp, clear vision used in reading and driving. When critical areas of the macula become swollen with excess fluid, vision may be so badly blurred that these activities become difficult or impossible.

Some people with diabetes develop an even more sight-threatening condition called *proliferative retinopathy*. It may occur in people who have macular edema, but also can develop in those who don't. In proliferative retinopathy, abnormal new blood vessels grow on the surface of the retina. These fragile new vessels can easily rupture and bleed into the middle of the eye, blocking vision. Scar tissue also may form near the retina, ultimately detaching it from the back of the eye. Severe visual loss, even permanent blindness, may result. But this happens in only a small minority of people with diabetes.

How Many Diabetics are Affected?

Approximately 40 percent of all people with diabetes have at least mild signs of diabetic retinopathy. About 3 percent have suffered severe visual loss because of this disease.

In general, the longer one has had diabetes, the greater one's chances of developing diabetic retinopathy.

What are the Symptoms of Diabetic Retinopathy?

As already indicated, diabetic retinopathy generally causes no symptoms in its earliest stages. For the person who develops macular edema, blurring of vision may provide a clue that something is wrong. But proliferative retinopathy can progress a long way without any warning signs. That is why a person with diabetes should make regular visits to an eye specialist, so any eye problems can be detected and treated if necessary.

How is Diabetic Retinopathy Treated?

Recently, scientists have found that laser treatment can prevent visual loss in many people with diabetic macular edema. In this treatment, called photocoagulation, powerful beams of light from a laser are aimed at leaking retinal blood vessels in the macula. The goal of treatment is to seal the vessels and prevent further leakage. In many patients, this treatment halts the decline in vision or even reverses it.

Research also has shown that laser photocoagulation can dramatically reduce the risk of blindness in people who have proliferative retinopathy. For these patients, the laser is used in a different way: It is not directed at the macula but is aimed at hundreds of spots in other parts of the retina. The purpose of the treatment is to destroy diseased tissue and stop the retinopathy from getting worse. In fact, the treatment can reduce the risk of severe visual loss by 60 percent.

The studies which proved the value of laser treatment for people with diabetic retinopathy were supported by the National Eye Institute. It is part of the National Institutes of Health, a component of the U.S. Department of Health and Human Services.

These studies also have helped ophthalmologists determine which diabetic patients need laser treatment and when to begin it.

Who Should Have Laser Treatment?

An ophthalmologist (a medical doctor who specializes in the care of eye conditions) usually will consider laser treatment when a person with diabetes has proliferative retinopathy or retinal signs that suggest this condition may soon develop. Also, people with a significant degree of macular edema would now be considered for laser treatment.

When deciding whether to recommend laser treatment to a particular patient, the ophthalmologist weighs the potential benefits—preventing or delaying severe visual loss—against the risk of unwanted side effects. These may include some loss of central or side vision.

Unfortunately, laser treatment cannot restore sight to the person who has already suffered severe retinal damage from diabetic retinopathy. Also, the laser generally is not used when bleeding inside the eye has made it difficult or impossible for the ophthalmologist to see the areas that need treatment.

What is Vitrectomy?

A few diabetic retinopathy patients—including some who have had photocoagulation—go blind from massive bleeding inside the eye. Now, ophthalmologists can remove the blood and scar tissue from the center of the eye. This procedure is known as vitrectomy. Following vitrectomy, patients can often see well enough to move around on their own. Occasionally, vision in the operated eye recovers enough for the patient to resume reading or driving.

What Research is Being Done on Diabetic Retinopathy?

The National Eye Institute is supporting a nationwide study to determine whether photocoagulation—used alone or in combination with aspirin—can benefit people who are still in the early stages of diabetic retinopathy. Almost 4,000 patients are enrolled in this 5-year clinical trial. It already has proven the value of photocoagulation for macular edema (see "How is diabetic retinopathy treated?"), and is expected to yield further valuable findings in the future.

Another clinical trial sponsored by the Institute and Pfizer, Inc., is evaluating a new drug called sorbinil to see if it can prevent eye and nerve damage in people with diabetes.

In addition to these clinical trials, the Institute is supporting an extensive program of research on the causes, detection, and treatment of diabetic retinopathy.

Who can Refer You to an Eye Care Specialist?

If you know you have diabetes, you are probably under the care of a physician who can refer you to an eye doctor for regular examinations and treatment, if needed. You may also request the name of an appropriate eye doctor from eye care centers affiliated with academic institutions, from a hospital, or from a diabetes clinic at a medical center.

You may obtain information on diabetes from the American Diabetes Association, 1660 Duke Street, Alexandria, Virginia 22314, telephone (703) 549–1500; and the Juvenile Diabetes Foundation, 432 Park Avenue South, 16th Floor, New York, New York 10016, telephone (212) 889–7575. Check your local telephone directory for their affiliates or chapters near you.

What Help is Available to the Person who has Already Lost Vision from Diabetic Retinopathy?

There are many useful devices that can help a partially sighted person to make the most of his or her remaining vision. Called low vision aids, these devices have special lenses or electronic systems that produce enlarged images of nearby objects.

If you need low vision aids, your eye care specialist can generally prescribe them. Often, he or she will be able to suggest further sources you might contact to get information about counseling, training and other special services for people with low vision. These may include a nearby school of medicine or optometry.

Chapter 41

Early Treatment Diabetic Retinopathy Study (ETDRS)

INFORMATION FOR PATIENTS

Conclusions of the Early Treatment Diabetic Retinopathy Study

Introduction

The 3,711 patients who participated in the Early Treatment Diabetic Retinopathy Study (ETDRS) have been vital to this landmark clinical trial in vision research. They, like the other members of the research team, were asked to make a long-term commitment to the study. Thanks to study patients' belief in the importance of scientific research, the ETDRS has now produced results that will benefit millions of people through the coming decades. Now that the study has ended, this explanation for patients has been prepared to give an overview of the study conclusions and to explain what they mean to people with diabetic retinopathy.

Background

Diabetic retinopathy is a frequent complication of diabetes, a disease that affects approximately 11 million Americans. It is a leading cause of blindness among young adults.

For patients with diabetes, regular, comprehensive eye examinations

---

This information was prepared by the Scientific Reporting Section of the National Eye Institute, National Institutes of Health. October, 1989.

through dilated pupils and careful followup are very important. Long before a patient notices blurring of vision from diabetic retinopathy, an eye examination can reveal abnormalities in the retina, such as hemorrhages (bleeding), closure of blood vessels, and leakage of fluid. This leakage may cause macular edema (swelling of the macula). The macula is the part of the retina that provides sharp, central vision.

If many retinal blood vessels become closed, new abnormal vessels and scar tissue tend to form on the surface of the retina. Hemorrhage from these vessels into the gel that fills the inside of the eye (vitreous) or retinal detachment caused by shrinkage of the scar tissue can lead to visual loss, even blindness.

Ophthalmologists use two types of laser treatment for diabetic retinopathy. In **focal photocoagulation treatment**, the laser beam is aimed at and seals the leaky retinal blood vessels that cause macular edema. In **scatter photocoagulation treatment**, the laser beam is used to produce many tiny burns scattered throughout the retina, sparing the macula. This slows the growth and development of new blood vessels and scar tissue.

Studies of Diabetic Retinopathy

In the 1970s, the National Eye Institute (NEI), part of the Federal Government's National Institutes of Health, sponsored the Diabetic Retinopathy Study (DRS), a nationwide clinical trial. This study evaluated whether scatter treatment would slow the progression of advanced diabetic retinopathy and prevent visual loss.

Data from the DRS demonstrated that scatter treatment was effective in preventing severe visual loss. Treatment was recommended for eyes with **high-risk proliferative retinopathy**, a stage of the disease likely to lead to severe visual loss if untreated.

In 1979, the NEI initiated the ETDRS to determine whether scatter treatment in earlier stages of diabetic retinopathy would reduce further the risk of blindness. The ETDRS also evaluated focal treatment because several clinical investigations had suggested that focal treatment might be an effective therapy for macular edema. The study was conducted at 22 medical centers throughout the United States.

The ETDRS asked three questions: (1) Is laser treatment effective for diabetic macular edema? (2) When in the course of the disease is the best time to begin laser treatment for diabetic retinopathy? (3) Does aspirin treatment alter the progression of diabetic retinopathy?

ETDRS Treatments

To evaluate the effect of laser treatment, one eye of each patient was randomly assigned to receive immediate treatment. The other eye initially was not treated, but was **carefully followed and evaluated every four months** and received laser treatment if the eye progressed to the high-risk stage.

Eyes selected for immediate treatment received one of four different combinations of focal and scatter treatment. By varying the amount of scatter treatment given and the time of initiation of focal treatment for macular edema, the study investigators hoped to find the best possible early treatment strategy.

To evaluate the effect of aspirin on diabetic retinopathy, all ETDRS patients were randomly assigned to either two tablets of aspirin per day (total daily dosage, 650 mg) or placebo, pills without active ingredients.

ETDRS ophthalmologists evaluated all patients through eye examinations every four months. They examined the majority of patients regularly for at least four years, and some patients for more than nine years.

The effectiveness of ETDRS treatments was measured by how well the patients maintained their vision and whether their retinopathy progressed.

ETDRS Conclusions and Recommendations

The ETDRS results will be published in the scientific literature. Based on these results, scientists have reported the following answers to the three ETDRS questions:

- *Focal treatment is effective for macular edema.*

Focal treatment for macular edema was so helpful in reducing the risk of visual loss that in 1985 ETDRS scientists changed the treatment plan. After that, every patient in the study was eligible for focal treatment if vision was threatened by macular edema. The final study results support these original findings.

On the other hand, scatter treatment was not effective for macular edema, and some patients had side effects such as mild decreases in central and/or peripheral vision following treatment.

- *Scatter laser treatment reduces the risk of severe visual loss. Rates of severe visual loss are low whether scatter treatment is given early or deferred until the development of high-risk proliferative retinopathy.*

The study results showed that the rates of severe visual loss were low for all patients in the ETDRS. Only 4 percent of eyes assigned to deferral of treatment (until high-risk proliferative retinopathy was observed) had severe visual loss after five years compared to 2.5 percent of eyes assigned to immediate treatment. However, about one-half of the eyes assigned to deferral of laser treatment never developed high-risk proliferative retinopathy during the seven years of followup. These eyes did not need scatter treatment and, therefore, avoided its side effects.

Provided careful followup can be maintained, it is safe to defer scatter treatment until retinopathy approaches or reaches the high-risk stage. In eyes with mild to moderate retinopathy, the rate of progression to this high-risk stage was very low. ETDRS results do not support early scatter treatment for these eyes.

- *Aspirin treatment does not alter the progression of diabetic retinopathy.*

The dosage of aspirin used in the ETDRS neither prevented the development of high-risk proliferative retinopathy nor increased the risk of vitreous hemorrhage. Aspirin did not affect vision in any way. Results indicate no reason for people with diabetes to avoid taking aspirin when it is needed for treatment of other problems.

Summary

The ETDRS has provided important results that can benefit people with diabetes. People who have not yet suffered visual loss from diabetic retinopathy have the most to gain from the ETDRS results. The risk of losing sharp central vision from macular edema can be reduced by focal treatment, and if retinopathy progresses toward the high-risk stage, scatter treatment can reduce the risk of blindness.

Regular eye examinations through dilated pupils are important for all people with diabetes. Early detection and appropriate treatment of diabetic retinopathy is the best way to maintain good vision.

Chapter 42

Cataracts

What is a Cataract?

A cataract is a cloudy or opaque area in the lens of the eye. The lens is located behind the pupil and iris. It helps focus light onto the retina, the light-sensitive tissue that lines the inside of the back of the eye. Usually, the lens is transparent. But if it becomes clouded, the passage of light is obstructed and vision may be impaired.

What Causes a Cataract?

When a cataract forms, there is a change in the chemical composition of the lens, but scientists do not know exactly what causes these chemical changes. The most common form of cataract is related to aging, although this type can occur at age 50 or even earlier. Cataracts also may be associated with diabetes, other systemic diseases, drugs, and eye injuries. Sometimes babies are born with congenital cataracts or develop them during the early years of life.

What are the Symptoms of a Cataract?

Cataracts usually develop gradually, without pain, redness, or tearing in the eye. Some cataracts never progress to the point where they seriously impair vision, whereas others eventually block most or all vision in the

---

NIH Pub. No. 93-201.

affected eye. The effect of a cataract on vision depends on several things: 1) its size, 2) its density, 3) its location within the lens.

Among the Signs that a Cataract may be Forming are:

- Hazy, fuzzy, or blurred vision. Double vision sometimes occurs, but this usually goes away as the cataract worsens.
- The need for frequent changes in eyeglass prescriptions. When the cataract progresses beyond a certain point, these changes no longer improve vision.
- A feeling of having a film over the eyes, or of looking through veils or a waterfall. The person with a cataract may blink a lot in an effort to see better.
- Changes in the color of the pupil, which is usually black. When the eye is examined, the pupil may look grey, yellow, or white, but color changes are not always noticeable.
- Problems with light. For example, night driving becomes harder because the cloudy part of the lens scatters the light from oncoming headlights, making these lights appear double or dazzling. Also, the person with a cataract may have trouble finding the right amount of light for reading or close work.
- "Second sight"—a temporary improvement in reading vision experienced by some people when their cataract reaches a certain stage of development. As the cataract progresses, vision again worsens.

None of these symptoms necessarily means that a person has a cataract, or if a cataract is present that it must be removed. However, people who have any of these symptoms should see an eye doctor.

When Should a Cataract be Removed?

A cataract should be removed surgically when it has progressed to the point where resulting vision problems interfere with one's daily activities. A second reason for cataract surgery, more urgent but less common than the first, is that the cataract has become completely opaque (mature). It is possible for a mature cataract to swell and even disintegrate inside the eye. Such changes can permanently endanger vision.

With congenital cataracts, it used to be standard practice to postpone surgery until the child was at least 6 months old. Recently, however, cataracts have been removed from the eyes of newborn infants with good results. Early removal of severe congenital cataract(s) is an important advance because it reduces the risk of visual loss resulting from the disuse of one or both eyes during childhood.

How are Cataracts Treated?

Treating cataracts really involves two steps. The first is removal of the clouded lens by an ophthalmologist. Surgery is the only method proven effective for removing cataracts. The second is finding an appropriate substitute for the natural lens. The decision about which substitute lens to use is usually made before surgery.

There are two general methods of removing a cataract: intracapsular and extracapsular extraction of the lens. Intracapsular extraction is sometimes used to remove senile cataracts. In this method, the entire lens, including its capsule, is removed.

Extracapsular extraction involves removal of most lens tissue but the back part of the lens capsule is left in place. In infants and young children, whose lenses are relatively soft, the lens tissue may be withdrawn through a hollow needle, a procedure called aspiration. A variety of extracapsular techniques are also used to remove the lens in adults.

One technique is called phacoemulsification. High-frequency sound vibrations (ultrasound) are used to soften and liquefy the lens so it can be aspirated through the needle.

Phacoemulsification should not be confused with another form of eye surgery, photocoagulation, in which laser light—not ultrasound—is used to treat some eye disorders other than cataract. A laser cannot remove a cloudy lens or make it clear again. However, some doctors may use a laser to open the front part of the lens capsule before removing the lens or to help patients who develop "after-cataract." (See "What happens after surgery?")

How Safe is Cataract Surgery?

Cataract surgery is one of the most successful operations done today—more than 90 percent of the people who have this surgery find that they can see better. Complications may occur, but most are treatable. Serious complications that threaten vision are rare.

Certain people may not benefit much from cataract surgery. They include people whose cataracts are not advanced enough to impair vision seriously and those whose vision is impaired by another eye disease as well.

In summary, each cataract patient should discuss the possibility of surgery with the doctor who examines his or her eyes to determine whether the potential benefits of cataract surgery outweigh the risks. It is also very important to decide in advance, with the help of the doctor, what form of substitute lens would be most suitable. Patients may want to get a second opinion on the advisability of surgery and on the most appropriate substitute lens to use after surgery.

What are the Choices for a Substitute Lens?

There are three options for replacing the natural lens removed in cataract surgery: eyeglasses, contact lenses, or an intraocular lens implant. Each has advantages and drawbacks.

Eyeglasses. This is a safe and time-proven solution to the problem of seeing without a natural lens. But cataract eyeglasses can have some unpleasant effects. Patients may be bothered by the fact that these glasses magnify objects 20–35 percent, affect depth perception until the person relearns how to judge distances, and limit side vision.

If only one eye requires cataract surgery, eyeglasses may well cause problems because the person is unable to fuse the different-sized images formed by the operated and unoperated eyes. Such patients are often advised before surgery that it would be best to use a contact lens, or have a lens implant.

Contact lenses. These usually provide better vision than eyeglasses and also are quite safe if handled and maintained properly. A contact lens may be especially helpful after cataract extraction in one eye. With a contact lens in the operated eye, the difference in the size of the images seen by the two eyes is much smaller. Soft contact lenses are commonly used for cataract patients.

Another option is the extended-wear contact lens. These lenses can be left in the eye for a longer period of time without being removed, even for sleep. They may be especially useful for people who have trouble inserting and removing a contact lens, because an eye care specialist can remove and clean them periodically. However, extended-wear lenses have some disadvantages: They are very fragile; some serious infections have been reported; their long-term safety is still being assessed; and they do require periodic removal, cleaning, and reinserting.

Intraocular lenses. These devices, sometimes called IOLs, are clear plastic lenses that are implanted in the eye during the cataract operation. Lens implants have certain advantages: They usually eliminate or minimize the problems with image size, side vision, and depth perception noted by people who wear cataract eyeglasses. Also, because lens implants remain in the eye and do not have to be removed, cleaned, and reinserted, they are more convenient than contact lenses. This is particularly true for people who have physical problems that would make it difficult for them to carry out the procedures involved in using contact lenses.

Because of these advantages, lens implants have been used with increasing frequency in recent years. About three-fourths of all people now undergoing cataract surgery have an IOL inserted at the same time, and the vast majority are very pleased with the results. Of course ophthalmologists will continue to study IOLs for many years in an effort to assess the long-term effects of implantation on the eye as well as the short-term complications.

What Happens After Surgery?

Most people who undergo cataract surgery are treated as outpatients and can go home the same day. For others, a stay in the hospital of 1–3 days may be required. In either case, during the early stages of recovery, patients need to take special care to avoid strenuous physical activity.

Sometimes people whose cataract surgery was performed by the extracapsular method develop a problem called "after-cataract." After the operation, the back part of the lens capsule left in the eye may become cloudy and interfere with passage of light to the retina.

The cloudy material must be cleared away, if possible, so that full vision can be restored. Ophthalmologists often treat after-cataract with an ophthalmic laser called the neodymium-YAG or "cold" laser. When this procedure is successful, the patient's vision is restored without additional eye surgery.

What Research is Being Done on Cataracts?

The National Eye Institute supports and conducts research on the eye and its disorders, including cataracts. The major goals of this research are to learn more about how and why cataracts develop, to find ways of preventing cataracts or slowing their progress, to evaluate the safety and effectiveness of techniques for treating cataracts, and to devise better methods of correcting vision after cataract surgery.

Chapter 43

Glaucoma

Why You Should Know the Facts about Glaucoma:

You may be among the two million adult Americans who have glaucoma. If you have this eye disease, you need treatment to prevent loss of vision. Although glaucoma cannot be cured, it can be controlled if detected and treated early.

Unfortunately, people who have glaucoma may not be aware that something is wrong with their eyes until it is too late to prevent visual impairment and even blindness. To guard against visual loss from glaucoma, people should have regular eye examinations—so their eye specialist can look for signs of this disease and determine if treatment is needed.

Regular eye check-ups are particularly important for people whose risk of glaucoma is higher than average. This includes black people, who are more likely than whites to develop glaucoma. It also includes everyone over 40, because glaucoma usually begins in middle age or later. Scientists do not yet know why aging makes a person more susceptible to glaucoma, but it is clear that the risk rises in the later decades of life. Also, there is an increased risk of glaucoma in people with diabetes or high blood pressure, and in those with a family history of glaucoma.

This brochure is mainly about the most common kind of glaucoma, which is called *open-angle glaucoma*. Other kinds of glaucoma are described briefly. In the back of the brochure, you will find out where to go for more information on glaucoma.

NIH Pub. No. 91-651.

What is Open-Angle Glaucoma?

In open-angle glaucoma, gradual changes within the eye lead to an internal fluid pressure that is high enough to damage delicate structures essential to vision. These changes occur in several stages:

- Fluid pressure inside the eye (*intraocular pressure*) begins to rise. This happens because the fluid that normally fills the inside of the eyeball flows in at the usual rate but drains too slowly. This fluid, called *aqueous humor*, is a clear liquid made continuously by cells inside the eye. Aqueous helps maintain the shape of the eyeball and bathes and nourishes the lens and cornea, transparent tissues located near the front of the eye (see Figure 43–1). Aqueous leaves the eye through a spongy meshwork of tissue located at the "angle" where the cornea and iris meet. When aqueous cannot exit fast enough, intraocular pressure rises. Why this happens is not known for certain, although scientists think the problem relates to changes in the drainage meshwork that are triggered by aging and by other factors that are still not understood. Although someone who has high intraocular pressure usually cannot feel it, an eye care specialist can detect and measure it with an instrument called a *tonometer*.
- Higher than normal intraocular pressure begins to destroy the tiny, delicate nerve fibers that make up the *optic nerve* at the back of the eye. Because the optic nerve relays visual messages from the eye to the brain—where seeing actually takes place—the health of this nerve is essential to sight.

Under prolonged high pressure, the optic nerve deteriorates and the patient's field of vision gradually gets narrower. Surprisingly, most people don't notice these changes until there is extensive loss of side vision.

- If optic nerve damage is not halted, glaucoma leads to tunnel vision and blindness. This can happen in just a few years. Glaucoma-induced vision loss is permanent and cannot be restored by treatment.

Therefore, to be fully effective, treatment must begin before there is serious damage to the optic nerve. That is why early detection is critical, for an eye specialist can detect what the glaucoma patient cannot: abnormalities of the optic nerve and subtle changes in the visual field. It is these key diagnostic signs, rather than elevated pressure, that indicate the presence of glaucoma. Although glaucoma is not contagious, if one eye is affected, the other eye will almost certainly develop the condition.

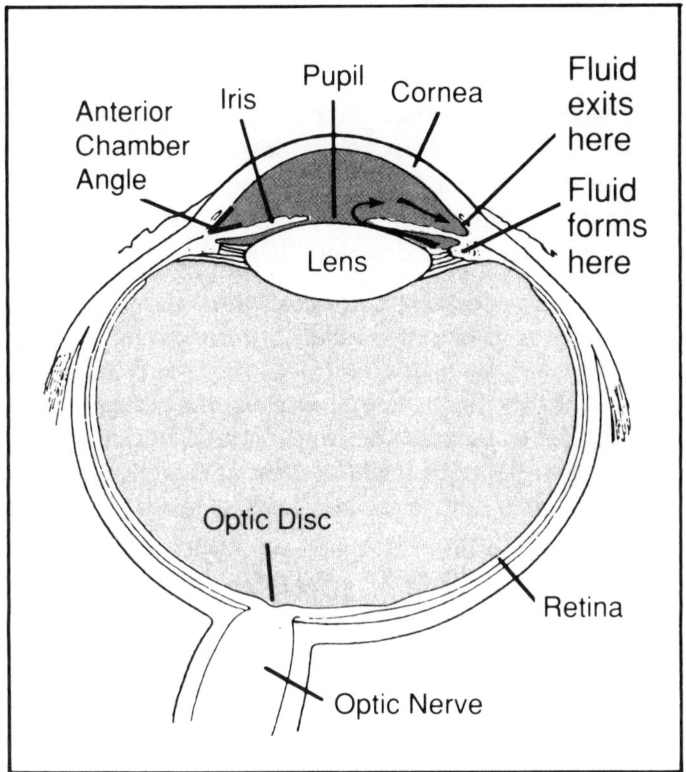

Figure 43-1.

How is Open-Angle Glaucoma Controlled?

The goal of treating open-angle glaucoma is to preserve vision by lowering intraocular pressure and preventing optic nerve damage. Here are some facts about the main forms of treatment in use today:

- Drugs for open-angle glaucoma are the most widely used method of treating this disease. These medications are taken as eyedrops or pills. Some improve fluid drainage, while others lower pressure by inhibiting fluid formation. Most cases of glaucoma can be controlled with one or more medications, and a majority of patients tolerate these drugs well.

However, in a few patients intraocular pressure is not adequately controlled by medications. Also, some people find that the drugs' side effects—such as stinging in the eye, blurred vision, or headaches—do not go away after the first few weeks of use but continue to be a problem. The patient may have trouble adhering to the prescribed dosage schedule and may be tempted to stop taking the medication or cut back on the dosage. In this situation, the patient should contact his or her eye doctor to discuss the problem and the best means of dealing with it. Changing the treatment plan without proper medical advice may allow intraocular pressure to rise again, and the patient may suffer needless visual loss as a result.

So, in spite of the fact that glaucoma can be controlled by medications in a majority of patients, other forms of treatment also play an important role in glaucoma therapy. These are described below:

- Conventional surgical techniques are intended to help fluid escape from the eye, and thus reduce pressure. Thirty years ago, before glaucoma drugs were available, surgery was the only effective treatment for glaucoma. Now ophthalmologists generally reserve surgery for patients whose glaucoma cannot be controlled by medications and for those who are unable to tolerate the side effects of these drugs. During the operation, the surgeon makes an opening to create a new drainage pathway so that aqueous can leave the eye more easily. After surgery, a few patients still need to use medication to keep their pressure under control and avoid loss of vision. And if the new drainage opening closes, a second operation may be needed.
- Argon laser surgery is an innovation in glaucoma treatment. The laser, a device that produces a high-energy beam of light, is used to make about 100 small burns in the drainage meshwork at the edge of the iris. Scientists think that the scars from these burns help stretch open the holes in the meshwork, making it easier for fluid to filter out. Laser surgery can be done in an ophthalmologist's office in a relatively short time. Usually, people who have this surgery must continue taking some glaucoma medication afterwards, although they may be able to lower the dosage and still keep intraocular pressure under control. However, the pressure lowering effect of the laser treatment may wear off eventually, and for this reason patients sometimes have a second or third treatment session.

What is Medical Science Doing About Open-Angle Glaucoma?

In the United States, most research on glaucoma is supported by the National Eye Institute (NEI). It is part of the National Institutes of Health, a component of the U.S. Department of Health and Human Services. The NEI is supporting a wide range of studies to learn more about the causes of glaucoma and improve its detection and treatment.

One major study now underway will further evaluate argon laser surgery for open-angle glaucoma. This nationwide study, called the Glaucoma Laser

Trial, is for people whose glaucoma was recently diagnosed. Its goal is to learn whether early laser treatment offers any advantages over treatment with medications alone. Another goal is to learn what disadvantages or risks may be associated with the new laser treatment. Findings from this research will help doctors determine the best approach to preserving the vision of people with open-angle glaucoma.

Clinical research on glaucoma drugs is aimed at improving their effectiveness, safety, and ease of use, and reducing their unpleasant side effects. Some scientists are searching for new—and better—drugs, while others are experimenting with new ways of delivering drugs to the eye.

Researchers are also studying different types of lasers, as well as ultrasonic devices, for treating open-angle glaucoma that does not respond to drugs or conventional surgery. In one study they are trying to find a way to improve the effectiveness of conventional glaucoma surgery. In addition, investigators are developing new diagnostic devices to improve the early detection of glaucoma, so that doctors will be better able to determine which patients need therapy.

Eye researchers are also trying to find out why black Americans appear to be particularly susceptible to open-angle glaucoma. In fact, some studies have suggested that the risk of glaucoma-induced blindness is several times higher for blacks than for whites. Scientists are attempting to identify the factors that might account for this difference. Their research is expected to yield important information that will lead to better ways of protecting black people from glaucoma.

Information that will help to improve glaucoma treatment is also expected to emerge from basic research on the eye. Such work includes studies of the changes that occur in the eye as it ages and the factors controlling production and drainage of aqueous humor.

What is Glaucoma Screening?

Many civic groups, hospitals, and community health centers in the United States offer glaucoma screening in an effort to identify people who are at high risk for glaucoma but don't know it. In screening programs, a health worker tests both eyes for increased pressure, using a tonometer. Tonometers may worry some people because part of the instrument touches the eye, but eyedrops can be used to numb the eye and the procedure is quick and painless. Some programs use non-contact tonometers which do not touch the eye, but instead measure the resistance to a puff of air blown at the eyeball.

The person who is found to have high intraocular pressure in a screening test is generally urged to make arrangements for a more thorough eye examination soon. This is because screening by tonometry can detect elevated intraocular pressure, but cannot reveal whether this condition has affected the optic nerve or side vision. To check for those key signs and thus learn whether glaucoma is present, doctors must examine the optic nerve and the field of vision. Intraocular pressure will be checked again to determine whether it is still elevated or whether it has dropped back to normal since the screening test. At the end of a complete eye examination, some people will learn that they have glaucoma and need treatment. Others will get the welcome news that they don't have the disease.

It is important to remember, however, that "passing" a screening test for glaucoma does not necessarily mean that you have no eye problems. Some cases of glaucoma are missed by screening, and other eye diseases may go undetected as well. So people who appear problem-free on the screening test should continue to have regular, thorough eye examinations to safeguard their visual health.

What is Ocular Hypertension?

Occasionally, eye examinations reveal that the pressure within one or both eyes is above normal, but the optic nerve and visual field are all right. This condition is called *ocular hypertension*. A person who has it is at risk of developing glaucoma; the higher the pressure, the greater the risk. If ocular hypertension is diagnosed, the eye care specialist will be able to advise whether it is better to begin treatment to lower the intraocular pressure right away, or whether it is preferable to wait, have regular eye check-ups, and consider treatment only if definite signs of open-angle glaucoma appear.

What are the Other Forms of Glaucoma?

- In *low-tension glaucoma*, optic nerve damage and restricted side vision occur unexpectedly in a person with normal intraocular pressure. The treatments used for this condition are the ones described in the section headed "How is open-angle glaucoma controlled?"
- In some people, an anatomical peculiarity of the eye, often inherited, makes the angle between the iris and cornea unusually narrow and easily closed off. This narrow angle can retard fluid drainage, causing numerous episodes of high pressure—a condition called *chronic narrow-angle glaucoma*. If the narrow angle closes suddenly and completely, fluid backs up fast and eye pressure goes up rapidly. This event, called *acute narrow-angle glaucoma* or *angle-closure glaucoma*, is a medical emergency. It causes severe pain and nausea as

well as redness of the eye and blurred vision. Unless the patient has treatment to improve the flow of fluid, the eye can become blind in as little as one or two days. Generally, surgery is needed to restore outflow of aqueous and prevent further angle-closure attacks. Lasers have been very helpful as an alternative to conventional surgery for treating narrow-angle glaucoma.

- Some infants are born with defects in the angle of the eye that slow the normal drainage of aqueous. This relatively rare *congenital glaucoma* is easily recognized in affected infants, who have cloudy eyes, are sensitive to light, and tear excessively. Surgery is usually indicated and can prevent loss of vision if it is done soon enough.
- Glaucoma can also develop as a complication of other medical conditions. These *secondary glaucomas* are sometimes associated with eye surgery or with advanced cataracts, eye injuries, some kinds of eye tumors, or uveitis (eye inflammations). A severe form of glaucoma, called neovascular glaucoma, is linked to diabetes. Also, corticosteroid drugs—used to treat eye inflammations and a variety of other diseases—can trigger glaucoma in a few people.

How Can People Learn More About Glaucoma?

If you are in one of the groups at special risk for glaucoma, as described in the first section of this pamphlet, you should ask your doctor about this disease. He or she can test your eyes for high intraocular pressure or refer you to an eye specialist for glaucoma tests. If you are older than age 40, you should have your eyes checked for glaucoma every two to three years.

For more information on glaucoma, check your public library, or a medical library if you live near a hospital or medical school. Also, you may wish to contact these organizations:

American Academy of Ophthalmology
655 Beach Street
P.O. Box 7424
San Francisco, California 94120–7424
(415) 561–8500

American Optometric Association
243 Lindbergh Boulevard
St. Louis, Missouri 63141
(314) 991–4100

American Foundation for the Blind
15 West 16th Street
New York, New York 10011
(212) 620–2000

National Society to Prevent Blindness
500 East Remington Road
Schaumburg, Illinois 60173
(312) 843–2020

Chapter 44

Periodontal Disease and Diabetes: A Guide for Patients

Periodontal diseases affect the soft tissues and bone that support the teeth. "Gingivitis," or inflamed gums, is the early form of periodontal disease. If left unchecked, gingivitis can progress to a more severe condition called "periodontitis." This infection, caused by harmful bacteria, eventually destroys the bone and ligament which hold the teeth in place. Sound teeth may become loose and, if untreated, can be lost.

For people with diabetes mellitus, periodontitis can be a major complication of their disease. Periodontal infection can upset blood sugar control, and loose or missing teeth can make eating the right foods difficult.

What Causes It?

Dental plaque plays a major role in the development of gingivitis and other periodontal diseases. Plaque, a sticky film containing millions of bacteria, attaches to the teeth. Only certain types of bacteria, however, are suspected of causing gum disease. Dental scientists are studying these and other harmful organisms to determine the exact roles they play in periodontal problems.

Other factors that contribute to gum diseases include poor nutrition, inherited defects in infection-fighting cells, hormonal changes in pregnancy, and certain diseases such as diabetes mellitus.

NIH Pub. No. 87-2946.

Who is Affected?

Periodontal diseases are a problem for many Americans. In fact, the majority of the U.S. population above the age of 40 probably has some form of the disease, ranging from mild gum inflammation to severe periodontal infection. Although most of the damage from gum disease occurs after the age of 35, dental scientists believe that the disorder has its beginnings in youth. Most U.S. school children have gingivitis, and some even have the more destructive form of periodontal disease.

Recent studies show that persons with diabetes, especially those whose blood sugar levels are poorly controlled, are at higher risk of developing gum infections. Because of diabetes, periodontal disease is often more frequent and more severe, and tends to appear at an earlier age than in nondiabetics.

Diabetes and Susceptibility to Gum Disease

Thickening of Blood Vessels

Changes in blood vessels, an early complication of diabetes, may be part of the reason for increased susceptibility to gum disorders. Blood vessels deliver oxygen and nourishment to all body tissues, including those in the mouth, and carry away waste products made by the cells. Diabetes causes blood vessels to thicken, slowing down the flow of vital nutrients and the removal of harmful wastes. This can weaken the resistance of gum and bone tissue to infection.

Bacteria

Many kinds of bacteria thrive on sugars, including glucose. When diabetes is poorly controlled, high glucose levels in mouth fluids may encourage the growth of harmful germs and set the stage for gum inflammation.

Diabetic Control

Diabetic control, particularly in adults with noninsulin-dependent diabetes mellitus (NIDDM), also appears to play a role in their susceptibility to gum disorders. In those with poor diabetic control, periodontal disease is more prevalent, more severe, and causes more tooth loss than in nondiabetics of the same age.

In children with insulin-dependent diabetes mellitus (IDDM), gingivitis becomes more frequent and more severe as they approach puberty. As many as 20 percent of 11 to 18-year-olds with IDDM have some form of periodontitis. When IDDM is uncontrolled, it is not unusual to find severe periodontal disease and abscesses (acute infections in the tooth or gum) in young people and adults.

How Periodontal Disease Develops

Gingivitis

Gingivitis, the first stage of periodontal disease, is commonly caused by poor brushing and flossing habits that allow plaque to accumulate on teeth near the gums. At first, there is mild inflammation—slight redness and swelling of the gum tissue around one or more of the teeth. Later, these symptoms worsen, and the gums tend to bleed easily. Bleeding while toothbrushing is one of the earliest signs of gum disease. During these changes, the gums may—or may not—be tender and sensitive. Because not everyone develops symptoms, there may be no warning that disease is present.

Periodontitis

Gingivitis can be controlled with regular cleanings by the dentist and good daily home care. If untreated, the condition may progress to destructive periodontitis. Over time, the plaque hardens into "calculus" and extends from the gum line down along the tooth root. The gums gradually detach from the teeth, forming pockets that may progress to one-half inch or more in depth. Pockets tend to occur between teeth where the toothbrush cannot reach.

Tooth Loss

As the infection spreads, these pockets may fill with pus and cause bad breath. Eventually, the ligaments that fasten the teeth to the bone are destroyed, and much of the bone socket slowly disintegrates. The tooth loosens and may be lost.

The pattern of periodontal disease is complicated and not yet well understood. One tooth may be affected, or several. A tooth may be lost to disease, while its neighbor remains healthy. Active destruction of connecting tissues or bone may be going on at one site at the same time that other diseased sites are healing. It is important to remember that much of this destructive process can take place with little or no discomfort. You cannot always tell that periodontal disease is developing.

How is it Treated?

Plaque Removal

Treatment of periodontitis depends on how far the disease has progressed. In the early stages, the dentist or periodontist (a specialist in gum disorders) will remove plaque, calculus and inflamed tissues from under the gums. This deep cleaning procedure, called root planing and curettage, eliminates infection and makes it possible for the gum to reattach to the teeth, closing up pockets that harbor harmful bacteria.

The key to the success of root planing and curettage in the dentist's office is the patient's oral health care program at home. Stopping and reversing early periodontal disease require a team effort. When patient and professional work together, this approach to treatment is often all that is needed.

Periodontal Surgery

When periodontitis is more advanced, gum surgery may be necessary. Most surgical techniques used today give the dentist better access to the problem areas around the tooth roots. These procedures allow the dentist or periodontist to carefully remove calculus and infected tissues, and to smooth the root surfaces that have been damaged by disease. These steps help to get rid of pockets by enabling the gum to reattach to the teeth.

Gum and bone tissue that have been destroyed by advanced periodontitis do not grow back. Special techniques are available, however, to replace or rebuild some of these supporting structures. Bone-like materials made in the laboratory and gingival grafts taken from healthy gum tissue are often used in these procedures.

If You Have Diabetes. . .

Persons with diabetes should be evaluated by their physician before scheduling treatment for periodontal disease. The dentist or periodontist should also consult the physician before gum surgery to be aware of the diabetic patient's general condition. Knowing about a diabetic's medical history, especially if there are any problems with infection or blood sugar control, helps the dentist and physician to decide if a patient should receive an antibiotic before dental treatment. The decision whether or not to pretreat with antibiotics should be made by the health care team, based on the special needs of each patient and the type of dental procedure planned.

Dental appointments should be scheduled in the morning, generally about an hour and a half after breakfast and the morning insulin. This will ensure that scheduled meals are not delayed or missed. Morning appointments also give the patient and the dentist time during the day to monitor any effects of gum surgery on blood sugar levels. Acute infections, however, such as abscesses, should be treated right away.

For the controlled diabetic, periodontal surgery can usually be done in the dentist's office. Persons with more severe diabetes should have surgery in a hospital where the patient can be monitored more easily during and after the procedure.

Because of diabetes, healing may take more time. But with good medical and dental care, complications after surgery are no more likely than in nondiabetic patients. Once the periodontal infection is successfully treated, persons with diabetes often find that it is easier to control blood sugar levels.

Other Oral Diseases

Dental Caries

Young people with IDDM have no more dental caries (cavities) than nondiabetic children. In fact, IDDM patients who are careful about their diet and take good care of their teeth often have fewer cavities than other children because they don't eat many foods that contain sugar.

Thrush

Thrush is a fungal infection that occurs in the mouth. People with diabetes may be more prone to thrush because high blood glucose levels in the saliva encourage a fungus, called *Candida albicans*, to grow. Factors such as smoking and wearing dentures, especially when they are worn continuously, can lead to fungal infection. Special antifungal medications are available if needed to help treat this type of infection. Good diabetic control, no smoking, and removing and cleaning dentures daily can help prevent thrush from developing.

Dry Mouth

Dry mouth, a condition called "xerostomia," is often a symptom of undetected and untreated diabetes. When there is not enough moisture in the mouth to protect the soft tissues, they may become sore and more prone to developing ulcers. Good blood glucose control helps to alleviate dry mouth.

Keep Your Teeth

Persons with diabetes should be especially mindful of the importance of keeping their natural teeth. The bone surrounding the teeth may sometimes be damaged by periodontal infection, causing changes in the shape of the gum tissues. This uneven ridge may make it difficult to fit dentures properly and comfortably. In addition, diabetic persons may not tolerate full dentures very well because of gum soreness and tenderness, and the need for frequent relining of the dentures to match the changing contours of the supporting tissues.

Dental disease, particularly severe periodontal disease, can also interfere with good diabetic control by making chewing painful or difficult. Such discomfort could lead diabetics to choose foods that are easier to chew, but that may not be appropriate for their diet. Every effort should be made to preserve healthy natural teeth so that persons with diabetes can help maintain good control through proper nutrition—comfortably and efficiently.

How to Protect Your Teeth and Gums

Prevention is sound advice for diabetic and nondiabetic persons alike. Harmful bacteria constantly attack the teeth and gums as long as plaque is allowed to accumulate. The important thing to do—and most of us can do it ourselves—is to break up the plaque formation by brushing and flossing thoroughly. If this is done each day, you can actually prevent the disease from starting.

Even when some disease has already developed, dentists find that many patients respond well to a good plaque removal program. Within a week or so, the inflammation usually subsides, and the swollen gum shrinks and grows firm. After a few weeks, loose teeth may become more stable. Good home care is essential, however, to keep the periodontal infection from returning. People who practice effective plaque removal regularly can usually avoid these problems in the first place.

Brushing

Brushing is an important step in plaque removal. It should be done carefully, at least twice a day, and not too vigorously. Use a soft nylon brush with rounded ends on its bristles.

One good way to brush is as follows: First, brush at a 45-degree angle where the teeth meet the gums. Next, brush the outside surfaces of all teeth with short back-and-forth strokes. Then brush the inside of the front teeth with an up-and-down motion. Finally, brush the inside of the back teeth and chewing surfaces with short back-and-forth strokes. It is also a good idea to brush the rough upper surface of the tongue where debris and bacteria tend to collect.

Flossing

Use dental floss once a day to remove bacteria from between the teeth where most pockets begin. Take about 18 inches of dental floss wrapped around the middle fingers of each hand and grasp the thread between the thumbs and forefingers, spaced about an inch and a half apart.

With a sawing motion, bring the floss gently through the tight place between the teeth. Do not let the floss cut the gum tissue. Curve the floss carefully around the neck of one tooth. "Scrape" gently from below the gum to the surface, then guide the floss up and down the side of the tooth that can't be reached with a brush. Do this several times. Then shift the loop to the adjacent tooth and repeat this procedure before removing the floss from between the teeth. Repeat on the next tooth, using a clean section of floss. Each tooth must be cleaned in this way to break up the plaque.

To get under the small collars of gum tissue around the teeth, especially at the back and between the teeth, takes time and care. Your dentist can show you how to get at some of the harder-to-reach spots. Special floss holders are also available to help make flossing easier.

Check Your Work

Occasionally, you will want to check on how well you are removing the plaque. Since the early film of bacteria is colorless, a harmless "disclosing solution" containing vegetable coloring may be applied to the teeth and gums. The solution, available in liquid or tablet form from your dentist or pharmacist, will stain any remaining plaque and show you what areas you have missed. Just brush and floss these areas more carefully. Finally, rinse the mouth well.

Dental Check-ups

People with diabetes should have a dental check-up at least every 6 months. *Be sure to tell your dentist that you are diabetic.* When you visit the dentist, any calculus that may have accumulated can be removed, and a simple, quick examination will reveal spots requiring special attention. Your dentist can also tell if your gums bleed easily or if there has been any detachment of gum tissue from the teeth.

Teamwork

Remember, successful prevention or control of periodontal disease depends on teamwork. A good, daily home care program to remove plaque from the teeth, combined with regular check-ups by the dentist are the best defense against this important complication of diabetes.

Chapter 45

Pancreatitis

Your pancreas is a large gland behind your stomach and close to your duodenum. The pancreas secretes powerful digestive enzymes that enter the small intestine through a duct. These enzymes help you digest fats, proteins, and carbohydrates. The pancreas also releases the hormones insulin and glucagon into the bloodstream. These hormones play an important part in metabolizing sugar.

Pancreatitis is a rare disease in which the pancreas becomes inflamed. Damage to the gland occurs when digestive enzymes are activated and begin attacking the pancreas. In severe cases, there may be bleeding into the gland, serious tissue damage, infection, and cysts. Enzymes and toxins may enter the bloodstream and seriously injure organs, such as the heart, lungs, and kidney.

There are two forms of pancreatitis. The acute form occurs suddenly and may be a severe, life-threatening illness with many complications. Usually, the patient recovers completely. If injury to the pancreas continues, such as when a patient persists in drinking alcohol, a chronic form of the disease may develop, bringing severe pain and reduced functioning of the pancreas that affects digestion and causes weight loss.

What Is Acute Pancreatitis?

An estimated 50,000 to 80,000 cases of acute pancreatitis occur in the United States each year. This disease occurs when the pancreas suddenly

---

NIH Pub. No. 92-1596

becomes inflamed and then gets better. Some patients have more than one attack but recover fully after each one. Most cases of acute pancreatitis are caused either by alcohol abuse or by gallstones. Other causes may be use of prescribed drugs, trauma or surgery to the abdomen, or abnormalities of the pancreas or intestine. In rare cases, the disease may result from infections, such as mumps. In about 15 percent of cases, the cause is unknown.

What Are the Symptoms of Acute Pancreatitis?

Acute pancreatitis usually begins with pain in the upper abdomen, that may last for a few days. The pain is often severe. It may be constant pain, just in the abdomen, or it may reach to the back and other areas. The pain may be sudden and intense, or it may begin as a mild pain that is aggravated by eating and slowly grows worse. The abdomen may be swollen and very tender. Other symptoms may include nausea, vomiting, fever, and an increased pulse rate. The person often feels and looks very sick.

About 20 percent of cases are severe. The patient may become dehydrated and have low blood pressure. Sometimes the patient's heart, lungs, or kidneys fail. In the most severe cases, bleeding can occur in the pancreas, leading to shock and sometimes death.

How Is Acute Pancreatitis Diagnosed?

During acute attacks, high levels of amylase (a digestive enzyme formed in the pancreas) are found in the blood. Changes also may occur in blood levels of calcium, magnesium, sodium, potassium, and bicarbonate. Patients may have high amounts of sugar and lipids (fats) in their blood too. These changes help the doctor diagnose pancreatitis. After the pancreas recovers, blood levels of these substances usually return to normal.

What Is the Treatment for Acute Pancreatitis?

The treatment a patient receives depends on how bad the attack is. Unless complications occur, acute pancreatitis usually gets better on its own, so treatment is supportive in most cases. Usually the patient goes into the hospital. The doctor prescribes fluids by vein to restore blood volume. The kidneys and lungs may be treated to prevent failure of those organs. Other problems, such as cysts in the pancreas, may need treatment too.

Sometimes a patient cannot control vomiting and needs to have a tube through the nose to the stomach to remove fluid and air. In mild cases, the patient may not have food for 3 or 4 days but is given fluids and pain relievers by vein. An acute attack usually lasts only a few days, unless the ducts are blocked by gallstones. In severe cases, the patient may be fed through the veins for 3 to 6 weeks while the pancreas slowly heals.

Antibiotics may be given if signs of infection arise. Surgery may be needed if complications such as infection, cysts, or bleeding occur. Attacks caused by gallstones may require removal of the gallbladder or surgery of the bile duct.

Surgery is sometimes needed for the doctor to be able to exclude other abdominal problems that can simulate pancreatitis or to treat acute pancreatitis. When there is severe injury with death of tissue, an operation may be done to remove the dead tissue.

After all signs of acute pancreatitis are gone, the doctor will determine the cause and try to prevent future attacks. In some patients the cause of the attack is clear, but in others further tests need to be done.

What If the Patient Has Gallstones?

Ultrasound is used to detect gallstones and sometimes can provide the doctor with an idea of how severe the pancreatitis is. When gallstones are found, surgery is usually needed to remove them. When they are removed depends on how severe the pancreatitis is. If it is mild, the gallstones often can be removed within a week or so. In more severe cases, the patient may wait a month or more, until he improves, before the stones are removed. The CAT (computer axial tomography) scan also may be used to find out what is happening in and around the pancreas and how severe the problem is. This is important information that the doctor needs to determine when to remove the gallstones. After the gallstones are removed and inflammation subsides, the pancreas usually returns to normal. Before patients leave the hospital, they are advised not to drink alcohol and not to eat large meals.

What Is Chronic Pancreatitis?

Chronic pancreatitis usually follows many years of alcohol abuse. It may develop after only one acute attack, especially if there is damage to the ducts of the pancreas. In the early stages, the doctor cannot always tell whether the patient has acute or chronic disease. The symptoms may be the same. Damage to the pancreas from drinking alcohol may cause no symptoms for many years, and then the patient suddenly has an attack of pancreatitis. In more than 90 percent of adult patients, chronic pancreatitis appears to be caused by alcoholism. This is more common in men than women and often develops between 30 and 40 years of age. In other cases, pancreatitis may be inherited. Scientists do not know why the inherited form occurs. Patients with chronic pancreatitis tend to have three kinds of problems: pain, malabsorption of food leading to weight loss, or diabetes.

Some patients do not have any pain, but most do. Pain may be constant in the back and abdomen, and for some patients, the pain attacks are disabling. In some cases, the abdominal pain goes away as the condition advances. Doctors think this happens because pancreatic enzymes are no longer being made by the pancreas.

Patients with this disease often lose weight, even when their appetite and eating habits are normal. This occurs because the body does not secrete enough pancreatic enzymes to break down food, so nutrients are not absorbed normally. Poor digestion leads to loss of fat, protein, and sugar into the stool. Diabetes may also develop at this stage if the insulin-producing cells of the pancreas (islet cells) have been damaged.

How Is Chronic Pancreatitis Diagnosed?

Diagnosis may be difficult but is aided by a number of new techniques. Pancreatic function tests help the physician decide if the pancreas still can make enough digestive enzymes. The doctor can see abnormalities in the pancreas using several techniques (ultrasonic imaging, endoscopic retrograde cholangiopancreatography (ERCP), and the CAT scan). In more advanced stages of the disease, when diabetes and malabsorption (a problem due to lack of enzymes) occur, the doctor can use a number of blood, urine, and stool tests to help in the diagnosis of chronic pancreatitis and to monitor the progression of the disorder.

How Is Chronic Pancreatitis Treated?

The doctor treats chronic pancreatitis by relieving pain and managing the nutritional and metabolic problems. The patient can reduce the amount of fat and protein lost in stools by cutting back on dietary fat and taking pills containing pancreatic enzymes. This will result in better nutrition and weight gain. Sometimes insulin or other drugs must be given to control the patient's blood sugar.

In some cases, surgery is needed to relieve pain by draining an enlarged pancreatic duct. Sometimes, part or most of the pancreas is removed in an attempt to relieve chronic pain.

Patients must stop drinking, adhere to their prescribed diets, and take the proper medications in order to have fewer and milder attacks.

Additional Reading

Banks PA, Frey CF, Greenberger NJ. The spectrum of chronic pancreatitis. *Patient Care,* 1989; 23(9): 163–96. This review article for physicians is written in technical language. Available in medical libraries.

Facts and Fallacies About Digestive Diseases. 1991. This fact sheet discusses commonly held beliefs about digestive diseases, including pancreatitis and gallbladder disease. Available from the National Digestive Diseases Information Clearinghouse, Box NDDIC, 9000 Rockville Pike, Bethesda, MD 20892. (301) 468–6344.

Clayman CB, ed. *The American Medical Association Encyclopedia of Medicine.* New York: Random House. 1989. Authoritative reference guide for patients with sections on irritable bowel syndrome and other disorders of the digestive system. Widely available in libraries and bookstores.

Frey CF, et al. Progress in acute pancreatitis. *Patient Care,* 1989; 23(5): 38–53. This review article for physicians is written in technical language. Available in medical libraries.

Chapter 46

Pancreas Transplantation

Clinical researchers engaged in long-term studies of type I, or insulin-dependent, diabetes report that pancreas transplants not only free diabetic patients from insulin injections or a pump, but also halt structural changes in the kidney that are associated with degenerative renal diseases.

Preliminary findings by physicians at the University of Minnesota General Clinical Research Center in Minneapolis indicate that diabetic recipients of pancreas transplants who first received kidney transplants have less pronounced structural changes in their transplanted kidneys than do patients in a control group who received kidney transplants but no pancreas transplants. The control patients relied on standard insulin injections to maintain glycemic control. The study and control groups were matched for sex, age, duration of diabetes, and length of survival of transplanted kidney.

In recipients of successful pancreas transplants, blood sugar levels stay within normal range, according to Dr. Michael Steffes, professor of pathology. Five University of Minnesota Medical School faculty members were involved in the studies, as was Dr. Rudolf W. Bilous of the University of Newcastle-upon-Tyne in the United Kingdom.

The establishment of normal glycemic control in patients with diabetes by an insulin-producing pancreas transplant contrasts with the imprecise control by insulin therapy. "Neither multiple insulin injections nor continuous subcutaneous insulin infusion has been able to normalize glycemia in the long term," the research team reports. The improved glycemic control combined with the reduced kidney damage found in this study supports the

---

Research Resources Reporter, May 1990.

hypothesis that preventing hyperglycemia halts the progression of diabetic kidney disease, the investigators say.

Changes in the structure of the kidneys are observed as diabetic kidney disease progresses. Glomeruli, the kidney's blood-filtering clusters of capillaries, are associated with supporting cells and tissues called mesangium and are surrounded by an epithelial basement membrane. Diabetic glomerulopathy is characterized by expansion of the mesangial tissue and thickening of the basement membrane.

Before performing pancreas transplantation on 12 insulin-dependent diabetic patients—9 women and 3 men, 24 to 35 years old—who had received kidney transplants 1 to 7 years earlier, Dr. Steffes and his colleagues examined biopsy specimens of the transplanted kidneys. The researchers reexamined the transplanted kidneys of the patients from 23 months to 10 years after transplanting either a whole or partial pancreas.

After pancreas transplantation mesangial expansion and glomerular basement membrane thickening in the transplanted kidneys of the study group was minimal and did not progress significantly during the course of the study. Transplants of both partial and whole pancreas thus were effective in preventing progression of glomerulopathy. In contrast, mesangial expansion in transplanted kidneys was significantly greater in patients who had not received a pancreas transplant.

In their ongoing studies of pancreas transplantation in diabetes, recipients of earlier kidney transplants are not the only group of interest to the Minnesota researchers.

"We also are reviewing data on patients who received kidney and pancreas transplants at the same time and on those who received pancreas transplants but kept their own kidneys," Dr. Steffes notes. "For some undetermined reason the combined kidney-pancreas transplants work more effectively to maintain pancreas function."

"Fewer are rejected," adds Dr. David Sutherland, a surgeon and member of the Minnesota research team, who has been involved in more than 300 pancreas transplants since 1978. "The success rate is 75 percent for simultaneous transplants and 60 percent for pancreas transplants alone."

No additional immunosuppression is required for a combined transplant beyond that necessary for a kidney transplant, the researchers point out. Considering the benefits of normal glycemic control and the apparent ability of pancreas transplants to prevent recurrence of kidney disease, "patients needing a kidney also should get a pancreas," Dr. Sutherland says.

For insulin-dependent diabetics not suffering from end-stage diabetic nephropathy, the choice of whether to perform a pancreas transplant alone is more difficult. The inconvenience and potential side effects of lifelong immunosuppressive therapy are major considerations.

"The drug cyclosporine causes structural damage and a decrease in glomerular filtration rate," Dr. Steffes says. The classic immunosuppressive drugs prednisone and azathioprine do not decrease filtration rates, but cyclosporine is a more effective immunosuppressant, he adds. Currently the three immunosuppressants are used together. Prednisone can sometimes cause osteoporosis, weakening of the bones; cyclosporine can cause interstitial fibrosis, as well as lesions and thickening of arteries.

"There is a trade-off between the side effects of immunosuppression and the benefits of improved glycemic control," Dr. Steffes says. "Right now kidney function is the major consideration. Pancreas transplantations are not something you do as routine therapy."

After nephropathy the most common serious secondary complications of insulin-dependent diabetes involve the retina (sometimes leading to blindness), the nervous system (neuropathy), and the blood vessels. Ideally, physicians would like to know individual susceptibility to these complications, as well as the potential for pancreas transplants to prevent them or halt their progress.

"It's not clear that pancreas transplants with immunosuppression will give the best outcome," Dr. Sutherland says. "Some individuals may be worse off, but right now we have no way of identifying them."

Retinal and nervous system complications often have been far advanced in patients who received both pancreas and kidney transplants in response to end-stage renal disease, and it is not certain whether the course of these complications has been different from that observed in patients who received only kidney transplants, Dr. Sutherland points out.

However, sensory and motor nerve conduction has shown improvement after successful pancreas transplantation, he notes. Preliminary data collected by the University of Minnesota group also indicate that the course of autonomic neuropathy may have improved in some patients without advanced kidney disease who received only pancreas transplants.

According to Dr. Steffes, "The work on neuropathy is not as clear-cut as our results on kidney disease, and published findings so far show no effect on eye lesions in diabetic retinopathy. However, eye lesions can be arrested with photocoagulation therapy."

The Minnesota transplant team follows guidelines suggested recently by the University of Michigan pancreas transplant evaluation committee, Dr. Sutherland says. Patients who have advanced nephropathy but not end-stage renal disease may be candidates for combined pancreas-kidney transplants. Patients with autonomic neuropathy, but without advanced nephropathy, who are at risk for heart failure or stomach paralysis, may be candidates for pancreas transplants alone, he says.

The Minnesota researchers emphasize that their research to date has not provided evidence of improved long-term patient survival and that there is much more to learn about the potential risk, costs, and benefits of pancreas transplants. The operation should be performed only in an investigational setting, they add.

Nonetheless, the researchers say, pancreas transplantation has already shown more promise for halting secondary complications of diabetes than have intensive efforts to control blood sugar level through multiple insulin injections or subcutaneous insulin pumps. And as transplant techniques and immunosuppressive regimens improve, the number of transplant candidates could expand.

Furthermore, unlike the unmet demand for kidneys, the foreseeable demand for pancreases can be met even by the current supply of donor organs, according to Dr. Sutherland. "There should be a pancreatic transplant for everyone who needs it," he says.

—Jeffrey Norris

Additional Reading:

1. Bilous, R. W., Mauer, S. M., Sutherland, D. E. R., Najarian, J. S., Goetz, F. C., and Steffes, M. W., The effects of pancreas transplantation on the glomerular structure of renal allografts in patients with insulin-dependent diabetes. *New England Journal of Medicine* 321:80–85, 1989.

2. Mauer, S. M., Goetz, F. C., McHugh, L. E., Sutherland, D. E. R., Barbosa, S., Najarian, J. S., and Steffes, M. W., Long-term study of normal kidneys transplanted into patients with type I diabetes. *Diabetes* 38:516–523, 1989.

3. Sutherland, D. E. R., Dunn, D. L., Goetz, F. C., Kennedy, W., Ramsay, R. C., Steffes, M. W., Mauer, S. M., Gruessner, R., Moudry-Munns, K. C., Morel, P., Viste, A., Robertson, R. P., and Najarian, J. S., A 10-year experience with 290 pancreas transplants at a single institution. *Annals of Surgery* 210:274–288, 1989.

4. University of Michigan Pancreas Transplant Evaluation Committee, Pancreatic transplantation as treatment for IDDM: Criteria before end-stage diabetic nephropathy. *Diabetes Care* 11:669–675, 1988.

5. Mauer, S. M., Steffes, M. W., Ellis, E. N., Sutherland, D. E. R., Brown, D. M., and Goetz, F. C., Structural-functional relationships in diabetic nephropathy. *Journal of Clinical Investigation* 74:1143–1155, 1984.

The studies described in this article were supported by the General Clinical Research Centers Program of the National Center for Research Resources, the National Institute of Diabetes and Digestive and Kidney Diseases, the Juvenile Diabetes Foundation International, and the Wellcome Foundation.

Chapter 47

End-Stage Renal Disease: Choosing A Treatment That's Right For You

Introduction

This booklet is for people whose kidneys fail to work. This condition is called end-stage renal disease (ESRD).

Today, there are new and better treatments for ESRD that replace the work of healthy kidneys. By learning about your treatment choices, you can work with your doctor to pick the one that's best for you. No matter which type of treatment you choose, there will be some changes in your life. But with the help of your health care team, family, and friends, you may be able to lead a full, active life.

This booklet describes the choices for treatment: hemodialysis, peritoneal dialysis, and kidney transplantation. It gives the pros and cons of each. It also discusses diet and paying for treatment. It gives tips for working with your doctor, nurses, and others who make up your health care team. It provides a list of groups that offer information and services to kidney patients. It also lists magazines, books, and brochures that you can read for more information about treatment.

You and your doctor will work together to choose a treatment that's best for you. This booklet can help you make that choice.

When Your Kidneys Fail

Healthy kidneys clean the blood by filtering out extra water and wastes. They also make hormones that keep your bones strong and blood healthy.

NIH Pub. No. 93-2412.

When both of your kidneys fail, your body holds fluid. Your blood pressure rises. Harmful wastes build up in your body. Your body doesn't make enough red blood cells. When this happens, you need treatment to replace the work of your failed kidneys.

Hemodialysis

Hemodialysis is a procedure that cleans and filters your blood. It rids your body of harmful wastes and extra salt and fluids. It also controls blood pressure and helps your body keep the proper balance of chemicals such as potassium, sodium, and chloride.

Hemodialysis uses a dialyzer, or special filter, to clean your blood. The dialyzer connects to a machine. During treatment, your blood travels through tubes into the dialyzer. The dialyzer filters out wastes and extra fluids. Then the newly cleaned blood flows through another set of tubes and back into your body.

Before your first treatment, an access to your bloodstream must be made. The access provides a way for blood to be carried from your body to the dialysis machine and then back into your body. The access can be internal (inside the body—usually under your skin) or external (outside the body).

Hemodialysis can be done at home or at a center. At a center, nurses or trained technicians perform the treatment. At home, you perform hemodialysis with the help of a family member or friend. If you decide to do home dialysis, you and your partner will receive special training.

Hemodialysis usually is done three times a week. Each treatment lasts from 2 to 4 hours. During treatment, you can read, write, sleep, talk, or watch TV.

Side effects can be caused by rapid changes in your body's fluid and chemical balance during treatment. Muscle cramps and hypotension are two common side effects. Hypotension, a sudden drop in blood pressure, can make you feel weak, dizzy, or sick to your stomach.

It usually takes a few months to adjust to hemodialysis. You can avoid many of the side effects if you follow the proper diet and take your medicines as directed. You should always report side effects to your doctor. They often can be treated quickly and easily.

Hemodialysis and a proper diet help reduce the wastes that build up in your blood. A dietitian can help you plan meals according to your doctor's orders. When choosing foods, you should remember to:

- Eat balanced amounts of foods high in protein such as meat and chicken. Animal protein is better used by your body than the protein found in vegetables and grains.

- Watch the amount of potassium you eat. Potassium is a mineral found in salt substitutes, some fruits, vegetables, milk, chocolate, and nuts. Too much or too little potassium can be harmful to your heart.
- Limit how much you drink. Fluids build up quickly in your body when your kidneys aren't working. Too much fluid makes your tissues swell. It also can cause high blood pressure and heart trouble.
- Avoid salt. Salty foods make you thirsty and cause your body to hold water.
- Limit foods such as milk, cheese, nuts, dried beans, and soft drinks. These foods contain the mineral phosphorus. Too much phosphorus in your blood causes calcium to be pulled from your bones. Calcium helps keep bones strong and healthy. To prevent bone problems, your doctor may give you special medicines. You must take these medicines everyday as directed.

Each person responds differently to similar situations. What may be a negative factor for one person may be positive for another. However, in general, the following are pros and cons for each type of hemodialysis.

In-Center Hemodialysis

Pros

- You have trained professionals with you at all times.
- You can get to know other patients.

Cons

- Treatments are scheduled by the center.
- You must travel to the center for treatment.

Home Hemodialysis

Pros

- You can do it at the hours you choose. (*But you still must do it as often as your doctor orders.*)
- You don't have to travel to a center.
- You gain a sense of independence and control over your treatment.

Cons

- Helping with treatments may be stressful to your family.

- You need training.
- You need space for storing the machine and supplies at home.

Questions You May Want To Ask:

- Is hemodialysis the best treatment choice for me? Why or why not?
- If I am treated at a center, can I go to the center of my choice?
- What does hemodialysis feel like? Does it hurt?
- What is self-care dialysis?
- How long does it take to learn home hemodialysis? Who will train my partner and me?
- What kind of blood access is best for me?
- As a hemodialysis patient, will I be able to keep working? Can I have treatments at night if I plan to keep working?
- How much should I exercise?
- Who will be on my health care team? How can they help me?
- Who can I talk with about sexuality, family problems, or money concerns?
- How/where can I talk to other people who have faced this decision?

Peritoneal Dialysis

Peritoneal dialysis is another procedure that replaces the work of your kidneys. It removes extra water, wastes, and chemicals from your body. This type of dialysis uses the lining of your abdomen to filter your blood. This lining is called the peritoneal membrane.

A cleansing solution, called dialysate, travels through a special tube into your abdomen. Fluid, wastes, and chemicals pass from tiny blood vessels in the peritoneal membrane into the dialysate. After several hours, the dialysate gets drained from your abdomen, taking the wastes from your blood with it. Then you fill your abdomen with fresh dialysate and the cleaning process begins again.

Before your first treatment, a surgeon places a small, soft tube called a catheter into your abdomen. This catheter always stays there. It helps transport the dialysate to and from your peritoneal membrane.

There are three types of peritoneal dialysis.

1. Continuous Ambulatory Peritoneal Dialysis (CAPD)

CAPD is the most common type of peritoneal dialysis. It needs no machine. It can be done in any clean, well-lit place. With CAPD, your blood is always being cleaned. The dialysate passes from a plastic bag through the catheter and into your abdomen. The dialysate stays in your abdomen with the catheter sealed. After several hours, you drain the solution back into the bag. Then you refill your abdomen with fresh solution through the same catheter. Now the cleaning process begins again. While the solution is in your body, you may fold the empty plastic bag and hide it under your clothes, around your waist, or in a pocket.

2. Continuous Cyclic Peritoneal Dialysis (CCPD)

CCPD is like CAPD except that a machine, which connects to your catheter, automatically fills and drains the dialysate from your abdomen. The machine does this at night while you sleep.

3. Intermittent Peritoneal Dialysis (IPD)

IPD uses the same type of machine as CCPD to add and drain the dialysate. IPD can be done at home, but it's usually done in the hospital. IPD treatments take longer than CCPD.

CAPD is a form of self-treatment. It needs no machine and no partner. However, with IPD and CCPD, you need a machine and the help of a partner (family member, friend, or health professional).

With CAPD, the dialysate stays in your abdomen for about 4 to 6 hours. The process of draining the dialysate and replacing fresh solution takes 30 to 40 minutes. Most people change the solution four times a day.

With CCPD, treatments last from 10 to 12 hours every night.

With IPD, treatments are done several times a week, for a total of 36 to 42 hours per week. Sessions may last up to 24 hours.

Peritonitis, or infection of the peritoneum, can occur if the opening where the catheter enters your body gets infected. You can also get it if there is a problem connecting or disconnecting the catheter from the bags. Peritonitis can make you feel sick. It can cause a fever and stomach pain.

To avoid peritonitis, you must be careful to follow the procedure exactly. You must know the early signs of peritonitis. Look for reddening or swelling around the catheter. You should also note if your dialysate looks cloudy. It is important to report these signs to your doctor so that the peritonitis can be treated quickly to avoid serious problems.

Diet for peritoneal dialysis is slightly different than diet for hemodialysis.

- You may be able to have more salt and fluids.

- You may eat more protein.
- You may have different potassium restrictions.
- You may need to cut back on the number of calories you eat. This limitation is because the sugar in the dialysate may cause you to gain weight.

There are pros and cons to each type of peritoneal dialysis.

CAPD

Pros

- You can perform treatment alone.
- You can do it at times you choose.
- You can do it in many locations.
- You don't need a machine.

Cons

- It disrupts your daily schedule.

CCPD

Pros

- You can do it at night, mainly while you sleep.

Cons

- You need a machine and help from a partner.

IPD

Pros

- Health professionals usually perform treatments.

Cons

- You may need to go to a hospital.
- It takes a lot of time.
- You need a machine.

Questions You May Want To Ask:

- Is peritoneal dialysis the best treatment choice for me? Why or why not? Which type?

- How long will it take me to learn peritoneal dialysis?
- What does peritoneal dialysis feel like? Does it hurt?
- How will peritoneal dialysis affect my blood pressure?
- How do I know if I have peritonitis? How is peritonitis treated?
- As a peritoneal dialysis patient, will I be able to continue working?
- How much should I exercise?
- Who will be on my health care team? How can they help me?
- Who can I talk with about sexuality, finances, or family concerns?
- How/where can I talk to other people who have faced this decision?

Dialysis Is Not a Cure

Hemodialysis and peritoneal dialysis are treatments that try to replace your failed kidneys. These treatments help you feel better and live longer, but they are not cures for ESRD. While patients with ESRD are now living longer than ever, ESRD can cause problems over the years. Some problems are bone disease, high blood pressure, nerve damage, and anemia (having too few red blood cells). Although these problems won't go away with dialysis, doctors now have new and better ways to treat or prevent them. You should discuss these treatments with your doctor.

Kidney Transplantation

Kidney transplantation is a procedure that places a healthy kidney from another person into your body. This one new kidney does all the work that your two failed kidneys cannot do.

A surgeon places the new kidney inside your body between your upper thigh and abdomen. The surgeon connects the artery and vein of the new kidney to your artery and vein. Your blood flows through the new kidney and makes urine, just like your own kidneys did when they were healthy. The new kidney may start working right away or may take up to a few weeks to make urine. Your own kidneys are left where they are, unless they are causing infection or high blood pressure.

You may receive a kidney from a member of your family. This kind of donor is called a living-related donor. You may receive a kidney from a person who has recently died. This type of donor is called a cadaver donor. Sometimes a spouse or very close friend may donate a kidney. This kind of donor is called a living-unrelated donor.

It is very important for the donor's blood and tissues to closely match yours. This match will help prevent your body's immune system from fighting off, or rejecting, the new kidney. A lab will do special tests on blood cells to find out if your body will accept the new kidney.

The time it takes to get a kidney varies. There are not enough cadaver donors for every person who needs a transplant. Because of this, you must be placed on a waiting list to receive a cadaver donor kidney. However, if a relative gives you a kidney, the transplant operation can be done sooner.

The surgery takes from 3 to 6 hours. The usual hospital stay may last from 10 to 14 days. After you leave the hospital, you will go to the clinic for regular followup visits.

If a relative or close friend gives you a kidney, he or she will probably stay in the hospital for one week or less.

Transplantation is not a cure. There is always a chance that your body will reject your new kidney, no matter how good the match. The chance of your body accepting the new kidney depends on your age, race, and medical condition.

Normally, 75 to 80 percent of transplants from cadaver donors are working one year after surgery. However, transplants from living relatives often work better than transplants from cadaver donors. This fact is because they are usually a closer match.

Your doctor will give you special drugs to help prevent rejection. These are called immunosuppressants. You will need to take these drugs every day for the rest of your life. Sometimes these drugs cannot stop your body from rejecting the new kidney. If this happens, you will go back to some form of dialysis and possibly wait for another transplant.

Treatment with these drugs may cause side effects. The most serious is that they weaken your immune system, making it easier for you to get infections. Some drugs also cause changes in how you look. Your face may get fuller. You may gain weight or develop acne or facial hair. Not all patients have these problems, and makeup and diet can help.

Some of these drugs may cause problems such as cataracts, extra stomach acid, and hip disease. In a smaller number of patients, these drugs also may cause liver or kidney damage when used for a long period of time.

Diet for transplant patients is less limiting than it is for dialysis patients. You may still have to cut back on some foods, though. Your diet probably will change as your medicines, blood values, weight, and blood pressure change.

- You may need to count calories. Your medicine may give you a bigger appetite and cause you to gain weight.
- You may have to limit eating salty foods. Your medications may cause salt to be held in your body, leading to high blood pressure.

- You may need to eat less protein. Some medications cause a higher level of wastes to build up in your bloodstream.

There are pros and cons to kidney transplantation.

Pros

- It works like a normal kidney.
- It helps you feel healthier.
- You have fewer diet restrictions.
- There's no need for dialysis.

Cons

- It requires major surgery.
- You may need to wait for a donor.
- One transplant may not last a lifetime. Your body may reject the new kidney.
- You will have to take drugs for the rest of your life.

Questions You May Want To Ask:

- Is transplantation the best treatment choice for me? Why or why not?
- What are my chances of having a successful transplant?
- How do I find out if a family member or friend can donate?
- What are the risks to a family member or friend if he or she donates?
- If a family member or friend doesn't donate, how do I get placed on a waiting list for a kidney? How long will I have to wait?
- What are the symptoms of rejection?
- Who will be on my health care team? How can they help me?
- Who can I talk to about sexuality, finances, or family concerns?
- How/where can I talk to other people who have faced this decision?

Conclusion

It's not always easy to decide which type of treatment is best for you. Your decision depends on your medical condition, lifestyle, and personal likes and dislikes. Discuss the pros and cons of each with your health care team. If you start one form of treatment and decide you'd like to try another, talk it over with your doctor. The key is to learn as much as you can about your choices. With that knowledge, you and your doctor will choose a treatment that suits you best.

Paying for Treatment

Treatment for ESRD is expensive, but the Federal Government helps pay for much of the cost. Often, private insurance or state programs pay the rest.

Medicare

Medicare pays for 80 percent of the cost of your dialysis treatments or transplant, no matter how old you are. To qualify,

- you must have worked long enough to be insured under Social Security (or be the child of someone who has) or
- you already must be receiving Social Security benefits.

You should apply for Medicare as soon as possible after beginning dialysis. Often, a social worker at your hospital or dialysis center will help you apply.

Private Insurance

Private insurance often pays for the entire cost of treatment. Or it may pay for the 20 percent that Medicare does not cover. Private insurance also may pay for your prescription drugs.

Medicaid

Medicaid is a state program. Your income must be below a certain level to receive Medicaid funds. Medicaid may pay for your treatments if you cannot receive Medicare. In some states, it also pays the 20 percent that Medicare does not cover. It also may pay for some of your medicines. To apply for Medicaid, talk with your social worker or contact your local health department.

Veterans Administration (VA) Benefits

If you are a veteran, the VA can help pay for treatment. Contact your local VA office for more information.

Social Security Income (SSI) and Social Security Disability Income (SSDI)

These benefits are available from the Social Security Administration. They assist you with the costs of daily living. To find out if you qualify, talk to your social worker or call your local Social Security office.

Organizations That Can Help

There are several groups that offer information and services to kidney patients. You may wish to contact the following:

American Kidney Fund
Suite 1010
6110 Executive Boulevard
Rockville, MD 20852
(800) 638–8299

American Association of Kidney Patients
Suite LL1
1 Davis Boulevard
Tampa, FL 33606
(813) 251–0725

National Kidney Foundation, Inc.
30 East 33rd Street
New York, NY 10016
(800) 622–9010

National Kidney and Urologic Diseases Information Clearinghouse
Box NKUDIC
9000 Rockville Pike
Bethesda, MD 20892
(301) 654–4415

Additional Reading

If you would like to learn more about ESRD and its treatment, you may be interested in reading:

Your New Life With Dialysis—A Patient Guide for Physical and Psychological Adjustment
Edith T. Oberley, M.A., and
Terry D. Oberley, M.D., Ph.D.

Fourth edition, 1991
Charles C. Thomas Publishers
2600 South First Street
Springfield, IL 62794–9265

Understanding Kidney Transplantation
Edith T. Oberley, M.A., and
Neal R. Glass, M.D., F.A.C.S.
Charles C. Thomas Publishers, 1987
2600 South First Street
Springfield, IL 62794–9265

Kidney Disease: A Guide for Patients and Their Families
American Kidney Fund
Suite 1010
6110 Executive Boulevard
Rockville, MD 20852
(800) 638–8299

National Kidney Foundation Patient Education Brochures
Includes information on treatment, diet, work, and exercise.
National Kidney Foundation, Inc.
30 East 33rd Street
New York, NY 10016
(800) 622–9010

Medicare Coverage of Kidney Dialysis and Kidney Transplant Services: A Supplement to Your Medicare Handbook
Publication Number HCFA-02183
U.S. Department of Health and Human Services
Health Care Financing Administration
Suite 500
1331 H Street, NW
Washington, DC 20005
(301) 966–7843

Renalife Magazine
American Association of Kidney Patients (AAKP)
Suite LL1
1 Davis Boulevard
Tampa, FL 33606

(813) 251–0725
Published quarterly.

Family Focus Newsletter
National Kidney Foundation, Inc.
30 East 33rd Street
New York, NY 10016
(800) 622–9010

For Patients Only Magazine
Suite 400
20335 Ventura Boulevard
Woodland Hills, CA 91364
(818) 704–5555
Published six times per year.

PART FOUR

RESEARCH IN DIABETES

Chapter 48

Diabetes Special Report

In 1991, diabetes affected between 13 million and 14 million Americans. Most of them are over 50 and many are minorities: Blacks, Hispanics, Native Americans and Native Hawaiians are disproportionately affected by the disease. More than half a million Americans develop diabetes every year, and the burden of this chronic disorder is increasing as the population ages and the number of Hispanic Americans grows. Diabetes is the sixth leading cause of disease-related death in the United States.

As common as diabetes is, approximately half the people who have the disease don't know it. Diabetes often goes undiagnosed until the heart, eye, nerve or kidney damage it can cause shows itself. Even with treatment, people who have diabetes are twice as likely to suffer stroke and heart disease and 15 times more likely to suffer a non-accident-related amputation than those without the disease. It is the leading cause of new blindness among Americans: 6,000 adults lose their sight each year as a result of diabetes.

Diabetes also is the single largest cause of kidney failure in the United States, accounting for 30 percent of new cases of end-stage renal disease. The Federal Government pays for 90 percent of the treatment for end-stage renal disease, a bill that came to $4.4 billion in 1987. Total costs for medical care and lost productivity resulting from diabetes are more than $40 billion every year. Yet, the impact of this chronic metabolic disease is often overlooked.

NIH Pub. No. 92-3422.

Diabetes Creates Metabolic Havoc

In a healthy body, digested food produces glucose (sugar), which enters the bloodstream. Insulin, a hormone secreted by the pancreas, converts glucose into energy. When diabetes occurs, the body does not make or use insulin properly, depriving the body of fuel. Glucose accumulates in the blood; over time this can damage the heart, kidneys, eyes, and nerves. Uncontrolled glucose levels can cause coma and death. As a result of previous research in cellular and molecular biology, it is now recognized that diabetes is not a single disease but a complex group of disorders that causes potentially lethal glucose imbalance. The primary forms of the disease are insulin-dependent diabetes mellitus (IDDM) and noninsulin-dependent diabetes mellitus (NIDDM).

The National Institute of Diabetes and Digestive and Kidney Diseases (NIDDK) and several other components of the National Institutes of Health (NIH), including the National Institute of Environmental Health Sciences, the National Center for Nursing Research and the Office of the Director, support research on the predictors and causes of diabetes as well as ways to prevent it and its complications.

Advances reported by NIDDK grantees in 1991 include work that should lead to a specific and simple screening test to predict IDDM and provide a clearer understanding of some predictors of the more prevalent NIDDM; the development of devices to improve the treatment and the quality of life for patients with IDDM; and the identification of a gene marker for one type of diabetes, a first step in understanding the complex pathology of glucose intolerance (the inability of the body to use glucose normally). Researchers are engaged in clinical trials using immunotherapy to delay or prevent IDDM, to improve techniques for islet cell transplantation, and to understand how intensive insulin therapy affects diabetic complications. NIDDK support also has furthered knowledge about factors that contribute to diabetic complications, as well as the effects of maternal metabolism on infant development.

Insulin-Dependent Diabetes Is an Autoimmune Disease

Insulin-dependent diabetes, also known as Type I or juvenile-onset diabetes, usually attacks those under 30; it affects approximately 750,000 Americans. IDDM occurs when the body's own immune system—which is meant to protect the body from foreign invaders—instead targets and destroys healthy, insulin-producing beta cells in the pancreas. Scientists do not yet understand precisely why this happens, but by the time the symptoms of diabetes occur, most of the body's ability to produce insulin is gone. Those with IDDM must have daily insulin injections to survive.

Cloning of Critical Protein Supports Early Identification of IDDM

In the last 20 years, researchers have established that diabetes can be predicted using blood tests for three markers: cytoplasmic islet cell autoantibody, insulin autoantibody, and the 64K autoantibody. Last year, NIDDK-supported researchers established that the 64K antigen was glutamic acid decarboxylase (GAD), a protein found in the beta cells and in the brain. This advance raised the prospect of the development of a simple blood test to screen high-risk individuals—and eventually the general population—for GAD antibodies, which appear up to 7 years before IDDM actually occurs. Researchers at the University of Washington in Seattle have now cloned the form of GAD found in beta cells and found that it has its own specific identity. GAD-1, found in the brain, is located on chromosome 2. The gene for GAD-2, or beta cell GAD, is located on chromosome 10, some distance from the nearly identical GAD-1. Now that scientists know the specific structure and "face" of GAD-2, they can begin searching for the elements in it that may trigger the antibodies that initiate beta cell destruction. Understanding GAD-2 may help explain the causes and pathology of IDDM.

Because GAD-2 is the earliest and best marker for beta cell destruction, its specific identity will support the design of simple, inexpensive screening tests for IDDM. Researchers now hope within a year to develop a test for early diagnosis of IDDM. Identifying the pre-symptomatic onset of the disease will allow intervention before significant beta cell destruction occurs, and perhaps even lead to prevention of disease.

Prevention of diabetes is the goal of several scientists involved in clinical trials of immunosuppressive drugs such as azathioprine (Imuran), which researchers hope will prevent autoimmune destruction of beta cells. By screening close relatives of patients already diagnosed with IDDM, these scientists are identifying people at highest risk of IDDM as potential participants for clinical trials now in progress.

IDDM May Begin with Viral Infection

In related research, scientists are examining viruses capable of mimicking the molecular makeup of other proteins to determine if they might contribute to the onset of IDDM. For example, the Coxsackie virus, known to cause respiratory infections, contains a protein resembling GAD. Scientists speculate that if a person susceptible to IDDM is infected with a Coxsackie or similar virus, the immune system may mistakenly also target GAD and begin destroying beta cells.

Beta Cell Transplants, Artificial Pancreas Show Promise

Other work is focused on replacing destroyed beta cells in people who have IDDM. For some time, NIDDK-supported researchers have been developing techniques for transplanting islet cells into IDDM patients and finding ways to protect these transplanted cells from being rejected by the body. Promising results seen in some patients last year have led to clinical trials at several islet cell transplantation centers around the country.

Other NIDDK-supported researchers, in conjunction with Biohybrid Technologies and W. R. Grace & Co., developed an artificial pancreas and successfully tested it in diabetic dogs. The biohybrid organ, so called because it is part plastic and part living cells, effectively regulated blood glucose levels in 6 of 10 diabetic dogs for several months. A semi-permeable plastic membrane inside the artificial pancreas allows blood to nourish implanted insulin-producing islet cells while protecting them from larger immune system cells that ordinarily would cause rejection.

Such transplants might prove superior to human pancreas transplants not only because the surgery is less traumatic but also because immunosuppression is not needed for survival of the islet cells. For these reasons, surgeons could substitute more readily available animal islets for human islet cells. Clinical trials in humans could begin in 2 years.

NIDDK Tests Non-Invasive Blood Glucose Monitor

To maintain strict control of their blond glucose, patients with IDDM must prick their fingers several times a day to measure glucose levels. NIDDK researchers are conducting trials of a non-invasive monitor developed by a Maryland biotechnology firm, Futrex. Based on agricultural technology, the monitor uses near-infrared light waves to measure the amount of glucose in the blood. If sufficient precision can be achieved, such a sensor could improve the quality of life for people with diabetes who depend on insulin to maintain proper glucose levels.

Noninsulin-Dependent Diabetes Results from Insulin Resistance

NIDDM is the most prevalent form of diabetes affecting, approximately 95 percent of the 14 million Americans who suffer from this chronic metabolic disorder. Also called adult-onset or Type II diabetes, NIDDM develops from insulin resistance. The body produces insulin, but for unknown reasons, doesn't use it well. Usually, NIDDM is controlled by diet, exercise, and oral drugs, which help boost the action of insulin. It is this form of diabetes that disproportionately affects Blacks, Hispanics, Native Americans and Native Hawaiians, although the reasons for this are not yet clear. Because insulin resistance is the abnormality most commonly found in people with diabetes, studying its source and mechanisms is a primary focus of NIDDK researchers and grantees.

Insulin Action is a Complex Biochemical Process

In an effort to understand what goes wrong when a defect in insulin action occurs, researchers have focused on deciphering the complex cascade of biochemical events that enables insulin to convert glucose to energy the body can use and store. Ordinarily, insulin binds to insulin receptors on the cell surfaces of a number of tissues, including muscle, fat, and liver tissue. This binding triggers tyrosine kinase activity, a catalyst for phosphorylation, a process whereby phosphate is added to the protein that makes up the insulin receptor, and an important biological switch. When insulin binding takes place, it recruits molecules to transport glucose from the blood and use it for fuel or convert it to glycogen or fat for storage in tissue.

In people with NIDDM, something in this process goes awry. The body responds by producing more insulin to compensate for inadequate glucose conversion. As long as the beta cells can secrete enough insulin to overcome the insulin resistance, glucose levels are balanced. But if beta cells can't sustain this over-production, NIDDM results.

NIDDM is Genetically Determined

Researchers know from longitudinal studies of the Pima Indians in Arizona and of children whose parents have diabetes that insulin resistance, and subsequent NIDDM, appears to run in families. Scientists are beginning to substantiate their belief that, as in IDDM, a genetic predisposition is a factor in NIDDM and the disease is triggered by environmental factors not fully understood. Research is making it clear that genes determine not only who gets diabetes but also when and how severely the disease develops, as well as who is likely to develop complications of diabetes, such as kidney disease.

More than half of the Pima Indians over 35 have NIDDM, the highest incidence of diabetes in the world. They have been geographically isolated for hundreds of years and are more genetically homogeneous than Caucasians. For these reasons, NIDDK researchers in Phoenix have studied the Pima Indians since 1965 to better understand NIDDM. These scientists have found that in this Indian population, major risk factors for NIDDM are insulin resistance and obesity linked to a low metabolic rate. By applying DNA linkage analysis to the phenotypes of these abnormal conditions (that is, by looking for genetic markers linked to physical traits), researchers hope to identify the genetic determinants of NIDDM.

NIDDM is Genetically Complex

Unlike cystic fibrosis, which has been found to begin with a mutation in a single gene, diabetes is a genetically complex disease. Insulin resistance is not only associated with NIDDM, but also with several other metabolic abnormalities, such as obesity, hypertension, dyslipidemia, and atherosclerotic cadiovascular disease. According to NIDDK researchers, it is possible that this syndrome represents a heterogeneous collection of distinct genetic diseases. This hypothesis means that in several different individuals, diabetes might be caused by not one but several genes, making it a particularly difficult genetic puzzle, or as one scientist has called it, "a geneticist's nightmare." However, with advances in the techniques of modern molecular genetics, scientists are beginning to identify mutations in the insulin receptor gene capable of causing a variety of missed connections or malfunctions in insulin binding. Investigators also are beginning to understand how a combination of risk factors may trigger the disease, rather than its being caused directly by a single factor. For instance, obesity alone can cause insulin resistance in non-diabetic individuals, and it increases the level of risk for those likely to develop NIDDM. NIDDK researchers have noted the possibility that mutations in the insulin receptor gene may constitute a genetic predisposition that exacerbates obesity-induced insulin resistance.

Researchers Identify Predictors of NIDDM

In related studies, Phoenix researchers and a research team supported by the National Heart, Lung and Blood Institute (NHLBI) found that hyperinsulinemia, a sign of insulin resistance, exists at a young age in Pima Indian children age 6 to 19.

Hyperinsulinemia, or excess insulin in the blood, initially acts to maintain blood glucose balance. If the insulin-producing beta cells are unable to meet the continuing need for increased production, NIDDM develops. Compared with a population of Caucasian children at low risk for NIDDM, Pima children had significantly higher levels of fasting hyperinsulinemia, an indicator of insulin resistance and a predictor of NIDDM.

Other NIDDK-supported researchers have identified hyperinsulinemia and a slow rate of glucose removal from the blood as primary defects in NIDDM and the best predictors of the disease in the children whose parents have diabetes. These defects have been found to be present at least 10 years before diagnosis and to precede the diminished insulin secretion that eventually occurs in people with NIDDM.

Scientists Find Gene Marker for Another Form of NIDDM

In 1991, NIDDK-supported scientists contributed to finding a gene marker for another form of NIDDM called mature onset diabetes of the young (MODY). Studying five generations of a family with MODY, scientists were able to identify a gene on the long arm of chromosome 20 that appears to be linked to diabetes in 40 members of the 275-member family. Because this marker occurs in a select population with a very specific form of the disease, it may not play a role in more common forms of diabetes. Nevertheless, the finding confirms that genetics is a factor in the development of NIDDM and is a critical first step in finding the genes that cause the more common forms of diabetes. Researchers hope this new marker will open the door to finding other genes that regulate insulin production and secretion. Identifying and understanding genetic variations and the complex ways they might combine to cause NIDDM may eventually enable screening and intervention before the onset of the disease, as well as lead to the development of potential therapies for specific manifestations of the disease.

Intensive Insulin Therapy Improves Glucose Uptake

In work supported by NIDDK and the General Clinical Research Centers Program of the National Center for Research Resources, scientists have found that a specific defect in some obese NIDDM patients with poor blood glucose control can be treated with intensive insulin therapy. In these patients, poorly controlled blood sugar made it difficult for tissue in skeletal muscle to take up glucose. The effectiveness of intensive insulin treatment suggests that the defect in tissue affinity for glucose is an acquired one.

Maternal Diabetes Affects Intellectual Development in Offspring

Another area of significant interest in diabetes research is the effect that a mother's diabetes may have on her child. Babies of mothers with preexisting diabetes are 5 times more likely to be born with birth defects than babies born to non-diabetic mothers, although recent studies have demonstrated that strict blood glucose control in diabetic women both prior to and during pregnancy reduces that risk to normal.

In related research supported by NIDDK, the National Institute of Child Health and Human Development, and the National Center for Research Resources, scientists correlated measures of glucose and lipid (fat) metabolism in pregnant diabetic and non-diabetic women with intellectual development in their children between the ages of 2 and 5. They concluded that maternal diabetes during pregnancy may affect the behavioral and intellectual development of a child. Lower I.Q. scores were associated with gestational ketonemia, excessive levels of potentially poisonous chemical bodies that build up in the mother's blood when insufficient insulin forces the body to break down fat for its energy. This research emphasizes the influence of maternal metabolism on the unborn child, and the need for careful monitoring and management of pregnant women with diabetes.

NIDDM Prevalence Found to Be High Among Hispanics

NIDDK also has laid the groundwork for understanding the future potential impact of NIDDM. An NIDDK epidemiological evaluation of the prevalence of NIDDM among Hispanics, based on the Hispanic Health and Nutrition Examination Survey (HHNES), illustrates that compared with whites, Cubans had diabetes rates 50 to 60 percent higher, and Mexican Americans and Puerto Ricans were 110 to 120 percent more likely to have NIDDM. The study, which used household interviews to identify diagnosed diabetes and an oral glucose tolerance test to determine undiagnosed diabetes, surveyed Mexican Americans in the southwest United States, Cuban Americans in the Miami, Florida area, and Puerto Ricans in the New York city area.

All these groups were from geographic areas previously unstudied. The prevalence of NIDDM was found to be 6.2 percent in whites, 9.3 percent in Cubans, 10.2 percent in Blacks, 13 percent in Mexican Americans, and 13.4 percent in Puerto Ricans. Diabetes was more prevalent among individuals who were older, obese, or who had family history of the disease.

National Cancer Institute

Researchers studying diabetes and cancer are interested in the regulation of cell growth and metabolism. Studies of one type of diabetes are relevant to understanding the role of insulin and related growth factors in the growth of certain tumors. In another type of diabetes, normal cells in the pancreas are destroyed, resulting in a decrease in insulin productions. The destruction may be caused by an autoimmune reaction. This research is relevant to understanding how the immune system distinguishes between normal and abnormal cells, such as tumor cells.

Cancer-related diabetes research in 1991 included a study using transgenic mice—mice whose chromosomes contain experimentally added genetic material. The added gene was *H-ras*, a gene frequently associated with cancer. Mice, in which the protein encoded by this gene was expressed, developed degeneration of the beta cells, and eventually, diabetes.

Other studies have shown that the onset of diabetes in rats results in both an increase in concentrations of specific nutrients in the blood and an uptake of these nutrients by malignant tumors. This relationship suggests that one or more of these nutrients (glycerol, fatty acids, triglycerides, and ketones) are required for tumor cells to divide and grow. Studies have shown that people with diabetes are more susceptible to pancreatic cancer, a connection that may be associated with this process.

National Heart, Lung, and Blood Institute

Research by the National Heart, Lung, and Blood Institute (NHLBI) on diabetes focuses on its role as a risk factor for cardiovascular diseases (CVD) and on its effects on the cardiovascular system. Among Americans with NIDDM, 60 percent of deaths are attributed to ischemic heart disease (coronary artery disease) and 20 percent to other diseases of the heart and blood vessels. Moreover, there is evidence that part of the increased risk of CVD associated with diabetes may develop in the prediabetic period, when glucose levels are normal or minimally elevated. Current data suggest that the impact of diabetes on the risk of vascular disease differs between men and women and among racial groups. NHLBI recently initiated a collaborative, multidisciplinary study to assess the relation between increasing concentrations of glucose and varying levels of insulin and insulin resistance and other CVD risk factors and to the presence of atherosclerotic vascular disease.

Meanwhile, NHLBI-supported basic researchers are making progress in their quest to determine the underlying cause of diabetes-induced vascular damage. One of the earliest events in diabetes is a change in the function of endothelial cells—the cells that line all blood vessels in the body. Under normal circumstances, endothelial cells produce relaxing factors, such as endothelial-derived relaxing factor (EDRF), prostaglandins, and enzymes that activate or break down regulatory hormones. These cells and their factors play a key role in maintaining normal functioning of the smooth muscles of the blood vessels. There must be balance between keeping blood vessels sufficiently open to allow passage of blood and having adequate muscle tone to maintain blood pressure that will facilitate blood flow. The integrity and functioning of the endothelial cell layer, however, become profoundly altered in humans (and animals) afflicted with diabetes. The high level of blood glucose characteristic of diabetes impairs the effectiveness of endothelial cells in regulating blood vessel relaxation, as has been demonstrated in animals. Recent NHLBI-supported studies have provided evidence that this impairment may be due to interference with a number of normal endothelial processes. Research findings suggest that a protein modifier, protein kinase C, may play a role in this process since inhibitors for this factor seem to prevent the detrimental effect of exposing normal arteries to high glucose levels. The normal response to another factor acetylcholine, also was shown to be impaired in a rabbit model of diabetes.

These basic research findings are intriguing because they indicate that the serious alterations in vascular function characteristic of diabetes can be initiated by simple changes in the endothelial cell's milieu, and that this alteration in function occurs long before any damage to blood vessels is evident. Future investigation of the mechanisms by which high blood glucose levels disrupt endothelium-dependent dilation of the blood vessels will likely provide direction for the development of therapeutic agents and other measures that will prevent and reduce the vascular effects of diabetes.

National Institute of Dental Research

The National Institute of Dental Research (NIDR) supports basic and clinical research on diabetes, a disease that has implications for oral health and function. NIDR intramural scientists are focusing on the role of the immune system in the development of insulin-dependent diabetes mellitus.

The investigators examined two classes of B cells, important components of the human immune system that produce IgM and IgG, two classes of antibodies. They found that healthy persons and patients with newly diagnosed IDDM had similar blood levels of IgM and that these antibodies reacted only mildly with a wide variety of cell proteins, including insulin.

Studies of IgG antibodies, however, told a different story. Like IgM, IgG antibody in healthy individuals also reacted weakly with insulin, as well as with other cellular proteins. But in patients with newly diagnosed IDDM, IgG reacted strongly, and only, with insulin, at levels 20 limes higher than in nondiabetic persons. Previously, it was believed that the strong IgG reaction was a response to injected insulin. The NIDR study revealed, however, that elevated IgG antibodies were detected in IDDM patients even before they were treated with insulin. The IgG response, therefore, was "self-directed" against the patient's own insulin. This finding offers insight into the autoimmune processes at work in the development IDDM and has diagnostic and treatment implications.

National Institute of Neurological Disorders and Stroke

Many Americans with diabetes also have some degree of nerve damage or diabetic neuropathy. This damage can be severe enough to cause pain, tingling sensations, and numbness. More threatening, however, is nerve damage that cuts off sensation and masks injuries, such as foot or leg ulcers. These can lead to infection and gangrene that may eventually lead to amputation. Among people with diabetes, neuropathy often is associated with other disabling complications such as eye or kidney disease and may play a role in sudden death.

Because there is a lack of reliable information on the extent of disability caused by diabetic neuropathy, the National Institute of Neurological Disorders and Stroke (NINDS) supports a comprehensive, long-term comparative study of a cross-section of diabetic patients and of individuals without diabetes. This study has developed accurate, reproducible methods to probe the frequency, severity, and symptoms of nerve damage over time.

The investigators are examining risk factors for the development and progression of diabetic neuropathy, including the control of blood sugar levels, age, duration of diabetes, regulation of high blood pressure, and smoking. These and other studies are increasing the understanding of the biological mechanisms involved in diabetic neuropathy, as well as helping scientists develop treatments and assess how control of risk factors may influence the disease.

National Institute of Allergy and Infectious Diseases

The National Institute of Allergy and Infectious Diseases (NIAID) conducts and supports research on the causes and treatment of a variety of disorders of the immune system, including autoimmune diseases such as NIDDM. Autoimmune disease results when the immune system mistakenly attacks the body's own tissues.

In persons with IDDM, the immune system mistakes insulin-producing islet cells for foreign matter capable of harming the body and then destroys these cells. Researchers have been examining the role that T cells, which are part of the immune system's arsenal, play in destroying islet cells. NIAID-supported scientists have shown how one type of T cells, CD4+ cells, may facilitate this destruction. CD4+ cells, also called helper T cells, initiate many immune system responses. The scientists found that CD4+ cells in non-obese, spontaneously diabetic mice may induce an inflammatory reaction that destroys the islet cells. Therefore, anti-inflammatory drugs may control the progress of IDDM in the body.

NIAID-supported scientists have developed a transgenic mouse model in which they reproduced manifestations of IDDM that are similar to those found in humans, such as low insulin and high blood sugar levels. A viral gene was inserted into the islet cells of the mice; the animals then developed diabetic symptoms when infected with the whole virus later in life. Studies in the transgenic mice of the types of immune cells that contribute to the destruction of islet cells should help scientists develop strategies to prevent or treat diabetes.

National Institute of General Medical Sciences

The National Institute of General Medical Sciences (NIGMS) supports basic research and research training that provide the foundation for a better understanding of fundamental life processes. This research contributes new knowledge and theories to the disease-targeted programs of other NIH components, including those related to diabetes.

NIGMS also supports a major resource for genetics researchers, the Human Genetic Mutant Cell Repository, which contains cell lines from patients with a wide variety of genetic disorders and from normal individuals whose cells are used as controls. Cell lines in the collection include those from individuals with various types of diabetes such as IDDM, NIDDM, MODY, and diabetes insipidus (a form of diabetes that results from abnormal pituitary or kidney function) with optic atrophy.

Among the diabetes-related research projects supported by NIGMS are studies of the regulation of the gene that codes for insulin; the transport of proteins, including insulin, within the cell; protein secretion by the cell; the structure and function of cell receptors for insulin and other proteins; basic metabolic processes at the cellular and molecular levels; and the effect of severe trauma and disease on glucose metabolism and insulin resistance.

National Institute of Child Health and Human Development

National Institute of Child Health and Human Development (NICHD) research on diabetes focuses on the impact of diabetes and glucose metabolism on pregnancy and the developing fetus.

NICHD grantees led by Dr. Barbara Stonestreet of the Women and Infants Hospital of Rhode Island in Providence have investigated glucose metabolism and insulin action in developing organisms. Infants born to diabetic mothers face an increased risk of polycythemia, an abnormal increase in the number of red blood cells. In addition, the blood of these infants clots more easily than normal blood, increasing their risk for small strokes and subsequent brain damage.

Recently, NICHD grantees tested the Pedersen hypothesis, which states that a fetus produces large quantities of insulin to process the glucose that passes through the placenta from its diabetic mother's circulation. The hypothesis contends that it is the extra insulin that results in the increased number of red blood cells, not the mother's high blood glucose levels.

The researchers infused insulin into the blood of fetal sheep for 11 days. Compared to the control animals, the fetal sheep had significantly elevated red blood cell levels, lending support to the Pedersen hypothesis.

In addition, NICHD studies have sought to discern the biochemical events involved in glucose metabolism early in life. This information may one day lead to treatment advances for infants born to diabetic mothers.

NICHD grantees led by Dr. Sherin Devaskar of the St. Louis University School of Medicine in Missouri investigated how glucose, essential for brain functioning, is transported into the fetal brain. Glucose first is transported into cells with the aid of a family of compounds known as glucose transporters, or GTs. The five major types of GTs (Glut 1, 2, 3, 4, and 5) reflect the different glucose needs of various tissues. In brain tissue, GT 1 and GT 3 are most active. The researchers found that, in rat brains, GT 1 constantly increases throughout gestation and during the new born period. Moreover, GT 1 increases in specialized brain areas.

Other NICHD grantees led by Dr. Rebecca A. Simmons of the University of California in San Francisco have determined that the need for glucose declines in fetal calf lung tissue shortly before birth. In fact, the need for glucose, as measured by lactate, a by-product of glucose metabolism, decreases by as much as 80 percent during this period.

National Eye Institute

Diabetic retinopathy—a disease that affects the delicate blood vessels of the retina—is a leading cause of new blindness in middle-aged Americans. Although NEI-supported research has led to treatment that reduces the risk of vision loss from advanced diabetic retinopathy (DR), the Institute still has two major goals: learning how the retinopathy develops and finding ways to slow or prevent early destructive changes in the blood vessels of the retina. The NEI-supported Wisconsin Epidemiologic Study of Diabetic Retinopathy has investigated whether blood pressure or serum levels of sugar and lipids (fats) affect the severity of the retinopathy and the hard exudates that often develop in the retinas of people with diabetes. Exudates consist of large molecules that escape from the blood through weakened retinal arteries. The lipids get trapped in the retina because they are too large to re-enter the bloodstream through retinal veins.

Recent findings from the Wisconsin population-based study support the current dietary management of diabetes, which includes control of blood lipids. In all patients in the study who used insulin, the severity of the development of hard exudates correlated with the levels of total blood cholesterol. The same correlation was not found in people with NIDDM who do not have to use insulin. The researchers suspect that triglycerides, another type of lipid, may be the source of exudates in the latter group. The findings suggest that the source of exudates in IDDM differs from that in people with NIDDM who do not need insulin injections. If further research confirms this, dietary control of lipids may need to differ for the two types of diabetes.

In other research, intramural scientists have inoculated bacterial cells with the DNA sequence that codes for the enzyme aldose reductase. Researchers believe that aldose reductase is implicated in the early cellular breakdown that leads to diabetic eye disease. The inoculated bacteria are yielding abundant amounts of active aldose reductase, which is valuable for use in studies aimed at the development of a safe and effective inhibitor of the enzyme.

NEI-funded scientists also are studying several growth factors (proteins) to determine whether they influence the development of new but weak blood vessels that proliferate in advanced diabetic retinopathy. Although no causal effect has been established, the researchers have found above-normal levels of two fibroblast growth factors in retinal tissues of people with proliferative diabetic retinopathy, the severe form of the disease. Fibroblast cells are an important part of blood vessel walls.

Other researchers have found that people with proliferative retinopathy have more insulin-like growth factor IGF in their blood than do those who have nonproliferataive retinopathy. IGF, which is produced outside the retina, may interact with other factors in a way that influences new blood vessel growth in the retina. If a causal relationship can be found for one or more of these growth proteins, scientists can focus on devising ways to halt their abnormal activity.

National Institute on Aging

The National Institute on Aging (NIA) conducts and supports research on the physiological mechanisms of diabetes, a frequently occurring disorder associated with old age. Older people are often less active and gain weight. The increase in body fat associated with this weight gain then interferes with insulin action and may contribute to diabetes.

Recent NIA-sponsored research measured the effect of regular physical exercise on the metabolic rate of sedentary and physically active younger and older men. The resting metabolic rate and the rate of calorie "burn-off" in a meal affect body composition. If calorie intake remains the same, a higher resting metabolic rate and a higher metabolic rate after meals help prevent the accumulation of body fat.

The study indicated that active older men burned calories more quickly after a meal and had a higher fasting metabolic rate than sedentary men. Physical activity helped control weight by increasing calories burned even at rest. The results suggest that physical activity helps slow age-associated gains in body fat and may prevent or delay the onset of diabetes—a beneficial impact of regular exercise on a chronic disease of older people.

National Center for Research Resources

Resource centers and shared research facilities provided by the National Center for Research Resources (NCRR) support a variety of studies focused on understanding, treating, and preventing diabetes.

Scientists in the General Clinical Research Center (GCRC) at Rockefeller University in New York City reported in 1991 that an excessive accumulation of proteins and peptides modified by glucose appears to be involved in the chronic complications of IDDM. These naturally occurring molecules are called advanced glycosylation end-products (AGEs). The researchers found that the AGE levels were significantly higher in tissues of diabetic patients than in those of normal individuals. Levels in patients with end-stage kidney disease were almost twice as high as in diabetic patients without kidney disease. AGE peptide levels in the blood of diabetic patients correlated with the severity of their kidney dysfunction. A patient who had undergone a kidney transplant and who had normal kidney function had an AGE peptide blood level similar to that of persons with diabetes but without end-stage kidney disease.

A substitute for injecting insulin would he a great boon for persons with IDDM. In a preliminary evaluation at the outpatient GCRC of Johns Hopkins University Hospital in Baltimore, Maryland, four outpatients with NIDDM and two non-diabetic persons received aerosolized insulin by inhaling through the mouth. The Hopkins researchers hypothesized that earlier inhalation trials gave poor results because of an inadequate dose of insulin, probably due to loss of drug before it reached the lungs, so they focused on developing a system that would maximize drug delivery there. They found that their technique could deliver the same dosage of insulin as an injection, and without any adverse effects. The researchers are particularly encouraged because the maximum levels of insulin in the blood were achieved much quicker by inhalation than they are by injection. Many other questions about aerosol insulin treatment, especially how long its effects last, remain to be answered, and studies addressing these questions are continuing at the GCRC.

Using tissue supplied by the National Disease Research Interchange, a resource center supported by NCRR's Biological Models and Materials Program, scientists at the Washington University School of Medicine GCRC in St. Louis, Missouri, have identified two techniques that appear to contribute to successful outcome of islet cell transplantation in IDDM patients:

cryopreservation (freezing and storing the cells) in order to pool tissue from several donors, and low-temperature culture of islet cells before transplantation to reduce those cells that are the targets for rejection by the recipient's immune system.

Outlook

Since 1921, when the discovery of insulin made it possible to save the lives of people with diabetes, tremendous strides in diabetes research have vastly improved quality of life for patients who, in an earlier time, would simply have wasted and died. Much of that progress has ensued because of the dedicated work of more than a dozen components of NIH. Researchers continue to conduct basic and clinical studies that steadily increase knowledge about this complex disease. An ever-broadening understanding of immunology, molecular biology, and genetics has spurred diabetes research in recent years. Today, biomedical researchers seek to understand the molecular nature and the complex interaction of multiple metabolic systems, which should aid in preventing and curing diabetes. The concerted commitment of NIH scientists from every discipline contributes daily to the realization of this goal.

Chapter 49

Diabetes Research

Highlights of Accomplishments and Opportunities in Diabetes Research

Congress implemented the recommendations of the National Commission on Diabetes by passing the National Diabetes Act (P.L. 93–354) and by significantly augmenting the NIH research budget in 1977. The resulting research accomplishments of the past decade have been truly remarkable. No member of the Commission or Congress could have envisioned or predicted the startling advances that have been made in the short span of 10 years. In some instances, entirely new concepts were developed that provided further insight into diabetes and also were applicable to other human diseases. As a result of advances in our understanding of the causes of diabetes and its complications, the next decade now holds real opportunities for the prevention and cure of diabetes and its complications. The opportunities cited below appear to be among the most promising and exciting. They should, however, be considered only as examples. The course of biomedical research is not always predictable; thus, approaches must remain flexible so that advantage may be taken of major break-throughs that may be occurring even as this report is being written. These research highlights are followed by the NDAB's recommendations for support of new and ongoing Federal research programs. Additional information about research advances and opportunities may be found in [Chapter 50 of this volume].

Excerpts from: *The National Long-Range Plan to Combat Diabetes.* NIH Pub. No. 88-1587.

Advances in Our Understanding of Insulin-Dependent Diabetes and Opportunities for Cure or Prevention

Genetic Factors of IDDM

Studies during the past decade have shown that patients with IDDM have genetic markers, called histocompatibility proteins, that are associated strongly with the development of insulin-dependent diabetes. Because these genetic markers are necessary but not sufficient for the development of IDDM, it appears that some additional, as yet unknown, environmental factors are required to cause the destruction of the beta cells and the development of diabetes. Environmental factors, either viruses or chemical agents, alter the beta cells to permit their immunologic destruction in genetically susceptible individuals. Antibodies to islet cells have been demonstrated in newly diagnosed IDDM patients. These islet cell antibodies or immune cells are believed to be responsible for the recognition and destruction of the altered beta cells.

Animal Models of IDDM

In 1975, few animal models of diabetes were available, and none resembled the human form of IDDM. In the past 10 years, two animal models (the BB rat and NOD mouse) have been developed that do resemble IDDM. In both, diabetes develops spontaneously and immunologic destruction of the beta cells occurs. In the BB rat, diabetes can be prevented by transfusion of normal white blood cells into the animals. Further immunologic studies on these two models should provide insight into the cause of IDDM and possible approaches to prevent diabetes in humans.

Prevention of Insulin-Dependent Diabetes

Identification of the prediabetic state in diabetes is essential to efforts to prevent the development of the disease. Perhaps the single most important advance of the past two decades in diabetes research has been recognition that autoimmune destruction of beta cells takes months or years to reach completion. Simple and inexpensive techniques are now available to identify the presence of the autoimmune state and to track the functional loss of beta cells resulting from their progressive destruction. Whereas currently the clinical diagnosis of diabetes is almost never made until the destructive process is nearly complete and insulin injections are required to prevent death, intervening before insulin-producing cells have been irreversibly destroyed may become a strategy to prevent progression of diabetes and its complications.

To identify those individuals in whom the destructive process has begun and who therefore are at high risk of developing IDDM, studies of relatives of persons with IDDM have been conducted. These studies have identified individuals who possess the genetic markers associated with IDDM and who also have islet cell antibodies, insulin antibodies, and slight impairment in the release of insulin from the beta cells following glucose stimulation. Because these changes may be present for months or years before a patient develops overt diabetes, it may become possible to develop strategies to thwart the subsequent development of diabetes in these individuals.

Immunosuppressive drugs have been administered to patients at the time of onset of IDDM, and this immunotherapy has produced a remission of diabetes in some patients. Unfortunately, the diabetic state returns when the immunosuppressive therapy is stopped. In addition, currently available immunosuppressive drugs have serious adverse side effects that preclude their prophylactic or prolonged use in persons at risk for diabetes. Research has shown that the interaction of white blood cells in an immune reaction results in the release of lymphokines, certain hormone-like substances that are responsible for stimulating the white blood cells to produce specific antibodies or to develop killer cells that will recognize and destroy altered or foreign cells. One of these lymphokines, Interleukin-1, inhibits glucose-induced insulin secretion from beta cells following exposure to the lymphokine for a few hours or destroys the beta cells if the exposure is extended to a few days. This important finding raises the possibility that certain lymphokines in IDDM may be responsible for the destruction of beta cells. These studies, in conjunction with the immunologic investigations of the two animal models of IDDM, may lead to specific therapeutic agents that could be used to prevent the development of overt diabetes in individuals who are identified as being genetically predisposed to develop the disease.

Many potentially effective interventions are being tested in rodent models of IDDM, and other interventions may soon be available. Evaluation of preventive interventions will require multicenter clinical trials. To prepare for such trials, a large high-risk population should be assembled for prospective studies of the natural history of prediabetes, employing and refining all available parameters and introducing new and more sensitive yardsticks of islet destruction and virological surveillance. Most of the techniques required are simple and inexpensive and can easily be applied by existing facilities in diabetes centers.

The prevention of IDDM seems potentially feasible given our present understanding of its natural history. Through additional fundamental research into the immunological processes underlying IDDM and subsequent clinical research into the techniques for interfering with its immunologic development, a cure for IDDM may become a reality.

Advances in Our Understanding of Noninsulin-Dependent Diabetes and Opportunities for Cure or Prevention

Insulin Synthesis, Secretion, and Action

The major defects in patients with NIDDM are a loss of sensitivity of the principal target tissues (liver, skeletal muscle, and fatty tissue) to insulin action and a decrease in the sensitivity of the beta cells to glucose resulting in a reduction in insulin release. Significant advances have been made in understanding the biochemical events involved in the formation of proinsulin in the insulin-producing beta cell following glucose stimulation, the conversion of proinsulin to insulin, and the stimulation of release of insulin granules from the beta cell by glucose and other stimulators. Molecular biologic studies of insulin synthesis have demonstrated abnormal forms of insulin that are the products of defective insulin synthesis in some patients with diabetes. These abnormal forms of insulin react abnormally with target cells; the result is diabetes. Studies of insulin secretion have shown that the beta cell requires the direct interaction of other cell types in the islets and their hormonal products for the beta cell to respond to glucose stimulation with normal insulin release.

A decade ago, the mechanisms by which insulin acted on target cells to permit the entry, metabolism, and storage of glucose and other nutrients into these cells were unknown. In the interim, specific receptors for insulin have been identified on the cell membranes of target tissues. Insulin receptors have been isolated, their chemical structure has been determined, and the gene responsible for their formation has been cloned. In addition, the signaling mechanisms initiated by the receptors are now being elucidated. These outstanding achievements make it possible to begin to understand the intracellular events following the interaction of insulin with its receptors. These basic investigations provide the fundamental information needed to determine the defect in insulin receptor and postreceptor action in people with NIDDM, and basic research in the mechanisms of insulin secretion and action has reached the point where it is realistic to expect that an understanding of the causes of NIDDM at the molecular level can be achieved within the next decade.

Prevention of Noninsulin-Dependent Diabetes

Recognition of the prediabetic state applies to NIDDM as well as to IDDM. NIDDM is now known to be a distinct entity with obesity, insulin resistance, and inability to increase insulin secretion as underlying causes. The development of insulin resistance appears to be a prerequisite for the development of impaired glucose tolerance and NIDDM. Environmental factors such as physical activity and intrauterine environment also appear to influence the development of NIDDM. Other suspected risk factors include diet, hypertension, and hyperlipoproteinemia. Although the exact role that genetics plays in the development of NIDDM is not known, studies of identical twins have shown that genetic factors play a role in the development of the disease. The rapid and continuing development of gene probes now offers an opportunity to elucidate the genetic determinants of NIDDM. Research to definitively identify the risk factors of NIDDM will lead ultimately to its prevention.

Dramatic progress has occurred in our understanding of the essential link between NIDDM and obesity. Nevertheless, effective control of obesity is still difficult in most patients with NIDDM. Further fundamental information has been developed on the role of diet and exercise in the control of blood glucose and insulin resistance in patients with NIDDM. However, additional basic and clinical research is needed to aid the understanding of the control of obesity, regulation of energy expenditure, and eating behaviors. We have the opportunity to "cure" most patients with NIDDM and obesity, but to achieve this "cure," more effective clinical approaches to the treatment of obesity must be developed.

Advances in the Therapy of Diabetes and Opportunities for Cure Through Transplantation or Artificial Pancreas

Human Insulin

One of the most remarkable accomplishments in the past 10 years was the isolation of the human insulin gene, determination of its structure, and the resultant production of human insulin by recombinant DNA technology. This achievement moved rapidly from the laboratory to the industrial production of human insulin, which is now available for treatment of patients with diabetes. In 1975, the National Commission on Diabetes was concerned that the demand for insulin throughout the world would soon exceed the supply of insulin extracted from beef and pig pancreases. The use of recombinant DNA technology for the production of human insulin has resolved this potentially catastrophic problem.

Insulin Pumps

A decade ago, large devices had been developed that could be used at the bedside of patients to deliver appropriate amounts of insulin to control blood sugar. In the interim, miniaturization of this type of device has led to the production of small insulin pumps for continuous variable delivery of insulin. These pumps can be programmed to meet expected requirements for insulin secretion, but current models lack a biocompatible glucose sensor for continuous measurement of the changing levels of blood sugar in the patients. The technology for the development of artificial glucose sensors has advanced considerably, but a reliable implantable glucose sensor still eludes us.

Transplantation

Segmental and whole pancreas transplantation has been performed successfully in a number of patients with diabetes. However, permanent immunosuppressive therapy is required to maintain the grafts and prevent rejection. For this reason, the transplants are done late in the course of diabetes and in patients who simultaneously receive a kidney transplant or will require a kidney transplant within 1 or 2 years. One problem with the procedure is the elimination of secretions from the exocrine portion of the pancreas. New surgical techniques developed in the past few years have helped to alleviate this difficulty. Segmental or whole pancreas transplants with continuous immunosuppressive therapy have produced normal levels of blood glucose in some patients with diabetes.

The ideal approach for treatment of a patient with IDDM would be to transplant normal islets as replacements for the damaged or destroyed beta cells. Ten years ago, transplants of islets in inbred strains of rats were shown to reverse the diabetic state to normal. The islet transplants also prevented or reversed early complications of diabetes that involved the eye and kidney in these animals. An unexpected and promising development occurred during the past decade when islets were successfully transplanted between strains of animals, without the use of immunosuppressive drugs, by treating the islets before transplant to destroy or alter the white blood cells (dendritic cells). This accomplishment raised the possibility that islet transplants could be attempted in patients with diabetes without the use of immunosuppressive therapy.

The development of methods for the isolation of large numbers of islets from the human pancreas, both adult and fetal, has made it possible to initiate clinical trials on islet transplantation in patients with diabetes. The early findings are encouraging, and studies are in progress at several institutions to determine whether islet transplantation can be used as a new therapeutic approach to diabetes.

The potential for curing diabetes using pancreas transplants, islet transplants, or an implantable artificial pancreas is real. Our advances in understanding in this area during the past decade have been phenomenal. Opportunities also exist for basic research into the causes of islet degeneration in diabetes and for additional clinical research into the techniques for the prevention of the destruction of transplanted islets.

Advances in Our Understanding of and Opportunities for the Prevention or Cure of the Complications of Diabetes

Extremely serious complications that affect the eye, kidney, cardiovascular system, peripheral nerves, and fetus can occur in patients with diabetes. Studies in experimental animals indicate that these diabetic complications may be due to elevated levels of blood glucose in diabetes. The multicenter Diabetes Control and Complications Trial has been initiated to assess the effect of glucose control in humans. The long-range approach to the prevention of the complications of diabetes is to prevent diabetes itself and to devise improved therapy, such as islet transplantation or an artificial beta cell, to maintain normal blood glucose levels at all times. While these long-term strategies are being pursued, other approaches have been developed to delay the development of, or to treat, these complications.

Eye Complications

Laser photocoagulation has been proved effective in the treatment of diabetic eye disease, and further trials are now under way to identify more precisely the best timing and techniques to prevent blindness. Treatment of damaged blood vessels with lasers in the early stages of diabetic retinopathy preserves vision and delays the development of further vascular damage. Vision loss caused by bleeding into the vitreous, the gel-like substance that fills the eyeball, now can be treated by a new surgical technique called vitrectomy that was developed during the past decade. When this procedure is performed soon after the hemorrhage occurs, vision usually is restored.

Studies in experimental animals have shown that abnormal increases in the blood sugar activate an enzyme system (aldose reductase system) that forms products that impair nerve function and may also damage small blood vessels in the eye. During the past decade, aldose reductase inhibitors have been developed to block this enzyme system and thereby prevent the accumulation of damaging products even though blood glucose levels are above normal. Studies using aldose reductase inhibitors are now in progress to determine whether diabetes-induced damage to blood vessels in the eye can be prevented or arrested.

Diabetes in Pregnancy

Women with diabetes risk serious complications of pregnancy and a threefold increased incidence of congenital anomalies in their babies. Clinical studies have shown that meticulous regulation of blood glucose during the second and third trimester of pregnancy reduces the frequency and severity of most complications of pregnancy to those associated with nondiabetic pregnancies. Preliminary studies suggest that careful control of diabetes before and during the initial 12 weeks of pregnancy, when the baby's organs are being formed, will reduce the occurrence of birth defects. The opportunity exists for more fundamental research into the causes of the increase in birth defects in infants of mothers with diabetes, now the most common cause of death in these babies.

In addition, 2 to 3 percent of all pregnancies in the United States are complicated by gestational diabetes, that is, carbohydrate intolerance first recognized during pregnancy. This diagnosis carrics a high probability for diabetes in the mother under nonpregnant conditions. More important, if unrecognized or untreated, it is accompanied by markedly increased obstetrical complications and morbidity.

Diabetic Kidney Disease

Kidney disease is an important cause of death and disability for individuals with diabetes. The degenerative changes in the small blood vessels that result from diabetes cause the kidneys to lose their ability to filter waste products from the blood. Studies during the past decade have demonstrated that some of these early changes in kidney function can be reversed or prevented by strict control of blood glucose levels and by treatment of kidney infections and hypertension. In addition, advances in kidney dialysis and in renal transplantation have enabled patients with diabetes to achieve survival rates approaching those of patients without diabetes also receiving such treatment.

The outlook for patients with diabetic renal disease has improved dramatically, but early diagnosis and prevention are still elusive. Additional basic information must be sought regarding the exact causes of diabetic renal disease. Careful evaluation is needed of new forms of early treatment such as the reduction in dietary protein and vigorous treatment of hypertension, particularly therapy using new pharmacologic agents such as angiotension-converting enzyme inhibitors.

Diabetic Neuropathy

Diabetic neuropathy has become better understood during the past decade, and now treatment strategies are being developed. Several promising leads are being pursued, including the role of aldose reductase inhibitors. Yet, basic research is still needed into the pathophysiology of diabetic neuropathy. Also needed is a good clinical definition of diabetic neuropathy to evaluate new therapeutic approaches. The opportunity to advance the understanding of diabetic neuropathy is real, and success will depend on increased cooperative efforts between the diabetes community and the various agencies within the NIH that are interested in the study of diabetes and neurologic diseases.

One of the effects of peripheral neuropathy is loss of sensation in the legs and feet. Repeated, unrecognized trauma to insensitive feet frequently leads to ulceration and infection. These infections may progress to gangrene when impaired circulation, resulting from diabetic peripheral vascular disease, limits the delivery of oxygen and antibiotics. When this cycle is not controlled, amputations must be performed to prevent death. Patient and professional education programs on proper foot care for persons with diabetes have been developed and need to be more widely implemented. A machine, the pedabarograph, has been devised that identifies pressure points on the foot; use of this device may help persons with diabetes recognize areas that need special care to prevent foot irritations and subsequent infection.

Cardiovascular Disease

Although the incidence of cardiovascular disease in patients with diabetes has declined during the past decade following the trend in the general population, this complication is still responsible for three-fourths of the deaths in patients with diabetes mellitus. Over the next decade, we will need to conduct both fundamental research into the causes of atherosclerosis and clinical research into the effect of controlling risk factors in patients with diabetes on the subsequent reduction of atherosclerotic morbidity and mortality.

Most patients with diabetes have multiple risk factors for cardiovascular disease in addition to the diabetes itself; these risk factors include cigarette smoking, high blood lipids, and hypertension. Growing evidence that intervention to reduce these factors reduces cardiovascular morbidity and mortality requires the development of more effective methods to assist patients in making lifelong changes in behavior and lifestyle. This effort will require collaboration between psychosocial and medical experts.

Advances in Our Understanding of the Epidemiology of Diabetes and Opportunities for Further Research

Epidemiologic research has led to much of the increased understanding of the etiology of IDDM and NIDDM and of the complex interrelationships between risk factors and complications of the disease. Results of this research have allowed us to learn more about the relationships among hypertension, lipids, physical activity, diet, obesity, genetics, and diabetes. During the next decade, we must develop an increased understanding of the complex interrelationships between genetic and environmental factors. This understanding can only be achieved by developing new data bases for important populations with diabetes, including minorities such as American Indians, blacks, and Hispanics. Establishing such data bases will provide reliable information on the relationship of current risks for the development of diabetes mellitus and its complications and the effect of therapeutic interventions on these risks.

Recommendations for New Research Programs

The diabetes research accomplishments of the past decade can be attributed in part to the implementation of the Commission's recommendations contained in the first long-range plan. The diabetes community and the general public recognize and applaud the leadership provided by Congress and the administration in implementing those recommendations. The new long-range plan includes recommendations for the continuation and strengthening of the ongoing diabetes research programs, including the research and manpower development programs of the NIDDK, the diabetes-related research activities by other NIH Institutes, the DERC's and DRTC's, and the Diabetes Control and Complications Trial.

The new long-range plan also contains additional programmatic research initiatives vital to continued progress toward the eventual prevention of diabetes and the reduction of its social and economic consequences. These new initiatives are designed to build on existing programs and improve the effectiveness and efficiency of those activities. These new initiatives include:

- *Diabetes Interdisciplinary Research Programs*, to promote the integration of new research methodologies developed by basic scientists into diabetes-related research programs.
- *Biologic Resource Bank for Studies on Diabetes*, to facilitate the sharing of valuable, expensive, and scarce biological research materials and to apply new research technologies from the basic sciences for the utilization and analysis of these materials.
- *Information and Data System for Diabetes Research*, to facilitate and encourage the sharing of diabetes research data between individual investigators. . . .

Recommendations for Current Research Programs

The recommendations for new research programs described above were designed expressly to complement and build on the successful research mechanisms that facilitated the exciting and promising research advances described in this report. Adequate support for the current programs is essential to achieve the goals of the next decade. Therefore, the NDAB has developed recommendations for (1) the individual research project program, the backbone of diabetes research; (2) the training and development of research personnel to arrest the decline in the number of qualified investigators and to facilitate the training of diabetes researchers in the new research methodologies developed in the basic sciences; (3) research centers to provide specialized research resources; and (4) clinical trials.

Individual Research Project Grants

The mainstay of the NIH extramural research program is the "R01," the individual research grant. The individual research grant remains the largest component of the NIH research program, accounting for 66 percent of the total NIH extramural research budget. Individual research grants support the best and the brightest of our Nation's scientists; through the individual research grant, the impressive scientific advances detailed in this report have been brought to fruition.

Individual research grants relating to diabetes are funded by all NIH Institutes. The NIDDK, the lead Institute for diabetes research, supports about 60 percent of all NIH individual diabetes research grants through its Division of Diabetes, Endocrinology, and Metabolic Diseases. The NIDDK provides grant support for investigator-initiated studies that cover a wide range of fundamental and clinical studies related to the etiology, pathogenesis, prevention, diagnosis, treatment, and cure of diabetes mellitus and its complications. . . .

Training and Development of Research Personnel

Remarkable progress has been made in the diabetes research program since the original long-range plan was developed in 1975. Exciting research opportunities now exist that offer the vision of even greater progress toward the prevention and treatment of diabetes and its complications during the next decade. However, these opportunities are appearing at a time when the number of trained investigators in diabetes-related areas is declining rapidly. The NDAB is deeply concerned about this trend.

It is clear that NIH manpower development programs were a major force in the expansion of the Nation's biomedical research capability over the past several decades. It is also quite clear, however, that these same NIH programs have markedly declined during the past decade due to fiscal constraints. The decline in the number of young investigators being trained in diabetes-related disciplines is a reflection of this broader trend.

A second set of problems relates to the extraordinary explosion of new knowledge and techniques in fields such as molecular biology, molecular virology, molecular genetics, immunology, protein chemistry, receptor signaling, growth control mechanisms, and gene engineering. Whereas the potential application of these basic science advances gives promise for fundamental advances in understanding the basic mechanisms responsible for diabetes and its complications, in developing better treatment, and indeed the possibility for preventing and curing diabetes and its complications, these advances also have created an unprecedented gap between the potential and the capabilities of many investigators currently involved in diabetes research and in the training of the next generation of diabetes researchers. Establishing the Diabetes Interdisciplinary Research Programs proposed by this long-range plan would address and respond to some of these problems by providing an appropriate training environment; however, funds for the training of these investigators will still need to be provided via NIH manpower programs.

Expenditures for diabetes-related manpower programs supported by the NIDDK have decreased from approximately $7.4 million to $6.1 million between fiscal year 1980 and fiscal year 1986. This decline is even greater when these expenditures are adjusted for inflation. As a result, the total number of individuals that could be supported has declined by 33 percent, from 312 to 214, during the same period. . . .

Diabetes Research Centers

The Diabetes Research Centers Program consists of two types of centers. The program was initiated in 1973–74 with the establishment of the DERC's. In 1975, the National Diabetes Commission (the predecessor of the NDAB) concluded that there was a significant and deleterious gap between the body of knowledge resulting from diabetes research and the quality of diabetes care generally available in the United States. To help close this gap, the Commission endorsed the creation of the DRTC's. DRTC's were subsequently established in 1977 as a result of legislative mandate (P.L. 93–354). Currently, there are 12 diabetes centers—6 DERC's and 6 DRTC's. The primary goal of both types of centers is the augmentation of ongoing basic and clinical biomedical research through the establishment of shared core resources, modest research enrichment programs, and the development of new research initiatives through support of pilot and feasibility projects. Each center was established after exhaustive peer review.

Each center is located at a research institution with an outstanding history of excellence in biomedical research and substantial ongoing high-quality research being conducted by NIH-funded investigators. These investigators come together because of a common interest in diabetes, but they come from many disciplines, programs, and departments. The shared core resources bring the investigators together in a milieu that provides for interactive, cooperative, and collaborative research. Many of the research advances discussed earlier in this long-range plan have come from funded investigators at DERC's and DRTC's. . . .

The Training Component of the Diabetes Research and Training Centers

In addition to their primary mission of providing support for diabetes research discussed above, DRTC's were initiated to develop new, innovative state-of-the-art training programs for health care professionals responsible for the care, management, and treatment of patients with diabetes. These primary health care professionals cover a broad spectrum of professions (physicians, nurses, dietitians, pharmacists, psychologists, podiatrists, social workers, etc.) in diverse stages of career development (students, interns, house staff, practicing professionals, specialists, etc.). The guidelines for the DRTC's were designed to encourage innovation and flexibility in developing programs to fill the gap between present practice and state-of-the-art approaches. In this regard, DRTC's have made major contributions in developing and validating programs and materials for primary health care professionals involved with persons with diabetes. . . .

Many opportunities now exist for DRTC's to expand their collaborative efforts with health professional societies and voluntary health agencies and with the new Diabetes Translation Center at the CDC. These increased collaborations should further the ability of the DRTC's to meet their original goal of improving the knowledge, attitudes, and skills of health care practitioners who deal with patients with diabetes mellitus. . . .

General Clinical Research Centers

The General Clinical Research Centers Program, funded by the DRR, supports 78 noncategorical clinical research facilities at academic medical institutions. GCRC's provide an ideal (and frequently the only) environment for controlled clinical investigation because they are discrete units with their own beds, nurses, dietitians, other support staff members, specialized laboratories, and a computer-based data management and analysis system. Research protocols related to a variety of diseases compete on the basis of scientific merit for the use of the facilities. It is noteworthy that 328 investigators supported by $52.8 million in NIH grants conducted 522 diabetes-related projects in these centers in fiscal year 1986. This degree of support and involvement attests to the high quality and importance of the GCRC's, not only to diabetes but to the entire spectrum of health problems.

The vast majority of all clinical investigation related to diabetes, including activities of the DRTC's, DERC's, the Diabetes Control and Complications Trial, and other diabetes research programs described earlier, is conducted in these facilities. Many of the major research advances directly applicable to the management of diabetes and its complications, including evaluation of insulin-delivery devices for regulation of blood glucose, elucidation of the role of newly discovered hormones in maintaining normal metabolism in humans, and the definition of the cause of insulin resistance in noninsulin-dependent diabetes, are the result of research conducted in GCRC's. Over the past decade, the budget for this important program has not kept pace with inflation. Despite small annual increases, the program has experienced a loss of six centers over the past 10 years and a decrease in the level of support, expressed in constant dollars, for each center. Unfortunately, because of the noncategorical nature of the program, no one specific disease constituency has felt the need to focus attention on this resource. However, it should be clearly recognized that a continued decline of this successful resource program will have a serious impact upon diabetes research progress. . . .

Diabetes in Pregnancy Research Centers

Considerable progress has been achieved in the field of diabetes and pregnancy in the last decade. Maternal mortality is now similar both for women with diabetes and for women in the general population, and fetal mortality has fallen significantly in the best centers devoted to care of women whose pregnancies are complicated by diabetes. However, higher incidences of congenital anomalies, macrosomia, late intrauterine death, and respiratory distress syndrome remain a significant problem in pregnant women with diabetes.

The NICHD supports a broad range of research related to the effects of diabetes on maternal and child health, including three multidisciplinary centers that focus on pregnancy in women with diabetes. These centers are providing important information on the prevention of perinatal morbidity and mortality related to diabetes.

Metabolic studies are providing insight into carbohydrate and protein metabolism of the newborn. Centers have examined the effects of the abnormal intrauterine environment in maternal diabetes, the effects of intrauterine exposure to insulin, and glucose production by newborn infants. Animal studies have shown that exposure to insulin accelerates fetal growth.

An important ongoing research project in one of the pregnancy centers is the development of an implantable open-loop insulin infusion system for treatment of IDDM. The system delivers insulin into the peritoneum in a preprogrammed fashion, which the patient can adjust according to periodic blood glucose measurement and anticipated caloric intake. The system is expected to facilitate strict metabolic control, which is especially important during pregnancy to reduce birth defects and excess infant mortality.

In some women, pregnancy can cause abnormalities of carbohydrate metabolism, known as gestational diabetes mellitus (GDM). A followup of 158 patients with GDM indicated that women who needed insulin in addition to their diet regimen were generally older than age 25 and delivered infants with a higher birth weight than women who could be controlled by diet alone. Obese patients with GDM had an even higher risk for neonatal macrosomia. . . .

Intramural Program

Major diabetes research efforts are under way within the intramural research program of the NIDDK and other NIH Institutes. Numerous research projects, including various combinations of laboratory, clinical, epidemiologic, and biometric investigations, are conducted by scientists in facilities in Bethesda, Maryland, and by the NIDDK in Phoenix, Arizona. Effective research strategies are ensured through close collaboration among scientists within the NIH and other Government agencies and at institutions throughout the United States and abroad. . . .

National Diabetes Data Group

The National Diabetes Data Group (NDDG) is an NIDDK advisory group consisting of Federal, academic, and lay representatives with interest and expertise in the epidemiologic and public health aspects of diabetes. In its 9-year history, the NDDG has spearheaded the effort to define, coordinate, and develop the statistical, epidemiologic, and public health aspects of diabetes, particularly in the research arena. The NDDG has sponsored national expert committees to standardize methodologies for classification and diagnosis of diabetes to ensure that data emanating from different research centers have a comparable basis. At the same time, these recommendations have provided the medical community with an internationally recognized set of standards by which to diagnose and classify patients. Other NDDG expert committees have addressed research methods to determine the scope and impact of diabetes and its complications. Areas of research that emerged as particularly important or problematic have received special attention. . . .

Diabetes Control and Complications Trial

. . . The Diabetes Control and Complications Trial (DCCT) is a large-scale long-term multicenter clinical trial that was designed to assess the effects of two forms of treatment for IDDM on the development and progression of the early vascular complications of IDDM. The effects of standard or conventional therapy for IDDM, consisting of one or two daily injections of mixed insulins with quarterly visits to a clinic, will be compared with those effects obtained by using a number of the newer technologies available for treating IDDM. These technologies include intensive self blood glucose monitoring, external insulin infusion pumps, and other injection devices, coupled with monthly visits to a clinic and frequent telephone contact. . . . [for a report on the results of the DCCT see Chapter 34].

Other Clinical Trials

On occasion, further progress in disease-related questions can be made only by the use of a clinical trial or multicenter study. This is the case when advances from basic science experimentation require validation by clinical application or when specific features of a disease cannot be duplicated in animal models. A number of questions in clinical diabetes have now progressed to this point. Representative examples include the primary prevention of IDDM using immunosuppression, the evaluation of various intervention strategies in gestational diabetes mellitus, the role of non-pharmacological therapies such as exercise in NIDDM, the use of low-protein diets in end-stage renal disease associated with diabetes, and studies of the effects of new pharmacological agents. Although clinical trials constitute a very expensive form of scientific enterprise, in appropriate circumstances, they can yield results that are unattainable by any other approach, and they may definitively prove the hypotheses of prior laboratory experimentation.

Clinical trials that examine the management of eye complications experienced by patients with diabetes and the complications of pregnancy are being conducted by the NEI and NICHD, respectively. The outcome of these trials will have a major impact on the prevention of diabetes-related vision loss and on the reduction of birth defects in infants of mothers with diabetes. . . .

Diabetes Mellitus Interagency Coordinating Committee

The Diabetes Mellitus Interagency Coordinating Committee (DMICC) initially was authorized by the National Diabetes Research and Education Act of 1974 (P.L. 93–3 54) and was reauthorized in subsequent legislation. In summary, the Committee's charges are as follows:

- To coordinate the research activities of the NIH that relate to diabetes mellitus and its complications.

- To coordinate those activities of all Federal programs that are related to diabetes mellitus and its complications.
- To provide a forum for communication and exchange of information necessary to coordinate related Federal activities.
- To prepare a report summarizing the Committee's activities for each fiscal year. . . .

National Diabetes Advisory Board

The major role of the NDAB over the next 5 years will be to advise Congress and the Secretary of the Department of Health and Human Services on diabetes issues while overseeing implementation of this plan. As in the past, the NDAB also will sponsor special conferences, identify areas that require special initiatives, report annually on the progress made in research and translation, and identify future opportunities and budgetary needs. . . .

Chapter 50

Summary of Accomplishments and Future Directions in Diabetes Research

Etiology of Insulin-Dependent Diabetes Mellitus

Accomplishments

The past 10 years have witnessed a remarkable increase in knowledge about the roles of genetic and autoimmune factors in the etiology of IDDM. In the mid-1970's, it was definitely demonstrated that IDDM (and not NIDDM) mainly affects individuals who have inherited certain factors belonging to the group of tissue antigens known as the HLA system. The presence of HLA factors or cells in the body's tissues is determined genetically by a complex of genes called the major histocompatibility complex (MHC) located on chromosome 6. This finding proved beyond a doubt that IDDM and NIDDM were separate entities that involved completely different genetic and pathogenic mechanisms. The biological function of MHC, as defined in very basic animal studies, led to the increasing focus on IDDM as a disease involving autoimmune processes.

There may be two different HLA factors (one termed DR3 and the other DR4), each of which predisposes to the development of IDDM by a separate, but apparently additive, mechanism. Ninety percent of patients with IDDM possess HLA-DR3 or DR4 (or both), compared with only about 25 percent of the general population. These observations clearly show HLA factors to be major genetic markers, but their presence does not serve to identify the specific population susceptible to the development of IDDM. While indi-

---

Excerpts from: *The National Long-Range Plan to Combat Diabetes.* NIH Pub. No. 88-1587.

viduals who have inherited DR3 or DR4 have a 3 percent risk of developing IDDM, an increased risk compared with the general population, the presence of these genetic markers does not permit selection of individuals for potential interventions. Family studies of HLA-haplotype (group of genes contributed by either parent) sharing among affected sib pairs have directly ruled out a dominant model of genetic susceptibility; the recessive model also seems unlikely on indirect grounds.

The accumulated weight of evidence gathered in the past 10 years strongly indicates that IDDM is an autoimmune disease. The observation that only approximately 30 percent of genetically identical twins both develop diabetes emphasizes the critical role of factors in the environment that trigger the active destruction of pancreatic beta cells in susceptible individuals. Moreover, it appears that the portion of the immune response concerned with the way foreign substances are recognized and processed may be most involved in this process.

Autoantibodies directed against pancreatic islet cells have been demonstrated in patients with newly diagnosed IDDM. Islet cell autoantibodies also may be found in otherwise healthy siblings of HLA-identical probands affected with diabetes; these are the siblings who appear to go on to develop IDDM. In addition, insulin autoantibodies have been detected in about one-third of the relatives of patients with IDDM.

In the pancreas of newly diagnosed patients with IDDM, investigators have demonstrated a process characterized by the presence of damaged beta cells surrounded by cell types involved in the physiologic immune response. This "insulitis" also was observed when a portion of pancreas from a nondiabetic individual was transplanted to his genetically identical but diabetic twin. The typical transplant rejection problem did not occur, but the islets of the transplanted pancreas appeared to be specifically attacked by the immune system of the host with diabetes. "Insulitis" was present on biopsy, islet cell antibodies appeared in the serum of the transplant recipient, and progressive loss of insulin-producing function was documented.

An animal model for IDDM has become available. The BB/Wor rat develops a spontaneous diabetic syndrome that resembles human IDDM and can be used for experiments that are not possible with human patients. For example, several laboratories have investigated the effect of therapy to suppress the immune system on the development of diabetes in the rat. Recent studies indicate that cyclosporin A can be administered intermittently and still be effective in preventing the onset of diabetes. This is important because continual cyclosporin A therapy can cause kidney damage, yet discontinuance of cyclosporin A leads to the recurrence of diabetes. Other studies showed that antidiabetic actions of cyclosporin A include preventing the release from the killer white cells of an agent that is toxic to beta cells and blocking the production of killer white cells that destroy the islet cells.

In another study, daily injections of insulin were made to BB/Wor rats that would normally go on to develop diabetes. Instead, when insulin therapy was discontinued, very few of the animals went on to develop diabetes. These studies suggest that insulin therapy of diabetes-prone animals may interrupt the activation of immune attack of beta cells or may help to render beta cells resistant to immune injury.

Future Research Directions

Despite advances in knowledge, a breakthrough has not yet occurred with regard to defining the etiology of IDDM. The challenges in this field for the next 10 years are formidable. Advances in basic research are vital in all areas of diabetes, but they are particularly important in any discussion of the genetics and etiology of IDDM because what appears today as basic research in immunology, genetics, virology, and other related fields may turn out to have direct implications for IDDM research. Identification of the specific genes that are responsible for the genetic susceptibility to IDDM will permit the use of more precise genetic markers to define susceptible populations. Definition of the actual gene products is essential to the investigation of the mechanism by which susceptibility is conferred. Knowledge of the nongenetic (environmental) factor or factors responsible for triggering beta cell destruction in susceptible individuals is vital to the development of vaccines for protection of susceptible individuals if a virus, for example, is involved. It is now recognized from both metabolic and immunologic data that the IDDM disease process usually begins years before the detection of the clinical disease and that insulin secretory capacity is impaired before hyperglycemia occurs. Immunologic markers for IDDM, such as islet cell antibodies and insulin antibodies, must be further evaluated and related to abnormal beta cell function. It may be that preclinical IDDM is not always a steady progressive process, but may be intermittent and probably cumulative. If this progression can be identified, it may be possible to identify those individuals at risk for developing clinical IDDM and to halt the onset of clinical disease. The precise mechanism by which the host's immune system participates in the process of beta cell destruction must be defined, including how the system is activated, which phases of the immune response are involved, and how the entire sequence is maintained in the activated state. These findings will be essential in the search for immunosuppressible agents that will be more specifically targeted and have fewer side effects than cyclosporin A.

Etiology of Noninsulin-Dependent Diabetes Mellitus

Accomplishments

Current evidence indicates that three factors contribute to the pathogenesis of noninsulin-dependent diabetes: genetic predisposition, insulin resistance, and impaired beta cell function. Studies of identical twins have shown that development of NIDDM is greatly influenced by heredity. In addition, genetic research is continuing to show evidence of an association between an increased risk of developing NIDDM when changes are present in the DNA flanking the insulin gene or other genes.

A variety of causes of insulin resistance have been documented in patients, including decreases in the binding of insulin to receptors located on the surface of target cells, a reduction in the ability of insulin to stimulate glucose transport and glucose utilization by isolated fat cells, and secretion of an abnormal insulin molecule. The events that occur after insulin binds to its receptors have been well documented, but at present, the mechanisms of these events are poorly understood. Abnormalities in various counter-regulatory hormones also may play a role. During the past decade, techniques have been developed to quantify the degree of insulin resistance separately in the liver and peripheral tissues and to separate receptor and postreceptor mechanisms.

Clinical research studies have shown that lowering blood glucose levels in patients with NIDDM can restore both insulin secretion and action toward normal. Weight loss, physical training, and refinement in diet management all have been found to contribute to the control of hyperglycemia of NIDDM. Pharmacologic research has provided evidence that sulfonylurea compounds enhance insulin action in the liver and peripheral tissues at several steps; thus, the ability of these drugs to lower plasma glucose may not be due totally to their ability to stimulate insulin secretion.

Future Research Directions

The precise nature of the multiple genetic-environmental interactions in the development of NIDDM remains to be determined. A better understanding of the normal regulation of carbohydrate, lipid, and protein metabolism might clarify the processes that underlie NIDDM. An intensive search should be initiated for genetic and physiologic markers that may facilitate identifying the prediabetic state and determining the mode of inheritance of each form of NIDDM. The genetic and physiologic significance of the restriction enzyme polymorphism in the DNA region flanking the insulin gene must be clarified, and a search must be conducted for other such polymorphisms in other genes that may play a role in diabetes.

Further information is needed on the natural history and predictive value of impaired glucose tolerance. Efforts also should be made to determine whether progression from impaired glucose tolerance to NIDDM can be prevented by weight control, drugs, dietary manipulations, or increases in physical activity or training. Understanding is needed of the mechanisms of the various combinations of impaired insulin action and insulin secretion.

Increased knowledge of insulin action at the cellular level is a prerequisite for defining the mechanism of insulin resistance in NIDDM. Prospective studies, both in selected populations and in families, must be conducted in an effort to define the relationship between the defect in insulin secretion and action in the pathogenesis of NIDDM.

In the area of therapy for NIDDM, more effective approaches to weight loss in obese patients who have NIDDM must be devised. Long-term studies of the effects of variations in the kind and amount of dietary carbohydrate and fiber on both lipid and carbohydrate metabolism must be performed. Because there is a close correlation between maximal aerobic capacity and the ability to dispose of dietary carbohydrate, attention should be given to improved physical training in NIDDM patients. There is also a need for elucidating further the effect at the cellular level of insulin itself, sulfonylureas, and other orally effective agents, particularly on post-binding steps in insulin action. Attempts should be made to characterize people who do and do not respond to sulfonylureas, either acutely or after several months of therapy, to better understand the reasons for therapeutic failures. In addition, the potential synergistic effect of those compounds in combination with other possible hypoglycemic agents should be explored. New pharmacologic approaches to improve insulin action and secretion are needed. The effects of intensive insulin therapy on subjects with NIDDM must be clarified.

Epidemiology

Accomplishments

Epidemiology integrates basic and clinical sciences at the population level, and it is useful for determining risk, identifying etiologic associations in diverse populations, testing new therapies, and evaluating health services programs. Accomplishments in the epidemiology of diabetes mellitus include clearer definitions of the risk of both IDDM and NIDDM; the characterization of the rates of complications of diabetes mellitus; the identification of high-risk ethnic groups for NIDDM internationally; and a better understanding of the role of obesity, physical inactivity, and racial admixture as risk factors for NIDDM. Glucose levels have been shown to have clear-cut bimodality in several populations, which, when coupled with other research on microvascular complications, have added to the evidence for the role of elevated blood sugar as a major risk factor.

Population-based registries of IDDM have been established in several countries, and international collaboration has been initiated. A spectrum of populations from low risk (0.5/100,000 a year) to high risk (30/100,000 a year) for IDDM has been identified, and studies are under way to determine the role genetic differences may play in the varying risks.

In the past 10 years, an explosion of quantitative data about diabetes incidence (number of new cases), prevalence (total number of existing cases of diabetes), risk factors, complications, and characteristics resulted in the largest compendium of epidemiologic data on diabetes ever published, *Diabetes in America* compiled by the National Diabetes Data Group. The National Diabetes Data Group and the World Health Organization prepared recommendations for the standardization of methods and diagnostic criteria for diabetes as a result of epidemiologic studies of several populations.

Future Research Directions

Research opportunities in the epidemiology of diabetes are vast. They interact with most fields of biomedical research aimed at identifying the etiology of diabetes and its complications, its prevention, and translation of research into practice.

Major new initiatives of the NDAB, including the Diabetes Interdisciplinary Research Programs, Biologic Resource Bank for Studies on Diabetes, Information and Data Systems for Diabetes Research, and the Diabetes Translation Center, all provide opportunities for the involvement of epidemiologists. Incorporation of the latest biologic markers into field studies of informative populations will be hastened by developing close working relations between laboratory and field researchers. Major population-based studies of both IDDM and NIDDM are collecting biologic samples that, under appropriate circumstances, should be shared with other investigators.

Genetic determinants that predispose to NIDDM, obesity, and hypertension appear to differ between racial and ethnic groups. Further studies in these populations are necessary to better understand the observed patterns. Newer methods to characterize insulin secretion and insulin sensitivity must be made usable for field studies so that large representative samples can be studied to allow the improved characterization of alterations in carbohydrate and lipid metabolism that occur with aging and with NIDDM.

Prospective studies of individuals with impaired glucose tolerance, a high-risk group for NIDDM, are crucial. These studies should include potential genetic markers as well as markers of insulin secretion and sensitivity and measures of changes in physical activity, diet, and weight.

The potential for primary prevention of NIDDM through controlled interventions in high-risk subjects based on overweight, positive family history, impaired glucose tolerance, minimal physical activity, and membership in an ethnic group with genetic predisposition should be seriously explored. Similarly, the potential for reversing hyperglycemia before the onset of micro- or macrovascular complications by combinations of pharmacologic and nonpharmacologic interventions must be pursued. Both the efficacy, or knowledge that a given intervention works in highly selected subjects, and the efficiency, which is the impact of an intervention in the community of patients with diabetes, must be established with carefully controlled studies.

The role of environmental factors in populations is the major challenge for epidemiologists interested in IDDM etiology. Major collaborative initiatives are needed to study potential agents in siblings of persons with IDDM who possess identical HLA factors. Further understanding of the natural history of IDDM in individuals older than 20 years of age also is needed. The proportion of older onset persons who have markers for IDDM (islet cell antibodies, anti-insulin antibodies) is largely unknown. Once the entire age-specific onset patterns are known, a better understanding of the time of exposure to environmental agents can be determined. These studies could be done using prospective investigations of IDDM siblings as well as in large health maintenance organizations where repeated screenings can occur. The primary prevention of IDDM through immunotherapy of islet cell antibody positive siblings and the reversal of incident IDDM via immunosuppression require epidemiologic input. The long-term prognosis from these interventions is currently unknown, so detailed followup of these cohorts is required across centers, each with small numbers of treated subjects. When benefit and toxicity can be determined, collaborative clinical trials must be conducted.

International registry activities in IDDM must be strengthened to allow for accurate comparative studies among informative populations. These registries can define the absolute risk and risk factors for acute and chronic complications and serve as the location for case-control studies in representative subjects for host and environmental factors. With more populations studied, those populations with differing risks for complications can be compared to identify locations where risk factor studies are needed and where new etiologic factors may be identified.

Standardization of clinical and laboratory definitions and methods used with diabetes complications is needed. Population-based information must be augmented on the incidence and risk factors for several complications, including autonomic and peripheral neuropathy, nephropathy, and infections. Studies of known risk factors (hypertension, lipid patterns, smoking) for macrovascular complications in varying populations is critical to an understanding of different environmental and genetic components of risk among persons with diabetes.

Prevention of complications in patients through interventions aimed at risk factors other than blood sugar requires a major investigation. The NHLBI in conjunction with the NIDDK should be encouraged to begin a major cardiovascular-diabetes initiative.

Studies aimed at determining the role that psychosocial, behavioral, and socioeconomic factors play in self-care and patient adherence need to be carried out using standardized measures of clinical course and acute and chronic complications.

Population-based studies of gestational diabetes are needed, emphasizing more efficient screening protocols and study of prognosis of both mother and infant. Intervention studies aimed at elucidating the proper role of diet and exercise in gestational diabetes are needed.

A mechanism must be established to evaluate new therapeutic techniques rapidly for persons with diabetes. Experience with the World Health Organization trial of insulin infusion pumps indicates that drug interventions and new technologies need clinical trials before widespread marketing is undertaken. Because other more sophisticated artificial insulin delivery systems are nearing human use, planning for clinical trials must be initiated.

Nutrition, Obesity, and Exercise

Accomplishments

Of the various environmental factors that affect glucose regulation in NIDDM, dietary modification, the treatment of obesity, and increased physical activity are the most important. With proper attention to these three areas, patients with NIDDM often can be managed successfully without the use of pharmacologic agents.

Most investigators now favor providing at least 50 percent of calories from carbohydrates in calorie-restricted diets. This prevents the development of ketosis and metabolic acidosis, allows preservation of muscle glycogen stores, and maintains the capacity for strenuous physical exercise. In addition, including carbohydrates in very low-calorie diets may have a protein-sparing effect with better preservation of nutritionally sensitive serum protein markers such as transferrin, thyroxin-binding prealbumin, and retinol-binding protein.

Although not yet proved, recent evidence suggests that high protein intakes may, over a long period, be injurious to renal function and may be contraindicated in persons with diabetes who are at increased risk for renal failure. The most prudent dietary recommendation would appear, therefore, to be to maintain protein intake at approximately 12 to 15 percent of total calories rather than the 20 percent formerly recommended in diets for people with diabetes.

During recent years, evidence has accumulated to support increasing the carbohydrate content of the diet while, at the same time, decreasing the fat content, particularly the amount of saturated fats. Current recommendations suggest that carbohydrates should make up 50 to 60 percent of total calories and that total intake of fats should be limited to 30 percent of calories. Because persons with diabetes are particularly susceptible to the development of macrovascular disease, the intake of saturated fats should be kept at less than 10 percent of calories and cholesterol intake restricted to 300 mg a day or less.

Increasing the carbohydrate content of the diet results in improved tissue sensitivity and responsiveness to insulin and may help to counteract the insulin resistance usually present in patients with NIDDM. On the other hand, some individuals may develop increased serum triglyceride concentrations on high carbohydrate diets, and this may pose an increased risk for the development of atherosclerosis in these patients. In this situation, carbohydrate intakes of 40 to 50 percent of calories may be more appropriate. Thus, it is important to individualize the dietary recommendation, with overall goals being to achieve the best possible regulation of blood glucose and to prevent both the micro- and macrovascular complications of the disease.

It is now clear that several factors influence the rate and magnitude of the rise in blood glucose that occurs following the ingestion of a carbohydrate-containing meal. A new concept, the "glycemic index," has been used by some researchers to describe the blood glucose response produced by ingestion of a specific food, expressed as a percentage of the response produced by an equivalent amount of glucose. Striking differences depending on the source and form of the carbohydrate have been found in the plasma glucose and insulin responses to orally administered simple and complex carbohydrates. Numerous studies have been conducted to determine the effects of the physical form of food, the effects of cooking, and the effects of combining carbohydrates with other nutrients or with fiber. At the present time, the general recommendation is to emphasize the use of complex carbohydrates and to restrict the use of sucrose to approximately 5 percent of calories.

Fructose, which is sweeter than sucrose and does not require insulin for its metabolism, has been recommended as a beneficial nutritive sweetener in diabetic diets. Following fructose ingestion, blood glucose and insulin responses are small, and fructose is readily taken up by the liver, where it is metabolized.

A number of benefits of increased dietary fiber have been identified but not conclusively proved for patients with NIDDM. Several studies have shown that high-carbohydrate, high-fiber diets are associated with lower blood glucose rises and lower plasma insulin concentrations in both normal individuals and patients with NIDDM. This is due, in part, to a slowing of carbohydrate digestion and absorption and possibly to other effects that are not yet well understood.

The hormonal and metabolic responses to exercise have now been studied extensively in both normal and diabetic humans and animals. It is now possible to design a rational approach to the use of exercise as a therapeutic tool and also to allow patients with diabetes to exercise safely.

The use of exercise in the treatment of persons with noninsulin-dependent diabetes has received considerable attention during the past several years. In both IDDM and NIDDM, a number of real and potential benefits of regular physical exercise have been identified. In addition to improved fitness and a general sense of well-being, several risk factors for the development of cardiovascular disease are reduced by physical training. These include a lowering of serum triglycerides and low-density lipoprotein cholesterol, increased high-density lipoprotein cholesterol, increase in blood vessels leading to the heart and in work efficiency of the heart, improved lung function, and lower blood pressure. In persons with NIDDM, insulin sensitivity is improved and plasma insulin concentrations are lower following physical training. In addition, exercise may be used as an adjunct to low-calorie diets to induce weight loss. Several studies in both humans and animals have confirmed that physical conditioning increases sensitivity to insulin, although the mechanism by which this occurs is still not well understood.

Despite these apparent benefits of exercise, there are also significant risks and limitations that must be considered. In addition to problems with blood glucose regulation, the capacity for aerobic exercise may be decreased in some persons with diabetes, and complications such as retinopathy, neuropathy, and nephropathy may be relative contraindications for exercise.

Future Research Directions

More knowledge is needed regarding basic nutrient requirements and the optimum composition of the diet for persons with diabetes. There is still controversy regarding the relative amounts of dietary carbohydrate and fat that should be recommended for these diets, particularly as they relate to serum cholesterol and triglyceride levels and the development of atherosclerosis and coronary artery disease. The roles of saturated and unsaturated fats in the diet and of specific fatty acids such as eicosopentanoic acid, found in high concentration in certain fish oils, in the pathogenesis or prevention of atherosclerosis are still poorly understood.

It is now clear that the glycemic response to various foods depends on the type of food, its physical state, and its interaction with other foods. The concept of using a glycemic index to plan diets for people with diabetes needs to be evaluated and validated in clinical trials. The role of dietary fiber in lowering blood glucose rises and lipid levels needs further study. Because not all dietary fiber has the same effect and because the amounts needed to produce significant improvement in blood glucose control are rather large (25 g a day or more), more studies are required to determine the exact usefulness of high fiber diets in the treatment of NIDDM. Further studies also are needed on the roles of fructose and nonnutritive sweeteners in the diabetic diet.

Many questions still remain regarding the role of exercise in the treatment of NIDDM. Good evidence exists to show that regular exercise is associated with increased tissue sensitivity to insulin and that glucose tolerance is improved significantly by weight reduction and physical training. However, the specific role of exercise in the prevention or treatment of NIDDM remains to be determined. Further studies are needed to determine the mechanism by which exercise stimulates glucose uptake and metabolism in skeletal muscle and how exercise and training result in increased insulin sensitivity. Studies also are needed to examine the capacity for exercise in patients with diabetes, particularly the effects of autonomic neuropathy on exercise performance and regulation of glucose metabolism. Potentially deleterious effects of exercise on the development or progression of complications from diabetes must be examined, and better regimens for the management of exercise in insulin-treated people with diabetes must be developed.

Aging, Glucose Intolerance, and Noninsulin-Dependent Diabetes Mellitus

Accomplishments

It has been known for at least 40 years that glucose tolerance declines with age and that NIDDM occurs more commonly as humans get older. However, only during the past few years have we begun to understand why defects in carbohydrate metabolism are associated with aging. Only recently has it become possible to begin speculating on how the deleterious metabolic effects of age can be attenuated and prevented.

Theoretically, glucose intolerance must be caused by defects in insulin secretion or insulin action, or both. Recent studies in rats have shown that glucose-stimulated insulin release per beta cell declines with age, and this loss of insulin secretory function seems to be an inexorable consequence of growing older. Because aging also is associated with an increase in beta cell mass, maximal glucose-induced insulin secretion per pancreas in older rats is not reduced when compared with young animals. These data strongly suggest that rats compensate for the age-associated reduction in insulin secretion per beta cell by making more beta cells, and it is this beta cell hyperplasia that enables older rats to secrete enough insulin to maintain near-normal glucose tolerance.

The ability of insulin to stimulate glucose uptake also declines with age, but the nature of this age-related change is different from the loss of insulin secretory function that occurs with aging. Resistance to insulin-stimulated glucose uptake, both in vivo and in the perfused muscle, is present in older rats. The decline in insulin action that occurs with age seems to be to a large extent secondary to the obesity and physical inactivity that occurs under laboratory conditions as rats grow older. The insulin resistance in the older, nonobese, and physically inactive rat undoubtedly provides a further stress to the beta cell and requires an even greater degree of beta cell hyperplasia than the concomitant loss of insulin secretion per beta cell that occurs with age.

The situation in humans appears to be remarkably similar to that described in the rats. For example, the glucose intolerance seen with aging is not associated with hypoinsulinemia but rather with ambient plasma insulin concentrations that are equal to or greater in absolute terms than those in younger individuals. Furthermore, a great deal of evidence exists to indicate that resistance to insulin-stimulated glucose uptake not only exists in older individuals, but also that it correlates with the presence of glucose intolerance. The impact of age-related environmental variables on carbohydrate metabolism is also readily seen in humans. These metabolic defects can be reduced markedly if individuals remain relatively healthy, nonobese, and physically active.

The fact that NIDDM increases in frequency with age has become more understandable as knowledge of both the pathogenesis of NIDDM and the effects of age and important age-related variables on carbohydrate metabolism has increased. Patients with either impaired glucose tolerance or NIDDM are resistant to the ability of insulin to stimulate glucose uptake. Patients with impaired glucose tolerance apparently do not develop diabetes as long as they can secrete enough insulin to overcome the insulin resistance. When the ability to sustain hyperinsulinemia begins to decline, the development of frank NIDDM occurs. Chronic disease, obesity, and physical inactivity exaggerate the magnitude of insulin resistance in any given individual, requiring an increased insulin secretory response. If the same progressive and inevitable decline in insulin secretion per beta cell seen in rats occurs in humans, it would be even harder for the pancreas to maintain the degree of hyperinsulinemia required to prevent NIDDM from developing. It appears that the degree to which this occurs is to a large extent determined by environmental events that can be regulated. If this point of view is supported by future research results, it is obvious that we have at our disposal effective measures to reduce the incidence of NIDDM in the elderly.

Future Research Directions

More information is needed to define the reasons insulin secretion and insulin action are reduced with age. In the case of the beta cell, understanding is needed of the cellular and molecular events that cause insulin secretion per beta cell to decline inexorably with age. Similarly, it is essential to further quantify the relative impact of age, obesity, and physical inactivity on the insulin resistance seen with aging as well as to learn how these changes come about.

The ability of the organism to maintain stable, normal levels of glucose in the face of increased insulin resistance, whether due to age, genetic factors, or environmental variables such as obesity and physical activity, is a function of the insulin secretory capacity of the pancreas. In this regard, it is essential to learn more about the factors that regulate both beta cell secretory function and beta cell hyperplasia. It is also essential that we learn more about the relationship between the changes in carbohydrate and lipoprotein metabolism that occur with age. Hyperinsulinemia, which is associated with glucose intolerance in older individuals, has been shown to be related to increases in plasma very low-density lipoprotein triglyceride (VLDL-TG) and decreases in high-density lipoprotein (HDL) cholesterol concentrations. VLDL-TG levels tend to rise with age and HDL cholesterol levels to fall, and both of these changes increase the risk of developing atherosclerosis.

More must be learned about how to modify age-related defects of carbohydrate metabolism by environmental manipulation. The effectiveness of weight loss and exercise training programs in improving glucose tolerance and insulin action when initiated after untoward metabolic changes have already taken place must be determined. Behavioral research must assess the proportion of older individuals who can change their behavior enough to demonstrate any benefit.

The critical cut points of plasma glucose levels for the diagnosis of diabetes remain uncertain. The determination of glucose concentrations that clearly indicate the presence of diabetes must be correlated with associated characteristic abnormalities of the diabetic state or of high likelihood of development of these abnormalities on followup. Critical levels may not be the same in young, middle-aged, and old adults. Misdiagnoses also weaken research studies by inaccurate assignment of subjects into diabetic and nondiabetic categories. Because both false positives and false negatives carry the potential for considerable harm to individuals, longitudinal studies in populations are essential. This long-term effort ultimately also will involve controlled therapeutic interventions to determine what level of glucose intolerance at specific ages will benefit from being labeled as diabetic and treated accordingly.

The interrelations of diabetes with other common diseases need to be given further attention, particularly in older persons in whom multiple disorders are often present concomitantly. Also, it is of interest that there may be a disassociation or lack of coexistence of diabetes and Alzheimer's disease.

Insulin Synthesis and Secretion

Accomplishments

The beta cell, which produces and secretes insulin, is of primary importance in regulating total body glucose metabolism. It is clear that derangements in both the amount and rate of insulin synthesis or secretion cause profound changes in glucose homeostasis. In turn, beta cell function is closely regulated by most nutrient, hormonal, and neural changes. Therefore, this cell is highly sensitive and responsive to global and rapid changes in total body activity.

Beta cell function is central to all forms of diabetes. In NIDDM, impaired beta cell function is a major factor, if not a primary defect. The influences on residual beta cell function by obesity, diet, inter-islet and circulating hormones and neurohormones, gut factors, brain peptides, etc., are highly relevant to the intensity of the disease. In IDDM, progressive destruction of the beta cell occurs. Impaired insulin secretion is detected in the prediabetic phase when circulating islet cell antibodies appear, well before the onset of detectable clinical diabetes. Antibodies, autoimmunity, viral attack, and possibly chemicals in the environment may be involved in both early and progressive damage to the membranes, organelles, and metabolism of the beta cell, resulting in impaired synthesis, storage, and secretion of insulin.

General Regulation. Use of insulin clearance rates and measurement of levels of c-peptide (a peptide secreted by the pancreas in equal amounts to insulin) in blood and urine are permitting a better evaluation of beta cell function in normal people and in people with diabetes. Research has shown that time-related (kinetic) changes in insulin secretion can vary in diabetic states and can be responsible for modifying insulin availability and function in target tissues. Hyperglycemia per se has been found to cause impaired insulin secretion in diabetes. This glucose-induced desensitization of the beta cell can be partially improved by reduction of glucose levels with insulin, sulfonylureas, or diet. Thus, some of the impaired insulin release associated with diabetes may be partially reversible.

Synthesis. The insulin gene has been isolated and its structure has been determined in a variety of species, including humans. Human insulin is now produced commercially by genetic engineering, providing an unlimited supply of the hormone. The same techniques can be applied for the synthesis of unique insulins with possibly advantageous biologic stability or activity.

Although rare, forms of diabetes caused by insulin gene mutations have been discovered that result in the secretion of inactive insulin or, depending on the site of mutation, poorly active proinsulin, which cannot be converted properly. Synthesis of insulin precursors coded by insulin genetic DNA has been shown to be highly regulable; for example, glucose can increase the production of proinsulin by increasing m-RNA synthesis (transcription) or stabilization and by increasing effectiveness of existing m-RNA (translation).

Certain DNA sequences near the insulin gene have been discovered that enhance expression of the gene in the beta or other cells. Regulation of these enhancing segments may be able to provide an important control mechanism for insulin synthesis.

A polymorphic (variable) region of the 5' flanking section of the human insulin gene has been characterized and is being analyzed in people with diabetes as a possible genetic marker for this and other diseases. The patterns of these different forms of DNA vary among ethnic groups and are often clustered within families that have a high rate of diabetes. The insulin gene has been transferred successfully into cells that normally do not produce insulin, with the resultant production of insulin. Corollary studies have resulted in the chemical synthesis of modified DNA, which contains directing portions of the insulin gene; on injection into ova, this modified DNA has resulted in animals with modified beta cell function (beta cell tumors). Thus, introduction of insulin genes into cells and mechanisms for directing genes to the beta cell itself are now possible and could form the basis for a future therapeutic approach.

Molecular biology techniques are being used to produce c-DNA libraries. A DNA library or gene library is a collection of DNA fragments that theoretically contain at least one copy of each gene of the organism from which the DNA was obtained. These libraries can provide probes and other genetic tools to establish the identity and significance of proteins involved in maintenance of beta cell integrity against immune or chemical attack or those involved in regulation of synthesis, transport, and storage of insulin.

Processing and Secretion. Understanding of the basic mechanisms by which glucose, amino acids, and lipids regulate insulin processing and secretion in the beta cell has expanded greatly. Several beta cell tumor cell lines have been developed that provide large amounts of easily studied tissue. Pure beta cells have been isolated, thereby permitting evaluation of beta cell function divorced from influences of adjacent cells in the islets. Results show that the beta cell is dependent not only on normal nutrient agents that stimulate secretion but also is controlled by other hormones and neurotransmitters.

Evidence indicates existence of "precursor" or "committed" cells that are capable of developing into mature beta cells. Maturation of these cells is regulable and may be increased by glucose and possibly by other metabolic substrates and general growth factors. Of great importance is the identification of the growth factor requirements and growth factor receptors on the beta cell itself. Thus, a potentially rich source of new beta cells may be developed in people with diabetes who have reduced beta cell number and mass.

The pancreatic islet now is recognized as a complex organ composed of at least four hormone-secreting cell types (insulin, glucagon, somatostatin, and pancreatic polypeptide), nerve endings that produce neurohormones, and central nervous system peptides. Insulin secretion from the beta cell is, in part, regulated by the paracrine (local) interactions of these islet products. The anatomical relationships and vasculature of the islet cell types now have been elucidated and semiquantitated.

The mechanisms for transport and processing of insulin and insulin precursors through the various organelles of the beta cell have been clarified. Results indicate that (1) conversion of insulin from its precursor, proinsulin, can be regulated by glucose and energy availability and can result in major changes in production of processed insulin; (2) sorting of proinsulin/insulin for routing to secretory granules may involve special receptors; (3) insulin may be stored in secretory granules that permit newly synthesized insulin to be released in preference to older storage forms, a process regulated by fuel substrates (glucose, amino acids); (4) the final steps in secretion can require specific granular receptors that may be involved in the sequence of granular fusion (provision of insulin to the secretory system) and granule lysis (insulin release); and (5) intracellular autodigestion (degradation) of insulin is normally a slow process but may become a significant factor if insulin storage is abnormal. The primary signals by which fuels cause insulin secretion have been found to depend on their metabolic products or changes induced by their metabolism.

A variety of cellular mechanisms have been implicated in the coupling of secretagogues and insulin release. Phospholipids are found in all cell membranes. Many agents acting on beta cells cause splitting of these phospholipids and formation of complicated metabolic intermediates (e.g., cyclooxygenase, epoxide, and leukotriene pathways), which cause profound inhibition or stimulation of the insulin-release process. In addition, ion uptake and distribution, phosphate potential, redox potential, organelle pH, and c-AMP have been described as modulating factors. Calcium entry and distribution in different organelle storage compartments play a prime role. The action of calcium is highly integrated and cross regulated with calmodulin, c-AMP, and c-kinase systems. These three systems, in turn, have been shown to activate a class of enzymes, the protein kinases. Activated protein kinases cause phosphorylation of several beta cell proteins, including some in the cytoskeletal structure (microtubules, microfilaments) and in the storage granules. Modifying these proteins appears to regulate the final steps in secretion (mobilization of granules and fusion with the surface membranes).

The storage and secretion forms of insulin have been partially elucidated. In most species, insulin is stored as a complex with zinc. During secretion, the zinc insulin complex is dissociated almost instantly; most probably, insulin reverts to, and circulates in, its monomeric form.

Future Research Directions

General Regulation. The growth in our understanding of beta cell function at both the molecular and biological levels provides a basis for major advances in our comprehension of beta cell function during the next few years. There is a continuing need for new in vivo methods to assess accurately islet cell function and control in subjects both with and without diabetes. Approaches may include (1) developing mathematical models to translate changes in glucose, insulin, and c-peptide into functional estimates of insulin secretory capacity and (2) designing better test challenge procedures (e.g., utilizing controlled and timed infusions, clamping of variables such as glucose or other circulating nutrients). It is also critical that relatively simple standardized methods be developed that are applicable to large populations with various ethnic, cultural, and social backgrounds.

The kinetics of insulin release, including phasic secretion, time-dependent potentiation, and oscillatory characteristics, can be used to better understand beta cell function and to develop more informative procedures for assessing insulin secretion.

The biology of beta cells should be intensively studied in terms of the growth factor requirements and growth factor receptors present. The process of glucose-induced desensitization, which contributes to beta cell impairment in diabetes, should be clarified and preventive pharmaceutical interventions developed.

Synthesis. Advances are forthcoming in defining the molecular and cellular mechanisms that underlie the synthesis and secretion of insulin and that may contribute to the pathophysiology of diabetes. These studies will address how the biosynthesis of insulin from the insulin gene is regulated and how proinsulin is processed by the beta cell.

The role and regulation-sensitive sites in the DNA structure, at or around the insulin gene, should be clarified. This can be accomplished by synthesizing mutant DNA's in the laboratory and possibly by studying naturally occurring insulin gene mutations. Techniques for inserting normal or modified insulin genes and associated DNA into beta or other cells to enhance their suitability for transplantation into people with diabetes now can be expanded. The introduction of DNA for insulin into the patient with diabetes, or implantation of other critical beta cell proteins required for processing and secretion, has exciting possibilities for future unique treatment modalities.

As DNA libraries are expanded, standard molecular cloning techniques should be applied to elucidate the structures of synthesis- and secretion-related proteins in the beta cell. Predictably, these will include: (1) receptor molecules on the beta cell membrane for agents and other hormones that influence growth, synthesis, and secretion; (2) antigen proteins, targets for immunologic attack on the beta cell; (3) proteins and enzymes required for regulated secretory events; and (4) proteins required for synthesis and maturation of secretory granules.

Because of their important role in beta cell regulation in diabetes, the genetic, functional, and structural relationships involved in production of other islet peptides (glucagon, somatostatin, and pancreatic polypeptide), central nervous system hormones, gastrointestinal tract peptides, and central nervous system peptides should be expanded.

Processing and Secretion. It is now possible to understand the mechanisms required for the differentiation of the prebeta cells into fully functioning insulin-producing cells. Enhancing this pool of cells and determining how their differentiation into functioning cells can be regulated can be of particular importance in renewal of beta cells in people with diabetes. Enhancing growth and functional maturation of fetal beta cells should be a related goal because large pools of fetal beta cells may become a major source of insulin-producing cells for transplantation. More information is needed about intrabeta cell communication and the relationship of beta cells to nerves and other cell types within the islet.

Methods should be expanded for preparing large quantities of viable islet material and for isolating pure beta and other islet cells. Isolating and purifying beta cell organelles (Golgi apparatus, different forms of granules, plasma membrane, etc.) and quantitating morphometric analysis at the electron microscopic level should be expanded to further our understanding of the mechanisms involved in transport of proinsulin from its site of synthesis through various cellular compartments to the eventual secretory process. Clarification is needed of the mechanism in which the converting enzyme acts to process proinsulin to insulin. Microtechniques should be further developed as an alternate to disruptive cell fractionation procedures to study dynamic compartmentalization of intermediates. Monoclonal antibodies now can be developed against islet membrane proteins to establish the membrane-protein interrelationships that affect insulin synthesis, packaging, and secretion.

Because IDDM is characterized by destruction of beta cells, further studies are required of the biochemical nature of attacks on beta cell integrity induced by chemicals, viruses, and components of the immune system. Agents that stimulate protective mechanisms within the beta cell (e.g., free radical scavengers, DNA repair systems) now can be further developed.

The processes that couple metabolism of sugars, amino acids, fatty acids, and ketones to regulation of insulin synthesis and secretion need to be clarified. In addition to metabolic intermediates of the nutrients that may serve as specific signals, the role of ions (such as calcium, potassium, and zinc), pH, energy, and redox state of the beta cell should be studied further. The metabolism that integrates the three major regulatory pathways affecting protein phosphorylation and subsequent insulin secretion can be further defined. Although stimulation of protein kinases and the subsequent phosphorylation of many beta cell proteins have been established, the importance of specific phosphorylated proteins in beta cell function requires further elaboration.

Tumor-cell lines are now available for studying insulin synthesis and processing at the molecular level; better characterized and more stable lines, particularly of human origin, are required. In addition, genetic animal models of diabetes are needed to establish the aberrations at the molecular level that can precipitate different forms or characteristics of diabetes.

Insulin Action

Accomplishments

In most tissues, insulin is a major hormone promoting the constructive metabolism of sugars, lipids, and amino acids. In target cells, insulin has three major sites of metabolic regulation. It increases the transport of glucose and other substrates across the cell membrane, it activates a number of intracellular enzymes in the cytoplasm and cell organelles, and it regulates the synthesis of RNA and DNA within the nucleus. At present, there is no single comprehensive theory that explains all of the actions of insulin.

Insulin action initially depends on insulin receptors, which are specific molecules on cell surfaces. Sophisticated biochemical, biophysical, molecular biological cloning, and morphologic techniques have permitted scientists to make substantial progress in defining the detailed structure and understanding the function of insulin receptors and the way in which glucose, insulin, and other hormones trigger cell activities via several signaling mechanisms. These molecular biological techniques are being used to elucidate the close relationship of the insulin receptor to other growth factor receptors and oncogenes (genes that produce a substance capable of transforming a normal cell into a malignant one) as well. The insulin receptor is composed of two different glycosylated protein subunits. The alpha subunit contains the insulin binding site, and the beta subunit contains tyrosine kinase, an enzyme that is activated by insulin. The total structure of the receptor subunits and their location across the plasma membrane has been established. The nature of the precursor protein and how it is processed to the active receptor also has been determined.

The insulin receptor shows extensive structural homology to the receptor for insulin-like growth factor I (IGF-I), which may account for some of the known growth-promoting activities of insulin. The gene for the insulin receptor has now been mapped to the short arm of chromosome 19, whereas the insulin gene itself is located on chromosome 11. The insulin receptor gene has been fully delineated.

Insulin has been shown to stimulate insulin receptor autophosphorylation and phosphorylation of other cellular proteins. It is probable that this phosphorylation of cellular proteins is an important mechanism by which insulin causes its many cellular activities. Tyrosine kinase catalyzes protein phosphorylation and is an integral part of the insulin receptor structure. The exact role of tyrosine kinase is still not clear, nor is it known which of the cellular phosphorylated proteins mediate insulin's action. The biological significance of tyrosine kinase has been established recently by selective mutation experiments, which demonstrated that when tyrosine kinase is impaired, insulin action is impaired. Decreased insulin receptor kinase activity has been reported in tissues from animals with diabetes and from patients with insulin resistance and NIDDM; however, this defect may reflect the altered metabolic state of patients rather than a basic genetic lesion.

A decrease in insulin receptor abundance or quality may contribute to insulin resistance in diabetes. In addition, postreceptor defects of the metabolic signals that mediate insulin's action also occur. The nature of these mediators of insulin's action has been partially characterized. Current studies suggest that, after interaction with its receptor on the plasma membrane, insulin stimulates an endogenous and specific phospholipase C. This enzyme then hydrolizes a membrane glycolipid or glycoprotein resulting in the generation of a complex carbohydrate phosphate-containing mediator that also may contain inositol and glucosamine. Insulin also has been found to increase cellular free calcium, possibly, although not necessarily, through its activation of phospholipase C, which is known to mobilize calcium from tissue sources. Elevated calcium, in turn, combines with calmodulin, which results in phosphorylation of cellular proteins and increased biological effects. Insulin also increases calcium binding and inhibits the activity of a calmodulin-sensitive ATPase in the plasma membrane. Some actions of insulin may require the interaction of the insulin receptor with both calcium and calmodulin.

Insulin has been shown to increase glucose transport in fat and muscle by inducing the translocation of glucose transporters to the plasma membrane from a large intracellular transport pool. Stimulation of transport can be caused by metabolic inhibitors that deplete ATP. Thus, some regulation by insulin may be related to this energy dependence of the glucose transport system. The structure of the glucose transporter has been shown to contain areas of activity that suggest either a glucose binding site or a membrane pore structure. The insulin receptor kinase also may regulate glucose transport by phosphorylation or dephosphorylation, thereby activating the glucose transporter protein.

Although a major action of insulin takes place when the hormone interacts with its receptor on the plasma membrane, insulin also may carry out some of its actions in the cell interior. Specific insulin binding sites have been identified in the Golgi apparatus, endoplasmic reticulum, nuclei, and nuclear envelopes. Insulin is now known to control mRNA accumulation in a wide variety of cells in both a positive and negative manner. Insulin also regulates mRNA synthesis (transcription) as well as efflux from isolated nuclei. The interaction of insulin with the nucleus and the resulting regulation of RNA metabolism and DNA synthesis may explain the growth-promoting characteristics of this hormone.

Future Research Directions

It is now possible to distinguish and characterize insulin receptor and postreceptor defects in patients with diabetes. Further studies are now practical for establishing which of the defects contribute to insulin resistance in obesity and NIDDM. At the mechanistic level, the developing data on the systems that mediate insulin's action between initial receptor binding and final biological effects should be expanded.

Alternative Insulin Delivery Systems

Accomplishments

The administration of insulin by subcutaneous injection has serious drawbacks that go beyond inconvenience and discomfort. Insulin absorption from the subcutaneous space varies greatly from day to day, depending on the depth of injection, tissue vascularity, local temperatures, subsequent exercise of the limb used as the site of injection, and other factors. Furthermore, subcutaneous insulin absorption is too slow to duplicate the normal rapid-phase release of insulin from the pancreas, and insulin is released into the peripheral circulation instead of the normal route into the portal vein. Finally, because absorption is insensitive to changes in blood glucose or other islet-active agents, it rarely achieves physiologic insulin/glucose dynamics. Multiple injections of insulin each day have provided improved control but are subject to the same limitations. Because it is likely that abnormal homeostasis contributes to diabetic complications, the continued development of systems that can deliver insulin more physiologically is of major importance.

Various approaches have been developed or suggested to improve methods of insulin delivery. External insulin infusion pumps with variable infusion rates determined by the patient are now in widespread use by an estimated 7,000 to 10,000 persons with diabetes. Constant-rate implantable insulin infusion pumps also have been developed, and external regulation is being attempted. Some promising results and considerable useful research data have been generated with these devices. However, all of these current infusion systems require considerable skill and attention on the part of both patients and health care professionals, and they are not suitable for all patients. A transcutaneously implanted needle-sensor that "reads" blood glucose values has been described but is not fully developed.

Future Research Directions

Without question, the most important long-term advance yet to be made is the development of a continuous blood glucose sensor. Such a sensor must be reliable, accurate, and capable of long-term function or be easily replaceable. If open-loop (without glucose sensing) implantable insulin pumps with sophisticated electronic control systems are developed, their interface with the signal generated by a continuous glucose sensor would be possible. The closed-loop implantable insulin infusion pump has the potential to normalize most metabolic abnormalities associated with diabetes and could dramatically reduce the peripheral disease that can be so disastrous for the person with diabetes.

Other approaches include the hybrid artificial pancreas, which involves the implantation of islet cells protected by a semipermeable membrane from humoral or cell-mediated rejection. Various polymers for the membrane have been suggested and tried, such as alginatepolylysine biocompatible membranes, and various implantation sites have been proposed.

The use of biodegradable materials that contain insulin that, as pellets, slowly release insulin needs further development. Similarly, development of membranes that permit the slow release of insulin from implanted reservoirs needs further investigation. If perfected, these devices could provide a continuous flow of insulin at a constant basal rate for relatively long periods. Such devices would be simple to implant and easy to remove; however, they currently are difficult to make sensitive to changes in ambient glucose and other secretagogues and potentially would require repeated surgical procedures (even if minor) over the years.

Other examples of possible methods to introduce glucose sensitivity include (1) incorporating glucose-sensitive lectins into insulin complexes which, in the presence of increased glucose, would release insulin and (2) using pH-sensitive membranes whose permeability to insulin would be increased when a glucose signal is enzymatically transposed into a pH change.

Various other approaches to the physiological delivery of insulin are in early stages of development. Among these approaches are iontophoresis, in which insulin is delivered from a reservoir under the control of an electric current passed transcutaneously, and dialysis systems, in which the insulin-containing solution to be dialyzed is implanted. In the future, the possibilities of introducing the insulin gene or novel cells engineered to express the insulin gene into subjects with diabetes should be explored.

To develop most insulin delivery devices, it will be necessary to overcome several obstacles, including prevention of insulin aggregation or precipitation in reservoirs or catheter tips; development of encasing, or encapsulating, materials with long-term compatibility with body tissues and fluids; and development of consistent and reliable signal systems to generate changes in insulin release on biological or patient demand.

Associated with the development of insulin delivery devices are the continued clinical studies required to determine the beneficial role of tight glucose control on diabetic peripheral disease. Studies in all these areas should be encouraged for the future development of insulin infusion devices.

Transplantation

Accomplishments

Transplants of islets within inbred strains of rodents have been shown to reverse experimentally induced diabetes, with maintenance of normoglycemia for their lifespan. Rodents with diabetes develop early complications involving the kidney, eye, peripheral nerves, cartilage, bone, and the heart that are similar to the early complications that occur in human diabetes. Transplants of islets in animals with diabetes prevents these complications from occurring. If islet transplantation occurs after the diabetic complications are established, the islet grafts either prevent the further progression of the complications or reverse them to normal.

A most significant development in the past few years is the demonstration that eliminating or altering lymphoid antigen-presenting cells in the islets before transplantation will prevent rejection of the islets without any requirement for immunosuppressive therapy of the recipients. A second important finding is that these islet pretreatment procedures also will prevent rejection of islets transplanted across a closely related species barrier (rat to mouse). Studies are in progress to determine whether rejection of islets across a wider species barrier (such as hamster to mouse or pig to mouse) can be prevented by these procedures. Methods have been developed for the mass isolation of canine and primate islets. Reversal of pancreatectomy-induced diabetes in both species can be accomplished by islet transplantation.

Although there have been a number of transplants of islet tissue in patients with diabetes in the past several years that have been called "islet transplants," these actually have been partially digested pancreatic fragment transplants that have not provided adequate responses. Recent technologic improvements in islet isolation methods are now producing better islet preparations that contain partially purified, viable isolated islets from cadaver donor pancreas. These advances have reached the point that islet transplantation clinical trials have been initiated in patients with advanced diabetes who require immunosuppression for maintenance of kidney grafts. The results indicate partial function in the majority of these islet transplant recipients, although none has become insulin independent.

Procedures to transplant either the whole pancreas or pancreatic segments have been refined and successfully performed, resulting in patients who are insulin independent after surgery. In 1985, 160 successful transplants were performed worldwide. Although immune rejection remains a major difficulty, the surgical techniques required for transplantation have been refined and are no longer an obstacle. Vascular anastomosis, a procedure that stitches blood vessels to each other, has been perfected, and the problem of pancreatic enzyme drainage has been solved by inserting the pancreatic duct into the bladder. Excellent results have been achieved at three centers (Iowa, Minnesota, and Wisconsin), and pancreas transplantation has now become a therapeutic, not investigative, procedure.

Improved methods for culturing and isolating islet tissue from the fetal pancreas also have made it possible to initiate clinical trials with transplants of fetal pancreas in patients with advanced diabetes who require immunosuppression for maintenance of kidney grafts. Current efforts of fetal islet research are focused on improving the isolation, culturing, and preservation of fetal islet tissue and improving conditions that permit islet replication and procurement of appropriate fetal pancreas for study.

Future Research Directions

Current research focused on studies to improve the quality and quantity of islet tissue for transplantation, the effects of immunosuppression on islet engraftment and function, and procurement and preservation of both the pancreas and isolated islets must be continued.

It is necessary to expand the procurement, preservation, and distribution by peer review of cadaver donor pancreases and develop the mechanisms and support for providing an adequate supply and distribution of islet tissue for research and clinical use. Until clinical endocrine pancreas transplantation becomes standardized, these activities should only be conducted at institutions with appropriate expertise, and these institutions should be adequately funded for this effort. The techniques of islet isolation and purification must be improved and standardized, and the availability of the standardized reagents required for endocrine pancreas transplantation must be secured.

The success of islet transplantation will require determining the optimal surgical technique for whole and segmental pancreas transplantation, including identifying the optimal immunosuppressive regimen, developing the techniques for immune monitoring of recipients for the early detection of graft rejection, and documenting thoroughly the effect that endocrine pancreas transplants have on the complications of diabetes. It is essential that funds be provided to support and expand clinical trials on human islet transplantation. Support also is needed for a worldwide central endocrine pancreas transplant registry that provides direct access to the data.

Basic research needs include defining the mechanisms leading to and maintaining islet graft acceptance and improving these methods of immunomodulating donor islet tissue and the recipient responses to the graft; defining the factors that determine the growth, replication, and differentiation of islet tissue after transplantation, including the effect of the diabetic state itself; investigating whether autoimmune change of implanted islets (exclusive of allograft rejection) limits effectiveness of transplantation and defining the mechanisms of this process and methods to avoid it; defining the effect of immunosuppressive therapy on islet tissue engraftment, replication, and function and the mechanism involved in graft rejection; and establishing effective islet cryopreservation techniques for adequate islet banking. It also will be necessary to develop the technology to provide effective immunoprotective devices for islet transplantation. To promote the expertise of clinicians, support should be provided to establish regular workshops on the immunobiology of the endocrine pancreas and to establish international short-term traineeships to develop special skills by individual investigators.

Alternative initiatives include enhancing the supply of transplantable beta cells and inducing insulin gene expression in cultured nonbeta cells obtained from the transplant recipient. The limited availability of transplantable islets now and in the future would be alleviated if replication of beta cells could be induced in culture, as is the case for cultured keratinocytes used in skin grafts. The problems that beset islet transplantation could be overcome if insulin production could be induced in nonbeta cells obtained from recipients with IDDM. Such tissue could be stimulated to proliferate and then reimplanted into the donor, obviating problems of rejection and recurrence.

Pancreatic transplantation (whole or isolated islets) is of course one approach to attempting physiologic delivery of insulin. The topic will not be further discussed here, however, because immunosuppression, transplant biology, and other problems of transplantation are considered elsewhere. Autologous transplantation, the harvesting and reimplantation of a patient's own islets during pancreatectomy, is a relatively straightforward approach that eliminates the need for immunosuppression. But even this procedure is not uniformly successful and requires further experimental development.

Pharmaceutical Agents

Accomplishments

NIDDM patients who cannot control their blood glucose with diet therapy are usually treated with oral hypoglycemic agents that increase insulin secretion and have other beneficial effects on carbohydrate utilization. New and more potent oral medications have been developed and now are approved for general use. These drugs have been shown to have insulin-enhancing actions in addition to their well-known actions to increase insulin secretion from the pancreas. Other drugs—aldose reductase inhibitors, which decrease sorbitol accumulation—are being tested clinically for their potential effects to improve eye and nerve complications.

Future Research Directions

Studies should be continued on the mechanism of action of therapeutic agents (e.g., sulfonylureas, prostaglandins, adrenergic agents) on the metabolic phenomena associated with insulin synthesis, packaging, and secretion. There should be a continued search for new hypoglycemic agents that may act either to enhance insulin action or insulin secretion, particularly those distinct from the sulfonylurea compounds.

Studies with B-pertussis toxin, which interacts with the adenyl cyclase system thereby activating the enzyme and insulin secretion, should focus on the development of derivatives that selectively stimulate insulin secretion. Continued work on the development of somatostatin derivatives should be expanded. Studies on long-term action of insulin-like agents (e.g., vanadate) to treat experimental diabetes in animals should be pursued.

The multiple pathways of phospholipid and arachidonic acid metabolism need further exploration, and the information needs to be integrated with development of novel hypoglycemic agents.

New agents that may act to inhibit aldose reductase or to prevent or reverse the accumulation of advanced end products of protein glycosylation should be sought. An example, aminoguanidine, currently is being tested experimentally in diabetic animal models.

Eye Complications

Accomplishments

Severe eye disease, particularly retinopathy, is a devastating complication of diabetes and is the leading cause of new cases of blindness among adults in the United States. Thus, its prevention is clearly a high priority in the treatment of patients with diabetes. It is unclear whether retinopathy is an inevitable consequence of diabetes, perhaps due to genetic factors inherent in the disease, or whether it can be prevented through manipulation of environmental factors such as blood glucose levels and degree of protein glycosylation. Recent research indicates that genetic factors do not play a role in the development of severe eye disease in patients with IDDM.

This lack of association with inherited factors is supported by the finding that macrovascular disease, which is known to be familial, did occur in siblings. These findings suggest that blindness is not an inevitable consequence of diabetes and possibly could be amenable to alteration of factors that have an impact on blood glucose levels and protein glycosylation.

Progress is continuing in treating and preventing eye complications in diabetes, both in clinical therapy and fundamental research. Long-term followup studies have confirmed earlier reports that photocoagulation (use of a laser beam that generates heat and coagulates vessels) can reduce the risk of blindness by 60 percent in patients who have severe stages of retinopathy. Vitrectomy, a surgical procedure to remove blood-clouded vitreous and scar tissue from the eye, is being evaluated in cases of very severe retinopathy.

Epidemiologic studies have demonstrated strong relationships between the severity of retinopathy and levels of glycemic control and blood pressure. A model similar to diabetic retinopathy has been developed in galactosemic dogs. This finding supports the hypothesis that an elevated glucose level itself may lead to retinopathy.

Additional evidence suggests the pathogenesis of diabetic retinopathy may be related to a defect in retinal vascular autoregulation. Functional insulin receptors have been identified on retinal endothelial cells and pericytes (the cells initially involved in diabetic retinopathy), and further progress has been made toward isolating the retinal factor that stimulates neovascularization.

Future Research Directions

The specific environmental and lifestyle factors that lead to retinopathy and blindness in diabetes, and possibly to other microvascular complications, are unknown. Continued support of these studies, and of the Diabetes Control and Complications Trial, should ensure that these factors are identified and that their contributions to the complications of diabetes are quantified. This research would provide a sound scientific basis for programs to reduce these risk factors in the population with diabetes.

Although important progress has been made in the treatment of diabetic retinopathy, current treatments do not help all patients nor do they resolve the fundamental problem of closure of retinal vessels that underlies progressive retinopathy. Greater investment in fundamental research is needed if treatment for diabetic retinopathy is to proceed beyond its current empirical stage and become more uniformly successful. The multiple pathways of investigation include intraocular changes in the progression of the disease process and their responses to therapy, relationship of eye changes to systemic conditions, more sophisticated methods of measuring these changes, and patient population studies.

Studies of early tissue changes should continue on the polyol pathway in which glucose is converted to sorbitol and fructose by an enzyme, aldose reductase, which is activated when blood sugar is not within normal limits. With accumulation of sorbitol in various cells and tissues, changes may occur that significantly affect function. Further testing of aldose reductase inhibitors may give clues to the importance of this metabolic pathway.

Investigation is needed of the impact of hyperglycemia on cell function and anatomy on both neurosensory and mesodermal structures, retinal endothelial cells, pericytes, and retinal pigment epithelial cells.

Blood-retinal barrier deterioration should be studied by developing animal models, more accurate methods of measurement of fluorescence, and ways of determining the course of anatomic and physiologic changes associated with the barrier breakdown. Culture of retinal, vascular, pigment epithelium, and neural cells will permit evaluation of their response to environmental stimuli and pharmacologic agents. Multiple aspects of retinal metabolism deserve further study, including energy requirements of specific cell types as related to their function, glucose transport through tissues, anaerobic and aerobic glucose metabolism in neurosensory retina, effects of metabolic by-products such as lactic acid, bicarbonate and pH on retinal vascular regulation, and oxygen gradients and utilization in the retina under normal and hyperglycemic conditions. Studies at the molecular genetics and molecular biology level of the basic pathogenesis of diabetic retinopathy should proceed in concert with the other investigations. The entire area of vasoproliferation is under intensive investigation, not only of the factors concerned with the incipience of new growth but also of growth inhibitors.

Vitreous changes at all stages of retinopathy have been grossly neglected except as a tissue to be cauterized or excised. Studies that pertain to the natural history of the relationship of the vitreoretinal interface, the shrinkage of the vitreous gel, and the effect of the gel on the neuroretinal and vasoproliferative tissue is miniscule when compared with the study of the retina over the past decade. Emphasis of study on anatomic, biochemical, and pathophysiologic changes in the vitreous gel as they relate to the retina and proliferative growth is a definite need. Increased commitment to a careful study of the vitreous by methods presently available or new technology (laser scanning ophthalmoscope) will reveal pertinent new relationships between the retina and the intact, partially detached, or completely detached posterior vitreous face. Such studies promise to afford significant new data in an important area, not only in regard to natural history but also in regard to the response of this tissue to established or new therapeutic modalities.

Therapeutic enhancements in the treatment of proliferative diabetic retinopathy and its sequelae remain a challenging area of further work. In addition to potential advantages of new intraocular surgical techniques, new laser technology may permit more precise intraocular surgery. New laser techniques include photodisruption (YAG laser) that can avoid entry into the eye. Eximer lasers, "cutting lasers" that permit precise incision without tugging on other tissues, may be developed as an intravitreous surgical device.

Another avenue of laboratory and clinical study is the inhibition of fibrous tissue formation, either in the natural course of late retinopathy or following vitrectomy surgery. Study of the various stages in the process of scar formation will be part of such a plan. Identification of systemic and local ocular factors that stimulate or inhibit intraocular fibrosis or activity of their precursors will be further areas to explore. Pharmacologic manipulation of these factors would be a logical subsequent step. Measurement of the systemic parameters that may create exacerbation of retinopathy represents a potentially worthwhile area of study. Conversely, alterations in the eye that occur with systemic abnormalities should be documented not only with the present clinical techniques of photography and fluorcscein angiography but also with newer techniques to measure blood flow and retinal oxygen consumption.

With the newer examination techniques, a more precise correlation between circulation to the fundus (posterior part of the eye) and general circulatory changes can be achieved. Because hormonal and humoral systemic changes may be associated with a rapid progression of retinopathy after years of stability, investigations in these areas could prove to be fruitful.

A continuance and expansion of epidemiologic studies should further refine knowledge of the natural course of the disease and the response to established treatments of various stages of retinopathy. Studies under way or soon to be implemented include the Early Treatment Diabetes Retinopathy Study, Diabetic Macula Edema Study, and the Diabetes Control and Complications Trial. Comparisons of different ethnically homogenous groups may reveal parameters that relate to the higher incidence of diabetes and associated problems in one ethnic group than in another.

Use of new techniques to verify data will be necessary to maximize the information obtained from present and future clinical studies. New methods of physical and psychophysical testing can give significantly more precise data than the standard visual acuities and fields, fundus photographs, and angiograms.

Subtle alterations in visual function occur in early retinopathy that are not discerned by present routine function tests. Psychophysical tests of many types are being developed that permit detection of early abnormality of retinal function and continuing evaluation as retinopathy progresses. Not only can they offer a more refined assessment of the natural history, but they also can monitor the response of the retina to various therapies. The use of laser doppler velocitometry, a technique of beaming laser light through the eye to record microvascular blood flow, permits precise measurements unachievable by angiographic techniques. Oximetry, a method of measuring the relative percentages of hemoglobin and oxyhemoglobin in the blood, when developed as a clinical test, will allow determination of oxygen consumption of retinal tissue. Anatomic studies with new technology will reveal previously undescribed microscopic and macroscopic abnormalities of the retina, as the laser scanning ophthalmoscope reveals vitreous abnormalities in a manner not previously described.

Diabetic Renal Complications

Accomplishments

Progress in this area over the past 10 years has been relatively modest, in part because of the small number of centers that have been engaged in this research. The more significant advances have included potential identification of patients who seem at highest risk for developing diabetic nephropathy in the future. These patients, although they appear in perfect health, are characterized by persistent microalbuminuria, glomerular hyperfiltration, and a modest blood pressure increase (although still within the normal range). Early evidence suggests that persistent microalbuminuria is reversible.

Clinical and experimental evidence indicates that glomerular hemodynamics are altered early in the course of diabetes with an increase in both pressure and flow rate. A reduction in glomerular pressure abrogates the glomerular and retinal microvascular lesions in experimental animals with streptozotocin-induced hyperglycemia. Similarly, preliminary clinical studies suggest that reduction in systemic hypertension may reduce the rate of deterioration of renal function in IDDM.

Future Research Directions

The pathophysiology of the glomerular changes in kidney disease of diabetes mellitus needs further investigation, and the underlying cause or causes of diabetic nephropathy must be defined. Investigation of normal glomerular/tubular structure and function at the cellular, biophysical, biochemical, and organ levels is a high priority. Studies in human and experimental models should be extended to determine the natural course of kidney disease of diabetes, including physiology, pathology, and biochemistry. Hemodynamic factors that require further investigation might include the effects of increased systemic pressure in kidney function and morphology; effects of modulation of glomerular hemodynamic factors at biochemical and biophysical levels; renal hypertrophy in response to hemodynamic factors; mechanisms of sodium excretion, control, and effects of hemodynamic characteristics; and neurologic control in hemodynamic regulation. Approaches include the possible effects of renal hyperfiltration in the initiation and progression of renal damage; the possible effects of intrarenal vasoactive substances; the possibility that decreased tissue myoinositol concentration may play a role in the kidney, perhaps by affecting endothelial responses; and the possible role of biochemical alterations in the glomerular filtration barrier, especially with regard to heparin sulfate and its turnover.

Factors that affect the rate of progression of microalbuminuria must be identified; these include the interrelationships between glomerular filtration rate, metabolic control, dietary factors, blood pressure, and smoking. In addition to microalbuminuria, markers must be identified that reliably predict the development of diabetic nephropathy but occur at a stage that is potentially reversible. The mechanisms linking the functional and structural changes in the diabetic nephron to the development of diabetic nephropathy must be determined.

Glomerular biochemistry is an area that deserves research attention. The biophysical and biochemical factors responsible for the organization and function of the glomerular filtration apparatus must be studied. Detailed analysis is needed of the regulation of the synthesis, metabolism, and degradation of the components of the glomerulus and mesangial matrix, including studies of heparin sulfate, type IV collagen, laminin, and fibronectin. The role of nonenzymatic glycosylation in these processes must be explored.

Investigations into glomerular cell biology should include studies of responses to insulin, insulin receptors, growth factors and cellular growth control mechanisms, and effects on physical properties and functions of the altered matrix. Research is needed on the synthesis of intrarenal neuroactive and vasoactive substances and the response to these substances of glomerular capillaries as well as other renal components. The properties of the glomerular cytoskeleton and glomerular cell interactions must be biochemically defined, particularly with regard to cell membrane related structures. These projects will require both in vivo and in vitro studies. The use of kidney biopsies should be encouraged whenever possible in these studies to define more precisely the structural and biochemical correlates.

Immune mechanisms in kidney disease of diabetes should be addressed in studies on the effect on the kidney of cellular and humoral immunologic mechanisms that are causal in the underlying diabetes mellitus and delineation of the effects of immunosuppressive agents on kidney function. Prevention of diabetic kidney disease using advances in immunology may now be investigated. Further studies also are needed on antigenicity of glycosylated proteins, genetic markers for glomerulosclerosis, and the genetics of hypertension.

Efforts to prevent diabetic nephropathy must be increased. This will require an increase in the research resources (investigators and money) devoted to the study of the underlying etiology of diabetic nephropathy and those factors that affect its onset and progression. The development of persistent proteinuria indicates that an irreversible stage of the disease has commenced. Because antihypertensive treatment only slows the inevitable descent into end-stage renal failure, efforts must be increased to identify potential diabetic nephropathy patients well before they reach this nonreversible point and to define interventions that can be effective.

Progress in the area of diabetic nephropathy also would be enhanced by funding centers for large animal kidney research with multi-investigator access. In addition, developing isolated and reconstructed glomerular cell systems is important to reproduce and study in vivo interactions.

At a clinical level, emphasis should be placed on prospective long-term early intervention trials designed to alter the hemodynamic and metabolic factors that appear to be involved in the development of diabetic nephropathy. These studies will provide extremely important information relative to issues such as which markers (or combinations thereof) have predictive value, the more precise definition of the stages prior to the onset of proteinuria and their potential reversibility, and the relative contribution of hemodynamic and metabolic factors to the developing pathology. These trials must document metabolic, physiologic, morphologic (biopsies), and functional events.

Other areas of clinical investigation of kidney disease of diabetes mellitus should include the epidemiology and natural history of the disease, the effects of anti-hypertensive agents, the relationship of glycemic control, and the effect of dietary modification on its course. Investigations are needed of interventional strategies other than blood pressure control, glycemic control, and dietary modification, and dialysis and transplantation studies should be started in persons with kidney disease of diabetes mellitus.

Hypertension, Diabetes, and the Kidney

Accomplishments

During the past several years, increasing attention has been directed to the relationship between carbohydrate metabolism, increased circulatory pressure, and the kidney. Two lines of scientific inquiry have developed that focus on these relationships. Recent experiments confirm that diabetic nephropathy may be initiated by an increase in glomerular capillary pressure, presumably secondary to an increase in glomerular filtration rate (GFR), which is present early in the natural history of diabetes and persists for years. Support for the view that altered glomerular function contributes to the glomerular injury of diabetes has been supported by studies of rats with experimental insulin deficiency. Micropuncture studies have demonstrated that this increase in GFR results from increases in hydraulic pressure and plasma flow rate in glomerular capillaries. The increased pressure and flow rate have been shown to promote glomerular injury in a number of different kidney disease models. These changes can develop in the absence of any increase in systemic arterial pressure. Progression of diabetic nephropathy to the point of hypertension seems to exacerbate this process.

However, increases in capillary pressure and flow do not seem to be the only factors responsible for glomerular injury in diabetes. Glomerular morphologic changes, including mesangial expansion, can develop in diabetic rats that do not exhibit increases in GFR. Other factors that may contribute to glomerular injury in diabetes include glycosylation of glomerular structural proteins, mesangial cell dysfunction with production of altered mesangial matrix material, glycosylation of circulating proteins that may then be deposited in the glomerulus, and altered platelet function leading to formation of microthrombi in glomerular capillaries.

The importance of the "hemodynamic" contribution to diabetic glomerulopathy derives from the fact that glomerular hemodynamic function has been altered in experimental animals and can presumably be altered in diabetic patients. Therapy to prevent development of diabetic nephropathy that does not depend on normalization of blood glucose is thus conceivably available.

Dietary protein restriction, which reduces capillary pressure and flow in the face of sustained hyperglycemia, has been shown to prevent development of glomerular sclerosis in diabetic rats. This latter observation is in accord with results of clinical studies that show that normalization of blood pressure slows the progression of human diabetic nephropathy.

A second line of investigation involves the relationship between carbohydrate metabolism and hypertension. Evidence exists that the common link between obesity and hypertension is the hyperinsulinemia frequently seen in obese individuals. Similarly, the fall in blood pressure following either weight loss or exercise training is associated closely with the fall in plasma insulin levels associated with these maneuvers. Finally, statistically significant relationships have been defined between level of blood pressure and plasma insulin concentrations. These data have led to the postulate that resistance to insulin-stimulated glucose uptake may be involved in the etiology of hypertension, presumably secondary to the hyperinsulinemia. Postulated mechanisms by which hyperinsulinemia may predispose to hypertension include increased renal sodium retention and enhanced sympathetic activity. Other lines of investigation have demonstrated promising leads. For example, in experimental animals with hypertension, an increased sensitivity of the vascular bed to vasoconstrictive agents is observed.

Future Research Directions

Many new and provocative ideas recently have been generated concerning the relationship among carbohydrate, hypertension, and renal function. There is an enormous need to pursue these various lines of investigation. For example, what are the stimuli responsible for altered glomerular function and kidney growth in diabetes? Do the same changes in glomerular filtration and pressure that have been demonstrated in animals with insulin-deficient diabetes and patients with IDDM also exist in NIDDM? What are the most effective ways to reduce the increased glomerular filtration and glomerular capillary pressure that occur in diabetes? Will these maneuvers effectively prevent progression of diabetic nephropathy? Is resistance to insulin-stimulated glucose uptake a common finding in hypertension? To what extent do changes in carbohydrate metabolism in hypertension contribute to hyperlipidemia in this situation? What are the causes of the increased sensitivity to vasoconstrictive agents? What are the possible alterations in the renin system in diabetes?

Atherosclerotic (Cardiovascular) Complications of Diabetes

Accomplishments

Although important advances have been made during the last 10 years in studying the etiology of atherosclerosis in the individual with diabetes, the mechanisms for the enhancement of atherosclerosis in diabetes remain obscure. Although people with diabetes tend to have an increased incidence of well-defined risk factors for atherosclerosis such as hypertension or obesity, diabetes exerts atherogenic effects that clearly are unrelated to other identified risk factors. It is not known whether this atherogenic effect works through independent mechanisms or through the amplification of the actions of other risk factors.

At least one-half of the excess coronary heart disease in women with diabetes has been shown recently to be independent of cardiovascular risk factors and hence may be due to diabetes per se. After statistical adjustment for the classic risk factors of hypertension, cholesterol, smoking, obesity, and family history, the risks remained excessively elevated—at threefold above women without diabetes. This research documents the excess rates of cardiovascular morbidity and mortality in women with diabetes. Hence, diabetes may be a major risk factor for cardiovascular disease in women, although metabolic pathways for this remain to be determined.

Many persons with diabetes display abnormalities in lipid and lipoprotein metabolism, most commonly an increased concentration of triglycerides and VLDL cholesterol. Some evidence exists that hypertriglyceridemia may be an independent risk factor in persons with diabetes. Abnormalities in the conversion of VLDL to low-density lipoproteins (LDL) also exist in the presence of diabetes. Untreated diabetes patients also tend to have reduced levels of the protective HDL and elevated levels of LDL, the most atherogenic lipoprotein. Clinical research has shown that achievement of excellent control of diabetes improves or corrects all of these abnormalities.

There is evidence, especially in experimental animals, that diabetes also changes the lipid and apoprotein composition of the lipoproteins. Because the apoproteins play essential roles in the activation of enzymes that metabolize lipoprotein lipids and in the interactions of lipoproteins with tissue cellular receptors, changes in the apoproteins may have adverse effects. Indeed, some studies have shown that persons with diabetes have decreased levels of an apoprotein required to activate lipoprotein lipase for the clearance of circulating triglycerides. The major apoproteins of LDL and HDL undergo excessive nonenzymatic glycosylation in diabetes: glycosylation affects the binding and uptake of these lipoproteins and may partly account for their altered concentrations.

Population studies in Japan suggest that strict control of risk factors may decrease the incidence of atherosclerotic complications. Improvements in plasma lipid concentrations and glycosylation of apoproteins can be achieved by strict control of diabetes. Present dietary recommendations for the management of diabetes also help to control lipid abnormalities. Active investigations are addressing the benefits of polyunsaturated fish oils in reducing platelet aggregation and lowering plasma triglycerides.

Diabetes may accelerate atherosclerosis through a number of effects unrelated to the standard risk factors. Platelet aggregation is enhanced in some patients with diabetes. Also implicated are alterations in the metabolism of arachidonic acid to thromboxanes and prostacyclins. Endothelial cell formation of prostacyclin, which prevents platelet aggregation and promotes vasodilatation, is reduced in patients and experimental animals with diabetes. Insulin treatment of animals reverses the decreased prostacyclin synthesis. One group has found that people with diabetes produce excessive amounts of two platelet factors, platelet-derived growth factor and epidermal growth factor, which may stimulate the proliferation of vascular smooth muscle cells in the atherosclerotic process.

Nonenzymatic glycosylation of several proteins may enhance atherogenesis. Advanced glycosylation end products (AGE) accumulate progressively on proteins such as collagen. AGE may increase lipid accumulation and stimulate platelet adhesion and aggregation. Changes in proteoglycan metabolism also may increase the trapping of atherogenic lipoproteins within the arterial wall.

Considerable debate has centered on the possible role of hyperinsulinemia as a promoter of atherosclerosis. Favoring a role for hyperinsulinism is the evidence for increased atherosclerosis in individuals who have impaired glucose tolerance and an elevated insulin response to a glucose load. Some studies also indicate that insulin stimulates lipid accumulation in and proliferation of vascular smooth muscle cells. On the other hand, improved diabetic control with insulin treatment obviously ameliorates a number of atherogenic factors. Although insulin is required for VLDL synthesis in the liver and hyperinsulinemia was shown by some to enhance VLDL production, adequate amounts of insulin are clearly required for the synthesis of lipoprotein lipase, an enzyme critical for VLDL removal.

Future Research Directions

Considerable work is needed to obtain a better understanding of the natural history of atherosclerotic changes in diabetes and the impact of various treatment modalities on these changes. Progress in the past has been hampered by the ability to follow only indirect manifestations of atherosclerosis (i.e., clinical effects) and the opportunity to examine tissue changes only at the time of surgery or autopsy. The development of a battery of powerful new noninvasive imaging techniques, such as computed axial tomography, ultrasound, magnetic resonance imaging, and positron emission tomography scanning, should soon make it possible to carry out prospective intervention studies on the prevention of atherosclerosis in patients with diabetes. Meanwhile, improved surgical techniques for the management of atherosclerotic complications provide an opportunity to obtain tissues for comparing blood vessels from patients with and without diabetes. Intensive studies are needed on the basic biology of endothelial and smooth muscle cells, particularly with reference to the effects of altered levels of glucose, insulin, lipids, and other factors, such as prostaglandins. The interaction of other cells such as platelets and macrophages with endothelial cells should be studied, and the levels of platelet-derived growth factors should be measured. Additional animal models suitable for studying the effects of diabetes on atherogenesis are needed.

Further clinical studies to evaluate the potential importance of hyperinsulinemia, glycosylated lipoproteins, and blood glucose in the genesis of atherosclerosis and of lipid abnormalities in diabetes should be performed. Because diabetes is known to affect small blood vessels in many parts of the body, it is important to determine if this process also occurs in the heart and, if so, to determine the functional consequence of such lesions.

Recent research results establish the need for medical strategies beyond routine management of coronary risk factors in women with diabetes. Further studies are needed to determine whether improved control of diabetes can reduce the morbidity and mortality from cardiovascular disease or whether having diabetes conveys an inherent risk for cardiovascular disease that cannot be reduced by currently known therapies. Efficacy of the newer therapies for heart disease should be tested in clinical trials in patients with diabetes, and cardiovascular risk factor reduction programs should be instigated in persons with diabetes to reduce the risk of cardiovascular disease attributed to these factors.

Neurologic Complications

Accomplishments

Complications of diabetes that involve the peripheral nervous system are a common problem in persons with diabetes. They can include pain, impaired sensory perception, muscle weakness, impotence, diabetic diarrhea, precipitous decreases in blood pressure, and impaired ability to recognize and counteract insulin-induced hypoglycemia. Studies in animal models of diabetes have shown that there is a dying back of nerve axons that first affects peripheral sensory nerves and then motor nerves. Morphologic studies of autonomic nerves that supply the small intestine have shown distinctive pathologic changes in rats with experimentally induced diabetes. These pathologic changes can be prevented by transplantation of pancreatic islets. Most important, maintenance of normoglycemia by islet transplants has been shown to reverse the pathologic changes to normal if the transplants are accomplished after the lesions have developed.

Biochemical studies have shown that the polyol pathway is activated in peripheral nerves in diabetes. As a result, certain metabolic abnormalities occur in these nerves. In addition, there is impairment in the transport of enzymes and proteins within the nerve fibers. These metabolic changes are responsible for impaired peripheral nerve function in diabetes early in the course of the disease. Later in the disease, it is believed that the small blood vessels that supply the peripheral nerves are damaged, resulting in impaired blood supply and decreased oxygen, which further injure the peripheral nerves.

In recent years, particular chemicals have been developed that will specifically block the activity of aldose reductase. Theoretically, blockage of this enzyme should interfere with the polyol pathway and thus prevent the early metabolic changes in peripheral nerves in diabetes. Studies in animals with diabetes have shown that administration of aldose reductase inhibitors or treatment with myoinositol will reverse these early metabolic changes to normal and prevent some of the abnormalities in nerve function. Clinical studies with aldose reductase inhibitors have been initiated to evaluate the effect of these agents on diabetic neuropathy.

In the person who does not have diabetes, metabolic studies have demonstrated that production of hypoglycemia with insulin will immediately trigger a response from the autonomic nervous system with release of epinephrine in conjunction with glucagon, which in turn releases glucose from the liver and restores the blood sugar to normal. In the patient with diabetes and autonomic neuropathy, this chain of events does not occur, and severe hypoglycemia may develop. In addition, the patient may not be aware of the hypoglycemia for reasons that are not understood at the present time.

Future Research Directions

Further research is needed to understand the basic mechanisms involved in the development of autonomic neuropathy and to develop corrective measures to overcome these defects. The NIH has in progress a multi-institutional clinical trial to determine whether tight control of the blood sugar in diabetes will affect the development of its complications. It is of great importance that studies on neurologic complications of diabetes be continued as a part of this long-term clinical trial to answer the question of the relationship of glycemic control to the development of diabetic neuropathy.

Basic studies should be expanded on the metabolic and biochemical changes in peripheral nerves in diabetes. The role of these metabolic changes and the effect of ischemia due to vascular disease on the development of diabetic neuropathy must be further investigated. Noninvasive techniques such as magnetic resonance imaging and positron emission techniques should be used to assess nerve function and metabolism. More basic scientists should be encouraged to enter the field of diabetic neuropathy research by providing workshops and establishing specialized diabetes centers to promote the interaction of basic and clinical scientists. Clinical tests for evaluation of autonomic nerve function in diabetes must be standardized. The support of primate centers must be continued to provide animal models of diabetes with a long lifespan so that studies on diabetic neuropathy can be accomplished in these animals. More studies are needed on the effect of acute and chronic hypoglycemia on the central and peripheral nervous systems. These studies are of particular importance at the present time because therapeutic attempts to improve blood glucose control undoubtedly will lead to increased incidences of hypoglycemia. More epidemiologic studies on the prevalence and morbidity of diabetes are needed to increase the awareness of the serious problems of diabetic neuropathy to both diabetologists and internists.

Very little information is available on the factors that lead to the development of impotence. It is presumed that diabetes produces changes in autonomic nerve fibers, which in turn lead to impotence. Further basic and clinical investigations are needed in this important area.

Complications of Pregnancy and Fetal Development

Accomplishments

The progress made over the past 10 years in the field of diabetes and pregnancy stands as a model for the possibilities for improvement in all areas of diabetes and its complications. Perinatal mortality in the best centers devoted to care of the pregnant woman with diabetes has fallen from 6.5 percent in the mid-1970's to 2 .1 percent in the mid-1980's. Because 50 percent of this perinatal mortality rate is attributable to major congenital malformations, the corrected perinatal mortality is approximately 1 percent, approaching that seen in the general population without diabetes. Pregnancy is the one area of human diabetes in which meticulous metabolic control has been conclusively shown to be effective.

The achievement of near-normal glucose profiles in pregnant women with IDDM has been made possible by new and improved technologies such as self blood glucose monitoring in the home setting and the development of optimal insulin delivery systems. The improvement in perinatal mortality is partially due to the development of better approaches to judge fetal maturation and, in particular, the ability of the neonate's lungs to permit survival. Overall, fetal maturation now is judged by a combination of electrocardiographic and ultrasonographic procedures, and improved techniques permit accurate assessment of pulmonary maturation. This combined approach has allowed the woman with diabetes to deliver the infant vaginally and close to term, thus decreasing the mortality and morbidity associated with respiratory distress syndrome, hypoglycemia, hypocalcemia, erythremia, and hyperbilirubinemia. The highly sophisticated technology now available in neonatal intensive care units also has aided survival in those infants born prematurely. Advances in respiratory equipment, for example, have allowed treatment for the respirator-dependent newborn infant without necessarily subjecting the baby to the risk of retrolental fibroplasia. The importance of gestational diabetes as a cause of stillbirths has led to the initiation of universal screening with glucose tolerance tests of all pregnant women in the third trimester. With improved case finding and strategies specific for the woman with gestational diabetes, improvement already has been noted in obstetrical outcome.

Future Research Directions

The remarkable improvements cited above should provide added incentive to the research needs for the next 10 years. Although not strictly a "research" issue, one clear priority is to bring to all women with diabetes that level of care that has been shown to afford the best possible prognosis. The Federal Government's role may be to designate specialized regional centers that are designed to encourage care of pregnant women with diabetes and to support public and professional education initiatives, with possible use of reimbursement formulas.

The preliminary findings that the incidence of congenital malformations can be reduced in infants born to women with diabetes if meticulous metabolic control is initiated *before* conception must be translated into common clinical practice. Reliable techniques to detect the presence of serious malformations in the fetus must be developed; this would permit rational counseling on the possibility of therapeutic abortion. Starting with suitable animal models, studies must be conducted to determine whether inadvertent but repeated hypoglycemia will have serious adverse effects on the fetus such as damage at the time of organogenesis or damage to the rapidly developing brain later in gestation. The mechanism by which the diabetic milieu causes abnormalities of overall fetal growth and development (including failure of fetal pulmonary maturation) needs to be defined in precise biochemical and physiologic terms. Evidence now is emerging that the pathway involves a functional deficiency of arachidonic acid during organogenesis, which may, in turn, be associated with a depletion of tissue myoinositol. These observations need to be confirmed and extended, because the myoinositol data would indicate that the mechanism for diabetic embryopathy is analogous to the putative pathway that is hypothesized to be responsible for diabetic neuropathy and retinopathy. Exploration should continue of alternate hypotheses such as the role of various metabolites and growth factors or inhibitors. Animal models would appear to be highly suitable for these studies, especially the use of the whole embryo culture technique. Progress in this area should be followed by clinical trials that use an intervention strategy based on more precise knowledge of the teratogenic mechanism.

Further improvements must be made in the treatment programs for women with diabetes. Complicated regimens for optimal insulin delivery need to be simplified and made more flexible. Explorations should be made of technologies such as glucose monitors with built-in memories and algorithms to guide insulin dose adjustment. Markers other than glycosylated hemoglobin to guide optimal pregnancy therapy need to be developed. The possible use of other glycosylated serum proteins with a shorter half-life may prove to be of use; standards and norms for pregnancy will need to be defined. For women with gestational diabetes, an improved, simplified approach to screening must be developed and validated to replace the time-consuming and costly method now used. Once the diagnosis of gestational diabetes is made, safe and simplified treatment programs must be devised and evaluated. Methods to validate these programs would include newer approaches to nutrition prescriptions, the evaluation of exercise as adjunct therapy, and the development and testing of safe oral hypoglycemic agents.

Closely related to the issue of pregnancy is the assessment of the safety and efficacy of contraception programs for women with diabetes. Giving the woman with diabetes a choice of contraceptive methods could help to plan pregnancy so as to achieve optimal metabolic control from preconception to delivery.

The long-term issues of diabetes in pregnancy should be explored. These issues include the effects of pregnancy on the diabetic woman's risk of development or progression of diabetic nephropathy and diabetic retinopathy. The possibilities have been raised that infants of mothers with diabetes are at increased risk for the development of obesity and neurologic dysfunction and for the future onset of diabetes.

Acute Complications

Accomplishments

The acute complications of diabetes include frequent, severe, or prolonged hypoglycemia, diabetic ketoacidosis, and nonketotic hyperosmolar coma. Research during the past decade has provided much new knowledge about these metabolic derangements.

With increased emphasis on maintenance of normal or near-normal blood glucose concentrations, the incidence and risks of hypoglycemia have increased. Some persons with diabetes are more prone to develop hypoglycemia than are others, and recovery from hypoglycemia may vary from one individual to another. Information is now available regarding the mechanisms of insulin-induced hypoglycemia and the glucose counter-regulatory system. When insulin is administered either subcutaneously or intravenously, glucose uptake and metabolism are stimulated in insulin-sensitive tissues (mainly skeletal muscle) and hepatic glucose production is inhibited. The maintenance of normal blood glucose levels is dependent on absorption of carbohydrates from the gastrointestinal tract. When food intake and plasma insulin concentrations are not coordinated, increased glucose utilization and decreased hepatic glucose production lead to hypoglycemia. Physical exercise potentiates the hypoglycemic effect of insulin by increasing glucose utilization in skeletal muscle and, to some extent, by enhancing insulin absorption from subcutaneous depots.

When insulin-induced hypoglycemia occurs, the glucose counter-regulatory system is activated and blood glucose levels are returned towards normal. In normal people, glucagon plays a primary role in promoting glucose recovery from insulin-induced hypoglycemia. Epinephrine appears to play a secondary role when glucagon response is normal; however, when glucagon secretion is deficient, epinephrine compensates for the lack of glucagon and returns blood glucose towards normal; if both hormones are absent, recovery from hypoglycemia fails to occur. Although both cortisol and growth hormone have anti-insulin effects in liver and peripheral tissues, respectively, and are increased in response to hypoglycemia, an increase in blood glucose is slow to occur. Thus, these two hormones do not play a significant role in the acute recovery from hypoglycemia but may be important in long-term regulation of blood glucose concentration.

Research has shown that many patients with diabetes mellitus have absent or blunted glucagon secretory responses to hypoglycemia. When this response is deficient, it frequently is compensated for by increased epinephrine secretion, and glucose recovery occurs. In some patients, both glucagon and epinephrine responses are deficient, resulting in frequent, severe, and prolonged hypoglycemia. The lack of normal glucagon and epinephrine responses to hypoglycemia appears to be secondary to the development of autonomic neuropathy. However, most patients with autonomic neuropathy who have impaired glucagon and epinephrine secretion develop severe unresponsive hypoglycemia, suggesting that other factors such as increased sensitivity to catecholamines and other as yet unidentified factors play a role in determining the frequency and severity of hypoglycemia reactions in patients with diabetes.

Major advances in the early recognition, understanding, and treatment of diabetic ketoacidosis during the past 10 years have led to decreased incidence, morbidity, and mortality of this life-threatening acute complication of diabetes mellitus. DKA may be the presenting manifestation of insulin-dependent diabetes in children and adults or may occur when insulin administration is discontinued or insulin requirements are increased by illness, injury, or stress. The exclusive use of short-acting insulin in patients using insulin-infusion devices or multiple daily injections has led to an increase in the incidence of DKA in these patients.

Advances in knowledge of the pathogenesis of DKA have included a better understanding of the regulation of hepatic ketogenesis and gluconeogenesis, the relative roles of insulin and glucagon in these processes, and the acid-base changes and fluid and electrolyte shifts that occur. The effects of altered glucose metabolism on red cell oxygen transport and release, the consequences of hypophosphatemia, hypokalemia, and hypocalcemia during treatment of DKA, and the effects of rapid rehydration and correction of acidosis by bicarbonate administration on central nervous system function are also now better understood. This understanding has led to significant improvements in therapy, including use of low-dose intravenous insulin infusions, proper replacement of fluid and electrolyte losses, administration of phosphates, and judicious use of intravenous bicarbonate solutions. These factors, along with improved monitoring and intensive care support, have resulted in reduced morbidity and mortality from DKA.

Like DKA, the pathophysiology of nonketotic hyperosmolar coma now is better understood, and as a consequence, treatment has improved. In this syndrome, insulin deficiency is not complete and ketosis is mild or absent. In many cases, hyperglycemia causes osmotic diuresis and dehydration, which in turn leads to worsening of the hyperglycemia, thus setting up a vicious cycle that ultimately leads to severe hyperglycemia, dehydration, and a hyperosmolar state. CNS function is impaired, often leading to focal seizures and coma. Treatment is similar to that of DKA, although smaller amounts of insulin are required and appropriate fluid and electrolyte replacement is the mainstay of treatment.

Future Research Directions

Additional knowledge of the counter-regulatory hormone responses in normal subjects and in those with diabetes, the role of autonomic neuropathy in the pathogenesis of severe hypoglycemia, and other factors that affect blood glucose regulation in insulin-treated diabetes is needed to further improve the care of individuals with diabetes and decrease the incidence and sequelae of hypoglycemia.

Investigators need to better understand central nervous system function in DKA and factors leading to brain edema, decreased function, and death. In addition, further knowledge is needed on regulation of glucose and lipid metabolism during insulin deficiency and of the hormonal responses and alterations in glucose regulation that occur in nonketotic hyperosmolar coma.

Dental Complications

Accomplishments

The oral and dental complications of diabetes mellitus include increased susceptibility to bacterial periodontal diseases and to fungus infections of the oral mucosa, reduced salivation, and diminished ability to taste and smell. The most important oral complication is the increased prevalence and severity of periodontal disease, in which the bone and soft connective tissues that hold the teeth firm in the jaws are destroyed slowly by bacterial infection, causing the teeth to become gradually loosened and lost. In the general population, periodontal disease is the principal cause of the loss of teeth in adults. During the past decade, epidemiologic data have been accumulated to verify the strong anecdotal belief that periodontal disease is more frequent and more severe in persons with diabetes than in the general population. Extension of a periodontal infection can be life threatening in a person with poorly controlled diabetes. Published case reports describe such serious complications as cavernous sinus thrombosis, a brain infection caused by direct extension from infected teeth, and recent clinical observations have included cases of severe peritonsillar abscesses with lockjaw, facial swelling, and ptosis of the eyelids in persons with diabetes.

In both IDDM and NIDDM, the most severe periodontal disease has been found in patients with poor metabolic control. In the IDDM group, periodontal disease was seen after puberty and affected 20 percent of the patients by age 18. Rapid bone loss was evident in many of these subjects, and the disease was associated with specific bacteria. In approximately 25 percent of the subjects with periodontal disease, there was reduced migratory ability in infection-fighting peripheral blood neutrophils. In Pima Indians with NIDDM, severe disease with rapid loss of tooth support was rampant, and the disease was associated with a particularly virulent form of *Bacteroides gingivalis*, the main pathogenic organism in adult periodontitis in the general population. The most striking finding in these patients was the high rate of tooth loss.

Another finding of great potential significance for both periodontal disease and diabetes was that the antibiotic tetracycline is effective against periodontal disease not only because of its antibacterial effect, but also because it reduces the high tissue levels of collagenase observed in persons with diabetes and in the diseased periodontal tissues of patients without diabetes. Collagenase is an enzyme that breaks down the connective tissue fibers that attach the teeth to the bone and keep them firmly in place.

Future Research Directions

In future research, strong emphasis should be placed on the reasons for the greater susceptibility of patients with diabetes to periodontal disease. Although the *B. gingivalis* organism appears to be the principal pathogen in rapidly progressing periodontal disease in adults who do not have diabetes, the strains isolated from patients who have diabetes are far more invasive and destructive than strains from persons who do not have diabetes. Therefore, the physiology of these highly virulent strains should be thoroughly studied, as well as the periodontal environment in which they grow and metabolize. It is equally important to characterize the immune response of patients with diabetes to this organism and its products.

Efforts should be generated to determine the true role of the reduced neutrophil chemotaxis sometimes manifest in diabetes. These efforts should parallel attempts to define the role of the abnormal collagen and connective tissue metabolism in periodontal disease susceptibility. Findings from both types of studies should be correlated with other medical complications such as retinopathy and osteoporosis.

Using a variety of in vitro and in vivo models, specific studies should examine the influence of insulin and other metabolic factors on bone formation and resorption. In view of preliminary findings that successful treatment of severe periodontal disease in juveniles with diabetes lowers insulin requirements, specific projects should be initiated to substantiate this finding. The Diabetes Control and Complications Trial should provide an opportunity to test the hypothesis that tight control of the blood glucose level is beneficial to periodontal health. Attempts also should be made to develop special therapeutic and preventive dental health regimens for patients with diabetes as a special risk group. Because the tetracycline family of compounds seems to exert not only an antibacterial effect but also a collagenase inhibition that may counteract the unfavorable effects of both diabetes and periodontal disease, further research in this area seems extremely promising.

Behavioral and Psychosocial Issues in Diabetes

Accomplishments

The management of diabetes requires that people with the disease significantly modify their lifestyle to adjust to a demanding treatment regimen. Long-term outcomes, including avoiding or minimizing complications, may be dependent on a complex series of interactions between biomedical and behavioral variables. An understanding of the dynamics of these interactions is required to devise and evaluate specific management strategies designed to improve the physical and emotional health of the person with diabetes. This understanding can best be achieved by coordinating the resources available from behavioral and biomedical sciences and by directing these resources to the specific problems of persons who have diabetes.

As health care providers continue to incorporate new technologies (such as self blood glucose monitoring) as part of sophisticated diabetes management, it has become increasingly clear that implementation of the medical regimen depends on the behavior of the patient. It is now quite obvious that while patient education is necessary, it is not sufficient in itself to guarantee behavior.

A growing concern exists for behavioral and psychosocial factors in diabetes mellitus as well as for recognition of the relationship between stress and deleterious medical outcomes. The behavioral sciences have made great strides over the past few decades, and there is now a sizable cadre of scientifically well-grounded behavioral research scientists. A body of work now is beginning to emerge that suggests ways in which behavioral sciences may contribute to clarifying the nature of many diabetes-related problems and lead to advances in treatment.

Some progress in this area has been made over the past 10 years. Advances include recognition of the idiosyncratic nature of patients' awareness of fluctuations in blood glucose levels; improvement in the research designs of psychosocial studies in diabetes, including the use of randomization and appropriate controls; improved understanding of developmental factors that play a role in the physical and psychological adaptation to diabetes; development of behavioral weight loss programs that have been shown to be effective in improving glycemic control in patients with NIDDM; beginning of a systematic exploration of how stress may affect glycemic control both directly (neuroendocrine and hormonal mediation) and indirectly (through changes in adherence to the regimen); and recognition of increased prevalence of depression both in patients with diabetes and their families and its effects on glycemic control. Short-term fluctuations in blood glucose levels have been shown to produce neuropsychological consequences, raising the question as to whether attempts at rigid control may have undesired effects on neuropsychological functions.

In recent years, the NIDDK funded a number of studies to develop optimal strategies for improving behavioral compliance as well as to determine relationships between psychological stress and fluctuations in blood glucose. Data resulting from these studies suggest that events that generate anxiety, specific intrapsychic conflicts, emotional deprivation, conscious and unconscious threats to security, and other unpleasant psychological experiences upset the control of diabetes. Two current studies are assessing behavioral techniques to control blood glucose fluctuations. Two other studies are exploring methods to control weight and to increase long-term adherence to diet and exercise.

Future Research Directions

Major opportunities and challenges exist for psychosocial research in diabetes. Behavioral research is needed to identify and measure the component skills involved in regimen adherence. These encompass cognitive factors, the linkages patients use in evaluating information and how they act on it, and problem-solving approaches in different subgroups. Advances in these fields could lead to specifically tailored programs that would foster problem-solving skills in individuals from diagnosis onwards and thus improve control of diabetes.

To achieve better self-care of diabetes, it is necessary to perform research designed to understand, predict, and alter patient behavior. In addition, key research questions concerning the effects of emotional factors on glucose control must be addressed. In a 5-year prospective study, 100 newly diagnosed children with diabetes, ages 8 to 13, are being assessed to determine the extent of depression in the child and in the parents. Still another ongoing longitudinal study is systematically assessing the impact of psychosocial and stress dimensions on outcome patterns of adolescents with diabetes. Another study will determine whether insulin-dependent diabetes significantly disrupts cognitive, perceptual, and motor functions in adolescents and adults. Previous studies have indicated the importance of factors such as individual coping resources, life stress, and family environment in the adaptation of a patient to a chronic illness. Few studies have rigorously evaluated the influence of these variables on favorable and unfavorable outcomes in IDDM.

Controlled studies of intervention in newly diagnosed children with IDDM and their families should be conducted. Preliminary research has identified "risk factors" that predict difficulties in future management. Well-designed studies, perhaps multicenter in scope, should be encouraged to explore health care interventions that might prevent or ameliorate predictable problems relating to diabetes control or to life crises.

Research needs to be expanded to include the environmental and psychosocial factors that can exert effects on glycemic control. Expansion involves the need to identify the neuroendocrine mechanism or mechanisms, whether there are specific biological or psychological markers for patients who appear at special risk (akin to the type A behavior pattern as a risk factor for cardiovascular disease), and behavioral techniques (such as relaxation) as possible therapeutic approaches. It should be emphasized here that psychosocial stimulation acting through the central nervous system may be an important hyperglycemic factor in NIDDM. Although it is included as an important outcome variable in the Diabetes Control and Complications Trial, further studies are needed to determine whether tight control impairs or improves neuropsychological function.

The systematic and rigorous examination of behavioral and psychosocial influences that affect the person with diabetes is still in its infancy. Each of the current and recently completed investigations will add to our understanding of all facets of this disease. Many more studies are needed before we can draw reliable conclusions.

Chapter 51

Recommendations for Biomedical Research Activities

Our increased understanding of the causes of diabetes and how it affects the body as well as the availability of improved diabetes management techniques such as laser surgery for diabetic eye disease is directly attributable to the biomedical research programs of the National Institutes of Health (NIH). Future progress in treatment and prevention strategies will depend on maintaining a strong biomedical research base.

In recent years the Board has become increasingly concerned about the future of diabetes research because NIH appropriations have not kept pace with the growing impact of this disease on society. Severe restrictions on budgets are placing many promising diabetes research initiatives in jeopardy. Diabetes is a major risk factor for heart disease and the single largest cause of kidney disease. It is the cause of most foot amputations, the leading cause of blindness among adults, and the leading cause of complications during pregnancy; therefore more resources must be allocated to the search for improved treatment and prevention of diabetes.

NATIONAL INSTITUTE OF DIABETES AND DIGESTIVE AND KIDNEY DISEASES

The National Institute of Diabetes and Digestive and Kidney Diseases (NIDDK), the lead agency at the NIH for diabetes research, is dedicated to the fight against diabetes and is prepared to initiate additional research projects on major causes of this disease and its complications, provided there

---

Taken from NIH Pub. No. 93-1587.

are funds to do so. Because of budget restrictions in FY 1993, the NIDDK is awarding grants to only 11 percent of all applicants compared with past years when more than 30 percent of applicants were funded. Having reviewed major diabetes programs at the NIH, the Board is concerned that many meritorious diabetes research proposals cannot be funded. Moreover, investigators can expect their grants to be reduced 25 percent from the amount deemed justified and approved by the reviewing study section. Unless this situation is alleviated, the prognosis for diabetes research that will lead to critical advances is poor.

By increasing the NIDDK's budget to the level that is commensurate with the burden of these diseases on society, Congress will stimulate diabetes research programs thereby providing new hope to the millions who suffer from diabetes and its complications.

The Board recommends that the total appropriation for the National Institute of Diabetes and Digestive and Kidney Diseases be increased to $835 million in FY 1994.

Diabetes Control and Complications Trial Followup

Carefully controlled clinical trials are essential for evaluating and investigating new approaches to disease management. They are an important step in the process of applying advances gained from research to improved patient care. Multicenter, cooperative clinical trials, involving large numbers of patients followed over time, are ideal for prospective investigations of the efficacy of a given approach to treatment. Such investigations allow clinical scientists to assess the feasibility and validity of a therapeutic approach in a variety of patient populations.

Ten years ago, the NIDDK initiated the DCCT to assess the impact of glycemic control on the microvascular complications of insulin-dependent diabetes mellitus (IDDM). The DCCT is approaching its originally projected termination date of December 31, 1993. Before beginning closeout of the formal trial and transferring its patients to other venues of care, the NIDDK should now consider what post-DCCT followup information ought to be obtained from this valuable group of patients after conclusion of the trial. By design, the primary outcome measurements of the DCCT will assess manifestations of early vascular disease and their relationship to blood glucose control. Ultimate morbidity and mortality from diabetic complications, particularly from clinical nephropathy (kidney failure), cardiovascular disease, and proliferative vision-threatening retinopathy will not be determined because relatively few such events are expected during the DCCT itself. Important information pertaining to those critical issues will be acquired after termination of the DCCT by further long-term observations of the patients in a less intensive and less costly manner.

The Board recommends that the Diabetes Control and Complications Trial and the National Institute of Diabetes and Digestive and Kidney Diseases staff work together to design and implement a suitable study of late vascular disease outcomes in IDDM, a study that takes full advantage of the valuable resource represented by the Diabetes Control and Complications Trial cohort.

NIDDM Clinical Trials

It cannot be assumed that the imminent findings of the DCCT will be directly applicable to NIDDM—a disease that has a different pathophysiological basis and predominantly affects an older population. Therefore, during 1992, the Board held a series of workshops to consider other important issues appropriate for large-scale clinical investigation. Board members solicited recommendations for potential clinical trials from a wide spectrum of professions within the diabetes community and then reviewed the state of the science in each proposed area. From these deliberations, several recommendations for additional clinical trials were forwarded to the NIDDK for consideration. After reviewing the NIDDK's decisions regarding such trials, the Board endorses the conclusions reached by the Institute.

The Board recommends that the National Institute of Diabetes and Digestive and Kidney Diseases initiate prospective randomized trials to test the efficacy of diet, exercise, and pharmacological agents: 1) in preventing the progression of impaired glucose tolerance (IGT) to NIDDM and 2) in preventing the development of subsequent cardiovascular disease in newly diagnosed patients with NIDDM. Minority groups at high risk for developing NIDDM and an appropriate balance of men and women should participate in these trials.

The Board recommends that Congress appropriate $15 million to the National Institute of Diabetes and Digestive and Kidney Diseases for FY 1994 to fund clinical trials in this area.

Search for the Diabetes Genes

Although scientists do not yet understand the specific cause or causes of diabetes, it is generally accepted that diabetes is a genetic disease with environmental determinants. For example, the fact that NIDDM can be present in varying frequencies among different racial groups all living in the same environment is most easily explained by a genetic basis for its presence. IDDM also appears to have a genetic basis. People with certain human leukocyte antigen (HLA) types are at increased risk for IDDM, and studies have shown that siblings of children with diabetes have a risk 7 to 18 times greater than children in the general population of developing IDDM.

During the past decade, scientists have isolated a number of genes responsible for serious diseases. However, the greatest challenge to diabetes genetic research arises from the fact that diabetes is not a single disease. The term encompasses a number of different conditions resulting in the diabetes syndrome; hence a number of different genes may be involved in the development of diabetes. Identifying a single genetic marker for diabetes, as has been accomplished for some disorders with straightforward inheritance patterns, seems unlikely.

The same problems and line of reasoning apply to the complications of diabetes. People with diabetes seem to differ in their susceptibility to complications of the disease, and it is suspected that a variety of genes may influence the development of long-term complications from diabetes.

The need to search for the genes involved in diabetes and its complications is urgent and requires collaboration among researchers from many disciplines. In its 1987 long-range plan, the Board stressed the need for interdisciplinary research collaboration and recommended that new mechanisms be established to support such broad-based projects. The NIDDK subsequently joined with the Juvenile Diabetes Foundation International (JDF) to issue a Request for Application (RFA) for new diabetes research programs that incorporate an interdisciplinary approach to the etiology and pathogenesis of IDDM and to the genetic susceptibility of the long-term complications of diabetes. This action represents a unique collaboration between a private health care agency and the Federal Government.

In the spring of 1992, the NIDDK and the JDF awarded "Program of Excellence" grants to six research centers in the United States and Canada, totaling $20 million. The research goals of these centers include: understanding why the immune system destroys insulin-producing cells in the pancreas, finding methods of protecting or regenerating insulin-producing islets under autoimmune attack, transplanting "surrogate" insulin-producing tissue, eliminating the body's rejection of these transplants, and growing insulin-producing cells outside of the body. The Board recognizes that this new program is a major step toward the goal of curing diabetes in this decade.

The Board recommends that Congress appropriate an additional $50 million to the National Institute of Diabetes and Digestive and Kidney Diseases to support activities related to the search for the diabetes genes.

Diabetes and Atherosclerotic Cardiovascular Disease

Atherosclerotic cardiovascular disease (CVD) is the leading cause of death in people with diabetes, as it is for all Americans (CVD caused 850,000 deaths in 1990). However, compared with the general population, people with diabetes are two to four times more likely to develop CVD; they develop it earlier in life and are twice as likely to die from it. This added risk is highest in individuals with diabetes who are age 45 and younger. Because of this increased risk and the relatively high prevalence of diabetes in the United States, diabetes contributes disproportionately to the Nation's high death rate from CVD.

Having diabetes makes a person more vulnerable to all of the major disorders affecting the large blood vessels, including peripheral vascular disease, cerebrovascular disease, and coronary artery disease. Ten percent of people with diabetes have peripheral vascular disease, which can result in amputation; strokes occur two to six times more often in people with diabetes, and their prognosis for recovery is poorer; and two-thirds to three-quarters of diabetes patients with lipoprotein abnormalities die of coronary artery disease at rates three to five times that of people without diabetes.

Moreover, compared with the general population, people with diabetes have more than twice the rate of hypertension and, at the same level of serum cholesterol, are three to five times more likely to develop coronary atherosclerosis. There is no question that diabetes is a significant added risk factor for atherosclerotic CVD.

Although there has been an explosion of knowledge about the cellular and molecular biology of atherosclerosis during the past decade, scientists know very little about how diabetes complicates the process or how to reduce the added effects of diabetes. Additional basic research to identify the causative factors and mechanisms that lead to increased atherosclerosis and cardiovascular mortality among people with diabetes urgently needs to be carried out.

In last year's report, the Board provided examples of promising areas of research and urged that $5 million in additional funds be appropriated to the National Heart, Lung, and Blood Institute (NHLBI) and the NIDDK to support a joint research program on the etiology and pathogenesis of atherosclerosis in diabetes. The NIDDK and the NHLBI also cosponsored a workshop on Diabetes and Mechanisms of Atherogenesis in 1992 where experts discussed scientific advances in vascular biology, lipid metabolism, thrombosis, and other areas that may contribute to understanding the interaction of atherosclerosis and diabetes. Several areas of basic and clinical science were identified for emphasis in future research such as molecular and cellular studies of the mechanisms that underlie the accelerated atherosclerosis seen in diabetes. The NIDDK and the NHLBI will continue to collaborate in these areas in the future.

The Board recommends that an additional $5 million be appropriated to the National Institute of Diabetes and Digestive and Kidney Diseases and the National Heart, Lung, and Blood Institute for a joint basic research program on the etiology and pathogenesis of atherosclerosis in diabetes.

Research Training

The future of diabetes research depends on the availability of biomedical scientists who are trained and experienced in this area. However, the number of qualified scientists with either a Ph.D. or an M.D. degree interested in pursuing careers in diabetes research is falling sharply. The number of applications for individual fellowships and career development awards in diabetes fell by *60 percent* between 1980 and 1990. This decline comes at a time when research discoveries in diabetes and related areas of medical science offer the potential for tremendous benefits and cost savings to society.

The Board recognizes that NIH support for research training has been reduced throughout all Institutes over the past 20 years. However, diabetes research training has been especially hard hit. To some degree, this decline reflects the fact that recent trainees are more concerned with fundamental biological questions than with disease-specific research. Similarly, the declining numbers of new physician-scientists can be attributed to a lack of exposure to diabetes issues in their formative career years as well as to the greater financial rewards for physicians who pursue clinical careers.

An aggressive approach to the diabetes research manpower problem is needed. Because most scientists are likely to continue their research careers in the same general area in which they were trained, the NIH must initiate funding mechanisms to attract Ph.D. and physician-scientists to diabetes-related areas of research early in their academic careers. With this in mind, the Board proposes two programs, both focused on the predoctoral level.

To train basic scientists for diabetes research, the Board recommends that the National Institute of Diabetes and Digestive and Kidney Diseases award grants to research institutions for predoctoral training of Ph.D. candidates in diabetes and related scientific disciplines. At least 10 such grants should be awarded. The Board recommends that Congress provide an additional $1.5 million in FY 1994 to initiate the diabetes Ph.D. training program. This appropriation should be increased to $3.1 million in FY 1995 and $4.8 million in FY 1996.

To attract physician-scientists into diabetes research, the Board recommends that the National Institute of Diabetes and Digestive and Kidney Diseases establish a training and career development program for medical students. The program should allow for 75 positions (25 new students per year for 3 years). The Board recommends that Congress provide an additional $1.25 million in FY 1994 to initiate the diabetes physician-scientist training program. This appropriation should be increased to $1.75 million in FY 1995 and $2.25 million in FY 1996.

Diabetes is recognized as a severe and growing health problem among minority populations, yet there is an acute shortage of minority scientists with career training in diabetes. The Board recognizes that the NIH has attempted to address this problem by developing programs that provide incentives and opportunities for minority research scientists and laboratories that recruit them. However, the effectiveness of these programs is hampered by several factors: (1) the limited number of minority applicants, (2) greater incentives for minorities as for all scientists to work in private industry or private practice, and (3) the overall decrease in interest in disease-specific research. The Board will continue to support NIH efforts to increase the participation of minorities in research programs and will make appropriate recommendations on minority research training as needed in the future.

Chapter 52

Advancing The Frontiers Of Diabetes Research And Treatment

by Calvin Pierce

Insulin-dependent diabetes, known for centuries as a potentially life-threatening condition, is finally giving up its secrets. Scientists are uncovering the mechanisms that cause diabetes, testing new drugs that may slow or even prevent the disease process, and developing new transplantation methods for treating diabetes. As investigators push forward in each of these areas, the goal of conquering diabetes continues to get closer.

Researchers at the University of Florida in Gainesville are helping pinpoint the genetic and autoimmune mechanisms that contribute to insulin-dependent (type I) diabetes. Led by Dr. Noel K. Maclaren, professor and chairman of the department of pathology, the researchers are developing screening tests that may help identify the one in 300 people who will later develop diabetes. Effective screening could make it possible eventually to intervene to prevent the onset of clinical diabetes, Dr. Maclaren says.

The work by the Florida investigators builds on a growing body of evidence that an autoimmune process is involved in the early stages of type I diabetes. At one time it was thought that diabetes arose suddenly as a result of an infection or a toxic chemical, since symptoms typically develop in a matter of days or weeks. But in the last two decades it has become clear that diabetes develops slowly, smoldering for years before the disease is diagnosed. "It's a completely different way of looking at the disease," Dr. Maclaren says.

In diabetes insulin-producing "beta-cells" in pancreatic islets are at-

National Center for Research Resources Reporter, April 1991.

tacked by the immune system. Insulin is a hormone crucial to the body's ability to make glucose in the blood available to tissues. As more and more beta-cells succumb to immunologic attack, a critical stage is eventually reached: the few beta-cells that remain cannot produce enough insulin to control blood sugar levels and maintain normal metabolism. Once diabetes is diagnosed, daily insulin injections are usually needed to prevent lethal elevations of blood sugar. Even with insulin therapy, however, patients often develop serious complications caused by damage to blood vessels, including stroke, heart disease, kidney failure, or blindness.

In the 1970's researchers found that many patients with newly diagnosed diabetes have self-directed antibodies, or autoantibodies, targeted at beta-cells and at insulin. "In the 'dark ages' when these antibodies were first being described, the focus was on trying to prove that the process was an autoimmune one," Dr. Maclaren says. "It took until the next decade before we began to wonder seriously how long these markers had been present" before the disease was diagnosed, he recalls.

Additional diabetes-related autoantibodies were discovered during the 1980's. Meanwhile, studies of relatives of diabetic patients showed that immunologic markers are present many years before the disease becomes apparent. There is now considerable evidence that the presence of such autoantibodies in nondiabetic people is a marker that predicts an increased risk of developing diabetes.

Dr. William Riley, a pediatrician in the University's department of pathology, worked with Dr. Maclaren's laboratory and with researchers at other medical centers in a decade-long study of more than 4,000 nondiabetic relatives of patients; most of the patients had developed insulin-dependent diabetes before age 21. Islet cell antibodies were present in the initial blood samples of 3 percent of the relatives. Of the 40 relatives who developed diabetes during followup, 32 had been positive initially for islet cell antibodies or had become positive by the time diabetes was diagnosed. The risk of diabetes was greatest for relatives who had the highest initial islet cell autoantibody levels, according to the researchers.

Dr. Mark Atkinson, another of Dr. Maclaren's associates at the University of Florida, has found evidence that a beta-cell protein having a molecular weight of 64,000 (64K) daltons may be the primary target of the autoimmune process. Blood tests for the anti-64K autoantibody showed that it was usually present in patients with diabetes and in high-risk relatives of diabetic patients. Relatives who tested positive for islet cell or insulin autoantibodies were considered high risk. The anti-64K autoantibodies were not found in any of the normal control subjects and were found only rarely in low-risk relatives of diabetic patients. In many of the subjects the anti-64K autoantibody was detected years before diabetes was diagnosed.

The function of the 64K protein in islet beta-cells is not known. Recently, however, the protein has been shown to be related to the enzyme glutamic acid decarboxylase, which promotes conversion of glutamic acid into the neurotransmitter called GABA. The Florida scientists believe that the anti-64K autoantibody may be the earliest and perhaps the best marker for impending diabetes yet found. Unfortunately, the method now used to detect this autoantibody is cumbersome and expensive. The assay, which currently depends on extraction of the 64K protein from islet cells, must be simplified if it is to be useful as a screening tool, Dr. Maclaren says. Researchers hope to determine the structure of the 64K protein and use recombinant DNA methods to produce large amounts of the protein.

Despite the apparent importance of the anti-64K autoantibody, efficient screening for diabetes is likely to involve tests for several different autoantibodies. The autoantibodies tend to appear in a sequence over several years, so tests may be selected according to the age of the person being screened, he says.

The risk of developing diabetes is influenced by genetic factors, particularly the genes coding for certain major histocompatibility complex (MHC) proteins. These cell surface proteins help the immune system distinguish the body's own normal cells from abnormal or foreign cells and microorganisms and are usually involved in cellular immune responses to bacteria, viruses, or other pathogens. The specific MHC proteins in patients with diabetes appear to contribute to abnormal activation of white blood cells that attack the beta-cells. In addition, a genetic defect in the immune system appears to prevent suppression of this immune response.

Genetic tests are unlikely to be useful for general screening, in part because the genetic studies are much more expensive than testing for autoantibodies. Another problem is that genes associated with diabetes are common even in people who never get the disease. "We know a lot about the genetics, and we know a lot about the process that causes the beta-cells to die. What we don't know is why only relatively few individuals with the genetic predisposition actually start the disease process," Dr. Maclaren says. Even in identical twins of whom one twin has diabetes, diabetes will develop in the other twin in only a minority of cases. "There must be some happenstance that we have not understood that triggers the disease," he says.

It appears that an infection or some other environmental factor is involved in the onset of type I diabetes. The Florida researchers suspect that the autoimmune process may be triggered in genetically susceptible people by a foreign protein introduced by an infection. The foreign protein may closely resemble a beta-cell protein, perhaps the 64K protein. This molecular mimicry may fool the immune system into carrying out a misguided attack against the body's own beta-cells. Such mimicry is known to be involved in other autoimmune disorders, including the rheumatic heart disease that can occur after a streptococcal throat infection, Dr. Maclaren notes.

Although molecular mimicry is a reasonable theory, "we're missing one piece of the puzzle—we haven't identified what the trigger is," Dr. Maclaren says. The search continues for a virus or other pathogen involved in the onset of diabetes. Once researchers know the amino acid sequence of the 64K protein—or perhaps some other protein that serves as the initial target of the autoimmune process—that sequence can be matched against the sequences of proteins produced during known infections. If an infection does trigger the autoimmune response, "we have to presume that it's something that's fairly common," he says. In theory, preventing the initial infection would prevent diabetes from developing later in life.

The Florida researchers, led by Dr. Riley and Dr. Jeff Krischer, are directing a multicenter clinical trial aimed at using the new knowledge about diabetes to prevent the disease in high-risk individuals with early signs of diabetes. In Gainesville, Boston, Denver, and Seattle investigators plan to screen up to 12,000 close relatives of patients with insulin-dependent diabetes. Some of the screening will be conducted at the University of Florida's General Clinical Research Center in Gainesville. The goal is to find about 100 subjects (mostly children and young adults) who test positive for islet cell autoantibodies and have decreased insulin production. "It's a completely different approach to diabetes," Dr. Riley says. "In the past, we've used insulin to treat the symptoms but have not treated the disease itself. What we're trying to do is get at the disease cause."

The subjects, who have approximately an 80-percent risk of becoming diabetic within 3 years, will be treated twice daily with an immunosuppressive drug called Imuran. In preliminary studies the Florida researchers found that Imuran protected beta-cells from further destruction in newly diagnosed diabetes patients. "We think it will almost certainly work to prevent or delay onset of diabetes," Dr. Maclaren says. In fact, daily treatment with the drug appears to have prevented diabetes in a 21-year-old Gainesville woman in whom marker antibodies for diabetes were detected 5 years ago.

The youngest subjects in the trial will be 7 years old. If the treatment proves useful it will later be used to treat even younger children at risk for diabetes. "The real tragedy is children who develop diabetes when they are 4 to 5 years old," Dr. Riley says. These children tend to develop the most severe complications of diabetes as they grow up, often needing kidney transplants by the time they reach their thirties.

Immunosuppressive therapy may be able to slow the disease process, but it has drawbacks. Currently available broad-acting drugs suppress the entire immune system and must be continued indefinitely; this exposes the patient to a potentially increased risk of infection and cancer. Although Imuran appears to be relatively safe in this regard, it will take years to determine whether the advantages of such therapy outweigh its disadvantages, Dr. Maclaren says. The Florida researchers hope that within the next 10 years it will be possible to design selective immunosuppressive agents that will eliminate only the small number of white blood cells that attack the beta-cells.

Researchers are studying other ways to block the autoimmune process in diabetes. One approach might be to use insulin therapy before the disease starts in an effort to prevent beta-cells from expressing molecules that provoke the immune reaction. Results from animal studies suggest, however, that this would require impractically high insulin doses. Another method might be to develop medications that scavenge the cell-destroying superoxides produced by white blood cells in connection with an autoimmune attack, since beta-cells cannot protect themselves against these compounds. In addition, there is evidence that dietary therapy, particularly protein restriction, could be used to modify insulin secretion and slow the disease process, Dr. Maclaren says.

Until specific preventive therapy becomes available, the most direct way to treat diabetes may be to transplant islets from cadavers. This approach has been limited, however, by inability to collect and transplant enough islets and by rejection of the donor islets by the recipient. Scientists at Washington University School of Medicine in St. Louis, Missouri, are developing methods to make islet transplantation a practical treatment for diabetes and to prevent the rejection process. Under the direction of Dr. Paul E. Lacy, the Robert L. Kroc Professor of Pathology, the researchers have developed new ways to isolate and store islets and have found that the rejection process is started by white blood cells present in donor islets.

The next step, now being tested in animal models, is to find ways to block the rejection process. "The key is to be able to transplant early in the course of diabetes, in the hope that the complications of the disease may be prevented, and to do it without continuous immunosuppression," Dr. Lacy says.

The potential value of islet transplantation was shown by Washington University surgeon Dr. David W. Scharp. In collaboration with Dr. Lacy, Dr. Scharp has performed 11 islet cell transplantations in a recent series of patients who had established kidney transplants and were already on immunosuppressive therapy. Nearly a million islets were isolated from cadaver donors using a low-temperature culture method and a cryopreservation process that allows islets from more than one donor to be collected and stored. Under local anesthesia, the islets were infused into the portal vein leading into the liver of patients at the university's General Clinical Research Center. One patient, who had had insulin-dependent diabetes for more than 30 years, has been able to stop insulin therapy for more than 9 months after receiving an islet transplant. Another patient was able to stop insulin therapy for several weeks. Such preliminary but encouraging results mark the first step toward determining whether islet transplantation is feasible, Dr. Scharp says.

Next, the investigators plan to transplant islets into patients who are simultaneously receiving a kidney transplant. "Right now we're only offering islet transplantation to patients with end-stage, multiorgan disease because we don't understand all the risk-benefit ratios yet," Dr. Scharp explains. "We hope to be able to expand these trials in the future to patients who are not immunosuppressed" by using new techniques that are being developed by Dr. Lacy and other scientists to prevent rejection, he says.

Widespread use of islet transplants could be limited by the inadequate supply of pancreases. There are about 2 million patients with insulin-dependent diabetes, but only 4,000 organ donors are available each year. Because islets are such a scarce resource, the St. Louis investigators distribute some of the islets they collect to about 30 other research centers. According to the researchers, the best prospect for expanding the supply of islets is to use an animal donor, perhaps the pig, together with techniques to prevent rejection. It is also possible to culture human fetal islet cells for transplantation, but Federal research in that area is banned, the investigators note.

Searching for ways to prevent islet rejection without immunosuppressive drugs, Dr. Lacy and his colleagues have found that macrophages and lymphocytes in islets from donor rats provoke an immune reaction in recipient rats. Altering or destroying these lymphoid cells in the donor islets can prevent rejection of islets transplanted from one strain of rat into another. Maintaining islets in low-temperature culture for several days, for example, causes islet lymphocytes to disappear and reduces the rejection response in recipient rats.

The St. Louis investigators recently showed that rejection is delayed when rat islet cells are treated with a substance called transforming growth factor—beta (TGF-beta) before being transplanted into diabetic mice. The researchers also combined TGF-beta treatment of the donor islets and treatment of the recipient mouse with a monoclonal antibody that blocks gamma-interferon. The combined treatment prevented islet rejection, producing indefinite survival of the transplanted islets. About half of the recipient mice actually became immunologically tolerant of the donated islets, showing no rejection of a later transplant of untreated rat islets from the same donor strain. Although it is not yet clear how TGF-beta and gamma-interferon prevent islet rejection both substances are known to influence immune function.

In future studies "we'll take the procedures used to prevent islet rejection in animals and see if we can use them to prevent human islet rejection without the continuous need for immunosuppression," Dr. Lacy explains. In initial human studies "we'll go first to the simplest procedures possible," including low-temperature culture of islets. Cryopreservation of islets from multiple human donors will minimize the immune reaction against islets from any single donor. Antilymphocyte antibody and the immunosuppressive drug cyclosporine also will be used for a short time to block rejection following transplantation.

If successful, such highly selective immunosuppressive therapy could obviate the need for potentially toxic, long-term immunosuppression. "We think, although we cannot prove it yet, that suppressor lymphocytes or mechanisms that cause immune unresponsiveness are reduced by conventional immunosuppressants. We don't want to give broad-acting agents that kill off all lymphocytes—we may be killing the ones we want," Dr. Lacy explains.

It should be clear within approximately 2 years whether this selective antirejection approach is effective. "If it doesn't work, then we'll add in other procedures" now being studied in animals, such as ultraviolet irradiation of islets or encapsulating islets to isolate them from the recipient's immune system. "On the basis of the animal work, I think there's a good chance of success, although it may take a while" to find the right combination of methods, Dr. Lacy says.

Another way to prevent islet rejection is under investigation by researchers at the University of Pennsylvania in Philadelphia. A team led by transplant surgeon and immunologist Dr. Ali Naji transplanted islets into the thymus of rats together with antibodies directed against the type of lymphocytes called T-cells. The transplanted islets survived indefinitely without the use of immunosuppressive therapy.

The key to this success appears to be the immunologically privileged status of the thymus, the organ where T-lymphocytes mature and learn to recognize foreign substances and to tolerate the particular body's own internal environment, or "self." New T-cells that matured in the presence of the transplanted islets learned to accept the islet cells as "self," according to the investigators. Thus rats that received islet transplants into the thymus did not reject islets that were later transplanted from the same donor into the kidney. Dr. Naji and his associates suggest that the technique could provide a new way to successfully transplant islets. They also speculate that the findings could eventually lead to methods to prevent rejection of other transplanted organs by manipulating immune responses.

Additional Reading:

1. Scharp, D. W., Lacy, P. E., Santiago, J. V., et al., Results of our first nine intraportal islet allografts in type I insulin-dependent diabetic patients. *Transplantation* 51:76–85, 1991.

2. Riley, W. J., Maclaren, N. K., Krischer, J., et al., A prospective study of the development of diabetes in relatives of patients with insulin-dependent diabetes. *New England Journal of Medicine* 323:1167–1172, 1990.

3. Atkinson, M. A., Maclaren, N. K., Scharp, D. W., et al., 64,000 M, autoantibodies as predictors of insulin-dependent diabetes. *Lancet* 335: 1357–1360, 1990.

4. Atkinson, M. A. and Maclaren, N. K., What causes diabetes? *Scientific American* 263:62–71, 1990.

5. Scharp, D. W., Lacy, P.E., Santiago, J. V., et al., Insulin independence after islet transplantation into type I diabetic patient. *Diabetes* 39:515–518, 1990.

6. Carel, J. C., Schreiber, R. D., Falqui, L., and Lacy, P. E., Transforming growth factor-beta decreases the immunogenicity of rat islet xenografts (rat to mouse) and prevents rejection in association with treatment of the recipient with a monoclonal antibody to interferon-gamma. *Proceedings of the National Academy of Science U.S.A.* 87:1591–1595, 1990.

7. Posselt, A. M., Barker, C. F., Tomaszewski, J. E., et al., Induction of donor-specific unresponsiveness by intrathymic islet transplantation. *Science* 249:1293–1295, 1990.

The research described in this article was supported by the General Clinical Research Centers Program of the National Center for Research Resources, the National Institute of Diabetes and Digestive and Kidney Diseases, the National Institute of Allergy and Infectious Diseases, the American Diabetes Association, and the Juvenile Diabetes Foundation.

Chapter 53

Diet and Exercise in Noninsulin-Dependent Diabetes Mellitus

Introduction

Diabetes mellitus is a major health problem. It is a leading cause of death. It is the chief reason for new blindness, kidney failure, and limb amputation. Dialysis for kidney failure from diabetes alone costs over $1 billion annually, and this is expected to double over the next few years. Moreover, diabetes is a major emotional burden for many families.

Noninsulin-dependent diabetes (NIDDM, also called adult-onset or Type II diabetes) affects about 10 million Americans, mid-age or older, or approximately 90 percent of all diabetic people. The cornerstone of therapy is a style of life centered around diet and supplemented, if needed, by insulin or oral agents. With the very high association of NIDDM with overnutrition and overweight (approximately 80 percent of patients), much dietary effort is directed to caloric reduction, with exercise as an auxiliary means to increase caloric loss and to assist in glucose regulation. The therapeutic aim is normalization of blood glucose and lipid levels with the hope of diminishing cardiovascular risk and preventing complications.

There has been much interest in recent years in clarifying the underlying relationships between NIDDM and obesity, heredity, nutrition, physical activity, and other factors. Much has been learned from clinical studies in individuals with and without NIDDM and from parallel studies in experimental animals. However, conflicting claims have emerged for the effectiveness of new dietary strategies and exercise programs. Many of these

---

NIH Consensus Development Conference Statement, Vol. 6, No. 8, December 10, 1986.

have been publicized in the professional and lay literature, and this has caused some concern and confusion. In an effort to resolve this problem, the National Institute of Diabetes and Digestive and Kidney Diseases (NIDDK) and the NIH Office of Medical Applications of Research, in collaboration with Institute National de la Santé et de la Récherche Médicale (INSERM), France, sponsored a Consensus Development Conference on Diet and Exercise in Noninsulin-Dependent Diabetes Mellitus, December 8–10, 1986.

The conference brought together researchers, clinicians, other health professionals, and representatives of the public. Following 2 days of presentations and discussion by invited experts and the audience, a consensus panel, drawn from the health care and diabetes-interested communities, weighed the scientific evidence and formulated a draft statement in response to several questions:

- What is the significance of excess body fat in the patient with noninsulin-dependent diabetes mellitus? How can weight reduction be achieved and maintained?
- What are the appropriate components of the dietary prescription for patients with noninsulin-dependent diabetes mellitus?
- What are the benefits and risks of exercise in patients with noninsulin-dependent diabetes mellitus? How should exercise be prescribed?
- What is the evidence that weight control, diet, and/or exercise can prevent noninsulin-dependent diabetes mellitus?
- What are the directions for future research?

1. What is the significance of excess body fat in the patient with noninsulin-dependent diabetes mellitus? How can weight reduction be achieved and maintained?

There is strong evidence that NIDDM is genetically determined. Based on considerable epidemiologic data, it is apparent that obesity and aging promote the development of the disease in susceptible individuals. The prevalence of the disease increases steadily from the fourth decade. Individuals who are 20 to 30 percent overweight are clearly at an increased risk for NIDDM, and the risk accelerates with increased body weight. Data suggest that in addition to the degree of obesity, an increasing duration of obesity and the specific distribution of excess body fat are associated with the development of NIDDM. With regard to fat distribution, upper body or android obesity appears to be more strongly associated with diabetes than lower body or gynoid obesity. Individuals with a family history of NIDDM may develop the disease when they have only modest excess of body fat. These people should be assessed routinely for the presence of carbohydrate intolerance and encouraged to maintain desirable body weight.

Extensive studies demonstrate that obesity is characterized by insulin resistance. In the obese nondiabetic individual, the principal target tissues for insulin (liver, skeletal muscle, and adipose tissue) do not respond appropriately to those levels of the hormone found in nonobese individuals. The obese nondiabetic person can compensate for this impairment of hormone action by secreting increased amounts of insulin. Weight reduction in these nondiabetic individuals leads to reversal of insulin resistance and the return to a normal pattern of insulin secretion.

Pancreatic beta-cell dysfunction and insulin resistance are the cardinal pathophysiologic features of NIDDM. Both of these cellular alterations may be genetically determined. Although insulin resistance is present in the nonobese patient with NIDDM, associated obesity further aggravates the severity of impaired hormone action. Weight loss in the obese diabetic, as in the nondiabetic, ameliorates insulin resistance, and usually there is accompanying improvement in carbohydrate tolerance. Frequently, hyperglycemia is reduced when a low calorie diet is employed even before there is much weight loss. Furthermore, some studies have also shown modest improvement in beta-cell function when the blood glucose is lowered by diet or other means.

Some investigators are concerned that the hyperinsulinemia in NIDDM may contribute to the increased incidence of macrovascular disease. This possibility arises from the observation that the two most common conditions of hyperinsulinemia (obesity and NIDDM) are independently associated with increased cardiovascular risks. There are also data suggesting that the actions of insulin are not uniformly impaired in hyperinsulinemic states. Thus, it is possible that certain insulin-regulated, atherogenic processes may be accelerated in NIDDM with or without obesity. At present, the relationship between hyperinsulinemia and cardiovascular disease is largely speculative, and more definitive answers await additional investigation.

The cellular mechanisms of insulin action have been partially elucidated. There is universal agreement that insulin initiates its actions by interacting with specific receptors located on the surface of the target cell. The possibility that there is a receptor deficiency in human obesity and NIDDM has been extensively investigated. Most studies have examined the receptor status in readily available circulating monocytes or erythrocytes. The number of insulin receptors is often decreased in these cells, but the relevance of these findings to the major target tissues (liver, muscle, fat) for insulin action is not known. In fact, results of studies of insulin receptors in fat cells from individuals with NIDDM are conflicting, and studies are just emerging using human muscle and liver. The majority of investigators agree that cellular alterations, other than decreased receptor number, contribute to the insulin resistance of both obesity and NIDDM. Current areas of investigation include (1) functions of the insulin receptor subsequent to hormone binding, (2) the glucose transport process in muscle and adipose tissue, and (3) the status of those factors that may be the intracellular mediators of insulin action. Although the cellular alterations responsible for insulin resistance and beta-cell dysfunction in NIDDM are poorly understood, future studies of the beta cell and insulin action should provide new insights into the pathophysiology of this disease.

Blood glucose usually returns toward normal as weight loss occurs in the obese diabetic patient. Weight loss also improves hypertension, hypertriglyceridemia, and hypercholesterolemia. Achieving the goal of desirable weight is not easy. Twenty-five years ago, one-quarter of the patients who needed to lose 20 to 40 pounds were successful, and merely 5 percent lost more than 40 pounds. At that time, weight loss programs generally emphasized moderated caloric restriction and dietary counseling. Recently, several more successful strategies for weight loss have been developed. All these approaches continue to rely on reduced calorie ingestion. Although moderate caloric restriction (500 to 1,000 kcal below daily requirements) is preferred, fasts of several days' duration and very low calorie diets (to 400–600 kcal intake per day) for several weeks have been successfully employed with careful medical supervision.

Other successful programs have utilized support groups, behavioral therapy, and/or exercise in combination with caloric restriction. In recent years, the public has become aware of the health hazards of obesity. Low calorie foods and beverages are readily available, and health clubs exist in many neighborhoods. While all of these benefit those who need or desire to lose weight, weight reduction continues to be difficult. Furthermore, most individuals who lose weight will regain some or all of the lost weight.

A greater understanding and resolution of the pathophysiology and behavioral determinants underlying altered eating behavior are needed. While acknowledging the poor prognosis for weight loss maintenance, the panel recommends that most obese patients with NIDDM be maintained on diets moderately restricted in calories. Ideally, this diet should be associated with behavior therapy, group support, and nutritional counseling. An intensive support program of considerable duration may improve the likelihood of maintaining a desirable weight. Increased physical activity and, if appropriate, structured exercise programs are also considered useful adjunctive therapy.

2. What are the appropriate components of the dietary prescription for patients with noninsulin-dependent diabetes mellitus?

In individuals with NIDDM, the primary goal for treatment is to reduce blood glucose levels to normal. The diet for all persons with NIDDM should be nutritionally sound, and it should satisfy the recommended dietary allowances (RDA) and follow the *Dietary Guidelines For Americans* (Home and Garden Bulletin #232, 2nd Edition, Washington, D.C.: USDA and HHS, 1985). Since most persons with NIDDM have excess body fat, the primary dietary treatment is reduction of weight through caloric restriction. Some people with NIDDM have additional medical problems (e.g., lipoprotein disorders and hypertension) that require additional dietary recommendations.

Calories

A weight-reducing diet should be nutritionally complete, using a variety of foods. Moderate caloric restriction of 500–1,000 kcal below daily requirements may be optimal in producing a gradual sustained weight loss. After the desired weight has been achieved, maintenance of that reduced weight may be sustained by adjusting the caloric intake. With low caloric intake, nutrient deficiencies should be avoided. For lean persons with NIDDM, caloric intake should be adequate to maintain body weight.

Fat and Carbohydrate

A diet reduced in total and saturated fat and cholesterol has been recommended for all Americans to decrease the risk of coronary heart disease (CHD). Patients with NIDDM are at increased risk for CHD by virtue of their diabetes. In addition, they frequently demonstrate blood lipid abnormalities, including reduced high density lipoprotein-cholesterol (HDL-C) and elevated triglyceride concentrations. The initial approach for normalizing serum lipids in the majority of patients with NIDDM is to reduce hyperglycemia because this will frequently increase HDL-C and reduce triglyceride concentrations. High carbohydrate diets (50–60 percent of total calories) may effect these changes in some patients by enhancing insulin sensitivity. When blood glucose is normalized, the panel recommends that patients with NIDDM should further attempt to reduce their risk of CHD by reducing low density lipoprotein-cholesterol. Present recommendations for the general population include a reduction of total fat intake to less than 30 percent of calories, with saturated fat comprising less than 10 percent of total calories. This may be suitable for some but not all NIDDM patients (as discussed below).

A reduction in calories from fat usually requires an increase in calories from carbohydrates. High carbohydrate diets may be harmful in some patients by reducing HDL-C and increasing triglycerides. These diets are less effective than weight loss in normalizing blood glucose and may represent a serious lifestyle alteration for many patients. Consequently, the panel suggests that patients' adherence to a regimen of caloric restriction for weight loss is more important than alterations in the macronutrient composition of the diet. Also, both serum lipid and glucose concentrations should be monitored to determine the effectiveness of any dietary changes.

Other Carbohydrate Issues

Sucrose (table sugar)

In the past, individuals with NIDDM have been advised to avoid sucrose. The use of sucrose as a taste additive in mixed meals is acceptable (up to 5 percent of carbohydrate calorie intake) in patients who are lean and do not have carbohydrate-aggravated hyperlipidemia. The advisability of added sucrose intake above 5 percent of carbohydrate calories requires further investigation.

Fiber

Dietary fiber is plant material that is resistant to enzymes produced by humans. Most Americans consume 13 to 19 grams of dietary fiber per day. Some studies have suggested that dietary fiber is effective in controlling blood glucose and reducing plasma cholesterol, especially when used in very high carbohydrate diets (greater than 50 percent of calories); however, the results of these studies are inconclusive. Furthermore, high fiber diets may be less palatable, may require substantial changes in traditional eating patterns, may have effects on other nutrients, and may be contraindicated in patients with autonomic neuropathy.

Therefore, the panel reaffirms that the primary dietary intervention in NIDDM is weight reduction. However, if individuals desire to increase the fiber content of their diet, foods high in soluble fiber could replace some other carbohydrates. The use of purified fiber supplements is not recommended at this time for diabetes therapy.

Glycemic Index

Individual foods containing carbohydrate can have a high, medium, or low impact on postprandial blood glucose. This response can be quantified as "glycemic index." Several problems have been identified with the application of this methodology to the design of general guidelines of a dietary prescription for patients with NIDDM.

Many factors contribute to a different glycemic response from the same food. These include processing, cooking, and food storage time. Other considerations include the variable degree of mastication in the elderly with dental problems, the diurnal variation in absorption, and racial and ethnic differences. Some studies have shown diminution of glycemic effects when foods are combined in a mixed meal. For these reasons at this time the panel does not recommend the use of specific glycemic indices in the dietary therapy of patients with NIDDM.

Protein

There is no need to change the standard 12 to 20 percent protein content of the diet, providing RDA requirements are met, except in those who have specific problems in which protein intake should be reduced (i.e., in people with NIDDM who have renal disease).

Education

Different educational methods will be appropriate for individual patients and for varying ethnic diets. Whatever plan is used, intensive and frequent follow up and support are needed until fasting euglycemia is achieved and maintained. Behavior modification and exercise may be combined with diet instruction to enhance weight loss efforts. Changes in diet need to be made gradually. No single educational tool can accommodate the needs of all individuals with NIDDM. When diet therapy alone is unsuccessful or unacceptable because of quality of life issues or failure to reduce hyperglycemia, then alternative euglycemic therapy is indicated.

3. What are the benefits and risks of exercise in patients with noninsulin-dependent diabetes mellitus? How should exercise be prescribed?

The effect of regular physical exercise alone on metabolic control in NIDDM is quite variable and frequently of small magnitude. Greater improvement in glucose homeostasis can usually be obtained by weight loss. Despite the relatively small impact of exercise demonstrated to date, regular physical exercise may be a therapeutic component supplementing diet in selected patients.

There is epidemiologic and clinical evidence that physical activity may reduce the incidence of coronary heart disease (CHD) in the general population. The risk-benefit ratio of exercise in NIDDM remains to be defined. Because many of the complications of NIDDM are related to atherosclerotic cardiovascular disease, an increase in physical activity for NIDDM patients appears prudent. This recommendation is made despite the absence of conclusive studies and with recognition that improvements in CHD risk factors may not occur in those with NIDDM. Furthermore, the consensus panel seeks to emphasize that the possible benefits of body fat reduction outweigh putative exercise effects.

Vigorous exercise appears to blunt the rise in blood glucose that follows carbohydrate ingestion. In addition, exercise training may increase insulin sensitivity, but this change appears to be an acute effect associated with recent exercise and is reversed within 2 to 3 days by physical inactivity. Physical activity may assist in reducing body fat, but exercise without caloric restriction appears ineffective. Patients who exercise regularly may negate its weight-reducing effects by curtailing their usual activities and by increasing caloric intake.

Complications of exercise in NIDDM patients include cardiac events (infarction, arrhythmias, and sudden death), bone and soft tissue injuries, and retinal damage in patients—particularly with proliferative retinopathy. The incidence of these complications with exercise has not been defined.

NIDDM patients should undergo a thorough medical evaluation prior to increasing physical activity. The components of the evaluation will vary depending on the severity and duration of the diabetes, the presence of complications, the likelihood of asymptomatic CHD, and the intensity of the activity.

Because of the possible risks of retinal detachment and vitreous hemorrhage during exercise in patients with retinopathy, exercise that requires straining and breath holding (such as weight lifting) should be discouraged. Special attention should also be given to care of the feet during exercise.

In planning and recommending an exercise program for NIDDM patients, health professionals should be aware of several factors. The threshold of energy expenditure required to reduce postprandial hyperglycemia and to enhance insulin sensitivity has not been defined. The same holds true for the use of physical activity in lowering the incidence of CHD. The panel believes that NIDDM patients should tailor an increase in their overall physical activity to their physical capacity, preferences, age, and lifestyle. Also, because many of the metabolic effects of exercise are short-lived, it is extremely important that NIDDM patients choose exercises that they are likely to engage in frequently and continue over their lifetimes.

4. What is the evidence that weight control, diet, and/or exercise can prevent noninsulin-dependent diabetes mellitus?

Approximately 80 percent of persons with NIDDM have excess body fat. Cross-sectional population-based studies show that the prevalence of NIDDM increases with increasing body weight and that the risk of NIDDM is particularly high among obese persons with a family history of this disorder. These relationships suggest that avoidance or elimination of obesity in people whose relatives have NIDDM may delay or prevent the development of NIDDM. Weight reduction is best achieved through the use of hypocaloric diets. In normal weight people, there is no evidence that manipulation of dietary constituents (e.g., reducing refined carbohydrates or increasing complex carbohydrates or increasing dietary fiber) influences the risk of NIDDM. The possibility that exercise may prevent NIDDM is suggested by the observation that prolonged strenuous exercise in individuals with NIDDM may normalize fasting blood glucose and glucose tolerance.

However, there are as yet no irrefutable data to demonstrate that weight control, dietary modification, or exercise are effective in preventing or delaying NIDDM. Nevertheless, in the opinion of the panel, it is prudent to maintain or achieve normal body weight in an attempt to minimize the risk of NIDDM in susceptible persons.

5. What are the directions for future research?

Many of the issues discussed in this consensus conference need further research in laboratory, clinic, and community-based settings. The following major topics are suggested:

Questions Related to Obesity

- What is the etiology of the insulin resistance in the obese state?
- What is the etiologic basis of the obesity itself, from genetic, environmental, behavioral, and nutritional aspects?
- What are effective strategies for therapy of the obese state, particularly as it relates to diabetes?

Questions Related to Diabetes and Its Prevention

- What is the etiology of the beta-cell deficiency in NIDDM?
- What is the pathophysiology of the insulin resistance in the diabetic state without obesity?
- What is the nature of the inherited component in NIDDM?
- What is the relative effectiveness of regular physical activity and/or weight control in the prevention and treatment of NIDDM and its complications?
- What are predictors for the eventual development of NIDDM?

Questions Related to Nutrition

- What is the relationship of particular diets such as high carbohydrate diets to glucose and lipid metabolism?
- What are the roles of other dietary alterations such as changes in fiber content, various carbohydrates, and other foods on carbohydrate and lipid homeostasis?
- What are the optimal strategies to improve acceptance of therapeutic regimens?

Questions Related to Exercise

- What are the potential mediators of exercise effects?
- Under what conditions and in which NIDDM patients is exercise likely to be effective in enhancing glucose homeostasis and reducing coronary heart disease?
- Under what conditions is exercise likely to be counterproductive?

Questions Related to Complications

- What are the contributions of hyperinsulinemia, obesity, and glucose control to the risk of complications in NIDDM?
- What are the relationships of the carbohydrate and lipoprotein abnormalities and their treatments to the risk of macrovascular disease in NIDDM?

Conclusion

Noninsulin-dependent diabetes mellitus (NIDDM or Type II diabetes) is a major health problem. It is highly correlated with obesity and, thereby, with overeating. Normal weight maintenance continues as the cornerstone of therapy with oral agents or insulin added, if needed, to maintain blood glucose normal or near normal. For overweight individuals, reduced-calorie diets should be prescribed and attempts made to alter lifestyle within an acceptable degree for any given patient to encourage weight reduction. These alterations include increased physical activity, perhaps as prescribed exercise regimens, with the recognition that exercise alone is usually ineffective for weight loss unless accompanied by an appropriate diet.

Weight loss diminishes hyperglycemia to or toward normal. Exercise itself may have a small but transient direct effect in lowering blood glucose and insulin resistance. Various food combinations, and even different processing or cooking of the same foods, may produce different glucose responses. Incomplete information on these and other factors that affect this phenomenon in individual subjects minimizes the role of the glycemic index in overall diabetes management. Similarly, foods high in soluble fiber may diminish glucose elevation after meals and may be of use in individual patients, but high-fiber foods appear to be less important than adhering to a calorie-restricted diet and achieving weight loss in the obese diabetic person. Approximately four out of five patients with NIDDM are significantly overweight, and the panel's attention was focused on this group throughout its deliberations. Specific recommendations for diet and activity in the normal-weight NIDDM patient were not addressed except for endorsement of a lifestyle that avoids the development of obesity.

Finally, it appears prudent to prevent or reverse obesity, especially in individuals with a family history of diabetes, in the hope that the onset of diabetes may be prevented or postponed.

Members of the consensus development panel were:

George F. Cahill, Jr., M.D.
Panel Chairman
Vice President
Howard Hughes Medical Institute
Bethesda, Maryland

Elsworth R. Buskirk, Ph.D.
Professor of Applied Physiology
Pennsylvania State University
University Park, Pennsylvania

Linda M. Delahanty, M.S., R.D.
Clinical Nutrition Specialist
Massachusetts General Hospital
Department of Dietetics
Boston, Massachusetts

Stefan S. Fajans, M.D.
Professor of Internal Medicine
Chief
Division of Endocrinology and Metabolism
University of Michigan Medical Center
Ann Arbor, Michigan

James B. Field, M.D.
Rutherford Professor of Medicine
Baylor College of Medicine
Houston, Texas

Harmon E. Holverson, M.D.
Diplomate, ABFP
Private Practice
Emmett, Idaho

Joan Williams Hoover
Director
Consumer Health Information
United Seniors Consumer Cooperative
Washington, D.C.

Ralph I. Horwitz, M.D.
Associate Professor of Medicine and Epidemiology
Yale University School of Medicine
New Haven, Connecticut

Kathryn Iacocca Hentz
President
Iacocca Foundation
New York, New York

John M. Lachin, Sc.D.
Professor of Statistics
Codirector, Biostatistics Center
Department of Statistics, Computer
and Information Systems
George Washington University
Rockville, Maryland

Dean H. Lockwood, M.D.
Professor of Medicine
Head
Endocrine Metabolism Unit
University of Rochester Medical Center
Rochester, New York

F. John Service, M.D., Ph.D.
Professor of Medicine
Mayo Medical School
Consultant in Endocrinology and Metabolism
Mayo Clinic
Rochester, Minnesota

Paul D. Thompson, M.D.
Associate Professor of Medicine
Brown University Program in Medicine
Miriam Hospital
Providence, Rhode Island

Madelyn L. Wheeler, M.S., R.D.
Coordinator Research Dietetics
Diabetes Research and Training Center
Indiana University Medical Center
Indianapolis, Indiana

Members of the planning committee were:

George F. Cahill, Jr., M.D.
Panel Chairman
Vice President
Howard Hughes Medical Institute
Bethesda, Maryland

Eveline Eschwege, M.D., M.P.H.
Directeur de l'Unité de Recherches Statistiques
INSERM
Villejuif
FRANCE

Phillip Gorden, M.D.
Director
National Institute of Diabetes and Digestive and
Kidney Diseases
National Institutes of Health
Bethesda, Maryland

Van S. Hubbard, M.D., Ph.D.
Director

Nutrient Metabolism
Obesity, Eating Disorders, and Energy
Regulation Programs
Division of Digestive Diseases and Nutrition
National Institute of Diabetes and Digestive and Kidney Diseases
National Institutes of Health
Bethesda, Maryland

F. Xavier Pi-Sunyer, M.D.
Director
Division of Endocrinology and Diabetes
St. Luke's - Roosevelt Hospital Center
Associate Professor of Medicine
Columbia University
New York, New York

Martin Rose, M.D., J.D.
Chief Medical Officer
Office of the Director
Office of Medical Applications of Research
National Institutes of Health
Bethesda, Maryland

Robert Sherwin, M.D.
Associate Professor of Medicine
Yale University School of Medicine
New Haven, Connecticut

Robert E. Silverman, M.D., Ph.D.
Chairperson
Chief
Diabetes Programs Branch
Division of Diabetes, Endocrinology, and Metabolic Diseases
National Institute of Diabetes and Digestive and
Kidney Diseases
National Institutes of Health
Bethesda, Maryland

Simeon I. Taylor, M.D., Ph.D.
Senior Investigator
Diabetes Branch

National Institute of Diabetes and Digestive and Kidney Diseases
National Institutes of Health
Bethesda, Maryland

Georges Tchobroutsky, M.D.
Professor
University Pierre et Marie Curie
Head
Department of Diabetology
Hotel-Dieu Hospital
Paris
FRANCE

Judith Wylie-Rosett, Ed.D.
Assistant Professor
Epidemiology and Social Medicine
Albert Einstein College of Medicine
Bronx, New York

Michael J. Bernstein
Director of Communications
Office of Medical Applications of Research
National Institutes of Health
Bethesda, Maryland

Charlotte Armstrong
Public Affairs Specialist
National Institute of Diabetes and Digestive and
Kidney Diseases
National Institutes of Health
Bethesda, Maryland

The conference was sponsored by:

National Institute of Diabetes and Digestive and Kidney Diseases
Phillip Gorden, M.D.
Director

NIH Office of Medical Applications of Research
Itzhak Jacoby, Ph.D.
Acting Director

Chapter 54

Implantable Insulin Pumps

An implanted programmable insulin pump may help people with insulin-dependent diabetes mellitus (IDDM) control their diabetes better and more conveniently. The pump, which was developed at the Johns Hopkins University in Baltimore, Maryland, is nicknamed PIMS-programmable implantable medication system—and works by delivering insulin automatically from an internal reservoir according to programming stored in its microprocessor.

About the size and shape of a hockey puck, PIMS is implanted in the left side of the abdomen. A catheter runs from the pump to the peritoneal space, where the insulin is actually released. "There is evidence that intraperitoneally released insulin is preferentially absorbed into the portal blood circulation system, which is similar to insulin delivery in a nondiabetic person," says principal investigator Dr. Christopher Saudek, director of the Johns Hopkins General Clinical Research Center. "This delivery site may simulate natural insulin delivery better than insulin delivery via veins."

So far, Dr. Saudek and his colleagues have implanted PIMS in 18 patients; 10 at Johns Hopkins and 8 at the University of California at Irvine. The first pump was implanted in 1986. The operation is performed under general anesthesia, although Dr. Saudek believes it might one day be done under local anesthesia. No surgical or skin complications have been seen.

Patients enrolled in this initial study of PIMS had to have insulin-dependent diabetes that was controlled successfully by insulin for at least 1 year, according to registered nurse Michelle Rubio, who worked on the

---

Research Resources Reporter, July 1990.

project at Hopkins as a research nurse before taking her current position as a diabetes educator at the Good Samaritan Hospital in Baltimore. "The patient had to have IDDM because we didn't want competitiveness between insulin made by the patient and that released by the pump," she says. "But sometime in the future we might also be able to use an implantable pump for patients with type II (non-insulin-dependent) diabetes."

Once in place, the pump was programmed to deliver insulin at the level the patient required before surgery. "The physician programs the basal rate, that is, how much insulin is delivered basally over a 24-hour period, and what we call 'prandial command' options, which are used by the patients at mealtimes to tell the pump how much insulin to deliver over a specified period of time at a specified rate," explains Dr. Saudek. "The patient can communicate with the pump via an external transmitter held over the pump itself to select the proper prandial command, to turn off the pump, or to change a command midway, but the basal rate the physician has programmed will recycle every 24 hours." This system of programming appears to work well. Data collected during the study showed that there were no severe hypoglycemic reactions or episodes of diabetic ketoacidosis—an accumulation of certain toxic metabolites in the blood. Good glycemic control was established with significantly reduced blood glucose fluctuations.

Dr. Saudek attributes much of the success of PIMS to the special type of insulin used in its reservoir. "Ever since pumps were developed, the insulin has aggregated in the lines," he says. "With an external pump that just means you have to change the catheter, but with this pump it means surgery. Our insulin contains a special surfactant (a compound that reduces surface tension) to keep it from aggregating." In addition, this is a much more concentrated insulin preparation, which allows the pump reservoir to be smaller and refills to be less frequent. According to Ms. Rubio, "Refills were one of the things the patients complained about—even having to come in only once every 2 months for a refill was something they'd like to see reduced. But imagine how much more often they'd have to come in if they used a less concentrated insulin."

Refilling the pump is actually a relatively simple procedure, but it does require aseptic conditions. After the skin over the pump is cleaned, a needle is inserted into the pump reservoir to withdraw the old insulin, and then the new insulin is put in. "This brings up one of the special features of this pump," says Dr. Saudek. "Since you are dealing with as much as 4,000 units of insulin, you must be very careful not to get any into the body outside the reservoir. The insulin reservoir is maintained at less than atmospheric pressure through a special diaphragm separating it from a Freon-filled chamber. Unless the needle is firmly in the reservoir, no insulin will flow into it. You don't inject the insulin at all—it flows in when the needle is in the proper place and exposed to the negative pressure, so there's no chance of getting the insulin into the wrong place." The entire procedure takes about 15 minutes. Although the procedure is not technically demanding, Dr. Saudek does not believe patients can be trained to do their own refills at home, unless trade-offs are made by using less concentrated insulin and refilling more often.

Another feature of the pump is its ability to store information. The device contains eight integrated circuit chips, including a microprocessor, and a total of 3,000 bytes of memory. "You can retrieve information from the pump that indicates how much insulin has been delivered daily for the last 60 days or an hourly delivery record for the last 21 days by placing a communications head attached to a computer over the pump," says Ms. Rubio. "I could tell right away if the patients went off their diets, because their insulin requirements were greater—but I also knew how closely each patient's diabetes was being controlled." PIMS is quite reliable; only one pump has malfunctioned because of a manufacturing defect.

So far, the major problem with the pump has been blockage of the insulin delivery catheter by fatty tissue, called omental tissue, normally found in the peritoneum. During the initial 2-year followup of PIMS four patients developed catheter blockage. Two of the patients withdrew from the study, and two had their catheters repaired successfully at reoperation. "However, now a little more time has gone by, and we're starting to see more blockage 2 to 3 years after implantation," Dr. Saudek says. "It's clear that this is a common complication that has to be considered. Whether it will turn out that all patients will have the blockage over time, I don't know." One advance in the treatment of blockages is the use of laparoscopy-insertion of a periscope-like instrument through the abdominal wall—which permits the physician to gain access to the catheter through a small incision instead of a large abdominal incision. Laparoscopy results in considerably less trauma for the patient, according to Dr. Saudek.

One other slight problem with PIMS has been initial patient acceptance. Ms. Rubio says that in women, who typically have more abdominal fat than men, the pump is virtually hidden. "But thin men look at themselves after the operation and say, 'Look at that thing—it's huge!' They had some problems with changing body image, but we were able to work through those difficulties."

Even if the problems with blockage and patient acceptance were solved right away, one stumbling block remains before implantable insulin pumps will be *the* way to control diabetes. "A practical glucose sensor for use with the pump is what keeps us from the perfect system—what we call a closed loop system," Dr. Saudek states. PIMS operates now in an open loop fashion; it delivers insulin according to preprogrammed instructions or patient instructions, which occasionally result in errors. A glucose sensor would allow PIMS to measure the amount of blood sugar and automatically adjust the insulin dose correctly, which is what the pancreas does for people who do not have diabetes.

Several hurdles stand in the way of a practical implantable glucose sensor, says Dr. Saudek. "The glucose oxidase system we use to measure blood glucose currently depends upon fresh enzyme and reaction conditions that are simply not compatible with body tissues. Another consideration is how to keep the sensor in the appropriate milieu to reflect blood sugar concentration in the body."

Patients who have PIMS now "close the loop" by measuring their own blood sugar concentrations and giving the pump appropriate instructions. Patients must, therefore, understand and be educated about their diabetes before they can be considered appropriate candidates for PIMS. "Education is the only way to successfully treat diabetes," insists Ms. Rubio. "Once patients are educated about their diabetes, one can teach them control with a variety of therapies—but without education, nothing, including implantable pumps, will work."

Dr. Saudek is about to begin another trial with a slightly modified PIMS. As for the future of implantable programmable insulin pumps, he says, "I would be happy if pumps became a therapeutic option, a choice people could make in consultation with their doctor. It would be wonderful if this approach someday could make life easier and treatment better for people with diabetes."

—M. Elisabeth Tracey

Additional reading:

1. Saudek, C. D., Selam, J. L., Pitt, H. A., Waxman, K., Rubio, M., Jeandidier, N., Turner, D., Fischell, R. E., and Charles, M. A., A preliminary trial of the programmable implantable medication system for insulin delivery. *New England Journal of Medicine* 321:574–579, 1989.

2. Point Study Group, One-year trial of a remote-controlled implantable insulin infusion system in type I diabetic patients. *Lancet* 2:866–869, 1988.

3. Grau, U. and Saudek, C. D., Stable insulin preparation for implanted insulin pumps: Laboratory and animal trials. *Diabetes* 36:1453–1459, 1987.

4. Saudek, C. D., Developing and assessing an implantable insulin infusion pump. *International Journal of Technology Assessment in Health Care* 2:471–482, 1982.

The studies described in this report were supported by the National Institute of Diabetes and Digestive and Kidney Diseases, the General Clinical Research

Centers Program of the National Center for Research Resources, the Orphan Products Program of the Food and Drug Administration, and the Juvenile Diabetes Foundation.

Chapter 55

Muscles Pinpointed As Site Of Diabetic Defect

Persons with non-insulin-dependent diabetes mellitus (NIDDM) convert glucose to its starch-like storage form glycogen at only half the rate of normal individuals, according to scientists at Yale University in New Haven, Connecticut, and the University of Texas Health Science Center in San Antonio. The researchers also report that in both normal and diabetic persons almost all of the glucose to glycogen conversion takes place in the muscles, a finding that confirms earlier conclusions that were based on indirect evidence.

"In the past, no one knew for certain where the glucose went," says Dr. Robert Shulman, professor of molecular biophysics and biochemistry at Yale. "Textbooks usually say that after a meal glucose is stored in the liver as extra glycogen. Other researchers, including our collaborator Dr. Ralph A. DeFronzo, concluded that glucose was not stored primarily in the liver but seemed to go to the rest of the body, presumably muscle."

The new, conclusive results were obtained by nuclear magnetic resonance (NMR) spectroscopy, a technique that enables researchers to monitor the chemical makeup of tissues and detect changes in composition that signal physiologic changes. (For more information about nuclear magnetic resonance spectroscopy, see the *Research Resources Reporter,* January 1990.)

Dr. Robert Shulman, Dr. Gerald I. Shulman, associate professor of medicine at Yale University School of Medicine (not a relative of Dr. Robert Shulman), Dr. DeFronzo, and their colleagues studied a group of 11

Research Resources Reporter, September 1990.

nonobese men. They monitored the metabolism of glucose by the whole body and measured how rapidly glucose was converted to glycogen in the muscles. Glycogen serves as an energy reserve for the body; when needed, it is converted back to glucose, which is "burned" to provide energy for a variety of body functions. The glucose used by the researchers was enriched with the nonradioactive isotope carbon-13 (C-13), which gives an NMR signal. Isotopes are variants of a chemical element, in this case carbon, that have different masses but the same atomic number (for more information about nonradioactive isotopes, see the *Research Resources Reporter,* July 1990).

Five of the 11 men in the study had NIDDM, and 6 were healthy men without a family history of diabetes, who were control subjects. The healthy men were matched in age and weight to the men with NIDDM. The study was conducted in the General Clinical Research Center at Yale, where the diabetic men were hospitalized overnight and given infusions of insulin into an arm vein to normalize the blood glucose level before the study began.

During the study the men were positioned within the NMR spectrometer with a leg resting on a part of the instrument that transmitted and received the NMR signal. Somatostatin, a hormone-like natural compound, was administered to prevent endogenous insulin secretion by the pancreas. The investigators continuously infused insulin and glucose enriched with C-13 to elevate the plasma insulin and glucose concentrations to levels typically observed after a heavy meal. The same high glucose and high insulin levels were maintained in the blood of both control subjects and diabetics. The infusion technique, called a hyperglycemic-hyperinsulinemic clamp, thus permitted measurement of metabolic changes from the same starting points.

By measuring how much glucose was required to maintain the constant blood glucose concentration during the study period (2 hours) the researchers estimated the total glucose metabolism in the body. After correcting this value for glucose that was oxidized, or "burned," to carbon dioxide and exhaled—and a small amount that was excreted in the urine—Dr. Robert Shulman and his colleagues knew the amount of glucose that was metabolized but not oxidized in the body. They found that normal subjects apparently metabolized twice as much glucose per minute as did diabetics. The NMR measurements told them what happened to the glucose. The direct measurement of glycogen synthesis in the leg muscles—measured by quantifying the distinctive C-13 spectrum recorded by the NMR spectrometer—showed that the lower rate of glucose metabolism in diabetic men was due to a lower rate of glycogen synthesis. The rate of glycogen formation in muscles of men with NIDDM was only 40 to 50 percent of the rate of glycogen formation in muscles of healthy men. The results of the study also allowed the investigators to conclude that 70 to 90 percent of the glucose consumed in the body under conditions simulating a meal was stored as muscle glycogen in both the diabetic and healthy men. There was no difference between diabetic and healthy men in the amount of glucose oxidized.

The study provides the first direct demonstration that intravenous glucose disposal is achieved primarily through glycogen synthesis in muscle tissue, says Dr. Gerald Shulman. "Until now we had been able to measure rates of glycogen synthesis only at extremely high glucose levels. At levels close to physiological concentrations it was beyond the capacity of a muscle biopsy, combined with biochemical assays, to detect any increment in the glycogen content of biopsied tissue," he says.

Dr. DeFronzo, now a professor of medicine and chief of the diabetes division at the University of Texas Health Science Center in San Antonio, describes the status of the research before NMR spectroscopy in this way:

"We put catheters into the hepatic vein and into the femoral artery and the femoral vein, and we directly measured the amount of glucose going into the liver and muscles. When glucose was given intravenously, we found that 80 to 90 percent went to muscles. When glucose was given orally, 60 to 70 percent of the glucose entering the gastrointestinal tract was transported to the muscles," he says.

But he and his colleagues were blocked, Dr. DeFronzo says, when they tried to see what happened to the glucose in the muscles. "Was it being oxidized and used for energy? Or was it being converted to glycogen? We suspected it was going to glycogen. But the body's muscle mass is so enormous compared with the amount of glucose going into glycogen that routine biochemical methods could not identify the increase in muscle glycogen concentration."

The solution presented itself, according to Dr. DeFronzo, when they added the skills of Dr. Robert Shulman, who had developed NMR spectroscopy to the point where it could detect very small changes in glycogen concentration. "We went ahead and combined the methodologies," says Dr. DeFronzo.

The University of Texas clinician says there may be two reasons for the slow rate of muscle glycogen synthesis in NIDDM diabetics. "First, we think they may have an inherited defect in glycogen synthase, the enzyme that converts glucose to glycogen. Our preliminary findings in a study of Mexican-American children with a high risk of diabetes supports this concept. There may also be a second defect at one of the very early steps in glucose metabolism—probably in the glucose transport system.

"So there may be two problems. Glucose may not get into the cell normally, and once it gets into the cell, it doesn't get converted to glycogen normally. Both may be reasons why diabetics with NIDDM don't make an appropriate amount of glycogen."

The ability of exercise to speed up the transport of glucose into muscle makes exercise one of the cornerstones, along with diet, of treating NIDDM, Dr. DeFronzo notes. "It's been shown that exercise improves the transport of glucose into muscle cells and activates the glucose transport system, probably in the same fashion that insulin normally does."

Although a diabetic's body responds to exercise, it doesn't respond normally to insulin activation of the glucose transport system, Dr. DeFronzo says. "Insulin resistance is the primary problem for these patients—their muscle tissue does not respond properly to insulin. This is what starts the problem. Later, the liver also fails to respond normally to insulin and begins to overproduce glucose. Thus, decreased glucose uptake by the muscle and excessive glucose production by the liver contribute to the rise in blood glucose level in diabetic patients. Consequently, the beta-cells in the pancreas, which respond to blood glucose levels, are forced to increase their secretion of insulin. And over a period of time the beta-cells—which are continuously overworking—can't keep up this high pace of insulin secretion, and they begin to fail. When the beta- cells start to fail we see overt diabetes," Dr. DeFronzo says.

Dr. DeFronzo plans to pursue research on the genetic origins of diabetes through his study of children and young adult offspring of Mexican-American diabetics. "If both parents have NIDDM, the children have a 70- to 80-percent chance of developing diabetes. We have been studying these children at a time when their glucose tolerance is normal. Nonetheless, with the use of the insulin/glucose clamp technique we can show they are severely insulin resistant. We think the inability to form glycogen may well be the primary inherited defect."

Why diabetics synthesize glycogen so much more slowly than nondiabetics will also be studied further by Dr. Gerald I. Shulman at Yale. "We are hoping to use the NMR technique with Dr. Robert Shulman and Dr. Douglas Rothman to distinguish between the two possibilities: a defect in the delivery of glucose into the muscle cells or a defect in one of the rate-limiting steps in the enzymatic conversion of glucose to glycogen.

"We are hoping that NMR will help us distinguish between these possibilities," Dr. Shulman says.

—Jane Collins

Additional Reading:

1. Shulman, G. I., Rothman, D. L., Jue, T., Stein, P., DeFronzo, R. A., and Shulman, R. G., Quantitation of muscle glycogen synthesis in normal subjects and subjects with noninsulin-dependent diabetes by C-13 nuclear

magnetic resonance spectroscopy. *New England Journal of Medicine* 322: 223–228, 1990.

2. Bogardus, C., Lillioja, S., Stone, K., and Mott, D., Correlation between muscle glycogen synthase activity and in vivo insulin action in man. *Journal of Clinical Investigation* 73:1185–1190, 1984.

3. DeFronzo, R. A., Jacot, E., Jequier, E., Maeder, E., Wahren, J., and Felber, J. P., The effect of insulin on the disposal of intravenous glucose: Results from indirect calorimetry and hepatic and femoral venous catheterization. *Diabetes* 30:1000–1007, 1981.

4. DeFronzo, R. A., Tobin, J. D., and Andres, R., Glucose clamp techniques: A method for quantifying insulin secretion and resistance. *American Journal of Physiology* 237:E214-E223, 1979.

The research described in this article was supported by the National Institute of Diabetes and Digestive and Kidney Diseases and the General Clinical Research Centers Program of the National Center for Research Resources.

Chapter 56

Cytomegalovirus in Diabetics

Dormant cytomegalovirus (CMV) may be present in the pancreas of individuals with non-insulin-dependent diabetes mellitus (NIDDM), according to investigators at the Research Institute of Scripps Clinic in La Jolla, California. The researchers found CMV-specific nucleic acid in postmortem specimens of pancreatic tissue from adults with NIDDM. Specimens from nondiabetic age- and sex-matched control individuals did not show the CMV-associated nucleic acid footprint.

"This is the first evidence of cytomegalovirus nucleic acid sequences in pancreatic tissue from diabetics," says Dr. Michael B. A. Oldstone, head of the virology division in the department of neuropharmacology at the Research Institute of Scripps Clinic. "What this might mean in the etiology of NIDDM we don't know; it could be a coincidence, but we think it would be worthwhile to evaluate that."

Dr. Oldstone and coinvestigator Dr. J. Matthias Löhr extracted RNA from 82 paraffin-embedded or fresh-frozen pancreatic specimens and found that the specimens from 14 of 32 (44 percent) diabetic patients reacted positively with specific probes for human CMV gene products; 1 of 50 non-diabetic control specimens gave a positive reaction. Dr. Oldstone notes that the new evidence is consistent with his hypothesis that certain viruses can exist symbiotically in cells and alter the cellular function—in this case by reducing the islet cells' normal production of insulin.

Cytomegalovirus infections are common in the United States and elsewhere; antibody to CMV is present in 80 percent of individuals who are over

---

National Center for Research Resources *Reporter*, December 1991.

35 years old. Infections appear to be most serious in the fetus and in newborn infants affected by cytomegalic inclusion disease, as well as in immunosuppressed persons such as transplant recipients, persons with AIDS, and immunosuppressed cancer patients, according to experts in viral infections. "After active infection, the CMV itself can be found in a latent state in peripheral blood mononuclear cells (monocytes and lymphocytes)," Dr. Oldstone says.

Drs. Oldstone and Löhr made molecular probes of complementary DNA (cDNA) for several viruses (human CMV, which is a double-stranded DNA herpesvirus, and RNA viruses like mumps, rubella, and coxsackie) that had been shown in vitro to replicate in the insulin-producing islet cells of the pancreas or were known to infect islet cells during acute infection. The investigators then extracted RNA from the pancreatic specimens of the diabetic and nondiabetic individuals and used molecular biology techniques to analyze the pancreatic RNA for a relationship to the suspect viruses. Evidence of human CMV was found only in material from diabetic individuals. The tissues positive for CMV gene expression were negative for mumps, rubella, and coxsackie viral nucleic acids.

Despite clear evidence of CMV in the specimens of diabetic pancreases, the investigators found no inflammatory cells in the islets of Langerhans nor any structural abnormalities or injuries in the islet cells or elsewhere in the pancreas when the tissues were examined by light microscopy.

Dr. Oldstone says that "the virus might compromise the machinery that produces insulin but not enough to cause disease. The addition of other factors—a sublethal dose of a toxin, dietary factors, or the presence of other viruses—together with persistent CMV virus in the islet cells, might produce NIDDM. Cumulatively, they might bring insulin production lower until the clinical disorder would become apparent." This cumulative effect of several environmental agents, including viruses, has been observed to cause diabetes experimentally, he adds.

In addition to the NIDDM specimens studied, Drs. Oldstone and Löhr also studied a limited number of tissue specimens from persons who had insulin-dependent, or type I, diabetes mellitus. In this limited sample none showed evidence of genetic information from CMV, he says.

—Jane Collins

Additional Reading:

1. Löhr, J. M. and Oldstone, M. B. A., Detection of cytomegalovirus nucleic acid sequences in pancreas in type 2 diabetes. *Lancet* 336:644–648, 1990.

2. Oldstone, M. B. A., Viral alteration of cell function. *Scientific American* 261:42–48, 1989.

3. Schrier, R. D., Nelson, J. A., and Oldstone, M. B. A., Detection of human cytomegalovirus in peripheral blood lymphocytes in a natural infection. *Science* 230:1048–1051, 1985.

4. Notkins, A. L. and Yoon, J. W., Virus-induced diabetes mellitus. In: *Concepts in Viral Pathogenesis* (Notkins, A. L. and Oldstone, M. B. A., eds.) New York, New York: Springer-Verlag, 1984, pp. 241–247.

5. Jawetz, E., Melnick, J. L., and Adelberg, E. A., *Review of Medical Microbiology*. Los Altos, California: Lange Medical Publications, 1984, pp. 475–476.

Research described in this article was supported by the General Clinical Research Centers Program of the National Center for Research Resources, the National Institute on Aging, the National Institute of Allergy and Infectious Diseases, and a Juvenile Diabetes Foundation Fellowship Avard (M. L.).

Chapter 57

Gestational Diabetes

Many women who develop gestational diabetes mellitus during a pregnancy may become diabetic later in life. Few of these women, however, have in their blood the pancreatic islet cell antibodies (ICA's) that are considered markers for patients at risk for insulin-dependent diabetes mellitus, according to researchers at Case Western Reserve University and the University of Vermont in Burlington.

"In our study of 187 Vermont women with a history of gestational diabetes, islet cell antibodies were found in only 3 women (1.6 percent), a result in sharp contrast to earlier studies that suggested an ICA incidence of 10 to 38 percent," says principal investigator Dr. Patrick Catalano of Case Western Reserve University in Cleveland, Ohio.

Dr. Catalano and his colleagues were studying ICA's in women who had had gestational diabetes to determine the incidence of ICA in women with gestational diabetes and whether monitoring these antibodies would provide an early indication of developing diabetes. The appearance of antibodies against the beta-cells of the islets of Langerhans of the pancreas appears to signal ongoing destruction of these cells, the producers of insulin, eventually resulting in insulin-dependent diabetes mellitus (IDDM). According to medical authorities, approximately 10 percent of all diabetics in the United States have IDDM, also known as type I diabetes. The other 90 percent have non-insulin-dependent diabetes mellitus (NIDDM or type II diabetes), which often affects older, overweight persons. In NIDDM the pancreas

---

National Center for Research Resources *Reporter*, March 1992.

produces some insulin but there is still a failure to regulate blood glucose for reasons that are not well-understood. The American Diabetes Association estimates that half of all diabetic Americans do not know that they are ill.

Gestational diabetes mellitus—glucose intolerance in pregnant women who never have had diabetes—occurs in approximately 2.5 to 5 percent of pregnancies, according to the investigators. Most of these women revert to a normal carbohydrate metabolism some time after giving birth, but have a high incidence of diabetes later in life. In one study, for example, 26 percent of nonobese women with prior gestational diabetes and 47 percent of obese women with prior gestational diabetes developed diabetes. In contrast, only 2 and 5 percent of nonobese and obese women, respectively, who did not have a history of gestational diabetes developed diabetes.

The women's risk of developing diabetes at some time after a pregnancy may be a greater risk of gestational diabetes than any immediate risk to their infants. In the United States the risk of perinatal mortality among offspring of women with gestational diabetes does not appear to differ from that of the nondiabetic population, according to Dr. Catalano. This may result at least partly from treatment to normalize blood glucose levels in gestational diabetes patients and close obstetrical followup. Development of type I diabetes in these children does not correlate with their mothers' prior gestational diabetes, although children of mothers with gestational diabetes have an increased risk of obesity as adolescents; the obesity places them at a higher risk for type II diabetes.

For the measurement of ICA's in serum, Dr. Catalano and his colleagues relied on an assay that was developed earlier by researchers at the Joslin Diabetes Center in Boston. The Joslin Diabetes Center cooperated in the study by performing the assay on serum samples sent from Vermont.

Like previous ICA assays, the Joslin monoclonal antibody method relies on immunofluorescence to detect antibodies to the beta-cells. In addition, the assay uses monoclonal antibody conjugated to the dye rhodamine to rapidly identify islets. "This test is a very specific test that decreases the chance of false positive results," Dr. Catalano says. According to Joslin researchers, the test procedure also decreases the number of false negative readings, resulting in more reliable data than the indirect immunofluorescence assays used in the earlier studies. The incidence of ICA in a control population indicated by the protein A MoAb method is only 0.45 percent.

Because so few women with previous gestational diabetes had developed ICA's, the researchers have decided to eliminate the ICA assay as a predictor of future diabetes mellitus in women with a history of gestational diabetes. The rarity of ICA's also alleviates concerns that they might pose a widespread threat to fetal health.

Nevertheless, the three women in the study whose serum contained ICA's all had impaired glucose tolerance when tested several months after delivery of their infants. Oral glucose tolerance was normal for the 11 ICA-negative women in two control groups chosen for detailed comparisons; five women had had normal pregnancies, and six had developed gestational diabetes during the pregnancy. The ICA-positive women also had significantly higher fasting plasma glucose levels than the women in the other two groups. Only the fasting plasma glucose levels were significantly elevated when the ICA-positive women were compared retrospectively with the ICA-negative group for glucose testing during their pregnancies. The ICA-positive women also produced significantly less insulin immediately after an injection of glucose. Their total insulin production capacity was not impaired compared with the two control groups.

In their report the researchers suggested additional studies to determine whether the prevalence of ICA's increases over time after gestational diabetes and to search for a possible effect of ICA's on fetal islet cells. However, according to the investigators, such studies would be difficult to carry out because the number of women with gestational diabetes who are ICA-positive is too low (approximately 0.07 to 0.15 percent of all pregnancies) to provide sufficient subjects for the proposed studies unless a very large-scale study is conducted.

Instead, Dr. Catalano has begun to investigate various aspects of carbohydrate metabolism, comparing pregnant women with and without gestational diabetes, using pregravid studies of each woman as her own baseline, to detect any changes with the passage of time. "None of the metabolic tests I am using is unique, but there are differences in my approach," says Dr. Catalano. Specifically, he is using two techniques relatively new to obstetrical research, and he is searching for patterns in a combined analysis of the results of several tests rather than looking at each test separately.

One of Dr. Catalano's techniques employs stable isotopes to measure hepatic glucose production. In the other technique he uses the glucose clamp procedure to measure changes in insulin resistance. The glucose clamp technique involves a continuous infusion of insulin to achieve a high physiological level of insulin while the plasma glucose level is maintained (clamped) at a set level by variable infusions of glucose. A lower rate of glucose infusion means a lower rate of glucose disposal, implying insulin resistance. Conversely, a higher rate of glucose infusion is associated with greater insulin sensitivity.

Other techniques Dr. Catalano uses to study carbohydrate metabolism include the intravenous glucose tolerance test to measure insulin release, underwater weighing for percentage of body fat in body composition studies, and indirect calorimetry to examine energy expenditure.

So far 20 women have participated in these studies; 10 to 15 additional women are expected to participate.

In preliminary results Dr. Catalano reports that the combination of tests appears to be more sensitive in detecting differences in carbohydrate metabolism than any individual test. When test results for women who are 12 to 14 weeks pregnant are compared with the results obtained before conception, signs of gestational diabetes can already be detected. "This is earlier than previously thought possible," says Dr. Catalano.

By detecting gestational diabetes earlier and understanding the metabolic changes better, scientists expect to find ways to improve the health of both mother and child, according to Dr. Catalano.

—Linda Silversmith, Ph.D.

Additional Reading:

1. Catalano, P. M., Tyzbir, E. D., and Sims, E. A. H., Incidence and significance of islet cell antibodies in women with previous gestational diabetes. *Diabetes Care* 13:478–482, 1990.

The research on islet cell antibodies described in this article was supported by the General Clinical Research Centers Program of the NIH National Center for Research Resources and a Diabetes Treatment Centers of America Clinical Research Award. The research on carbohydrate metabolism is supported by the National Institute of Child Health and Human Development.

Chapter 58

Blood Sugar Analysis Without The Finger Prick

by Greg Pearson

A new procedure to measure blood glucose, or blood sugar, without drawing blood has the potential to significantly improve the quality of life for many diabetics, according to researchers at the University of New Mexico School of Medicine (UNMSM) and Sandia National Laboratories, both in Albuquerque.

To keep tabs on glucose levels in their bodies, insulin-dependent diabetics have to prick their fingers several times a day to draw blood, which they then analyze for glucose content using a test kit. Approximately 2 million people in the United States have insulin-dependent diabetes. This new procedure, which utilizes infrared (IR) spectroscopy, may be a more appealing alternative to the finger prick method because it uses a painless beam of light to measure blood sugar. "Our indications suggest that this noninvasive technique can be as good as invasive, chemically based determination of blood glucose," says Dr. R. Philip Eaton, chief of endocrinology and metabolism at UNMSM and director of the UNMSM General Clinical Research Center. Dr. Eaton and his coworkers have evaluated several spectrometers to determine how well they detect changes in blood glucose concentrations.

In an initial set of studies, involving three diabetic patients, the investigators tested two different types of spectrometers with three different types

---

National Center for Research Resources *Reporter*, January/February 1993.

of detectors. The researchers used two sophisticated multivariate calibration techniques to develop empirical models that relate changes in the calibration spectra to changes in blood glucose concentrations measured in blood samples.

In the experiments fasting patients ate a meal of pancakes and, 2 hours later, received three to five units of regular insulin. Blood samples were drawn at 10- to 30-minute intervals beginning with the meal and ending 3 hours after insulin administration. The measured glucose concentrations in the blood samples served as the reference values for the spectral modeling. The investigators obtained the IR spectral data by shining the infrared light through the finger after each blood sample had been taken.

The researchers also measured finger temperatures to rule out the possibility that a change in body temperature brought on by changes in blood sugar was influencing the noninvasive glucose measurement. "Often when people become profoundly hypoglycemic they sweat and become cold and clammy," notes Dr. M. Ries Robinson, a postdoctoral scientist at Sandia and a resident in the department of medicine at the University of New Mexico School of Medicine.

Over the study period the accuracy of the spectrometric method of glucose measurement in the three patients approached that required for clinical application, according to Drs. Eaton and Robinson. Both caution, however, that more patients must be studied before definitive statements can be made about the relative accuracy of the different spectrometer configurations.

One limitation of this early set of studies, the researchers note, is that a calibration model had to be developed for each patient. "We now have developed a more robust model that allows any unknown patient to be analyzed without having his or her blood drawn," says Dr. Eaton. The results of this work, based on more recent research involving 60 diabetic patients, have not yet been published but are in line with the results from the initial three patients, according to Dr. Robinson.

Another complicating factor is the wide segment (500 to 1,000 nanometers) of the IR spectral band being used by the investigators. Approximately 120 discrete wavelengths are being scanned and separated by the IR detectors, according to Dr. Eaton. "To make this a simpler and less expensive home instrument, we would like to select fewer wavelengths of the spectrum," he says.

The use of IR spectroscopy as a tool for monitoring blood glucose levels is made possible by the timely convergence of newly developed methods of multivariate analysis and the computational speed provided by the current generation of personal computers. "Infrared spectroscopy has been around for decades, but the mathematics involved in extracting information from very small squiggles has not," explains Dr. Eaton, adding that "even after the math had been developed, it could not be applied practically without the use of the 486 personal computer." Dr. Eaton credits Sandia scientists Drs. David Haaland and Edward Thomas with providing much of the mathematical underpinnings of the research.

Despite the existence of sophisticated multivariate analysis and powerful computing capacity, identifying and accurately measuring levels of glucose in the blood is quite difficult, the investigators say. Part of the problem is that many chemical compounds circulating in the bloodstream absorb light in the same spectral range as glucose. Dr. Robinson compares the challenge of trans-finger IR spectroscopy to "trying to find a little tiny needle in a very big haystack."

The New Mexico researchers are now working to increase the accuracy of the glucose-monitoring technique and improve the computational methodology. Another focus of ongoing research is the reproducibility of finger-sampling. One particular problem, for example, is that the position and stability of the finger within the testing device varies from test to test. This variability can affect the accuracy of test results.

Additional Reading:

1. Robinson, M. R., Eaton, R. P., Haaland, D. M., et al., Noninvasive glucose monitoring in diabetic patients, a preliminary evaluation. *Clinical Chemistry* 38:1618–1622, 1992.

2. Heise, H. M., Marbach R., Koschinsky, T., and Gries, F. A., Multivariate determination of blood substrates in human plasma by FTNIR spectroscopy. In *Eighth International Conference on Fourier Transform Spectroscopy* (Heise, H. M., Korte, E. H., Siesler, H. W., eds.). *Proceedings of the Society of Photo-Optical Instrumentation Engineers* 1575:507–508, 1992.

3. Janatsch, G., Kruse-Jarres, J. D., Marbach, R., and Heise, H. M., Multivariate calibration for assays in clinical chemistry using attenuated total reflection spectra of human blood plasma. *Analytical Chemistry* 61:2016–2023, 1989.

4. Zeller, H., Novak, P., and Landgraf, R., Blood glucose measurement by infrared spectroscopy. *International Journal of Artificial Organs* 12:129–135, 1989.

The research described in this article was supported by the General Clinical Research Centers Program of the National Center for Research Resources and by the U.S. Department of Energy.

Chapter 59

Hypoglycemia and Driving Performance

Investigators have tried to evaluate whether hypoglycemia, or low blood sugar, makes it more difficult for a diabetic person to control an automobile, but different researchers have reached different conclusions partly because of their inability to simulate and reproduce true driving conditions. Now Dr. Daniel J. Cox and his associates Drs. William Clarke and Linda Gonder-Frederick at the University of Virginia Health Sciences Center in Charlottesville report that, under realistic driving conditions in a driving simulator, hypoglycemia does affect people's driving performance. Diabetics can become hypoglycemic if they do not eat regularly or overtreat with insulin.

"Our study is the first one to use a driving simulator," says Dr. Cox, who is professor of behavioral medicine and psychiatry at the University of Virginia. "No other study has directly observed driving and hypoglycemia in diabetic patients." Other investigators studied databases in motor vehicle departments or asked diabetic drivers how many accidents or motor vehicle violations they had been involved in.

The University of Virginia scientists tested the driving performance of 13 women and 12 men (average age 36 years) who had had insulin-dependent diabetes mellitus for an average of almost 15 years. The objective, standardized evaluation of an individual's driving performance was made possible by a newly developed driving simulator from the Atari Company that contains such realistic features as a life-sized steering wheel and gas and brake pedals. The driver watches a 25-inch color graphics screen that updates

---

NCRR *Reporter*, July/August 1993.

20 times per second and shows eight versions of a 4-mile course, including stop signs and lights; oncoming, same-lane, and cross traffic; realistic road obstacles; and posted changes in speed limits. The driver also hears engine, wind, road, and traffic noises. The system tracks 112 driving variables simultaneously 20 times per second and can simulate the steering, braking, acceleration, and suspension characteristics of different vehicles.

The volunteers were admitted to the university's General Clinical Research Center the evening before the 2-day study and were then allowed to drive the simulator for 30 minutes. During the next 2 days the participants did eight 4-minute runs on the driving simulator, six while they had normal blood sugar concentrations (6.4 ± O.67 mM), and two while they had mild (mean blood sugar 3.6 ± 0.33 mM) and moderate hypoglycemia (mean blood sugar 2.6 ± 0.28 mM), respectively. Each driving test was complemented by a 30-minute evaluation of reaction time and memory. The patients knew that their hypoglycemic driving performance was being evaluated, but were not told when their blood sugar was abnormal. During each test two driving parameters were evaluated: Steering and speed control.

The researchers controlled the patients' blood sugar concentrations by connecting them to an insulin/glucose infusion system that measured blood sugar concentrations and automatically administered insulin or glucose to maintain preset values.

During moderate hypoglycemia the diabetic volunteers swerved more, spun more, and spent more time over the midline and off the road than when they had normal blood sugar or were only mildly hypoglycemic. Moderate hypoglycemia also induced the patients to drive significantly slower than the posted speed limits. "I think they perceived that they were unable to maneuver as well as when they had normal blood sugar concentrations and therefore compensated by driving slower," says coinvestigator Dr. William Clarke, professor of pediatrics at the University of Virginia. "It is not pleasant to be hypoglycemic. I have been hypoglycemic, and my personal impression of it is that one has a feeling of heaviness and an inability to move rapidly." Overall, during mild hypoglycemia only two persons (8 percent) showed a decreased driving performance. During moderate hypoglycemia 35 percent of the patients were affected.

During moderate hypoglycemia many patients (58 percent) said before the driving test that they would not want to drive if they could choose. In contrast, 77 percent of the patients realized after the test that they would not want to drive. However, only 50 percent of patients who did the worst driving anticipated their poor performances, and after the test 25 percent of these said they were still willing to drive. Most people recovered quickly when their blood sugar was restored to normal. "We tested them approximately 25 minutes after their blood sugar had returned to normal, and the group data indicated that they recovered right away, but the individual data showed that a couple of people did not recover immediately," says Dr. Cox.

The researchers emphasize that since the tests lasted only 4 minutes, longer driving periods might be expected to affect mild hypoglycemic periods as well. "We now have a new, more sophisticated simulator with a wraparound screen, so the driver can see traffic coming from either side or from behind. In the new simulator we plan to test drivers for 25 to 30 minutes," says Dr. Cox.

The researchers stress that diabetics should always check their blood sugar before driving and pay attention to how they feel and what they think their blood sugar level might be. "People should ask themselves 'How am I functioning right now?' and use the answer to evaluate what their blood sugar level might be. They should not just depend on physical symptoms," Dr. Cox explains.

Dr. Clark advises diabetic drivers to never miss a meal. "They should not drive past meal or snack times, and they should carry food and blood sugar monitoring supplies with them in the car," he says.

—Ole Henriksen, Ph.D.

Additional Reading

1. Cox, D. J., Gonder-Frederick, L., and Clarke, W., Driving decrements in type I diabetes during moderate hypoglycemia. *Diabetes* 42:239–243, 1993.

This research was supported by the General Clinical Research Centers Program of the National Center for Research Resources, the National Institute of Diabetes and Digestive and Kidney Diseases, and the American Automobile Association for Traffic Safety.

Chapter 60

Research Opportunities and Programs in the Division of Diabetes, Endocrinology, and Metabolic Diseases

Division of Diabetes, Endocrinology, and Metabolic Diseases

The National Institute of Diabetes and Digestive and Kidney Diseases (NIDDK) was established in 1950 to further the mission of the National Institutes of Health (NIH) to improve human health through biomedical research. The NIH, the largest biomedical research center in the world, is the research arm of the Public Health Service within the U.S. Department of Health and Human Services.

The NIDDK conducts and supports research and research training related to a broad array of diseases that are characterized by chronicity and long-term disabling effects. The Division of Diabetes, Endocrinology, and Metabolic Diseases (DDEM), NIDDK, has responsibility for extramural programs related to diabetes mellitus and its complications; to endocrinology and a variety of endocrine disorders; and to metabolism and metabolic diseases, including cystic fibrosis.

Through the DDEM, the Institute provides approximately $300,000,000 to scientists in medical schools; universities; and other research institutions throughout the country, including private industry. Support for basic and clinical biomedical research, as well as epidemiologic and behavioral studies and clinical trials, is provided through investigator-initiated research grants, new investigator awards, program project and center grants, cooperative agreements and Small Business Innovative Research awards. The division also supports a variety of career development awards as well as a limited

---

NIDDK, May 1993 (in part)

number of resource and research and development contracts. In addition, the division provides leadership in coordinating activities throughout the NIH and various other Federal agencies.

Brief descriptions follow for each of the division's major program areas. Additional information regarding specific programs may be obtained directly from each program office.

Richard C. Eastman, M.D.
Director, Division of Diabetes,
Endocrinology, and Metabolic Diseases
Donna Belcher, Secretary
Building 31, Room 9A16
Bethesda, MD 20892
(301) 496–7348
FAX (301) 496–2380

Diabetes Programs Branch

Judith E. Fradkin, M.D.
Acting Chief, Diabetes Programs Branch
Gayla Elder-Leak
Lead Grants Technical Assistant
Westwood Building, Room 621
Bethesda, MD 20892
(301) 594–7567
FAX (301) 594–9011

Insulin Dependent Diabetes Mellitus (IDDM) Research Program

This program emphasizes support of investigator-initiated basic and clinical research relating to IDDM, pancreatic secretion of insulin, and islet transplantation. Studies focus on: (1) the etiology, pathogenesis, prevention, diagnosis, treatment and cure of IDDM; (2) the immunobiology of autoimmune diseases as it relates to IDDM; (3) the genetic basis of IDDM and identification of specific markers that characterize individuals predisposed to IDDM; (4) the viral etiology of IDDM; (5) the environmental factors that relate to pathogenesis of IDDM; (6) the growth and differentiation of the beta cell; (7) physiologic regulation of pancreatic secretion of insulin; (8) molecular mechanisms of the beta cell response to glucose and other secretogogues; (9) identification of individuals at risk of IDDM and development of methods to prevent IDDM in high risk individuals; (10) beta cell, islet or pancreas transplantation; (11) the development of other approaches to achieve euglycemia; (12) the development and utilization of animal models for IDDM to further our understanding of this disease; and (13) IDDM in minority populations.

For further information, contact:

Joan T. Harmon, Ph.D.
Chief, Diabetes Research Section Director, IDDM Research Program
Janie F. Brown
Grants Technical Assistant
Westwood Building, Room 622
Bethesda, MD 20892
(301) 594–7565
FAX (301) 594–9011

Noninsulin-Dependent Diabetes Mellitus (NIDDM) Research Program

The NIDDM Research Program supports investigator-initiated basic and clinical research in NIDDM, impaired glucose tolerance and insulin resistance. The majority of individuals who suffer from diabetes have NIDDM (Type II). NIDDM affects approximately 13 million Americans. The disease severely impacts on African Americans, Hispanic Americans, Native Americans, Native Hawaiians, and Asian Americans. Identification of genetic and environmental factors underlying NIDDM is a major goal of the NIDDM Research Program. Studies focus on: (1) the etiology, pathogenesis, prevention, diagnosis, treatment, and cure of NIDDM; (2) why American minority populations are so severely impacted by NIDDM; (3) the identification of genetic and environmental factors underlying NIDDM; (4) the biochemistry and cell biology of glucose intolerance, glucose resistance and NIDDM; (5) the mechanisms of action of insulin and insulinmimetic agents; (6) the insulin receptor structure and function, post-receptor signalling and insulin-dependent regulation of cellular processes; (7) the glucose transporters; (8) the cellular uptake of other sugars, amino acids, and macromolecules relevant to diabetes; (9) the metabolism of carbohydrate and protein in relation to diabetes including mathematical models of metabolism; (10) the relationship of exercise and obesity to diabetes; (11) the relationship of gestational diabetes to NIDDM; (12) prevention of impaired glucose tolerance and NIDDM particularly in high risk populations; and (13) the development and utilization of animal models to further our understanding of NIDDM.

For further information, contact:

Joan T. Harmon, Ph.D.
Chief, Diabetes Research Section
Acting Director NIDDM Research Program
Gayla Elder-Leak
Lead Grants Technical Assistant
Westwood Building, Room 626
Bethesda, MD 20892
(301) 594–7565
FAX (301) 594–9011

Diabetes Epidemiology Research Program

The Diabetes Epidemiology Research Program provides research grant and contract support for studies on the epidemiology of diabetes and its complications. This research focuses on the study of the distribution and determinants of diabetes in specified populations, including community-based populations and the general population. It includes studies on the patterns of diabetes demography, geographic and temporal variations in the disease, and variations in disease frequency by race, socioeconomic status, metabolic factors, and other determinants; studies on the etiology of diabetes including identification of risk factors determining susceptibility to diabetes and variations in the distribution of risk factors within populations and within individuals; and research on the etiology and pathogenesis of diabetes complications in well-defined populations to define and quantitate the complications of diabetes and factors that predispose diabetics to complications.

For further information, contact:

Maureen I. Harris, Ph.D., M.P.H.
Director, Diabetes Epidemiology
Research Program
Sharon D. Frazier
Grants Technical Assistant
Westwood Building, Room 620
Bethesda, MD 20892
(301) 594–7559
FAX (301) 594–9011

Diabetes Complications Research Program

This program focuses on research related to diabetic complications and to the effects of diabetes on organ systems, including but not limited to: the kidney, eye, nervous system, vascular system, and reproductive system. Areas of interest include the acute as well as the chronic complications of diabetes and includes fetal development in diabetes. The key areas related to pathogenesis encompass, but are not limited to: (1) the genetic factors influencing susceptibility to complications; (2) the interplay between diabetes and risk factors such as hypertension and smoking in pathogenesis of complications; (3) the polyol pathway, and nonenzymatic glycation of proteins; and (4) use of aldose reductase inhibitors, aminoguanidines, and other agents to prevent complications. Research on mechanical methods of insulin administration, including glucose sensors, pumps, and integrators, also constitute a focus of this program. In addition, efforts are supported to investigate the link between behavior and physical health as related to diabetes, including bio-behavioral mechanisms; identification and distribution of psychosocial risk factors in populations; and change of health-related behaviors and social interventions to prevent diabetes or its complications.

Not only does diabetes mellitus significantly affect minority populations, but its complications are disproportionately increased in minorities. A particular emphasis is placed on the need to understand the etiology, complications, and sequelae of diabetes in minority populations. The Diabetes Research Section encourages research on these issues in representative affected minority populations.

For further information, contact:

Charles A. Wells, Ph.D.
Director, Diabetes Complications
Research Program
Westwood Building, Room 620
Bethesda, MD 20892
Janie F. Brown
Grants Technical Assistant
(301) 594–7505
FAX (301) 594–9011

Diabetes Centers Program

Two types of center awards are offered: the Diabetes-Endocrinology Research Centers (DERC) and the Diabetes Research and Training Centers (DRTC). An existing base of high quality diabetes-related research is a primary requirement for establishment of either type of center. Through shared resources (core facilities), both types of center grants provide a mechanism for integrating, coordinating, and fostering in a cost effective way, the interdisciplinary cooperation of a group of established investigators conducting programs of active, high-quality research in diabetes and related endocrine and metabolic disorders. While direct funding for major research projects *per se* is not included in these center grant awards, limited funding for small research projects, pilot and feasibility studies, is included.

The essential difference between the two types of centers is that while the focus for the DERC's is entirely on biomedical research, the DRTC's have, as a required addition, a Demonstration and Education component. The activities supported by this component encompass translation research. This includes research related to the translation of state-of-the-art diabetes treatment and management methods to the diabetes community, including health care professionals and individuals with diabetes.

Specific guidelines relating to these centers are available from the Diabetes Centers Program Director. Advance consultation with program staff before submitting an application is strongly advised. Applications are accepted only in response to the issuance of specific Requests For Applications (RFA).

For further information, contact:

Sanford A. Garfield, Ph.D.
Director, Diabetes Special Programs
Gayla Elder-Leak
Lead Grants Technical Assistant
Westwood Building, Room 626
Bethesda, MD 20892
(301) 594–7535
FAX (301) 594–9011

Diabetes Clinical Trials Programs

Clinical trials in diabetes are supported by multiple mechanisms. Small investigator-initiated clinical trials are supported under regular grant mechanisms, and inquiries should be directed to the appropriate diabetes research program director listed above. Large clinical trials that involve multiple centers and significant resources require advance planning in consultation with Institute staff. Trials such as these are supported through special mechanisms. An example is the Diabetes Control and Complications Trial (DCCT), an ongoing study of early vascular complications of insulin-dependent diabetes mellitus (IDDM). This trial involves 1441 subjects recruited and followed over a ten-year period in 29 institutions in the U.S. and Canada. It is funded via cooperative agreement and research contract awards. Other multicenter clinical trials are currently under consideration including one related to prevention of noninsulin-dependent diabetes (NIDDM) and one on prevention of IDDM.

For further information, contact:

Sanford A. Garfield, Ph.D.
Director
NIDDM Clinical Trials Program
Gayla Elder-Leak
Lead Grants Technical Assistant
Westwood Building, Room 626
Bethesda, MD 20892
(301) 594–7535
FAX (301) 594–9011

Carolyn Siebert, MPH
Director
IDDM Clinical Trials Program
Terry Pike
Grants Technical Assistant
Westwood Building, Room 628
Bethesda, MD 20892
(301) 594–7561
FAX (301) 594–9011

National Diabetes Data Group

The National Diabetes Data Group (NDDG) serves as the major Federal focus for the collection, analysis, and dissemination of data on diabetes and its complications. Drawing upon the expertise of the research, medical and lay communities, the NDDG initiates efforts to: (1) define the data needed to address the scientific and public health issues in diabetes; (2) foster and coordinate the collection of these data from multiple sources; (3) promote the timely availability of reliable data to pertinent scientific, medical, and public organizations; (4) modify data reporting systems to identify and categorize more appropriately the medical and socioeconomic impact of diabetes; and (5) promote the standardization of data collection and terminology in clinical and epidemiologic research. In addition, the NDDG staff works closely with members of the scientific community to stimulate development of new investigator-initiated research programs in diabetes epidemiology.

For further information, contact:

Maureen I. Harris, Ph.D., M.P.H.
Director, National Diabetes Data Group
Sharon D. Frazier
Grants Technical Assistant
Westwood Building, Room 620
Bethesda, MD 20892
(301) 594–7559
FAX (301) 954–9011

. . .

Mechanisms of Research Support

Research Project Grant

These investigator-initiated research grants are awarded to public and private organizations and institutions, governments and their agencies (including other Federal institutions), foreign institutions, and international organizations, to provide support for a discrete, specified research project to be performed by a named principal investigator. Detailed information and eligibility criteria may be found in the *Grants Policy Statement* which is generally available in the grants and contracts office of the institution or can be obtained from the Division of Research Grants, National Institutes of Health, Westwood Building, Room 449, Bethesda, MD 20892.

MERIT Award

Investigators who have demonstrated superior competence and outstanding productivity during their previous research endeavors may be selected to extend an initial 5-year research project grant award for an additional 3 years based on an expedited review. The Method To Extend Research In Time (MERIT) Awards are selected by NIH staff in consultation with the National Advisory Councils, from competing research applications. **Investigators May Not Apply for Merit Awards.**

FIRST Award

The objective of the First Independent Research Support and Transition (FIRST) Award is to provide a sufficient initial period of research support for newly independent biomedical investigators to develop their research capabilities and demonstrate the merit of their research ideas. These grants are intended to underwrite the first independent investigator efforts of an individual; to provide a reasonable opportunity for him/her to demonstrate creativity, productivity, and further promise; and to help effect a transition toward the traditional types of NIH research project grants. The principal features are (1) new investigators may receive awards for a period of up to 5 years; (2) the maximum level for these awards is $350,000 for a 5-year period; and (3) the award will permit optional carry-over of unobligated balances from one budget period to the next.

Small Business Innovations Research Program

An amendment to the Small Business Act now requires certain Federal agencies, including the NIH, to set aside funds to promote technological innovation within the American small business community. The purpose of the new legislation is to give small business an increased role in the Federal research and development (R&D) efforts as well as to attract private capital to commercialize the results of federally funded research.

The Small Business Innovation Research, or SBIR, program consists of three phases: phase I—the establishment of the technical merit and feasibility of research and development ideas that may lead to commercial products or services (up to 6 months); phase II—the in-depth development of research and development ideas proposed in phase I (up to 5 years); and phase III—the promotion of commercialization of the results of the R&D funded by Federal agencies or use of non-SBIR contracting for products or processes as developed for use by the U.S. Government.

The implementation of this program is principally through the research grant mechanism. Applications will be considered in any area within the mission of the division, although special programmatic interests have been developed as guidelines for those interested in applying for support.

Program Project Grant

This grant provides support for a broadly based, multidisciplinary, often long-term targeted research program consisting of coordinated research activities and projects led by established investigators. Program projects are directed toward well defined research goals and generally involve the organized efforts of a number of individuals who are conducting research projects designed to elucidate various aspects or components of a central theme. The program project grant can provide support for certain basic resources used by groups in the program, including clinical components, the sharing of which facilitates the total research effort. Eligibility criteria are the same as for the traditional research project grant. Specific guidelines are available from the appropriate research program directors. Consultations with program staff prior to submission of an application are highly recommended.

Center Grant

Core Center grants supported by the Division are based on the concept of providing shared resources (cores) for a group of established investigators who are conducting independent programs of active, high-quality research. The center grant provides a mechanism for integrating, coordinating, and fostering interdisciplinary research among these investigators. Centers also provide funding for shared resources, limited support for pilot and feasibility studies, and funds for program enrichment. The pilot and feasibility studies are small research projects of limited duration. Their purpose is to enable investigators who are new to the program area to become independent or to support new research directions for established investigators. Core Centers are supported in the Diabetes Centers Program and the Cystic Fibrosis Program. The Cystic Fibrosis Program also supports Specialized Centers for Research (SCOR). SCOR's support a full spectrum of research in a given area, from very basic to clinical, and represent a multidisciplinary attack on a specific disease or question in biomedical research. Applications for center grants are usually accepted only in response to Requests For Applications (RFA).

Cooperative Agreement

A cooperative agreement reflects an assistance relationship between the NIH and a recipient, but with substantial programmatic involvement by the NIH. The NIH assists, supports, or stimulates the recipients, and is involved substantially with recipients in conducting projects similar in program intent to those for grants, with the NIH playing a partner role in the effort. Applications for Cooperative Agreements are accepted only in response to Requests For Applications.

Training and Career Development Opportunities

National Research Service Awards

Three types of awards are available under this program: institutional training grants, individual postdoctoral fellowships, and senior research fellowship awards.

Training grants are awarded to domestic nonprofit, private, and non-Federal public institutions to support costs of training students in biomedical research at the predoctoral and postdoctoral levels. A predoctoral program must offer the opportunity for individuals to broaden their scientific backgrounds. These awards are, however, not made to support study leading to the M.D., D.O., D.D.S., or similar professional degrees nor are they to support nonresearch clinical training.

Postdoctoral fellowship awards are made directly to qualified individuals who have received a Ph.D., M.D., or equivalent degree for specified research training programs. The award provides the opportunity to carry out supervised research to enable biomedical scientists, clinicians, and others to broaden their scientific backgrounds and expand their potential for research in health-related areas. Prior to submission, an applicant must arrange for an appointment to an appropriate institution and acceptance by a sponsor who will supervise the training and research experience. The institutional setting may be a domestic or foreign nonprofit, private or public institution, including the NIH.

Senior fellowships provide the opportunity for experienced scientists to make major changes in the direction of their research careers, to broaden their research capabilities, or to enlarge their command of an allied research field. Candidates must have received a doctoral (Ph.D., Sc.D., D. Eng., M.D., D.D.S., D.O., D.V.M., O.D.), or equivalent degree, foreign or domestic, and must have had at least 7 subsequent years of relevant research or professional experience by the time the award is made. Senior fellowships will normally be awarded for a period of 12 months. Continued support beyond the first year is contingent upon the research training plan, satisfactory progress, and the availability of funds. The total period of the award will not exceed 24 months. These awards are not made for study leading to any of the professional degrees (M.D., O.D., D.D.S., etc.) or for residency or other nonclinical training.

Physician Scientist Award

The Physician Scientist Award provides a first research experience for newly trained clinicians to develop independent research skills and experience in a fundamental science. Candidates will ordinarily have completed at least 1 postgraduate year of clinical training by the time the award is made. This award will enable physicians with clinical training to undertake up to 5 years of special study in basic science with a supervised research experience. Consultation with program/Institute staff is recommended before submitting an application.

Clinical Investigator Award

The Clinical Investigator Award (CIA) is directed toward clinically trained individuals with demonstrated aptitude in research and provides them with the opportunity to develop into independent biomedical investigators. The award is intended to facilitate transition from postdoctoral training to a career as an independent investigator. Five years of salary support and a limited budget for research expenses are provided. Generally, candidates (M.D. or equivalent) must have 2 years of clinical experience and at least 2 years of postdoctoral by the time the award is made.

Research Career Development Award

The Research Career Development Award (RCDA) is a special 5-year salary grant to enable investigators who have demonstrated outstanding research potential to further develop their research careers. RCDA's are available for persons who have demonstrated independent research accomplishments but who need additional time in a productive scientific environment. The division will accept RCDA applications only from applicants who are principal investigators on a regular research grant supported by this division. Alternatively, an applicant may submit a regular research grant application and an RCDA application concurrently. The RCDA is not intended for the untried investigator nor for those already established as independent investigators. Neither is the award intended simply to substitute one source of salary support for another for an individual who is already conducting full-time research or as a mechanism for providing institutional support.

For further information, contact:

Ronald N. Margolis, Ph.D.
Acting Director
Training and Careers Program
Sharon D. Frazier
Grants Technical Assistant
Westwood Building, Room 620
Bethesda, MD 20892
(301) 594–7549
FAX (301) 594–9011

Additional Information

Applications and general information regarding NIH grants policy and procedure can be obtained from the Office of Grants Inquiries, Division of Research Grants, Westwood Building, Room 449, Bethesda, MD 20892.

Advisory Support and Information Services

National Diabetes Advisory Board

The National Diabetes Advisory Board was established by Congress in 1976 to review and evaluate the implementation of the national Long-Range Plan to Combat Diabetes and to periodically update the plan to ensure its continuing relevance; to advise and make recommendations to Congress, the Secretary of Health and Human Services, and the heads of other appropriate Federal agencies for the implementation and revision of the plan; and to report its findings annually.

Raymond M. Kuehne
Executive Director
Information available from:
NDAB
1801 Rockville Pike
Suite 500
Rockville, MD 20852
(301) 496–6045

Diabetes Mellitus Interagency Coordinating Committee

The Diabetes Mellitus Interagency Coordinating Committee (DMICC) was established by Congress in the fall of 1974. The committee includes representatives from all Federal departments and agencies whose programs involve health functions and responsibilities relevant to diabetes mellitus and its complications. Functions of the DMICC are to coordinate the research activities of the NIH and those activities of other Federal programs that are related to diabetes mellitus and its complications; to contribute to ensuring the adequacy and soundness of these activities; and to provide a forum for communication and exchange of information necessary to maintain coordination of these activities.

Richard C. Eastman, M.D.
Chair
(301) 496–7348
FAX (301) 496–2830

Sanford A. Garfield, Ph.D.
Executive Secretary
(301) 594–7535
FAX (301) 594–9011

Building 31, Room 9A16
Bethesda, MD 20892

National Diabetes Information Clearinghouse

The National Diabetes Information Clearinghouse functions as the central point for the collection and dissemination of information about educational and scientific materials, programs, and resources relevant to diabetes. The clearinghouse works closely with the Diabetes Research and Training Centers, local and national diabetes organizations, professional groups, state departments of health, and other Federal and state agencies. The overall goals of the clearinghouse are to increase knowledge and understanding about diabetes among patients, health professionals, and the public, and to function as a catalyst in assisting and enhancing the efforts of these various groups in the development and exchange of educational materials and diabetes information.

Elizabeth H. Singer
Director
Carmen L. Robinson, Secretary
Building 31, Room 9A04
Bethesda, MD 20892
(301) 496–3583

World Health Organization (WHO) Collaborating Center for Diabetes

This center, sponsored by DDEM, solicits and provides guidance in developing international research about diabetes through NIH research grants and contracts; promotes interchange of scientific and health information among WHO member countries; and provides expert advice and consultation to WHO and other international committees and agencies.

Maureen I. Harris, Ph.D., M.P.H.
WHO Center Director
Joan T. Harmon, Ph.D.
Basic Sciences Program Director
Judith E. Fradkin, M.D.
Acting Clinical Sciences
Program Director
Ronald N. Margolis, Ph.D.
Acting Information and Education

Program Director
Westwood Building, Room 620
Bethesda, MD 20892
(301) 594–7559
FAX (301) 594–9011

APPENDIX

WHERE TO GO FOR MORE HELP AND INFORMATION

Chapter 61

Directory of Diabetes Organizations

This directory lists some major voluntary, governmental, and private organizations involved in diabetes-related activities. Some organizations offer educational and other types of services to people with diabetes and their families and friends; others primarily serve health care professionals.

American Association of Diabetes Educators (AADE)
444 N. Michigan Avenue, Suite 1240
Chicago, IL 60611
(312) 644–2233 or 1–800-338–3633

The AADE is a multidisciplinary organization, with state and regional chapters, for health professionals involved in diabetes patient education. It sponsors beginning- and advanced-level continuing education programs and a certification program for diabetes educators and provides grants, scholarships, and awards for educational research and teaching activities. AADE's annual meeting features continuing education programs in areas relevant to diabetes treatment and education.

Publications: The AADE publishes a bimonthly journal, *The Diabetes Educator,* curriculum guides, consensus statements, self-study programs, and other print and nonprint resources for diabetes educators.

NDIC, November 1993

American Diabetes Association (ADA)
ADA National Service Center
1660 Duke Street
Alexandria, VA 22314
(703) 549–1500 or 1–800-232–3472

The ADA is both a professional association and a private, nonprofit, voluntary organization with state and local affiliates and chapters. It serves people with diabetes, their families and friends, and health professionals and research scientists involved in diabetes-related activities. The organization funds diabetes research and education activities; sponsors educational programs, including an annual meeting, postgraduate courses, consensus meetings, and special symposia; administers a recognition program for diabetes outpatient education; develops professional guidelines for diabetes care; and serves as an advocate for diabetes on social, medical, and research issues in the legislative and public health arenas. Local ADA affiliates often sponsor educational programs and support groups for persons with diabetes and their families.

Publications: The ADA publishes monthly and quarterly magazines for patients, including *Diabetes Forecast*; professional journals focusing on basic and clinical research, including *Diabetes*, *Diabetes Care*, *Diabetes Spectrum*, and *Diabetes Reviews*; other publications, including cookbooks, meal planning guides, pamphlets, brochures, and books for patients; and clinical manuals, nutritional guides, audiovisuals, statistical reports, and curriculum guides for professionals.

Diabetes Care and Education Practice Group (DCEPG), The American Diabetic Association
216 W. Jackson Blvd, Suite 800
Chicago, IL 60606–6995
(312) 899–0040, ext. 4813

The DCEPG, a special interest group within The American Dietetic Association, is composed of Registered Dietitians and other professionals who provide diabetes nutrition care and education services. The group promotes professional standards to strengthen and expand the role of the professional dietitian in diabetes practice; responds to the needs of diabetes organizations and industry with regard to diabetes nutrition issues; promotes clinical and educational research to improve diabetes management; develops guidelines for the nutritional management of diabetes; and maintains a network of practicing dietitians available for consultation services to health professionals and people with diabetes.

Publications: The DCEPG publishes two newsletters, *Newsflash* and *On the Cutting Edge,* review papers and bibliographic resources in the area of diabetes and nutrition, nutrition guides for professionals and patients, an exercise kit for patients, and nutrition guides for ethnic and regional foods.

Diabetes Research and Education Foundation

P.O. Box 6168
Bridgewater, NJ 08807–9998
(908) 658–9322 (Tuesday-Thursday Only)

The foundation, which is funded by Hoechst-Roussel Pharmaceuticals, Inc., offers grants in the form of "seed money" to support novel initiatives in diabetes research and education. The foundation's Board of Trustees includes specialists in diabetes research, clinical practice, pharmacy, and patient education.

Publications: Annual Report

Diabetes Research and Training Centers (DRTCs)

The six DRTCs supported by the National Institute of Diabetes and Digestive and Kidney Diseases offer continuing education, seminars, and workshops in state-of-the-art diabetes management for health care professionals; an array of tested evaluation and assessment instruments; and professional expertise in developing and implementing diabetes programs in a variety of settings. The centers are located at major medical centers affiliated with universities and also offer patient referral services.

Publications: Individual centers produce a variety of educational materials, including audiovisuals, that are available to health care professionals. Persons desiring additional information about materials and programs should contact individual centers listed below.

Einstein/Montefiore DRTC
1300 Morris Park Avenue
Belfer 1308
Bronx, NY 10461
(718) 430–2908 or 430–3345 (epidemiologist)

Indiana University DRTC
Regenstrief Institute, 5th Floor
1001 West 10th Street
Indianapolis, IN 46202
(317) 630–6375

Michigan DRTC
G1205 Towsley Center, Box 0201
University of Michigan Medical School
Ann Arbor, MI 48109–0201
(313) 763–1426

University of Chicago DRTC
Center for Research in Medical Education and Health Care
5841 S. Maryland Avenue, MC 6091
Chicago, IL 60637
(312) 753–1310

Vanderbilt University DRTC
Vanderbilt Medical Center
305 Medical Arts Building
Nashville, TN 37232–2230
(615) 322–4257 or 322–6001 (answering service)

Washington University DRTC
Diabetes Education Center
33 S. Euclid Boulevard
St. Louis, MO 63108
(314) 361–4808

Division of Diabetes Translation, Centers for Disease Control and Prevention (CDC)
National Center for Chronic Disease Prevention and Health Promotion
TISB Mail Stop K-13
4770 Buford Highway, NE
Atlanta, GA 30341–3724
(404) 488–5080

An agency of the Public Health Service, Department of Health and Human Services, the CDC is responsible for developing public health approaches to reduce the burden of diabetes in the United States. The agency supports diabetes control programs in 26 states and 1 territory; carries out state and national surveillance activities to assess the prevalence and impact of diabetes and possible contributing factors; develops consensus guidelines for clinical and public health practice; supports community-based preventive programs for minority populations and the elderly; and coordinates Federal activities related to translating research findings into clinical practice, including issues related to cost and reimbursement practices, disability, and quality of life.

Publications: The CDC has developed a practice manual for primary care practitioners and a companion guide for patients, surveillance reports, and guidelines relating to patient education and educational reimbursement and maternal and child health. Individual state programs also have developed patient and professional publications.

Indian Health Service (IHS)
IHS Headquarters West
Central Diabetes Program
2401 12th Street, N.W., Room 211N
Albuquerque, NM 87102
(505) 766–3980

An agency of the Public Health Service, Department of Health and Human Services, the IHS supports 17 model Diabetes Health Care Programs serving Native Americans and Alaskans at existing IHS health care facilities to develop and evaluate effective and culturally accepted prevention and treatment methods for diabetes and its complications. Diabetes control officers in each IHS region provide surveillance, training, and other services to promote the use of techniques piloted at model sites.

Publications: The model programs and the IHS headquarters program have developed culturally relevant publications for native populations, including nutrition guides, complication-specific educational materials, and guides for professionals. Publications are available only to persons working with Native American or Alaskan populations.

International Diabetes Center (IDC)
5000 West 39th Street
Minneapolis, MN 55416
(612) 927–3393

A division of the Park Nicollet Medical Foundation, the IDC offers a year-round schedule of diabetes education classes for people with diabetes and educational programs in team management of diabetes for health professionals, provides inpatient and outpatient treatment services in adult and pediatric clinics, supports clinical research to assess new diabetes care systems and approaches, conducts psychosocial research, and supports a network of IDC satellite centers that offer specialized programs in diabetes. The IDC has been designated as a World Health Organization Collaborating Center For Diabetes Education and Training.

Publications: The organization publishes *Living Well With Diabetes,* a quarterly magazine for people with diabetes. Other publications include management and nutrition guides for patients, low-literacy level patient education booklets, guides for health professionals, audiovisuals, and general publications related to chronic health problems and nutrition.

For publications/mail order pharmacy services:
Chronimed
P.O. Box 47945
Minneapolis, MN 55447–9727
1–800-876–6540 or 1–800-477–6388 (In MN) (612) 546–1146

International Diabetes Federation (IDF)
40 Rue Washington
1050 Brussels, Belgium
32–2/647–4414

In collaboration with more than 100 member associations in over 80 countries, the World Health Organization, and other affiliated organizations and individuals, the IDF is engaged in a global effort to ensure the availability of quality care, essential drugs, education, and appropriate modes of treatment for people with diabetes.

Publications: The IDF publishes the *IDF Bulletin,* a journal, and a newsletter; *Directory 1991, A Guide to the Activities of Member Diabetes Associations;* and other publications.

International Diabetic Athletes Association (IDAA)
6829 N. 12th Street
Suite 205
Phoenix, AZ 85014
(602) 230–8155

The IDAA is a nonprofit, membership organization for persons with diabetes who participate in fitness activities at all levels. The organization sponsors workshops, conferences, and other events and offers educational programs for active individuals with diabetes and their families and friends and for diabetes educators, coaches, school nurses, recreation workers, and other professionals who interact with people with diabetes in a recreational setting. The organization's board of directors includes well-known athletes with diabetes, physicians, and other health professionals who are experts in diabetes and sports.

Publications: The IDAA publishes the quarterly newsletter, *The Challenge,* which includes helpful articles about managing diabetes during athletic activities and stories about people with diabetes who participate in sports events.

Joslin Diabetes Center
One Joslin Place
Boston, MA 02215
(617) 732–2400

The Joslin Diabetes Center offers inpatient and outpatient treatment, education, and other support services to adults and children with diabetes; provides professional medical education; sponsors camps for children with diabetes; and supports research to improve treatment and find a cure for diabetes and its complications. The center is affiliated with Harvard Medical School and a number of hospitals in the Boston area and operates affiliated clinics in several states. The Joslin Diabetes Center is one of six Diabetes Endocrinology Research Centers supported by the National Institute of Diabetes and Digestive and Kidney Diseases.

Publications: Joslin publishes a variety of educational materials for patients and professionals, including manuals, nutrition guides, materials for children with diabetes, and films. The *Joslin Magazine* is issued quarterly to members of the Joslin Society.

Juvenile Diabetes Foundation (JDF) International
432 Park Avenue South
New York, NY 10016–8013
(212) 889–7575 or 1–800-223–1138

The JDF, a private, nonprofit, voluntary organization with chapters throughout the United States and the world, raises funds to support research on the cause, cure, treatment, and prevention of diabetes and its complications. The organization awards research grants for laboratory and clinical investigations and sponsors a variety of career development and research training programs for new and established investigators. The JDF also sponsors international workshops and conferences for biomedical researchers, and individual chapters offer support groups and other activities for families.

Publications: The JDF publishes the quarterly journal *Countdown* and a series of patient education brochures about insulin-dependent and non-insulin-dependent diabetes.

National Diabetes Information Clearinghouse (NDIC)
Box NDIC, 9000 Rockville Pike
Bethesda, MD 20892
(301) 654–3327

The NDIC is a service of the National Institute of Diabetes and Digestive and Kidney Diseases, which is the government's lead agency for diabetes research. The NDIC functions as an information, educational, and referral resource for health professionals, people with diabetes, and the general public.

Publications: The NDIC offers a variety of publications for the general public, people with diabetes, and health professionals, including guides for patients and professionals, bibliographies, reports, and fact sheets. The clearinghouse also publishes the newsletter *Diabetes Dateline* and maintains the diabetes subfile on the Combined Health Information Database, available through BRS Online.

National Eye Institute (NEI)
National Eye Health Education Program
Box 20/20
Bethesda, MD 20892
1–800-869–2020 or (301) 496–5248

The NEI, one of the National Institutes of Health, supports basic and clinical research to develop effective treatments for diabetic eye disease. The institute's National Eye Health Education Program promotes public and professional awareness of the importance of early diagnosis and treatment of diabetic eye disease.

Publications: The NEI produces patient and professional education materials related to diabetic eye disease and its treatment, including literature for patients, guides for health professionals, and community education kits for community health workers and for pharmacists.

Pennsylvania Diabetes Academy
777 East Park Drive, Box 8820
Harrisburg, PA 17105–8820
(717) 558–7750
1–800-228–7823, ext. 271 (AA Medical Society)

The academy is a nonprofit organization affiliated with the Pennsylvania Medical Society. It operates as a cooperative venture with the state's Department of Health and the Pennsylvania Diabetes Task Force. The academy offers education, training, and consultation services to health care professionals in the state of Pennsylvania.

Publications: The academy publishes a newsletter and has developed self-study modules for physicians and low-literacy teaching aids for diabetes educators, which are available nationwide.

Chapter 62

NDIC (National Diabetes Information Clearinghouse)

What It Is

The National Diabetes Information Clearinghouse (NDIC) was established in 1978 to increase knowledge and understanding about diabetes among patients, health professionals, and the public. To carry out this mission, NDIC works closely with the diabetes community, forming a network that identifies and responds to informational needs about diabetes and its care.

Included in the NDIC network are the Diabetes Research and Training Centers; the Centers for Disease Control and its Diabetes Control Programs; other Federal agencies; voluntary organizations on the national, regional, and local levels; professional groups; and state departments of health. NDIC, working with a coordinating panel of representatives from these organizations, provides a forum for stimulating the development and exchange of diabetes information.

What It Does

Responses to Inquiries

NDIC responds to requests for information about diabetes and its complications and distributes information appropriate to health professionals, people with diabetes and their families, and the general public. Responses span a wide range of topics, from information about available patient ed-

NIDDK, August 1990.

ucation materials to statistical data from the National Diabetes Data Group about clinical and epidemiological characteristics of diabetes.

Publications

Topical bibliographies, listing a bibliographic citation, an abstract, and information about price, source, and availability for each item. Some citations include the reading level of the material. Readers must order the materials directly from the producer or publisher.

Diabetes Dateline, a current awareness newsletter that features news about diabetes research and announces meetings, special events, and new publications of interest to health care professionals.

The Diabetes Dictionary, an illustrated glossary of over 300 diabetes-related terms. The dictionary provides basic information for people who have diabetes and for their families and friends.

Other publications, including patient booklets about insulin-dependent and noninsulin-dependent diabetes, conference proceedings, monographs, reprints, and materials developed by the National Institutes of Health about various aspects of diabetes research and care.

Technical Guidance

To encourage health professionals and staffs of health organizations to develop high-quality educational materials and programs about diabetes, NDIC distributes resource materials for planning and implementing educational programs and evaluating educational materials. Included are guidelines and standards for educational programs recommended by national diabetes organizations.

Online Data Base

NDIC maintains an automated file of brochures, audiovisual materials, books, articles, teaching manuals, factsheets, and other educational materials on the Combined Health Information Database (CHID). People in the diabetes community have online access to this file through Maxwell Online and thus have readily available such information as bibliographic citations, abstracts, and price and ordering information for every item in the NDIC collection.

Several other health-related organizations have joined NDIC in creating CHID, which incorporates patient and professional materials and information about a number of chronic diseases and about health education issues in general.

How You Can Help

People and organizations who use NDIC are also its best sources of information. By sending descriptions of your educational activities, programs, and materials, you keep NDIC up to date and improve its services. Please send information about your activities and identify your informational needs. Also, add NDIC to your mailing list and tell others about its services. The Clearinghouse welcomes all inquiries. You may write or call:

National Diabetes Information Clearinghouse
Box NDIC
9000 Rockville Pike
Bethesda, Maryland 20892
(301) 468–2162

Chapter 63

DRTC's: Education Activities

The Diabetes Research and Training Centers (DRTC's) are an invaluable resource for diabetes educators and other health professionals involved in treating or counseling people with diabetes.

The DRTC's offer continuing education, seminars, and workshops in state-of-the-art diabetes management for professionals; an array of tested evaluation and assessment instruments; and professional expertise in developing and implementing diabetes programs in a variety of settings.

The DRTC program was established in 1977 by the Diabetes Research and Education Act (P.L. 91–354) in response to a recommendation of the National Commission on Diabetes. Currently, six DRTC's are supported by the National Institute of Diabetes and Digestive and Kidney Diseases (NIDDK). The centers are located at major academic institutions in New York, Illinois, Indiana, Michigan, Tennessee, and Missouri.

DRTC Demonstration and Education Activities

In addition to carrying out basic and clinical research, each DRTC includes a Demonstration and Education Division that focuses on issues related to diabetes translation, including patient education, professional training, and community outreach. DRTC researchers seek to develop and demonstrate innovative approaches to providing quality diabetes care. Many center programs are carried out onsite in model demonstration units, and many take place in community settings. The DRTC's have developed link-

---

NIH Pub. No. 93-3267.

ages with major diabetes professional and voluntary organizations as well as with groups in the communities served by the centers.

Each center also offers a range of educational materials, including videotapes, curricula, and program guides for health professionals. Following are examples of current DRTC demonstration and education activities.

Albert Einstein DRTC

Demonstration and education activities of the Albert Einstein College of Medicine DRTC in Bronx, New York, are under the direction of Dr. Judith Wylie-Rosett. Many of these activities target prevention and treatment of complications of diabetes, and several focus on minority populations.

The Einstein DRTC staff and Columbia University are collaborating on a clinical trial to evaluate a telephone-based consultation model to increase eye screening in Black Americans with diabetes. In another collaboration with the American Diabetes Association (ADA), DRTC staff produced a Spanish-language video, "Diabetes and You: Responsible de du Salud," which is being distributed by ADA.

Working with the Division of Diabetes Translation, Centers for Disease Control and Prevention (CDC), DRTC staff developed and evaluated a problem-based learning curriculum based on the CDC manual The Prevention and Treatment of Five Complications of Diabetes: A Guide for Primary Care Practitioners. Copies of the curriculum and the manual are available from CDC. [For your convenience, the updated version of this manual, *The Prevention and Treatment of Complications of Diabetes*, is reproduced in Chapter 35.]

The Einstein DRTC also offers diabetes specialty training for students at the masters and doctoral levels in conjunction with Yale University School of Nursing, Ferkauf Graduate School of Psychology of Yeshiva University, and the Health Education Program of Teachers College of Columbia University. Students can develop skills related to medical management, patient education, and health care research.

Chicago DRTC

The Demonstration and Education Division of the Chicago DRTC, based at The University of Chicago, is directed by Dr. Wylie McNabb. Many of the programs focus on minority health issues. PATHWAYS, a weight loss program developed by the center for Black American women with diabetes, is being implemented in inner-city churches by lay volunteers. A Spanish-language version of the program is being pilot tested in a Hispanic/Latino neighborhood clinic.

The center recently conducted a diabetes health and wellness survey of more than 3,500 minority individuals in the inner city. The information from the survey will be used to develop community-based interventions for health promotion and disease prevention.

Other programs developed by the DRTC include "From the Basics Forward," a comprehensive continuing education program for diabetes educators, which is being disseminated nationally by the American Association of Diabetes Educators; "In Control," a clinical patient education program for young children with diabetes and their parents; and "Get Going," an exercise program for women with diabetes who live in the inner city.

Indiana DRTC

The Demonstration and Education Division of the Indiana University DRTC, located in Indianapolis, is directed by Dr. David Marrero. The division has developed model programs relating to pregnancy and diabetes, adolescents and diabetes, and low income and minority populations. Many of the programs incorporate computer and telecommunications technology to assist in patient care.

Following a survey of primary care physicians in the state to assess community-based standards of care, Indiana DRTC staff developed several postgraduate medical education courses on principles of intensive diabetes management and the detection and treatment of secondary complications associated with Type I and Type II diabetes. Materials produced in conjunction with these activities include treatment algorithms, study guides, slide and audio programs, and computer-based patient simulations and Hypermedia education programs.

Michigan DRTC

Under the direction of Dr. Roland G. Hiss, the Demonstration and Education Division of the Michigan DRTC at the University of Michigan in Ann Arbor develops model clinical and educational programs relating to the complications of diabetes, adolescents, minority persons, and older adults, as well as educational programs and materials for health professionals and patients in general. Many of the center's programs focus on communities and community organizations for patient education and empowerment.

The Michigan DRTC also develops and evaluates programs and instructional materials and evaluation instruments to measure knowledge and self-care skills and practices of patients. The center offers an undergraduate course for students at the University of Michigan, a teaching and counseling skills course, and basic and advanced symposia for health professionals.

The DRTC publishes a series of outlines entitled "Life with Diabetes" for use in diabetes patient education programs and curricula for use in educational programs for adolescents and for adults with noninsulin-dependent diabetes. A series of 21 patient education booklets, videotapes, and other print materials has also been produced. These materials and instruments are available from the center.

Vanderbilt University DRTC

Directed by Dr. Rodney Lorenz, the Demonstration and Education Division of the Vanderbilt University DRTC in Nashville, Tennessee, has assumed a leading role in improving the teaching skills of health professionals involved in diabetes education. The center's Effective Patient Teaching courses and workshops are widely attended. The courses were recently expanded to include adherence counseling skills, home study formats, and training of trainers.

Vanderbilt DRTC staff have produced videos for problem-based patient learning. Other materials developed by the center include patient education checklists; knowledge and assessment questionnaires for patients and professionals; and interviewing, teaching, and adherence promotion skills manuals.

Washington University DRTC

The Diabetes Education Center of the Washington University DRTC in St. Louis, Missouri, under the direction of Dr. Debra Haire-Joshu, offers graduate courses for multidisciplinary professionals in the development and evaluation of diabetes health care services. A variety of courses and materials is available from the center. Other current activities focus on the translation of results of the Diabetes Control and Complications Trial and collaboration with professional organizations in developing diabetes curricula for dietitians.

The center also conducts intervention studies to educate health professionals in smoking cessation skills, with protocols to be implemented as an ongoing component of training programs. In addition, cultural influences in diabetes are addressed in studies that characterize societal, subcultural, and family factors associated with adherence and metabolic control among Black American youths with insulin-dependent diabetes. Consultants from these studies are available to assist diabetes practitioners who work with minority families.

Guidelines for optimal treatment of diabetes call for integrated care provided by a multidisciplinary team of health care professionals. The Washington DRTC conducts studies to identify organizational characteristics and processes that may influence the development of networks for integrated diabetes care, particularly in rural communities.

Diabetes Research and Training Centers Demonstration and Education Divisions

Judith Wylie-Rosett, Ed.D., R.D.
Albert Einstein College of Medicine
Belfer 1308
1300 Morris Park Avenue
Bronx, NY 10461
(718) 430–2646 or 430–3345
Fax (718) 828–9125

David Marrero, Ph.D.
Indiana University School of Medicine
Regenstrief Institute, 5th Floor
1001 West 10th Street
Indianapolis, IN 46038
(317) 630–6375, Fax (317) 630–6962

Roland G. Hiss, M.D.
Michigan Diabetes Research and Training Center
G1205 Towsley Center, Box 0201
University of Michigan Medical School
Ann Arbor, Ml 48109–0201
(313) 763–1426
Fax (313) 936–1641

Debra Haire-Joshu, Ph.D., R.N.
Washington University School of Medicine,
Diabetes Education Center
33 South Euclid Boulevard
St. Louis, MO 63108
(314) 361–4808, Fax (314) 361–8295

Wylie L. McNabb, Ed.D.
Center for Research in Medical Education and Health Care
University of Chicago
Department of Medicine
5841 South Maryland Avenue, MC 6091
Chicago, IL 60637
(312) 753–1310, Fax (312) 753–1316

Rodney Lorenz, M.D.
Diabetes Research and Training Center
Vanderbilt Medical Center
305 Medical Arts Building
Nashville, TN 37232
(615) 322–4257 or 322–6001
Fax (615) 322–2198

Chapter 64

Diabetes Aids and Resources For People With Visual or Physical Impairment

Products for People with Vision Problems

American Foundation for the Blind
15 W. 16th Street
New York, NY 10011
Telephone: 1–800-232–5463 or (212) 620–2000

National Library Service for the Blind and Physically Handicapped
The Library of Congress
1291 Taylor Street, NW
Washington, DC 20542
Telephone: (202) 707–5100
(Distributes a minibibliography of diabetes-related materials recorded on tape or in braille.)

Resources for Rehabilitation
33 Bedford Street, Suite 19A
Lexington, MA 02173
Telephone: (617) 862–6455
(Distributes various guides and manuals for professionals and large-print materials for people with impaired vision.)

NDIC, September 1992.

National Association for the Visually Handicapped
22 W. 21st St.
New York, NY 10010
(212) 889–3141
(Resource for information about products for people with diabetes and impaired vision.)

The NDIC is a service of the National Institute of Diabetes and Digestive and Kidney Diseases, National Institutes of Health. All products listed in this search are from the NDIC subfile of the Combined Health Information Database (CHID), an on-line database available through BRS/Maxwell Online, Inc. The database is updated quarterly. As new products are identified by NDIC staff, information about them is entered on the database. The database also lists pamphlets, books, articles, brochures, films, cookbooks, and other educational materials for people with diabetes and health professionals.

Chapter 65

Books for Blind and Physically Handicapped Individuals

A free national library program of braille and recorded materials for blind and physically handicapped persons is administered by the National Library Service for the Blind and Physically Handicapped (NLS), Library of Congress. With the cooperation of authors and publishers who grant permission to use copyrighted works, NLS selects and produces full-length books and magazines in braille and on recorded disc and cassette. Reading materials are distributed to a cooperating network of regional and subregional (local) libraries where they are circulated to eligible borrowers. Reading materials and playback machines are sent to borrowers and returned to libraries by postage-free mail. Established by an act of Congress in 1931 to serve blind adults, the program was expanded in 1952 to include children, in 1962 to provide music materials, and again in 1966 to include individuals with other physical impairments that prevent the reading of standard print.

Funding

The NLS program is funded annually by Congress. The fiscal year 1992 appropriation was $42,184,000. Regional and subregional libraries receive funding from state, local, and federal sources. The combined expenditure for the program is approximately $79,000,000.

Eligibility

Anyone who is unable to read or use standard printed materials as a result of temporary or permanent visual or physical limitations may receive

---

Taken from Library of Congress Pub. No. 73-146 (rev. 1/93).

service. A survey sponsored by NLS found that two million persons with some type of visual impairment may be eligible and another million with physical conditions such as paralysis, missing arms or hands, lack of muscle coordination, or prolonged weakness could benefit from the use of reading materials in recorded form.

Book Collection

Books are selected on the basis of their appeal to a wide range of interests. Bestsellers, biographies, fiction, and how-to books are in great demand. Titles expected to be extremely popular are produced on flexible disc in several thousand copies and circulated to borrowers within several months of their publication in print form. A limited number of titles are produced in Spanish and other languages for readers whose primary language is not English. Registered borrowers learn of new books added to the collection through two bimonthly publications, *Braille Book Review* and *Talking Book Topics*. Through a union catalog available on microfiche and in computerized form, every network library has access to the entire NLS book collection and to the resources of several cooperating agencies.

Magazines

Almost seventy magazines on disc and in braille are offered through the program. Readers may request free subscriptions to *U.S. News and World Report*, *National Geographic*, *Consumer Reports*, *Good Housekeeping*, *Sports Illustrated*, *Jack and Jill*, and many other popular magazines. Current issues are mailed to readers at the same time the print issues appear, or shortly thereafter. Magazines are selected for the program in response to demonstrated reader interest.

Equipment and Accessories

Playback equipment is loaned free to readers for as long as recorded materials provided by NLS and its cooperating libraries are being borrowed. Talking-book machines are designed to play disc recorded books and magazines at 8 rpm and 16 rpm; cassette machines are designed for cassettes recorded at 15/16 ips and the standard speed of 1 7/8 ips on 2 and 4 sides. Readers with very limited mobility may request a remote-control unit; hearing impaired readers may be eligible for an auxiliary amplifier for use with headphones. A cassette machine designed primarily for elderly persons is also available.

Music Services

Persons interested in music materials may receive them directly from the Music Section of NLS. The collection consists of scores in braille and large print; textbooks and books about music in braille and large print; and elementary instruction for voice, piano, organ, guitar, recorder, accordion, banjo, and harmonica in recorded form.

Volunteer Services

Free correspondence courses leading to certification in braille transcribing (literary, music, and mathematics braille) and braille proofreading are offered. Voice auditions and informal training are given to volunteer tape narrators affiliated with local recording groups. A directory of volunteer groups that produce books for libraries and individuals is published frequently. Volunteers may call on NLS staff for their expertise in braille transcription and recording techniques.

Information Services

Questions on various aspects of blindness and physical disabilities may be sent to NLS or to any network library. This service is available without charge to individuals, organizations, and libraries. Publications of interest to people with disabilities and service providers are free on request.

Consumer Relations

The consumer relations officer maintains regular contact with consumer groups and individual users of the program to identify and resolve service problems and to assure that users' needs are being met. Participating in surveys, evaluating new equipment, and serving on advisory committees are some of the ways in which consumers contribute to program development.

Research and Development

The NLS research program is directed toward improving the quality of reading materials and playback equipment, controlling program costs, and reducing the time required to deliver services to users. Current research activities include (1) the study of the centralization of the storage and delivery of braille books and NLS audio playback equipment, (2) the development of new mailing containers for braille books, (3) the application of digital techniques to NLS recorded material, and (4) the use of the latest advances in computer technology to provide automated communications links among NLS, all participating libraries, book and magazine producers, and distribution centers.

For Further Information

Ask your local public librarian for more information about the program and how to apply for service.

Chapter 66

Cookbooks for People with Diabetes: Selected Annotations

Preface

The National Diabetes Information Clearinghouse (NDIC) has prepared this bibliography as an information resource for people with diabetes and their families and for health care providers, health educators, and others involved in patient, public, and professional education. No attempt has been made to assess the educational value of the items listed, and their inclusion does not imply endorsement by the National Institute of Diabetes and Digestive and Kidney Diseases.

NDIC staff members have tried to identify all available cookbooks published since 1976 that emphasize recipes for people with diabetes. This publication indicates many of the books that incorporate the revised Exchange Lists for Meal Planning, which the American Diabetes Association and the American Dietetic Association updated in 1986. Most of the cookbooks published before 1986 are based on the 1976 exchange lists, unless otherwise noted. A companion bibliography that some of our readers may be interested in is "Diet and Nutrition for People with Diabetes."

Cookbooks are listed alphabetically by title. An author index and a subject index listing cookbooks by type also are included at the end of this bibliography.

The clearinghouse does not distribute the cookbooks listed in this bibliography. Please contact the source given for each book. Information about price and availability has been verified recently, but prices are subject to

---

NIH Pub. No. 88-2177.

change. [Please contact source for current price information.] Your comments and inquiries and also additional materials on the subject are welcomed. Please send these to the following address:

NATIONAL DIABETES INFORMATION CLEARINGHOUSE
Box NDIC
Bethesda, MD 20892
(301) 468–2162

COOKBOOKS FOR PEOPLE WITH DIABETES: SELECTED ANNOTATIONS

1.

American Diabetes Association/American Dietetic Association Family Cookbook. Vol. I. American Diabetes Association/American Dietetic Association. Prentice-Hall; Rev. 1987. 391 p.

Nutrition guides and about 250 recipes are presented in this cookbook for people with diabetes or others who must limit their intake of calories. The recipes were tested by dietetic students at Madonna College in Michigan and by volunteers who had family members with diabetes. For each recipe, exchange values (based on the 1986 exchange lists) and the estimated values in grams of carbohydrate, protein, and fat, along with milligram amounts of sodium and potassium, are listed for one serving. Appendixes contain additional information on exchanges, nutrition and physiology, cooking terms, common measurements, and recommended daily allowances. An index is included.

Price: $19.45 (nonmembers), $15.95 (ADA members).

Source: Contact local American Diabetes Association Affiliates (listed in telephone directories) or call 1–800-ADA-DISC.

2.

American Diabetes Association/American Dietetic Association Family Cookbook. Vol. II. American Diabetes Association/American Dietetic Association. Prentice-Hall; Rev. 1987. 448 p.

This cookbook, a sequel to the well-received volume I, was designed to enhance meal planning for people with diabetes and others concerned with healthy eating. It presents dietary information and more than 200 recipes, including several for ethnic dishes such as enchiladas and Oriental stirfry.

Each recipe includes a listing of exchange values (based on the 1986 exchange lists) and nutrients per serving. Narrative sections discuss weight control and exercise; glycemic response; living with diabetes; reducing sugar, calories, and food cost; and the use of protein-rich tofu in meal preparation.

Price: $19.45 (nonmembers), $15.95 (ADA members).

Source: Contact local American Diabetes Association Affiliates (listed in telephone directories) or call 1–800-ADA-DISC.

3.
American Diabetes Association/American Dietetic Association Family Cookbook. Vol. III. American Diabetes Association/American Dietetic Association. Prentice-Hall; 1987. 416 p.

This third volume in the cookbook series includes microwave adaptations for half of the recipes. It also presents microwaving tips and recipes for various ethnic dishes. Exchange information is based on the 1986 exchange lists.

Price: $19.45 (nonmembers), $15.95 (ADA members).

Source: Contact local American Diabetes Association Affiliates (listed in telephone directories) or call 1–800-ADA-DISC.

4.
Apricots: A Food That Fits. California Apricot Advisory Board; 1982. 7 p.

This pamphlet identifies the benefits of apricots for people on a diabetic diet. Serving ideas and recipes that use apricots are provided.

Price: Free.

Source: California Apricot Advisory Board; 1280 Boulevard Way; Walnut Creek, CA 94595. (415) 937–3660.

5.
The Art of Cooking for the Diabetic. K. Middleton, M.A. Hess. Contemporary Books; 1978. 372 p.

The 300 fully calculated recipes are based on ADA's list of food exchanges. A short glossary precedes an explanation of the diabetic diet. A section entitled "Living with Diabetes" offers information about sugar substitutes, food shopping, eating out, and physical activity.

Price: $11.95/paperback, $15.95/hardback.

Source: Contemporary Books, Inc.; 180 North Michigan Avenue; Chicago, IL 60601. (312) 782–9181.

6.

Basic Diabetic Meal Pattern. L. Kasala-Fredenberg. American Diabetes Association, Montana Affiliate, Inc.; 1982. 16 p.

The menus in this booklet are designed for a basic 1,200-calorie diabetic meal plan. Developed with cost considerations in mind, the menus meet the recommended dietary allowances for healthy adults. Cooking, shopping, and money-saving guidelines are included, and recipes for selected menu items are provided.

Price: $1.

Source: American Diabetes Association; Montana Affiliate. Inc.; Box 2411; Great Falls, MT 59403. (406) 761–0908.

7.

Basic Diabetic Menu Plan. Change of Menu; Rev. 1986. 48 p.

These diet plans provide menus for 8 weeks for 1,000-, 1,200-, 1,500-, 1,800-, and 2,400-calorie diets. Recipes, shopping lists, preparation hints, and a section of gourmet meals are included. This volume can be used with the monthly supplement to vary meal plans. The supplement can be purchased alone for $14 for a year's subscription. Exchange values are based on the 1986 exchange lists.

Price: $29.95; with monthly supplement, $39.95.

Source: Change of Menu; P.O. Box 544; Sylvania, OH 43560–0544. (419) 841–7821.

8.

Better Meals for You: The Microwave Way. R. Frank, ed. Diabetes Association of Greater Cleveland; 1981. 56 p.

These 33 recipes, developed and tested for use in 600- to 700-watt microwave ovens, have been adapted for people with diabetes from recipes initially published in Bon Appetit magazine. Directions for calculating food exchanges and a sample calculation form are included. The booklet includes the number of calories for each recipe, a weights and measures chart, and guidelines for the use of most seasonings.

Price: $2 plus $0.50 postage and handling (Ohio residents add 5 percent sales tax).

Source: Diabetes Association of Greater Cleveland; 2022 Lee Road; Cleveland, OH 44118. (216) 371–3301.

9.

Better Meals for You With Low-Calorie Gourmet Recipes. J. James, B. Kraus. Diabetes Association of Greater Cleveland; 1977. 48 p.

This booklet contains 87 popular gourmet recipes that have been revised as low-calorie dishes. They contain no added sugar and no artificial ingredients or sweeteners. A natural sweetener made with raisins and water and a "sour cream" made with cottage cheese and lemon juice are used in some recipes. The caloric count and diabetic exchanges have been calculated for each recipe, and the recipes are color coded according to basic food groups. Also included are a sample meal plan, diet guidelines, and a list of free foods.

Price: $2.95 plus $0.50 postage and handling (Ohio residents add 5 percent sales tax).

Source: Diabetes Association of Greater Cleveland; 2022 Lee Road; Cleveland, OH 44118. (216) 371–3301.

10.

Birthday Bonanza. I. Lockerbie, J. Eno. Rev. ed. Canadian Diabetes Association; 1981. 3 p.

This leaflet includes ideas for adapting cake mixes, icings, shortcakes, and ice cream; a recipe for chocolate syrup; and some additional tips for children's parties.

Price: Free.

Source: Canadian Diabetes Association; 562 Eglinton Avenue East; Suite 313; Toronto, Ontario M4P lB9. (416) 488–8871.

11.

Breakfast Ideas: Meal Planning With Exchanges. Dietary Department, University of Iowa Hospitals and Clinics; 1981. 13 p.

The 20 breakfast recipes presented in this booklet include information about exchanges and the total number of calories for each recipe.

Price: $0.40.

Source: University of Iowa Hospitals and Clinics: Dietary Department; Iowa City, IA 52242. (319) 356–2692.

12.

The Calculating Cook: A Gourmet Cookbook for Diabetics and Dieters. J. Jones. 101 Productions; 1977. 192 p.

Gourmet recipes for people with diabetes and for dieters are provided in this illustrated cookbook. Included are directions for adapted versions of many of the classic French sauces as well as several recipes for spicy (Mexican and curry) dishes. Information about the exchange system and lists of substitutes for each category are given.

Price: $6.95/paperback.

Source: MacMillan Publishing Company; Front and Brown Streets; Riverside, NJ 08075. (212) 702–2000. Order Number: ISBN 091–2238-232.

13.

Canning and Freezing with Low Salt and No Added Sugar. B. Wedman. Betty Wedman Services; 1979. 127 p.

This guide provides general canning and freezing information for preserving foods without adding sugar. It also includes recipes for jellies and jams, vegetables, and fruit preserves. Calorie counts and exchanges are given for each serving.

Price: $2.

Source: NAFCO; 901 Janesville Avenue; Fort Atkinson, WI 53538. 1–800-558–9595.

14.

Choice Cooking: For Those Who Care About Their Health and Enjoy Good Food. Canadian Diabetes Association. NC Press; 1982. 223 p.

This cookbook offers recipes for appetizers, beverages, sauces, soups, salads, vegetables, meats, fish, poultry, one-dish meals, meatless meals, breads, desserts, and preserves and pickles. The book has full-color photographs and is bound as a spiral notebook. The food group system, a Canadian form of the exchange system, is presented. Examples of menus for a variety of meals using the book's recipes are given.

Price: $12.15 (Canadian) plus $1.50 postage.

Source: Canadian Diabetes Association: 562 Eglinton Avenue East; Suite 313; Toronto, Ontario M4P lB9. (416) 488–8871. Order Number: ISBN 0–919601–69-3.

15.

The Complete Diabetic Cookbook. M.J. Finsand. Sterling Publications; 1980. 192 p.

More than 250 recipes, ranging from sandwich spreads and snacks to gourmet dishes, are featured in this cookbook. Regular and metric measurements are given for each ingredient, and every recipe shows the yield in total servings and the calorie count and food exchange equivalents for single portions. Directions for both range/oven and microwave cooking are given. Food exchange lists are based on the 1976 exchange lists. The book also lists calorie counts and exchange values for alcoholic beverages and many commercially prepared foods. The recipes are indexed.

Price: $8.95.

Source: Sterling Publishing Company, Inc.; Two Park Avenue; New York, NY 10016. (212) 532–7160.

16.

Cookbook for Diabetics and Their Families. University of Alabama Hospitals. Oxmoor House; 1986. 201 p.

The recipes in this book are designed so that individuals with diabetes and their families can eat the same foods. Basic nutrition concepts and exchange lists for meal planning are presented. Tips for selecting and purchasing foods are included, and nutrition labeling is explained. Recipes for beverages, breads, eggs and cheeses, meats, fish, potatoes and rice, salad dressings, and vegetables are presented.

Price: $10.95 plus $1 postage.

Source: University of Alabama Hospital; Department of Dietetics; 619 South l9th Street; Birmingham, AL 35233. (205) 934–4011.

17.

Cooking for Diabetics at Home and Away: A Diabetic's Easy Guide on How to Enjoy Life. W.A. Rhodes. Charles C. Thomas; 1976. 240 p.

This book contains information about food exchanges and calories per serving and the number of servings for each recipe. Advice is given about making choices when dining in restaurants, going to parties and picnics, or traveling. Recipes are included for beverages, appetizers and snacks, desserts, breads, meats and meat substitutes, poultry, seafood, soups and sandwiches, salads and salad dressings, and vegetables.

Price: $23.

Source: Charles C. Thomas, Publisher; 2600 South First Street; Springfield, IL 62794–9265. (217) 789–8980.

18.

Cooking for Love and Life. Vol. 1. P.S. Jamison. Recipes for Life; 1979. 272 p.

Information about exchanges, calories, carbohydrates, proteins, and fats per serving is included for each of the 300 recipes in this cookbook. Southern-style cooking (mostly Creole) is featured. Metric measurements, canning and freezing information, and a method for determining ideal weight are also included.

Price: $12.95 plus $1 postage (Louisiana residents add 5 percent sales tax).

Source: Recipes for Life, Inc.: P.O. Box 4718; Lafayette, LA 70502. (318) 234–2505.

19.

Cooking for the Health of It. G.L. Becker. Cumberland Packing Corporation; 1981. 159 p.

Recipes that use Sweet 'N Low® sugar substitute, Butter Buds® margarine substitute, and Nu-Salt® salt substitute are provided. Per-serving values of calories, protein, carbohydrates, fat, and sodium are given with each recipe.

Price: $3.95.

Source: Cumberland Packing Corporation; Two Cumberland Street; Brooklyn, NY 11205. 1–800-336–0363 or (718) 858–4200.

20.

Cooking With Care. American Diabetes Association, Colorado Affiliate; 1988.

Features low-fat, low-cholesterol, and sugarless recipes, and most are low in sodium. The book was prepared in conjunction with the affiliate's

"Celebrity Cookoff" event, and the recipes of well-known media personalities and other celebrities in Colorado are featured. Calorie, sodium, and cholesterol information is provided for recipes. Exchange list equivalents are based on the 1986 exchange lists. An introduction provides general information about diabetes and nutrition and exercise in diabetes management.

Price: $8.50 including postage; purchase may be considered a tax-deductible gift to ADA.

Source: American Diabetes Association; Colorado Affiliate; 2450 South Downing Street; Denver, C0 80210. (303) 778–7556.

21.
Cooking with "Catfish" Hunter: Tasty Recipes for People with Diabetes. J. Hunter. Upjohn Company; 1987. 20 p.

This booklet presents recipes and menus named in honor of Catfish Hunter's former profession—baseball. Examples of recipes included are Seventh Game Soup, World Series Stew, and Pitcher's Mound Pie. Nutritional information is provided for each recipe, and sample menus and a discussion of nutrition for people with diabetes are featured.

Price: Free.

Source: Cooking with "Catfish" Hunter; P.0. Box 307-C; Coventry, CT 06238.

22.
Cooking With Sweet 'N Low®: Take Your Pick of the Many Forms. Cumberland Packing Corporation; 1986. 20 p.

Recipes for substituting Sweet 'N Low® in place of granulated sugar and brown sugar are provided. Each recipe lists the calories per serving, number of servings per recipe, and number of calories saved by using Sweet 'N Low® instead of sugar. A Sweet 'N Low® conversion chart is provided for both granulated and brown sugar substitutes.

Price: $0.50.

Source: Sweet 'N Low®; Department A; Two Cumberland Street; Brooklyn, NY 11205. 1–800-336–0363 or (718) 858–4200.

23.
Creative Cooking for the Diabetic. L. Payne, I. Rapp. Deaconess Hospital; 1988.

The introduction of this manual identifies the goals of the diabetic diet, offers rules to aid in diabetes control, and reviews the main nutrients required for health. Subsequent chapters discuss cholesterol and fat in the diet, the amounts of protein and fiber found in meatless meals, the effects of exercise, and liquid diets. Suggestions are made for dining out, alcohol use, holiday and party menus, and brown bag lunches. Food exchange lists and fast food exchanges are included, as are a number of recipes, all of which have been kitchen-tested. Appendixes present sample meal patterns, convenience foods and their exchange values, and a listing of cookbooks.

Price: $9 plus $2 postage.

Source: Diabetes Information Center; Deaconess Hospital; West 800 Fifth Avenue; Spokane, WA 99210. (509) 458–7142.

24.

Creole Recipes for People With Diabetes. [anon.]. American Diabetes Association, Greater New Orleans Affiliate; 1985. 60 p.

To enhance daily meal planning by persons who have diabetes, Creole recipes were compiled by the New Orleans Dietetic Association in conjunction with the New Orleans chapter of ADA. The recipes include soups and appetizers, salads, entrees, sauces, starches and vegetables, and desserts. Skim milk is the basis for the milk exchange. Equivalents of artificial sweetener to refined sugar are listed for Sugar Twin®, Sugar Twin Brown®, Sweet 'N Low®, Adolph's Sugar Substitute®, and Sweet Magic®.

Price: $5 plus $1 postage.

Source: American Diabetes Association; Greater New Orleans Chapter, Inc.; 3101 West Napoleon Avenue; Suite 238; Metairie, LA 70001 (504) 837–2900.

25.

Delectable Dining for Diabetics. [anon.]. Rogue Valley Memorial Hospital; 1980. 201 p.

This cookbook contains recipes for appetizers, beverages, breads, cheeses and eggs, crock pot dishes, desserts, meat/fish/poultry, salads and salad dressings, sandwiches, sauces and relishes, soups, and vegetables. Food exchanges and carbohydrates, protein, and fat contents are listed for each recipe. Guidelines are given for the use of dietetic foods and sweeteners such as xylitol, mannitol, and sorbitol. Hints to aid food preparation and suggestions for dining out and holiday meals are offered. The cookbook concludes with recipes featuring low-cost foods, tips on home freezing and canning, instructions for making jams and jellies, the 1976 exchange lists, and a recipe index.

Price: $4.60 plus $0.70 postage.

Source: Rogue Valley Medical Center, Dietary Department; 2825 Barnett; Medford, OR 97501. (503) 773–6281.

26.

Delightful Diabetic Dining Cookbook. Shadyside Hospital Dietetic Interns. Shadyside Hospital; 1980. 57 p.

Recipes with cooking instructions and some general tips to make following a diet easier are incorporated in this cookbook. To facilitate meal planning, exchange values (1976) are given for entrees, vegetables, sauces and soups, salads, and desserts and also for special lunch box, picnic, party, and holiday recipes. Tips to help one follow a diet and suggestions for eating out are offered. An expanded exchange list, a list of dietary source books, and a recipe index are included.

Price: $5 plus $1 postage.

Source: Dietetic Education; Shadyside Hospital; 5230 Centre Avenue; Pittsburgh, PA 15232. (412) 622–2429.

27.

Diabetes Control and the Kosher Diet. A.P. Kahn. Wordscope Associates; 1985.

This book addresses the basic concerns of people with diabetes who keep kosher kitchens or who just enjoy traditional kosher foods. The book's 32 recipes for traditional and nontraditional Jewish foods for religious holidays and other meals were developed and tested by Teila Lechtman, R.D. Each recipe gives exchange values and nutritional information per serving. The book also includes chapters about diabetes and its management, diabetes and the kosher diet, and kosher convenience foods. A list of resources and a glossary are included. Members of the Chicago Rabbinical Council reviewed and contributed to the book, and all recipes and nutrition advice conform to the rules of Kashrut.

Price: $9.95 plus $1.55 postage.

Source: Wordscope Associates; P.O. Box 1594; Skokie, IL 60076.

28.

Diabetes Meal Planning and Recipes. B. Wedman. Betty Wedman Services; 1977. 36 p.

This booklet focuses on diabetes meal planning, with basic information given on menu planning, including modifications for traveling and illness. A number of recipes for several food groups are included along with holiday menus. Exchanges (1976) are listed for convenience soups and some Chinese and Mexican foods.

Price: $2.

Source: NAFCO; 901 Janesville Avenue; Fort Atkinson, WI 53538. 1–800-558–9595.

29.

Diabetes Over 60: Meals to Serve You Well. Canadian Diabetes Association; 1986. 28 p.

This booklet was developed to help older people with diabetes prepare satisfying and interesting meals. It contains sample menu suggestions, recipes for one or two servings, shopping and food storage ideas, tips on food preparation, and hints for "pepping up" meals. Foods to keep on an "emergency shelf" are listed, and precautions with respect to sugar, sodium, and cholesterol are spelled out. The booklet is also available in French.

Price: Free.

Source: Canadian Diabetes Association; 562 Eglinton Avenue East; Suite 313; Toronto, Ontario M4P lB9. (416) 488–8871.

30.

Diabetic Breakfast & Brunch Cookbook. M.J. Finsand. Sterling Publishing Company, Inc.; 1987. 160 p.

A variety of recipes for breakfasts and brunches are presented. Although directed to people on diabetic diets, the meals are meant to be enjoyed by the whole family. Breakfast and brunch suggestions feature foods from all of the basic food groups and include recipes for a variety of occasions: microwave recipes for one person, some breakfast recipes for children, and recipes for leisurely mornings. Each recipe includes calories and food exchanges for each serving, and measurements are provided in both metric and U.S. equivalents.

Price: $8.95.

Source: Sterling Publishing Company, Inc.; Two Park Avenue; New York, NY 10016. (212) 532–7160.

31.

Diabetic Cakes, Pies & Other Scrumptious Desserts. M.J. Finsand. Sterling Publishing Company, Inc.; 1988. 160 p.

Recipes for more than 200 low-calorie desserts made with sugar replacements are provided in this cookbook for people with diabetes and others on calorie-restricted diets. Included are recipes for pies, cakes, puddings, cookies, soufflés, ice cream and other frozen desserts, crusts, and toppings. Nutrition information and exchange values are provided for each recipe. Other features of the book include a discussion of various types of artificial sweeteners; recipe conversion guides; lists of flavorings, extracts, spices, and herbs; a discussion of the new exchange lists; and Weight Watchers® food product information.

Price: $8.95

Source: Sterling Publishing Company, Inc.; Two Park Avenue; New York, NY 10016. (212) 532–7160.

32.

Diabetic Candy, Cookie, and Dessert Cookbook. M.J. Finsand. Sterling Publications; 1982. 160 p.

The more than 250 recipes for candies, cookies, and desserts included in this volume use substitutes for sugar, syrups, toppings, puddings, and gelatins. The author identifies artificial sweeteners and other sugar replacements and describes their most appropriate uses. General cooking/baking instructions and nutritional information for various prepared dietetic foods are listed.

Price: $7.95.

Source: Sterling Publishing Company, Inc.; Two Park Avenue; New York, NY 10016. (212) 532–7160. Order Number: ISBN 0–8069-7586–5.

33.

The Diabetic Chocolate Cookbook. M.J. Finsand. Sterling Publications; 1984.

This cookbook offers low-calorie recipes for more than 200 desserts, including chocolate butter creams, French fudge, and creamy chocolate mousse. The cookbook contains sections on candy and fudge; cookies, bars, and brownies; cakes, pies, and pastries; chilled desserts; and syrups, beverages, and toppings. Each recipe includes calorie and food exchange information. The cookbook includes a discussion of sweeteners and sugar replacements and different kinds of chocolate and carob. The appendix includes the 1976 exchange lists, nutritional information about product labels, and a selected bibliography.

Price: $8.95 plus $1.50 postage/paperback only.

Source: Sterling Publishing Company, Inc.; Two Park Avenue; New York, NY 10016. (212) 532–7160.

34.

Diabetic Cooking for One or Two. Vols. 1 and 2. Change of Menu; 1986. 124 p. each volume.

Each volume includes more than 200 recipes for dishes that serve one or two people. Recipes are given for appetizers; sauces, dressings, and stocks; salads and soups; fruits and vegetables; fish, chicken, meat, dairy, and vegetarian main dishes; breads, pasta, rice, and potatoes; desserts; and beverages. Recipes use commonly available ingredients, and each includes nutrition information and exchange values based on the 1986 exchange lists. A shopping list of foods and spices to keep on hand and guidelines for cooking in small quantities are included.

Price: $12.95 for each volume.

Source: Change of Menu; Box 544; Sylvania, OH 43560–0544.

(419) 841–7821.

35.

Diabetic Dining. O. Kronschnabel. Reiman Publications; 1979. 98 p.

More than 150 recipes are included for people with diabetes and others who must follow special diets. Most of the recipes are tailored for those who cook for only two people.

Price: $3.95 plus $1.25 postage.

Source: The Country Store; P.O. Box 572; Milwaukee, WI 53201.

National: 1–800-558–1013; Wisconsin: (414) 423–0175. Specify Part No. 0453 when ordering.

36.

The Diabetic Gourmet. A.J. Bowen. Rev. ed. Harper and Row; 1980. 193 p.

Meal planning procedures and recipes to adapt a family's meals to the needs of a member with diabetes are provided. Types of diabetic diets—exchange, weighed, sugar-free, and altered-fat—are compared in terms of convenience and applicability to individual needs. Recipes include weights of carbohydrates, protein, and fats and the exchange values for each serving.

Price: $5.50/paperback, $13.45/hardback.

Source: Harper and Row; Keystone Industrial Park; Scranton, PA 18512. 1–800-638–3030 or 1–800-242–7737.

37.

The Diabetic Gourmet Cookbook. M.J. Finsand. Sterling Publications; 1986.

This cookbook includes more than 250 easy-to-understand recipes for dishes like lobster Newburg, vichyssoise, and chicken Kiev. This cookbook features a wide variety of reduced-calorie, low-sugar recipes for gourmet appetizers, beverages, entrees, soups and stews, pastas, sauces, breads, vegetables, and desserts. Each recipe lists calorie, carbohydrate, and food exchange information for each serving. Food exchange lists are based on the 1986 exchange lists.

Price: $19.95 plus $1.50 postage/hardback, $8.95 plus $1.50 postage/paperback.

Source: Sterling Publishing Company, Inc.; Two Park Avenue; New York, NY 10016. (212) 532–7160.

38.

Diabetic High-Fiber Cookbook. M.J. Finsand. Sterling Publishing Company, Inc.; 1985. 160 p.

Recipes in this book focus on ways to increase dietary fiber without sacrificing taste or changing calorie counts. More than 250 recipes using ingredients high in fiber such as whole-grain cereals and bran products; beans and other legumes, seeds, and nuts; and vegetables and fruits are presented. Recipes are provided for breakfast, appetizers and snacks, salads, vegetables, entrees, casseroles, breads, and desserts, and one chapter provides recipes and instructions for making homemade sausages. Every recipe includes calorie counts and diabetic exchanges, and some include microwave instructions. Measurements are provided in both metric and U.S. equivalents.

Cost: $8.95.

Source: Sterling Publishing Company, lnc.; Two Park Avenue; New York, NY 10016. (212) 532–7160.

39.

Diabetic Snack & Appetizer Cookbook. M.J. Finsand. Sterling Publishing Company, Inc.; 1987. 160 p.

Suggestions and recipes for quick, easy-to-fix, and healthy snack foods are provided. Included are recipes for soups, salads, sandwiches, fruity beverages, meats, sweets, frozen treats, and convenience foods. One chapter, entitled "Kids' Stuff," features recipes that youngsters can make and enjoy. Every recipe includes exchange values, calorie and carbohydrate counts, and yield. One section of the book lists foods to keep in stock, and another provides nutritional information about a number of brand-name food products. A discussion of the 1986 exchange lists also is included.

Price: $8.95.

Source: Sterling Publishing Company, Inc.; Two Park Avenue; New York, NY 10016. (212) 532–7160.

40.

Diet for a Healthy Heart. Nabisco Brands, Inc.; 1985. 45 p.

Recipes stressing low cholesterol and reduced saturated fat content are featured. Many of the recipes use Egg Beaters® in place of eggs. Sample meal plans and tables for diets based on certain calorie levels are included along with a table providing nutrient information for major food groups. Although they are not directed specifically to diabetic diets, recipes include exchange values. Recipes feature Fleischmann's products.

Price: Free.

Source: Nabisco Brands, Inc.; East Hanover, NJ 07936. (201) 503–2000.

41.

Dining with Your Diabetic Child. C. Briggs. Kerry and Christy Briggs; 1978. 79 p.

Six weeks of complete dinner plans are designed to enable families of children who have diabetes to eat according to the child's diet without loss of variety, nutrition, or enjoyment. Fifty recipes include soups, casseroles, salads, meat dishes, seafood, chicken, syrups, and gelatins. The recipes are approved by the patient education committee of the ADA, Utah Affiliate, Inc.

Price: $6.95 plus $1.50 postage.

Source: Ms. Christy Briggs; 433 East Deepdale Road; Phoenix, AZ 85022. (602) 993–8215.

42.
Equal® Low-Calorie Sweetener. Searle Consumer Products, Division of Searle Pharmaceuticals, Inc; 1987. 8 p.

This pamphlet, produced by the manufacturer of Equal®, discusses the sweetener's taste and caloric content, identifies its composition, and compares it with other available sweetening agents. The pamphlet includes suggestions on the use of Equal®, and contains two beverage and two dessert recipes.

Price: Free.

Source: Equal®; Box 8517; Chicago, IL 60680. (312) 470–9710.

43.
Fabulous Fiber Cookbook. J. Jones. Third ed. 101 Productions; 1985. 192 p.

This cookbook contains several hundred high-fiber recipes for dishes that are also low in calories. None of the ingredients used includes processed or refined foods or chemical additives. Exchanges are given for each recipe as well as calories and grams of fiber per serving. Extensive exchanges based on the 1976 exchange lists are included. The fiber content of the various exchange list foods is also given. References and an index are provided.

Price: $7.95/paperback.

Source: 101 Productions; 834 Mission Street; San Francisco, CA 94103. (415) 495–6040.

44.
Feast on a Diabetic Diet. E. Gibbons, J. Gibbons. Rev. ed. Fawcett; 1978. 314 p.

Recipes for people with diabetes and for nondiabetic individuals are included in chapters on topics such as "Vegetables, Salads, and Herbs";

"Main Dish Delights"; "To Exercise Your Sweet Tooth"; and the "Diabetic Camper". With the aid of a gram scale and a food table, people with diabetes are shown how to develop menus and adapt recipes in standard cookbooks to comply with the prescribed diet. There is also an appendix describing books, equipment, and supplies.

Price: $2.95/paperback.

Source: Fawcett Books; 400 Hawn Road; Westminster, MD 21157. (301) 751–2600; 1–800-638–6460: or 1–800-492–0782.

45.

Food for Survival and Other Helpful Hints for Living With Diabetes. J. Kenien, B.C. Stanislao. Fargo Diabetes Education Center; 1982. 39 p.

This illustrated booklet discusses nutrition management for diabetes and explains the exchange lists and their use. Additions to the exchange lists and the use of Heinz products in diabetic meals are listed. Instructions and a worksheet show how to figure exchange equivalents using nutrition labeling. The authors also present guidance about dietetic foods, meals during illness, the sweetening power of common artificial sweeteners or sugar substitutes, freezing and canning, and dining out. The booklet includes recipes and a recipe conversion worksheet, exchange values for fast-food restaurant fare, activity guidelines, and references.

Price: $2.50 plus $0.75 postage.

Source: Fargo Diabetes Education Center; Box 5364; NDSU Station; Fargo, ND 58105. (701) 293–4152 or 280–5570.

46.

Food Service Recipes. California Apricot Advisory Board. 3 p.

Three 5- by 8-inch cards provide recipes for using apricots in food service operations. Each of the five recipes lists the food exchanges and provides calorie, carbohydrate, fat, protein, and sodium information for one serving. A guide to availability, nutritional value, storage, and use of apricots is provided on the back of one recipe card.

Price: Free.

Source: California Apricot Advisory Board; 1280 Boulevard Way; Walnut Creek, CA 94598. (415) 937–3660.

47.

The Fruitsweet Cookbook. J.A. Pentico. American Diabetes Association, Iowa Affiliate; 1979. 26 p.

Recipes for desserts made from fruits, fruit juices, and fruit butters without adding sugar are provided. They are designed for dieters, people with diabetes, and others who wish to avoid "empty calories." The exchanges are given for single servings.

Price: $2.50 plus $0.45 postage.

Source: American Diabetes Association; Iowa Affiliate; 888 10th Street, Marion, IA 53302. (319) 373–0530.

48.

Gourmet Recipes for Diabetics. Perigee Books 1987. 232 p.

A sequel to "Recipes for Diabetics," this cookbook provides gourmet recipes for main courses, appetizers, soups, salads, desserts, and drinks. Many of the recipes are low in calories, fat, and cholesterol and contain plenty of fruits and vegetables. One chapter addresses how to compute food exchanges from nutrition labeling. The 1976 exchange lists and a daily menu guide are included along with a list of resources, a table giving diabetic exchanges for brand-name foods, metric conversion information, a buying guide for fruits and vegetables, and an index.

Price: $8.95.

Source: The Putnam Publishing Group; One Grosset Drive; Kirkwood, NY 13795.

49.

The Guiltless Gourmet. J. Gilliard, J. Kirkpatrick. Diabetes Center, Inc.; 1987. 170 p.

Recipes, menus, and nutrition information are presented especially for dieters, people with diabetes, and people on sodium-restricted or cholesterol-restricted diets. Cookbook recipes are designed to be simple, inexpensive, and low in calories, fat, cholesterol, and salt. Listed for each food serving are the number of calories; the amount of protein, carbohydrates, fat, cholesterol, sodium, and dietary fiber; and the exchange values computed by ADA. Reading Level: 10.

Price: $9.95.

Source: Diabetes Center, Inc.; P.O. Box 739; Wayzata, MN 55391. 1–800-848–2793.

50.

Healthy Holiday Recipes from Sweet 'N Low®. Cumberland Packing Corporation; 1986. 29 p.

This brochure provides 20 recipes (liquids and solid foods) for holiday foods that are low in sugar. Each recipe lists the calories saved by substituting saccharine sweeteners for granulated sugar. Tips on healthy holiday entertaining are provided as well as a Sweet 'N Low® conversion chart for both granulated sugar and brown sugar.

Price: $0.50.

Source: Sweet 'N Low®; Department A; Two Cumberland Street; Brooklyn, NY 11205. 1–800-336–0363 or (718) 858–4200.

51.

The High-Fiber Cookbook for Diabetics. M. Cavaiani. Perigee Books; 1987. 208 p.

Written by a registered dietitian who has diabetes, this cookbook provides more than 100 high-fiber recipes. The recipes are grouped into nine categories: soups, entrees, vegetables, salads, yeast breads, hot breads, cookies, pies, and puddings. Exchanges and nutritive values are listed per serving for each recipe. The book presents general information about diabetes, the benefits of fiber, and explanations of the 1986 exchange lists. Useful cooking and nutritional information is included as well as tips for lowering the sodium and cholesterol level of recipes.

Price: $8.95.

Source: The Putnam Publishing Group; One Grosset Drive; Kirkwood, NY 13795.

52.

High Fiber Delights. D. Willcox. Humana Hospital-Lucerne; 1984. 82 p.

Recipes are offered in the categories of entrees, vegetables, salads, breads and sandwiches, breakfast ideas, and desserts. According to the author, all recipes in the looseleaf binder are "low in fat, low in salt, sugar free, high in carbohydrate, and high in fiber." The food exchange values, calories, and amounts of protein, carbohydrates, and fat for a single serving are listed for each recipe. The food exchange system used is the high-carbohydrate, high-fiber (HCF) diet system, consisting of 10 food exchange groups.

Price: $8.

Source: Humana Hospital-Lucerne; Diabetes Care Center; 818 South Main Lane; Orlando, FL 32801. (305) 237–6111.

53.

Holiday Cookbook. B. Wedman. Prentice-Hall Press: 1986 219 p.

Traditional and nontraditional holiday recipes are featured in this cookbook for people with diabetes and their families. Each recipe contains food exchange values based on the 1986 exchange lists. This cookbook, written by a registered dietitian, provides the number of calories and grams of protein, fat, and carbohydrates per serving. It also includes sections about basic nutrition and diabetes, how to adjust favorite recipes to meet specific dietary requirements, and general meal planning information.

Price: $14.95 plus $1.50 postage.

Source: American Diabetes Association; National Service Center; 1660 Duke Street; Alexandria, VA 22314. 1–800-232–3472. In the Washington, DC, metropolitan area, (703) 549–1500.

54.

Holiday Cooking for the Diabetic. P. Nelson. Northeast Community Hospital; 1987. 33 p., revised yearly.

This annual cookbook published by Northeast Community Hospital provides caloric content and exchange information for each recipe. It contains traditional low-calorie, exchange-compatible holiday recipes such as turkey and dressing and nontraditional recipes such as Italian broiled cod. Short sections about breads, breakfasts, desserts, lunches, main dishes, salads, soups, and vegetables are included.

Price: $7.50.

Source: Northeast Community Hospital; Community Relations Department; 1301 Airport Freeway; Bedford, TX 76021. (817) 282–9211.

55.

The International Menu Diabetic Cookbook. B. Marks, L.H. Schechter. Contemporary Books; 1985. 364 p.

This cookbook features more than 300 international dishes for people with diabetes who are restricted to a low-fat, low-sodium, high-fiber, and sugarless diet. Based on ADA's recommendations for the diabetic diet, the recipes are easy to follow and have food exchange values and calculations. All have been approved by a registered dietitian.

Price: $14.95.

Source: Contemporary Books; 180 North Michigan Avenue; Chicago, IL 60601. (312) 782–9181. Order Number: ISBN 0–8092-5390–9.

56.

The Joy of Snacks. N. Cooper. Diabetes Center, Inc.; 1987. 269 p.

Recipes for more than 200 snack foods in 12 categories are given. Included are recipes for popcorn snacks, appetizers, muffins/breads, and a special chapter giving recipes that children will enjoy. Each recipe includes nutritional information as well as exchange values per serving. Similar information is listed for commercial snacks, including exchange values.

Price: $12.95.

Source: Diabetes Center, Inc.; P.O. Box 739; Wayzata, MN 55391. 1–800-848–2793. In Minnesota, 1–612-541–0239, collect.

57.

Just Delicious and Sugar Free. I. Ellenson. Juvenile Diabetes Foundation International; 1977. 20 p.

In this cookbook are sugar-free recipes for pies, cookies, cakes, breads and muffins, and other desserts and sauces. Sugar substitutes are used in some of the recipes, but most of them specify natural sweeteners such as unsweetened fruit or fruit juices. Each recipe provides the number of exchanges for a single serving.

Price: $4.

Source: Juvenile Diabetes Foundation International; Southeastern Michigan Chapter; 29350 Southfield Road, Room 38; Southfield, MI 48076. (313) 569–6171.

58.

Just Desserts: A Collection of De"Lite"ful Recipes. Rochester Regional Chapter of the American Diabetes Association: 1985.

The recipes listed in this cookbook are made primarily with low-fat, sugar-free ingredients. The selection of desserts found in the cookbook ranges from recipes for cakes, cookies, and pastries to those for puddings, muffins, and pies. Exchange values and caloric and nutritional information (for carbohydrates, proteins, and sodium) are listed for each recipe.

Price: $7.95 plus $1 postage.

Source: American Diabetes Association; Rochester Regional Chapter; 797 Elmwood Avenue; Rochester, NY 14620. (716) 271–1260.

59.

Kids, Food, and Diabetes: A Book of Recipes, Menus and Practical Advice. G. Loring. 1986.

Part I of this book for parents of children with diabetes offers basic exchange information and guidance for making daily food choices. Various menu ideas and recipes are included in part II. The last section, entitled the "Copebook," discusses how diabetes affects the stages of child development. This section also includes suggestions for helping parents effectively deal with diabetes-related psychological problems as well as a list of organizations that disseminate information about diabetes.

Price: $17.95 plus postage and handling/hardcover, $11.95 plus postage and handling/paperback.

Source: Contemporary Books, Inc.; 180 North Michigan Avenue; Chicago, IL 60601. (312) 782–9181.

60.

The Lowfat Lifestyle. V. Parker, R. Gates. LFL Associates; 1986. 261 p.

The recipes in this book focus on foods and ingredients that are low in fat. Although not specifically directed to people with diabetes, the nutrition guidelines presented stress weight loss and cardiovascular health, both of which are important to people with diabetes. This book includes recipes for all kinds of foods, hints about kitchen tools and ingredients, health and fitness tips, and keep-trim exercises. LFL also produces a monthly newsletter, LowFat Lifeline, available by subscription, and other cookbooks as well as nutrition posters, calipers, and audiovisual materials for nutrition educators.

Price: $9.95 plus $0.50 postage/paperback, $11.95 plus $0.50 postage/comb-bound.

Source: Lowfat Lifestyle; 52 Condolea Court; Lake Oswego, OR 97035. (503) 636–1559.

61.

Low Sodium, Low Cholesterol Diabetic Menu Plan: Easy Meal Planning for the Sodium/Cholesterol-Restricted Diabetic. Change of Menu; 1984. 48 p.

Menus are provided for 4 weeks for people with diabetes who also are on restricted sodium and cholesterol diets. Daily meal plans in chart form indicate portion sizes for diets ranging from 1,000 to 2,400 calories per day. Recipes, shopping lists, preparation hints, and a selection of gourmet meals are included.

Price: $19.95.

Source: Change of Menu; P.O. Box 544; Sylvania, OH 43560–0544. (419) 841–7821.

62.

Meal Challenge Cookbook. Roerig, Division of Pfizer Pharmaceuticals; 1988. 88 p.

This book features winning recipes from a national recipe contest sponsored by Roerig, a division of Pfizer Pharmaceuticals. Included are first-, second-, and third-place winners in each of five categories: appetizers, breads/soups/salads, side dishes, entrees, and desserts. Each recipe includes food exchange values based on the 1986 exchange lists and a nutritional analysis per portion.

Price: Free.

Source: Pfizer Pharmaceuticals; 235 East 42nd Street; New York, NY 10017. (212) 573–3178.

63.

Meal Management: A Diabetes Handbook. B. Billette, P. Orvidas. Portland Diabetes Center and Good Samaritan Hospital and Medical Center; 1984. 40 p.

Seven guidelines for following a diabetic diet are given as an introduction to a listing of foods and their exchange values. The booklet includes 10 recipes and a brief glossary.

Price: $5.

Source: Portland Diabetes Center; Diabetes Treatment Unit; 2282 Northwest Northrup Avenue; Portland, OR 97210. (503) 229–7227.

64.
Microwave Cooking for Diabetics. Change of Menu; 1988.

This book includes more than 125 recipes for preparing a variety of foods, from one-dish meals to desserts and appetizers, in a microwave oven. Information about microwaves and tips for microwave cooking are provided. Each recipe lists nutrient contents and exchange values based on the 1986 exchange lists.

Price: $12.95.

Source: Change of Menu; P.O. Box 54; Sylvania, OH 43560–0544. (419) 841–7821.

65.
Microwaving Light and Healthy. B. Methven. Cy DeCosse Inc.; 1985. 159 p.

Recipes for preparing healthy dishes in a microwave oven are provided. The recipes feature use of low-fat, high-fiber ingredients, and nutrient and exchange values are provided per portion for each recipe. The book is well illustrated and includes recipes for soups and appetizers; poultry, fish and seafood, beef, pork, and meatless dishes; vegetables, pasta, and grains; and baking and desserts. Advantages of microwave cookery are outlined, and directions are given for cooking healthy meals in a microwave oven. The importance of changing dietary habits and maintaining them for a lifetime is stressed.

Price: $14.95 plus postage. (Preview copies and educational discounts available.)

Source: Cy DeCosse; 5900 Green Oaks Drive; Minnetonka, MN 55343. 1–800-328–0590.

66.
Microwaving on a Diet. B. Methven. Publication Arts; 1981. 160 p.

Designed to show the use of a microwave oven to make diet foods flavorful, nutritious, attractive, and easy to prepare, this cookbook includes information about nutrition, the exchange system, and menu planning. It provides breakfast, lunch, and dinner menus with recipes for appetizers, soups, beverages, entrees, vegetables, fruits, breads, and desserts. Each recipe lists the per-serving measurement of calories, sodium, cholesterol, and exchanges.

Price: $14.95 plus postage. (Preview copies and educational discounts available.)

Source: Cy DeCosse; 5900 Green Oaks Drive; Minnetonka, MN 55343. 1–800-328–0590.

67.

More Calculated Cooking. J. Jones. 101 Productions; 1981. 192 p.

One of the purposes of this cookbook, written by the author of The Calculating Cook, is to show that the diabetic exchange diet does not have to be limited or dull. The author gives variations for each recipe to prime the reader's imagination to create variations by substituting or combining ingredients in new ways. The book features recipes in major food categories (soups and gravies, salads, vegetables, fish and meats, etc.), with international, ethnic, and vegetarian dishes well represented. Also included are an explanation of the exchange diet, exchange lists, and a "calculated hints" section on miscellaneous topics such as a kitchen vocabulary and how to "cure" an iron skillet.

Price: $6.95.

Source: MacMillan Publishing Company; Front and Bacon Streets; Riverside, NJ 08075. (212) 702–2000. Order Number: ISBN 086–61840-ISBNH.

68.

The New Diabetic Cookbook. M. Cavaiani. Contemporary Books, Inc.; 1984. 303 p.

Recipes for low-fat, low-sugar, low-cholesterol, low-salt, and high-fiber dishes are featured. Each recipe includes nutrient and exchange value information and tips for reducing the sodium content of the dish. Individual chapters discuss food exchanges and how to calculate exchange values, planning for special menus, cholesterol and fiber in the diet, canning and freezing foods, and equipment and ingredients to keep on hand. The book includes tables that provide nutrient analyses for all major types of foods.

Price: $9.95 plus $1 postage.

Source: Contemporary Books, Inc.; 180 North Michigan Ave.; Chicago, IL 60601. (312) 782–9189. In Canada, Beaverbrooks, Ltd.; 195 Allstate Parkway; Valleywood Business Park; Markham, Ontario L3R 4T8.

69.

Not Just Cheesecake! The Low-Fat, Low-Cholesterol, Low-Calorie Great Dessert Cookbook. M. Stone, S. Melvin, C. Crawford. Triad Publishing Company Publishing Company; 1988. 142 p.

Includes recipes for cheesecakes, baked pies, no-bake pies, mousses, ice cream, rice pudding, and other desserts that are made with yogurt cheese. The cheese is used as a substitute for commercial cream cheese and other commercial products. Instructions for separating cheese from low-fat yogurt are provided. Included in the recipes are directions for preparing low-calorie banana cream pie, peanut butter pie, marble cheesecake, lemon chiffon pie, cherry chocolate brownie bars, and key lime ice cream.

Price: $9.95 plus $2 postage.

Source: Triad Publishing Company; 1110 Northwest Eighth Avenue; Gainesville, FL 32601. (904) 373–5800.

70.

Oat Meals! Quaker Oats Company; 1988. 13 p.

Ten recipes for foods using oatmeal as an ingredient are provided. The booklet includes recipes for muffins, fruit bars, biscuits, main dishes, and a yogurt dessert. Nutrition information, including diabetic exchanges, is provided for each recipe as well as microwaving and freezing instructions when appropriate. The recipes use low-calorie, low-fat ingredients and are designed to be high in fiber.

Price: Free.

Source: Consumer Affairs Center; Quaker Oats Company; Chicago, IL 60604–9001.

71.

On the Light Side, Healthy Recipes for International-Style Entertaining. G.L. Becker. Cumberland Packing Corporation; 1988. 184 p.

This book features recipes for international and regional dishes using low-salt, low-cholesterol, low-fat ingredients. Recipes are provided for such dishes as Swedish meatballs, oysters Rockefeller, Boston brown bread, Indian-spiced scrambled eggs, lamb shish kebab, colcannon, falafel, and other exotic dishes. Exchanges are based on the 1986 exchange lists, and nutrient analyses are given for each recipe as well as information about calories, fat, and sodium saved by using recommended dietary ingredients.

Price: $7.95.

Source: Cumberland Packing Corporation; Two Cumberland Street; Brooklyn, NY 11205. 1–800-336–0363 or (718) 858–4200.

72.

Oriental Cooking for the Diabetic. D. Revell. Kodansha International/USA; 1981. 176 p.

This cookbook features 300 recipes ranging from exotic dishes to family fare and festive meals. It also contains comprehensive explanations of Oriental cooking, focusing on Chinese and Japanese; detailed information about nutrition; and sample diets for people with diabetes. Each recipe includes exchange values, calorie content, and milligrams of sodium per serving.

Price: $9.95/paperback

Source: Harper and Row; Keystone Industrial Park; Scranton, PA 18512. 1–800-638–3030, 1–800-242–7737.

73.

Pass the Pepper Please! International Diabetes Center; 1988. 66 p.

This guide for people on sodium-restricted diets features recipes for salt substitutes, prototype meal plans for diets of various sodium levels, tips for desalting recipes, information about sodium levels in common food products, and suggestions for shopping and cooking the low-sodium way. The first half offers general information about hypertension, hypertensive drugs, and the importance of controlling high blood pressure in people with diabetes. An appendix explains the 1986 exchange lists. The guide was developed by Diane Reader and Marion Franz, dietitians at the center, and features an introduction by Dr. Richard Bergenstal.

Price: $3.95 plus $1.50 postage.

Source: Diabetes Center, Inc.; P.O. Box 739; Wayzata, MN 55391. 1–800-848–2793. In Minnesota, 1–612-541–0239, collect.

74.

Potluck 1. Change of Menu; 1984. 78 p.

The book offers recipes, menus, and a few simple directions; extraneous information has been omitted deliberately to keep the book small. Recipes and menus are cross-referenced, and each recipe lists exchange values and nutrient quantities per serving. Menu charts list the quantities of each food item that meet requirements for diets in five categories, from 1,000 to 2,400 calories per day. Low-sodium and low-cholesterol meals are noted.

Price: $16.95.

Source: Change of Menu; P.O. Box 544; Sylvania, OH 43560–0544. (419) 841–7821.

75.

Recipes for Diabetics. B. Little. Bantam Books; 1985. 288 p.

This cookbook contains recipes and menu guides for planning meals that are low in calories, fat, and cholesterol and include plenty of fruits and vegetables. Exchange group breakdowns and calorie counts for measured individual servings are provided along with guides for using nutrition labeling to compute exchanges, dining out, buying and storing produce, and using recipes in the microwave. The book also contains recommended daily allowance tables for protein, vitamins, and minerals; a list of resources; and an index.

Price: $3.95.

Source: Bantam Books, Inc.; 666 Fifth Avenue; New York, NY 13795.

76.

Recipes for Diabetics (and Others Who Enjoy Good Food). Texas Department of Agriculture; 1981. 21 p.

This cookbook was prepared to facilitate the dietary management of diabetes. Exchange list values used in the recipes are those established by the ADA and the American Dietetic Association. There are approximately 30 recipes that include main dishes, vegetables, and breads. Brief consideration is given to nutritional labeling, eating out, and mobile meals or "brown bagging." A chart illustrates how herbs and spices can add variety to meals. Available in English or Spanish.

Price: Free in reasonable quantities.

Source: Library, Texas Department of Agriculture; P.O. Box 12847; Austin, TX 78711. (512) 463–7476.

77.

Snips and Spice and All That is Nice. J. Betschart, L. Siminerio, L. Steranchak, T. Yeager. Children's Hospital of Pittsburgh; 1987. 80 p.

This booklet offers food and activity ideas for parents of preschool-age children with diabetes. Recipes for substitutes for traditional party and holiday foods are provided along with tips for decorating foods for special occasions.

Price: $5.95 plus $1 postage.

Source: American Diabetes Association; Western Pennsylvania Affiliate, Inc.; 4617 Winthrop Street; Pittsburgh, PA 15213.

78.

Sodium Smart: The Campbell Plan for Low-Sodium Eating. Campbell Soup Company; 1984. 21 p.

A low-sodium diet plan based on eight food exchange lists is presented to help people who must restrict their sodium intake. The carbohydrate, protein, fat, calorie, and sodium content for each exchange is listed. Daily plans for dietary sodium levels from 1,000 to 3,000 milligrams are offered. A sample menu and a dozen recipes are included.

Price: Free.

Source: Consumer Nutrition Center; Campbell Soup Company; Campbell Place; Camden, NJ 08101. (609) 342–4800.

79.

Special Recipes for Special Diets: For Weight Control and Diabetic Diets. R. Glover. Glover Enterprises; 1981. 16 p.

The recipes for salads, entrees, vegetables, and desserts included in this booklet are designed to inspire creative cooking when preparing meals for individuals who are controlling their weight or following a diabetic diet.

Price: $3.

Source: American Diabetes Association; Cincinnati Affiliate, Inc.; 4055 Executive Park Drive; Cincinnati, OH 45241. (513) 733–8881.

80.

Stuffin' Muffin: Muffin Pan Cooking for Kids. S. Scherie. Young People's Press; 1981. 91 p.

Directed to children between 8 and 14 years old who have diabetes, this beginner cookbook uses the muffin pan to teach healthful gourmet cooking. It presents easy-to-follow, step-by-step directions to encourage experimentation with cooking techniques and foods. The cookbook includes more than 30 child-tested recipes for eggs; cheese; noodles and rice; salads and vegetables; potatoes and grains; meat, poultry, and fish; desserts; and "stuffin' muffins." All recipes represent alternatives to sweet, salty, processed, and artificial foods, and each provides food exchange equivalents. This cookbook also provides information about using the muffin pan, choosing ingredients, increasing recipes, freezing foods, cooking with friends, preparing to cook, safety procedures, measuring and measurements, and kitchen tools.

Price: $8.95.

Source: Young People's Press; Box 1005; Avon, CT 06001.

81.

Sugar Free: Creative Cooking for Diabetics and Their Families. C. Weiss, A.S. Uslander. Rev. ed. Budlong Press; 1988. 181 p.

Recipes low in fat, sugar, and salt content are presented in this cookbook, which can be used by the weight-conscious person as well as by the person with diabetes. The ADA 1986 exchange lists and extensive exchange lists for commercially prepared foods are given. Chapters include recipes for hors d'oeuvres, soups, main courses and vegetables; sugar-free desserts; and quiches, crepes, omelets, and souffles. Directions for many traditional American dishes and for several Chinese stirfried specialties are given.

Price: Write for complete information.

Source: Budlong Press Co.; P.O. Box 31032; Chicago, IL 60631–1032. (312) 763–7720.

82.

Sugar Free . . . Good and Easy. J.S. Majors. Apple Press; 1986. 128 p.

The focus of this cookbook is on recipes that are easy to prepare. Directions are provided for all kinds of foods, from appetizers to desserts, and nutritional information and exchange values are provided for each recipe. The publisher plans to update the book to conform to the 1986 exchange lists.

Price: $5.95.

Source: American Diabetes Association; Hawaiian Affiliate, Inc.; 510 South Beretania Street; Honolulu, HI 96813. (808) 521–5677. American Diabetes Association; Oregon Affiliate, Inc.; 3607 Southwest Corbett; Portland, OR 97201. (503) 228–0849. Apple Press, 5536 Southeast Harlow, Milwaukie, OR 97222. (503) 659–2475.

83.

Sugar Free . . . Goodies. J.S. Majors. Apple Press; 1988. 128 p.

Sugar-free recipes for a variety of dessert and snack foods are provided in this cookbook. Included are recipes for ice cream, jams, jellies, cookies, pies, cakes, and other dessert items. The exchange values provided for each recipe are based on the 1986 exchange lists.

Price: $6.95.

Source: American Diabetes Association; Hawaiian Affiliate, Inc.; 510 South Beretania Street; Honolulu, HI 96813. (808) 521–5677. American Diabetes Association; Oregon Affiliate, Inc.; 3607 Southwest Corbett; Portland, OR 97201. (503) 228–0849. Apple Press; 5536 Southeast Harlow; Milwaukie, OR 97222. (503) 659–2475.

84.

Sugar Free . . . Hawaiian Cookery. J.S. Majors. Apple Press: 1988. 128 p.

This cookbook provides more than 100 recipes for typical Hawaiian dishes, including fish, fruits, salads, and other light foods. The recipes emphasize use of fresh and natural ingredients. Exchange values provided for each recipe are based on the 1986 exchange lists.

Price: $6.95.

Source: American Diabetes Association; Hawaiian Affiliate, Inc.; 510 South Beretania Street; Honolulu, HI 96813. (808) 521–5677. American Diabetes Association; Oregon Affiliate, Inc.; 3607 Southwest Corbett; Portland, OR 97201. (503) 228–0849. Apple Press; 5536 Southeast Harlow; Milwaukie, OR 97222. (503) 659–2475.

85.

Sugar Free . . . Kid's Cookery. J.S. Majors. Apple Press; 1987. 128 p.

This book is a collection of sugar-free recipes designed for use by a young cook. Information about exchange lists, cooking techniques, artificial sweeteners, and cooking terms is presented in a simple style. For each recipe, the number of calories, the exchanges, and the nutritional content are given. Exchanges are based on the 1986 exchange lists.

Price: $6.95.

Source: American Diabetes Association; Oregon Affiliate, Inc.; 3607 Southwest Corbett; Portland, OR 97201. (503) 228–0849. American

Diabetes Association; Hawaiian Affiliate, Inc.; 510 South Beretania Street; Honolulu, HI 96813. (808) 521–5677. Apple Press; 5536 Southeast Harlow; Milwaukie, OR 97222. (503) 659–2475.

86.

Sugar Free . . . Microwavery. J.S. Majors. Apple Press; 1980. 168 p.

Sugar-free recipes for microwave cooking are featured in this cookbook. Recipes are included for appetizers and beverages, eggs and light fare, side dishes, soups, salads, sandwiches, main dishes, and sweets and treats. General rules for using microwave ovens and a recipe index are included.

Price: $6.95.

Source: American Diabetes Association; Oregon Affiliate, Inc.; 3607 Southwest Corbett; Portland, OR 97201. (503) 228–0849. American Diabetes Association; Hawaiian Affiliate, Inc.; 510 South Beretania Street; Honolulu, HI 96813. (808) 521–5677. Apple Press; 5536 Southeast Harlow; Milwaukie, OR 97222. (503) 659–2475.

87.

Sugar Free . . . Sweets and Treats. J.S. Majors. Apple Press; 1982. 111 p.

Recipes are provided for desserts and other sweets using fruit and fruit juices as the sweetening agent. The exchange system is explained, and exchanges are provided for foods used in the cookbook. Each recipe gives the number of grams of carbohydrates, protein, and fat in the finished product; the number of calories; and the exchange values.

Price: $6.95.

Source: American Diabetes Association; Oregon Affiliate, Inc.; 3607 Southwest Corbett; Portland, OR 97201. (503) 228–0849. American Diabetes Association; Hawaiian Affiliate, Inc.; 510 South Beretania Street; Honolulu, HI 96813. (808) 521–5677. Apple Press; 5536 Southeast Harlow; Milwaukie, OR 97222. (503) 659–2475.

88.

Sugar Free . . . That's Me. J.S. Majors. Apple Press; 1978. 200 p.

This cookbook contains recipes that have been calculated in terms of diabetic exchanges. It is divided into sections on breakfast foods, appetizers, main dishes, salads, sauces, breads, and soups. Noncaloric artificial sweeteners are substituted for sugar in the recipes. A brief explanation of the use of exchange lists is provided.

Price: $6.95.

Source: American Diabetes Association, Oregon Affiliate, Inc.; 3607 Southwest Corbett; Portland, OR 97201. (503) 228–0849. American Diabetes Association; Hawaiian Affiliate, Inc.; 510 South Beretania Street; Honolulu, HI 96813. (808) 521–5677. Apple Press; 5536 Southeast Harlow; Milwaukie, OR 97222. (503) 659–2475.

89.

Sweet and Natural: Desserts Without Sugar, Honey, Molasses, or Artificial Sweeteners. J. Warrington. The Crossing Press; 1982. 143 p.

This cookbook includes recipes for desserts made without sugar, honey, molasses, or artificial sweeteners. The author reviews some nutrition basics, including discussions about carbohydrates, fats, protein, meal planning, and food exchanges.

Price: $8.95 paperback.

Source: The Crossing Press; P.O. Box 1048; Freedom, CA 95019. (408) 722–0711.

90.

Sweet and Sugarfree: An All-Natural Fruit-Sweetened Dessert Cookbook. K.E. Barkie. St. Martin's Press; 1982. 160 p.

Recipes contained in this dessert cookbook are sweetened with fruit rather than with sugar or honey. Appendixes include hints about baking with fruits; information about exchanging whole grain flours for white flour; a comparison of the caloric values of sugar, honey, and fresh fruits; baking equivalents and substitutions; and charts of the nutritional values of unsweetened fruit juices, dried fruits, and raw fruits.

Price: $5.95 plus $1.50 postage/paperback.

Source: St. Martin's Press; 175 Fifth Avenue; New York, NY 10010. Attn: Cash Sales. (212) 674–5151. Order Number: ISBN-0–312-78066–4.

91.

Sweet 'N Low® Just Desserts. Cumberland Packing Corporation; 1986. 29 p.

This collection contains recipes with reduced sugar, fat, and salt levels that maintain the attractive appearance and good taste, texture, and volume of foods. The selection includes a variety of cakes, pies, and other desserts made with artificial sweeteners.

Price: $0.50.

Source: Sweet 'N Low®; Department A; Two Cumberland Street; Brooklyn, NY 11205. 1–800-336–0363 or (718) 858–4200.

92.

34 Ways to Cheat on Your Sugar With Sweet 'N Low®: Home Canning, Freezing, and Preserving Recipes. Cumberland Packing Corporation; 1982. 26 p.

Recipes for canning, freezing, and preserving foods using Sweet 'N Low® in place of sugar are provided. Tips for home freezing and canning and for making jams and spreads are given as well as a Sweet 'N Low® conversion chart for granulated sugar. Each recipe lists the calorie content.

Price: $0.50.

Source: Sweet 'N Low® Department A; Two Cumberland Street; Brooklyn, NY 11205. 1–800-336–0363 or (718) 858–4200.

93.

Vegetarian Cooking for Diabetics. P. Mozzer. The Book Publishing Company; 1987.

This book features recipes and information based on ovo-lacto vegetarianism. The first section begins with an explanation of the different types of vegetarianism and the different philosophies behind vegetarianism. It continues with a discussion of nutrition and covers protein, carbohydrates, fat, minerals, and vitamins; nutritional information; and advice about vegetarian foods such as vegetables, nuts and seeds, grains and flours, cheeses, fruits, and butter and margarine. This section also includes an explanation of the exchange system, converting to a vegetarian exchange system, diet and shopping tips, combining proteins, and a sample 2-day ovo-lacto vegetarian menu with calories and exchanges given. The second section of the book features recipes for breakfasts, breads, salads and salad dressings, soups and sandwiches, main dishes, and snacks. Each recipe includes a nutritional analysis for protein, carbohydrates, and fat as well as the specific diabetic exchanges based on the 1986 exchange lists.

Price: $9.95.

Source: The Book Publishing Company; P.O. Box 99; Summertown, TN 38483. (615) 964–3571.

AUTHOR/PRODUCER INDEX

Author/Producer (Item Number)

SUBJECT INDEX

General, Basic Cookbooks (Item Number)

Sugar Free: Creative Cooking for Diabetics and Their Families (81)
Sugar Free . . . Good and Easy (82)
Sugar Free . . . That's Me (88)

Gourmet/Ethnic Cookbooks

American Diabetes Association/American Dietetic Association Family Cookbook, Volume II (2)
Better Meals for You with Low Calorie Gourmet Recipes (9)
The Calculating Cook: A Gourmet Cookbook for Diabetics and Dieters (12)
Cooking For Love and Life (18)
Creole Recipes for People with Diabetes (24)
Diabetes Control and the Kosher Diet (27)
The Diabetic Gourmet (36)
The Diabetic Gourmet Cookbook (37)
Gourmet Recipes for Diabetics (48)
The Guiltless Gourmet (49)
The International Menu Diabetic Cookbook (55)
On the Light Side, Healthy Recipes for International-Style Entertaining (71)
Oriental Cooking for the Diabetic (72)
Sugar Free . . . Hawaiian Cookery (84)

Microwave Cookbooks

American Diabetes Association/American Dietetic Association Family Cookbook, Volume III (3)
Better Meals for You: The Microwave Way (8)
Microwave Cooking for Diabetics (64)
Microwaving Light and Healthy (65)
Microwaving on a Diet (66)
Sugar Free . . . Microwavery (86)

Canning/Freezing Cookbooks

Canning and Freezing with Low Salt and No Added Sugar (13)
34 Ways to Cheat on Your Sugar with Sweet 'N Low®: Home Canning, Freezing and Preserving Recipes (92)

Special Occasion Cookbooks

Birthday Bonanza (10)
Diabetic Snack & Appetizer Cookbook (39)
Healthy Holiday Recipes from Sweet 'N Low® (50)
Holiday Cookbook (53)
Holiday Cooking for the Diabetic (54)
The Joy of Snacks (56)

Dessert Cookbooks

Diabetic Cakes, Pies & Other Scrumptious Desserts (31)
Diabetic Candy, Cookie and Dessert Cookbook (32)
The Diabetic Chocolate Cookbook (33)
The Fruitsweet Cookbook (47)
Just Delicious and Sugar Free (57)
Just Desserts: A Collection of De"Lite"ful Recipes (58)
Not Just Cheesecake! The Low-Fat, Low-Cholesterol, Low-Calorie Great Dessert Cookbook (69)
Sugar Free . . . Goodies (83)
Sugar Free . . . Sweets and Treats (87)
Sweet and Natural: Desserts Without Sugar, Honey, Molasses, or Artificial Sweeteners (89)
Sweet and Sugarfree: An All-Natural, Fruit-Sweetened Dessert Cookbook (90)
Sweet 'N Low® Just Desserts (91)

Children's Cookbooks

Dining with Your Diabetic Child (41)
Kids, Food, and Diabetes: A Book of Recipes, Menus, and Practical Advice (59)
Snips and Spice and All That is Nice (77)
Stuffin' Muffin: Muffin Pan Cooking for Kids (80)
Sugar Free . . . Kid's Cookery (85)

Special Diet Cookbooks

Cooking for the Health of It (19)
Diabetic High Fiber Cookbook (38)
Diet for a Healthy Heart (40)
Fabulous Fiber Cookbook (43)
The High Fiber Cookbook for Diabetics (51)
High Fiber Delights (52)

The Lowfat Lifestyle (60)
Low Sodium, Low Cholesterol Diabetic Menu Plan: Easy Meal Planning for the Sodium/Cholesterol-Restricted Diabetic (61)
Oat Meals! (70)
Pass The Pepper Please! (73)
Sodium Smart: The Campbell Plan for Low-Sodium Eating (78)
Vegetarian Cooking for Diabetics (93)

Chapter 67

Diabetes-Related Programs for Black Americans: A Resource Guide

Introduction

Diabetes mellitus is a major health problem in black Americans. In 1986, the Task Force on Black and Minority Health, appointed by the Secretary of the Department of Health and Human Services (DHHS), cited diabetes as one of six health problems responsible for excess mortality among U.S. minority populations.

According to the U.S. Bureau of the Census, black Americans composed 12.2 percent of the U.S. population in 1988. Some 29.3 million Americans are black, 14 percent more than in 1980. Census figures document that blacks have higher rates of poverty and unemployment than do whites. They also have higher rates of noninsulin-dependent diabetes.

Relatively uncommon among black Americans at the beginning of this century, diabetes is now the third leading cause of death by disease in this population. A report issued by the National Center for Health Statistics (NCHS) in 1987 noted that the prevalence of diagnosed diabetes in black Americans has increased fourfold in just over two decades, from 228,000 in 1963 to approximately 1 million in 1985. This is almost double the rate of increase among white, non-Hispanic Americans. Another 1 million blacks are estimated to have undiagnosed diabetes.

The National Diabetes Data Group (NDDG) of the National Institutes of Health reports that the rate of noninsulin-dependent diabetes among black Americans is 50 to 60 percent higher than it is among white non-

---

NIH Pub. No. 90-1585.

Hispanic Americans. Blacks have higher rates of diabetes at all adult age levels, and among those 65 to 74 years of age, one in four has diabetes. Among black women diabetes can almost be termed epidemic: One in four black women older than 55 has diabetes—double the rate in white women.

Black Americans also experience higher rates of at least three of the serious complications of diabetes: blindness, amputation, and end-stage renal disease (ESRD). The rates of severe visual impairment are 40 percent higher in black patients with diabetes than in white patients. Black patients undergo twice as many amputations as do whites, and a study in Michigan found that the rate of ESRD was four times higher in blacks with diabetes.

According to the NCHS report, the higher diabetes rate in black Americans prevails across all major sociodemographic parameters—age, sex, educational level, marital status, living arrangement, and regional category. The prevalence of diabetes is highest in women, older people, the less educated, the formerly married, persons living alone, and persons in families with low incomes. In addition, diabetes is more prevalent among black people living in the central city and those living in the western United States.

Defining the Problem

In September 1988, the first of two national conferences was held to define issues and priority areas for activities to reduce the impact of diabetes on black Americans. Both conferences were chaired by Dr. Louis W. Sullivan, now Secretary of DHHS. Sponsors included the National Institute of Diabetes and Digestive and Kidney Diseases (NIDDK), the Office of Minority Health, the Centers for Disease Control (CDC), the American Diabetes Association (ADA), and the National Black Nurses' Association. The first conference focused on epidemiological and research findings relevant to diabetes and its complications in blacks, and the second on how to increase diabetes awareness within the professional and black lay communities.

Some major findings noted at the first conference were:

- Black people have a higher prevalence of obesity, a strong risk factor for NIDDM. Among people with diagnosed diabetes, 82 percent of adult black women are obese compared with 62 percent of white women; among men, 45 percent of blacks are obese compared with 39 percent of whites.

- Black Americans are known to have a high prevalence of hypertension, which is associated with retinopathy and renal and cardiovascular complications, major complications in black patients. Studies are needed to elucidate the disease processes involved in these conditions in black patients and to develop better methods of prevention and treatment.

- Studies of dietary habits of black Americans indicate that they consume less fiber and more cholesterol-rich foods than do whites, although their total calorie consumption and fat intake are lower.
- Black people tend to have less access to financial, social, health, and educational resources that would help improve their health status and health awareness.
- Educational resources, including materials and programs, oriented to black patients are needed that take into account black lifestyles, interests, and cultural and economic considerations.

In summing up the conference, Dr. James R. Gavin III, chief of the diabetes section at the University of Oklahoma Health Sciences Center, cited the need for a variety of scientific, behavioral, and social investigations to address the diabetes problem, which he said was "ravaging the black population." He particularly called for studies to define the genetic pedigree of diabetes in blacks, studies to determine the nature and role of fat distribution in blacks and its relationship to diabetes, research to assess the influence of socioeconomic and psychosocial factors in the black population, research to develop optimum treatment strategies for the complications of diabetes and for hypertension in blacks, behavioral studies on dietary and cultural influences in the black community, and development of educational resources that are relevant to black concerns and lifestyles. He also urged collaborative efforts by multiple institutions in affected communities and involving black community leaders to raise the level of awareness about diabetes among black Americans.

These issues were addressed at the second conference held in March 1989, "Diabetes in the Black Population: Imperatives for Action." The conference targeted two critical audiences for diabetes awareness activities: health professionals and the black community itself.

Speakers at the conference called for increased physician awareness of diabetes as a serious disease; increased screening activities, especially among high-risk minority patients; and increased education of black patients in modern diabetes management techniques. The need to involve the black community in health promotion activities, especially among black women, was stressed.

The two conferences succeeded in calling attention to the seriousness of the diabetes problem in blacks and in defining research and educational needs to address this crisis.

The Resource Guide

To facilitate this effort, the National Diabetes Information Clearinghouse (NDIC) has compiled this directory of programs and other resources for diabetes awareness and education in the black community. The purpose of the directory is to help health educators, public health officials, community leaders, and others in developing educational programs for black Americans.

The guide includes descriptions of diabetes-related programs that are targeted to black people or that serve communities with substantial black populations. To identify relevant programs, NDIC staff contacted health departments of states with CDC-funded diabetes control programs, ADA affiliates, Diabetes Research and Training Centers supported by NIDDK, and major black health-related organizations. There are 33 programs listed in this directory. They include general health awareness activities, as well as diabetes screening and treatment programs and projects focusing on complications and allied conditions such as hypertension. Continuing education and training programs for professionals working with black populations also are listed. Materials developed in conjunction with programs are noted in the description if they are available to other programs.

Programs are listed alphabetically by name of sponsoring organization. Each program profile contains the following information:

- Name of program
- Other sponsoring organization (if applicable)
- Type of program
- Audience
- Year program established (if known)
- Materials available
- Comments
- Name, address, and telephone number of contact person for additional information about the program.

The programs included in this guide do not represent an exhaustive list. NDIC encourages health professionals involved in diabetes-related programs for black people to provide information about their programs to the clearinghouse so that they may be included in future updates of this guide. A brief form is included at the end of the guide for this purpose. Completed forms may be sent to:

National Diabetes Information Clearinghouse
Box NDIC 9000
Rockville Pike
Bethesda, Maryland 20892.

The guide also includes a reading list of articles from the professional and popular media focusing on research and educational issues pertinent to diabetes in the black population. Some reference materials also are cited in the reading list.

Other Resources

A number of organizations are engaged in activities that relate directly or indirectly to diabetes awareness in the black community. These organizations are listed below with a brief description of their major activities and services.

Ad Hoc Committee on Minority Populations (AHC)
National Heart, Lung, and Blood Institute
Minority Program
Information Center
4733 Bethesda Avenue, Suite 530
Bethesda, MD 20814
(301) 951–3260

The Ad Hoc Committee on Minority Populations is a program of the National Heart, Lung, and Blood Institute (NHLBI), National Institutes of Health. The committee works with NHLBI to improve the health status of U.S. minority populations, with particular concern for the areas of hypertension, cardiovascular and pulmonary diseases, cholesterol, and smoking. The committee comprises 15 members, all health professionals, who represent Asian-Americans, black Americans, Native Hawaiians, Hispanics, and American Indians. AHC activities include development of the *Directory of Cardiovascular Resources for Minority Populations* and sponsorship of roundtable discussions on cholesterol and blood pressure control. The committee also is involved in the development of program activities and tools to help reduce CVD and related factors in minority populations.

The Alabama Cooperative Extension Service
United States Department of Agriculture
Duncan Hall, Room 220-B
Auburn University, AL 36849–5621
(205) 844–2224

The Alabama Cooperative Extension Service has developed a number of innovative community-level programs to teach nutrition and healthy food preparation and eating concepts. The program includes cooking and nutrition classes for families as well as for specific groups such as young people, a newsletter, followup services, and programs on local radio and television. In conjunction with the program, the staff has developed slide sets and videotape programs for low literacy and minority audiences.

Black Caucus Health Braintrust
Congressman Louis Stokes
2365 Rayburn House Office Building
Washington, DC 20515
(202) 225–7032

The Black Caucus Health Braintrust monitors and focuses on issues relevant to health needs of the black population. The group sponsors an annual legislative program that is open to the public and during the year sponsors workshops and symposiums on issues that affect the health of black people.

Black Health Research Foundation
128 E. 56th Street
New York, NY 10022
(201) 837–0690

The foundation has three main objectives: Funding of research into health problems that affect Afro-Americans, programs to increase the number of Afro-Americans in the health professions, and support for professional and community education programs.

Cancer Prevention Awareness Program for Black Americans
Office of Cancer Communications
National Cancer Institute
National Institutes of Health
Building 31, Room 4B47
9000 Rockville Pike
Bethesda, MD 20892
(301) 496–6792

The National Cancer Institute's Office of Cancer Communications has developed special educational materials for black Americans and, working through intermediary organizations, helps with the development and implementation of programs in the black community to promote awareness of cancer prevention.

Hypertension Control Program
Louisiana Office of Public Health
P.O. Box 60630
New Orleans, LA 70160
Janice Boatner-Burchelle, R.N., B.S.N.
(504) 568–7210

The Louisiana Office of Public Health sponsors an outreach program in cooperation with local black churches. The program initially focused on blood pressure control; today the program includes many risk-factor initiatives, such as weight control, smoking, and diet, with plans to include mammography in the near future.

Minority Initiative Project
American Diabetes Association (ADA)
1660 Duke Street
Alexandria, VA 22314
1–800-232–3472
(703) 549–1500

The ADA works with its affiliates to create networks between the ADA and key minority organizations in the community to identify the needs of minority organizations in relation to diabetes and to develop creative, workable programs to be implemented through the minority community itself. ADA programs involve community organizations, clergy and church leaders, representatives from schools, politicians, and social organizations, along with ADA staff and diabetes health professionals. The ADA has developed educational materials to be used with minority populations.

National Black Nurses' Association, Inc.
1012 Tenth Street, NW
Washington, DC 20001
(202) 393–6870

The National Black Nurses' Association is committed to providing quality health care services to black communities throughout the Nation. The association's 45 chapters conduct screenings and sponsor education programs, often in collaboration with other community groups and organizations. The association also seeks to influence public policy on minority health-related issues through lobbying efforts.

National Black Women's Health Project
1237 Gordon Street, SW
Atlanta, GA 30310
(404) 753–0916

Through a network of 98 state groups, the National Black Women's Health Project seeks to promote health awareness and mutual and self help activism on the community level to reduce health problems especially prevalent among black women. The organization maintains a database and speakers' bureau and plans to establish black women's self help centers and an Empowerment Through Wellness curriculum. Its newsletter, *Vital Signs*, is published three times a year.

National Medical Association (NMA)
1012 10th Street, NW
Washington, DC 20001
(202) 347–1895

This professional society for black physicians was established in 1895. It supports 32 state groups and 62 local groups and maintains 19 sections representing the major specialties of medicine. The organization conducts workshops and symposia and plans to establish a library and physician placement service. Its two publications are the *Journal of the National Medication Association* (monthly) and *National Medical Association Newsletter* (quarterly).

Network of Blacks in Dietetics and Nutrition
426 NW Ninth Avenue
Fort Lauderdale, FL 33311
(305) 463–6378

The Network of Blacks in Dietetics and Nutrition is a professional organization for dietitians. It works to promote the professional growth of its members and interest black health professionals in the field of dietetics as a career. The organization also functions as a network with other professionals in health education activities. A current focus of the network involves efforts to foster development of community-based health promotion and awareness programs among the black population.

Office of Minority Health Resource Center (OMH-RC)
P.O. Box 37337
Washington, DC 20013–7337
1-800-444-6472
(301) 587–1938

The OMH-RC is an information and referral resource for consumers and professionals in the area of minority health. The center, which is a service of the Office of Minority Health within DHHS, focuses on major health areas designated by OMH as critical issues in minority health: diabetes; cancer; cardiovascular and cerebrovascular diseases; infant mortality; substance abuse; AIDS; and homicide, suicide, and unintentional injury. Target populations include black Americans, Hispanics, Native Americans, Asians, and Pacific Islanders. The center offers traditional information and referral services as well as technical assistance in the priority health areas, including technical guidance in development of program and materials and other resources for health education activities.

Universal Health Associates, Inc.
1701 K Street, NW, Suite 600
P.O. Box 65465
Washington, DC 20035–5465
(202) 429–9506

Universal Health Associates, Inc., is a private organization specializing in audiovisuals for health education, with a special focus on materials directed to minority audiences. The organization functions as a clearinghouse for minority-appropriate health education audiovisuals. The organization distributes a number of educational videos on health topics, including diabetes, which are directed specifically to minority patients. Staff also work with educators and producers of educational films in identifying needs and offer technical expertise in the development and evaluation of materials. A special emphasis of University Health Associates is development of quality, low-cost educational films.

Program Listings

Note: This section lists programs that are target specifically to black Americans as well as those that include a substantial number of black patients in the client population served by the program.

Albert Einstein Diabetes Research and Training Center

1300 Morris Park Avenue
Bldg BEL, Room 1308
Bronx, NY 10461

Name of Program:
Diabetes Program Development for Neighborhood Family Care Clinics

Type of Program:
Diabetes education
Diabetes screening
Weight management

Audience:
People with diagnosed diabetes
Health professionals
General population

Year Program Established:
1988

Materials Available:
No (Materials in pilot testing)

Other Minority Groups Served:
Hispanics

Comments:

The Neighborhood Family Care Clinic diabetes project is designed to help primary care clinics with limited resources meet current diabetes care and education standards. Professional and patient modules have been developed with podiatry and weight control components. These are being tested. A protocol is being developed for complication screening and will be tested in spring 1990. The clinics participating in the pilot study are in minority communities with a large Hispanic population. Diabetes educational materials for Hispanics, including videotapes, are being planned for a project in collaboration with the Downstate New York affiliate of the American Diabetes Association.

Contact:
Judith Wylie-Rosett, R.D., Ed.D.
Program Coordinator
Albert Einstein DRTC
1300 Morris Park Avenue
Bronx, NY 10461
(212) 430–2646

American Diabetes Association—Ohio Affiliate, Inc.

225 West Exchange Street
Akron, OH 44302

Name of Program:
Health Services Advocacy Program

Type of Program:
General health promotion
Diabetes education
Diabetes screening
Weight management

Audience:
People with diagnosed diabetes
General population

Year Program Established:
1976

Materials Available:
Yes
ADA materials

Other Minority Groups Served:
Hispanics

Contact:
Yvonne Sebastian
American Diabetes Association—Ohio Affiliate, Inc.
225 West Exchange Street
Akron, OH 44302
(216) 762–7487

American Diabetes Association—Northern Illinois Affiliate, Inc.

6 North Michigan Avenue
Suite 1818
Chicago, IL 60602

Name of Program:
Southside Illinois Chapter of the American Diabetes Association

Type of Program:
General health promotion
Diabetes education
Nutrition

Support group
Continuing education/training
Foot care

Audience:
People with diagnosed diabetes
General population
Health professionals

Year Program Established:
1987

Materials Available:
Yes
ADA materials

Other Minority Groups Served:
Hispanics

Contact:
Ms. Marvin T. Smith
Community Relations Director
Southside Illinois Chapter of the American Diabetes Association
6 North Michigan Avenue, Suite 1818
Chicago, IL 60602
(312) 346–1805

Area Agency on Aging for North Florida, Inc.

Cedars Executive Center
North Monroe Street
Tallahassee, FL 32303

Name of Program:
Health Promotion for Citizens in Jackson County

Type of Program:
Weight management
Nutrition
Exercise

Audience:
General population

Year Program Established:
1988

Materials Available:
Yes

Contact:
Greg Harris
Area Agency on Aging for North Florida, Inc.
Health Promotion for Citizens in Jackson County
Cedars Executive Center
North Monroe Street
Tallahassee, FL 32303
(904) 488–0055

Center for Research in Medical Education and Health Care University of Chicago Diabetes Research and Training Center

Box 410
5841 South Maryland Avenue
Chicago, IL 60637

Name of Program:
Pathways

Type of Program:
Weight management
Nutrition
Exercise

Audience:
People with diagnosed diabetes

Year Program Established:
1990

Materials Available:
Yes
A manual for health professionals to use with patients is being developed.

Other Minority Groups Served:
Hispanics
Orientals
Children

Comments:

This 12-week pilot program focuses on weight management techniques for people with diagnosed diabetes. It involves 16 black women from the inner city, who meet weekly. Sessions focus on food selection, meal planning, cooking, and exercise. Participants get hands-on experience in all class activities. At the conclusion of the 12 weeks, additional sites will be sought to expand the program.

Contact:
Dr. Wylie McNabb
Principal Investigator
Center for Research in Medical Education and Health Care University of Chicago Diabetes Research and Training Center
Box 410
5841 South Maryland Avenue
Chicago, IL 60637
(312) 753–1310

Central Seattle Community Health Centers

105 14th Avenue
Suite 2C
Seattle, WA 98122

Name of Program:
Sound Heart

Type of Program:
Weight management
Nutrition
Exercise
Hypertension screening
Cholesterol screening

Audience:
Men and women, ages 18 to 59 years

Year Program Established:
1979

Materials Available:
Yes

Other Minority Groups Served:
Program serves minorities in general

Contact:
Amy S. Duggan
Director, Sound Heart
Central Seattle Community Health Centers
105 14th Avenue - Suite 2C
Seattle, WA 98122
(206) 461–6900

Colorado Department of Health Division of Prevention Programs

4210 East 11th Avenue
Denver, CO 80220

Name of Program:
Colorado Diabetes Control Program

Type of Program:
Eye screening
Hypertension screening
Prenatal care

Audience:
People with diagnosed diabetes

Year Program Established:
1977

Materials Available:
Yes
"Diabetes and Your Feet"
Brochures, posters, flipcharts

Other Minority Groups Served:
Hispanics

Comments:

The minority populations served by the Colorado DCP are primary users of the Denver Health and Hospitals public delivery system.

Interventions in Denver are not targeted at minority groups per se, but such subgroups compose the majority of system users.

Contact:
Sharon Michael
Colorado Department of Health
Division of Prevention Programs
4210 East 11th Avenue

Denver, CO 80220
(303) 331–8300

Community Outreach Misericordia Hospital

54th Street and Cedar Avenue
Philadelphia, PA 19143

Name of Program:
Diabetes Education Program

Type of Program:
General health promotion
Diabetes education
Diabetes screening
Weight management
Nutrition
Support group
Hypertension screening
Foot care education

Audience:
People with diagnosed diabetes
General population

Year Program Established:
1980

Materials Available:
Yes

Comments:

This program is a one-to-one counseling program based on the individual's ability. The approach is based on a needs assessment for each individual. All aspects of diabetes medication are covered, including insulin administration, education, and self glucose monitoring on an outpatient basis. The group support program begins every 5 weeks from September through June. In addition, screenings are held two to three times a year.

Contact:
Kay Stephens, R.N., CDE
Coordinator
Community Outreach
Misericordia Hospital
54th Street and Cedar Avenue
Philadelphia, PA 19143
(215) 748–9420

Florida Department of Health and Rehabilitative Services

Jefferson County Public Health Unit
275 North Mulberry Street
P.O. Box 156
Monticello, FL 32344

Name of Program:
Special Diabetic Program

Type of Program:
General health promotion
Diabetes education
Diabetes screening
Weight management
Nutrition
Exercise
Support
Continuing education/training
Eye screening
Hypertension screening
Foot care
Prenatal care

Audience:
People with diagnosed diabetes
General population
Health professionals

Materials Available:
Yes

Comments:

We serve a population of 70 percent black, 30 percent white, with occasional other nationalities. We have a general program for people with diabetes that includes return monitoring visits and further teaching. A major focus of our program is to improve patients' compliance, progress, and understanding of diabetes and diabetes control.

Contact:
P. Watkins, R.N., CHN
Diabetes Coordinator
Florida Department of Health and Rehabilitative Services
Jefferson County Public Health Unit
275 North Mulberry Street

P.O. Box 156
Monticello, FL 32344
(904) 997–5422

Florida Department of Health and Rehabilitative Services

Leon County Public Health Unit
2965 Municipal Way
Tallahassee, FL 32304

Name of Program:
Leon County Public Health Unit

Type of Program:
General health promotion
Diabetes education
Diabetes screening
Nutrition
Continuing education/training
Hypertension screening
Foot care
Referrals
Sick days guidelines

Audience:
People with diagnosed diabetes
General population
Health professionals

Materials Available:
No

Contact:
P. Snead, CHNS
Florida Department of Health and Rehabilitative Services
Leon County Public Health Unit
2965 Municipal Way
Tallahassee, FL 32304
(904) 487–3186

Grace Hill Neighborhood Health Center

2600 Hadley Street
St. Louis, MO 63106

Name of Program:
Health Promotion/Wellness Program

Type of Program:
General health promotion
Diabetes screening
Nutrition
Eye screening
Hypertension screening
Foot care
Prenatal care

Audience:
People with diagnosed diabetes
General population

Year Program Established:
1970's

Comments:
Grace Hill Neighborhood Health Center is a community health center. Comprehensive primary care services are provided on a sliding fee scale. Emphasis is placed on public health nursing, health promotion, and prevention/wellness. Diabetes education is incorporated into nutrition education sessions for the general community as well as for wellness leadership training programs.

Contact:
Villie A. Koenig
Managing Director - Primary Care
Grace Hill Neighborhood Health Center
2600 Hadley Street
St. Louis, MO 63106
(314) 241–2200

Grady Memorial Hospital

96 Armstrong Street
Atlanta, GA 30303

Name of Program:
Grady Diabetes Unit

Type of Program:
Diabetes education
Diabetes screening

Weight management
Nutrition
Continuing education/training
Hypertension screening
Foot care
Renal monitoring
Cardiac monitoring

Audience:
People with diagnosed diabetes
Licensed health care providers

Year Program Established:
1971

Materials Available:
Yes
"Diabetes Guidebook: Diet Section"
Price: $17. Available from: Davicone, Inc.,
1075 Lullwater Rd., NE, Atlanta, GA 30307

Other Minority Groups Served:
Hispanics
Vietnamese
Hearing-impaired

Comments:

We have 18,000 patients who have completed our Diabetes Detection and Control Center program since 1968. The initial visit is an 8-hour day of evaluation and education by a team comprising a nurse practitioner, physician, dietitian, and podiatrist on an outpatient basis. Then, patients are seen in the followup clinic as indicated. The team approach is critical to the success of the program. A mini residency for health professionals, "Modern Methods of Diagnosing and Treating Diabetes Mellitus and Its Complications," also is offered at the Unit through the Emory University School of Medicine.

Contact:
Daniel L. Gallina, M.D.
Grady Diabetes Unit
Grady Memorial Hospital
96 Armstrong Street
Atlanta, GA 30303
(404) 589–3716

Health Promotion Council of Southeastern Pennsylvania

311 South Juniper Street
Room 308
Philadelphia, PA 19107–5803

Name of Program:
Diabetes Identification and Follow-Up Program

Type of Program:
Hypertension screening
Counseling and followup of complications of diabetes and uncontrolled hypertension

Audience:
People with diagnosed diabetes

Year Program Established:
1987

Materials Available:
Yes
"Danger: Diabetes and High Blood Pressure"
Available as a brochure, standup poster, and wall poster

Comments:

Through our hypertension screening, we identify individuals who are already diabetic. We will briefly counsel them on the risks of having uncontrolled high blood pressure and/or diabetes and emphasize that the best prevention is control of both blood pressure and diabetes. We also emphasize regular eye and foot exams to prevent both retinopathy and neuropathy. If we are unable to counsel clients at screening, we will call them on the telephone. Three attempts are made to contact. If we cannot contact by telephone, a letter is then sent. After 1 year, we will recontact the client to determine his or her latest blood pressure and encourage continued control of diabetes and blood pressure.

Contact:
Thomas A. Elder
Program Coordinator
Health Promotion Council of SE Pennsylvania
311 South Juniper Street, Room 308
Philadelphia, PA 19107–5803
(215) 546–1276

Health Promotion Council of Southeastern Pennsylvania

311 South Juniper Street
Room 308
Philadelphia, PA 19107–5803

Name of Program:
Health Literacy Project

Type of Program:
General health promotion
Diabetes education
Weight management
Nutrition
Exercise
Continuing education/training

Audience:
People with diagnosed diabetes
General population
Health professionals
Low income African-American and Hispanic families

Year Program Established:
1987

Materials Available:
Yes
1. "Put Away Your Frying Pan." Videotape, VHS, 10 minutes, $15.
2. "Get Up and Move." Videotape, VHS, 10 minutes, $25.
3. Pamphlet masters for duplication:
    - Put Away Your Frying Pan
    - It's Making Me Sick: Alcohol and High Blood Pressure
    - I'm Doing It for Me: Mr. Hudson Goes on a Diet
    - The Odette Winters Show: Exercise Is for You Too.
4. "Improving Patient Compliance—Health Education for Non-readers." Videotape, VHS, 17 minutes, $35 (for staff development)

Other Minority Groups Served:

Our newly established Hispanic Health Literacy Project may choose to focus on nutrition issues appropriate for people with diabetes.

Contact:
Sarah Furnas, R.N.
Director
Professional Support Services

Health Promotion Council of SE Pennsylvania
311 South Juniper Street, Room 308
Philadelphia, PA 19107–5803
(215) 546–1276

HEALTH WATCH

Information and Promotion Service
3020 Glenwood Road
Brooklyn, NY 11210

Name of Program:
HEALTH WATCH

Type of Program:
General health promotion
Diabetes education
Weight management
Nutrition
Support group
Continuing education/training
Cardiovascular risk reduction
Hypertension screening
Cholesterol screening

Audience:
People with diagnosed diabetes
General population
Health professionals

Year Program Established:
1987

Materials Available:
No (see Comments)

Comments:
We are developing a videotape on the early detection and control of hypertension. The program will be directed to a general audience and its projected completion date is June 1990. HEALTH WATCH also sponsors conferences and community forums.

Contact:
Norma J. Goodwin, M.D.
President
HEALTH WATCH

3020 Glenwood Road
Brooklyn, NY 11210
(718) 434–5411

Henry J. Austin Health Center

321 North Warren Street
Trenton, NJ 08618

Name of Program:
Diabetes Classes

Type of Program:
Diabetes education
Nutrition

Audience:
People with diagnosed diabetes

Year Program Established:
1985

Materials Available:
No

Contact:
Ruth Rouse, R.N., C.D.E.
Henry J. Austin Health Center
321 North Warren Street
Trenton, NJ 08616
(609) 695–3349

Howard University Hospital

2041 Georgia Avenue, NW
Washington, DC 20060

Name of Program:
Diabetes Support Group

Type of Program:
Diabetes education
Support group

Audience:
People with diagnosed diabetes and their relatives

Year Program Established:
1989

Materials Available:
No

Contact:
Howard University Hospital
2041 Georgia Avenue, NW
Washington, DC 20060
Cynthia Barclay
(202) 483–2701
Juanita A. Archer, M.D.
(202) 865–1516
(202) 865–1947

Kansas Department of Health and Environment
900 SW Jackson Street
10th Floor
Topeka, KS 66612–1290

Name of Program:
Kansas Diabetes Control Program

Type of Program:
Diabetes education
Nutrition
Continuing education/training
Eye screening
Hypertension screening
Foot care
Prenatal care

Audience:
People with diagnosed diabetes

Year Program Established:
1987

Materials Available:
Yes
Diabetes "Owners Manual"
"Diabetes Passport"
(Additional materials in development)

Comments:

The Kansas Diabetes Control Program is funded by the Diabetes Translation Center of CDC and addresses the diagnosed diabetic population in Kansas. It is not limited to the black population; however, program efforts are currently concentrated in the most densely populated areas of the state, which also have the highest percentage of blacks in the population. Program components include comprehensive screening, referral, and care for people with identified diabetes to prevent four of the complications: eye disease, hypertension, lower extremity amputation, and adverse outcomes of pregnancy.

Contact:

Paula F. Marmet, M.S., R.D.
Program Administrator
Kansas Diabetes Control Program
Kansas Department of Health and Environment
900 SW Jackson Street - 10th Floor
Topeka, KS 66612–1290
(913) 296–1207

Kings County Hospital

451 Clarkson Avenue
Brooklyn, NY 11203

Name of Program:

Outpatient Diabetic Clinic

Type of Program:

Diabetes education
Weight management
Exercise
Eye screening
Hypertension screening
Foot care
Prenatal care
Nutrition

Audience:

People with diagnosed diabetes

Year Program Established:

1981

Materials Available:

Yes

Materials developed include exchange lists for Caribbean foods, other ethnic exchange lists, a diabetes diet guide, and measure kit. A diet guide for use in hospitals and private practice is planned.

Other Minority Groups Served:
Caribbean

Comments:
This program in a large municipal hospital serving a predominantly minority population offers a wide range of diabetes educational services. The program ties in with a cardiovascular risk reduction program in the same hospital, and patients are referred to the other program for aerobic exercise and other support services.

Contact:
Eunice Lewis, R.D.
Kings County Hospital
451 Clarkson Avenue
Brooklyn, NY 11203
(718) 735–2372

Liberty Medical Center

2600 Liberty Heights Avenue
Baltimore, MD 21215

Name of Program:
Community Health Awareness Monitoring Program (CHAMP)

Type of Program:
General health promotion
Diabetes education
Diabetes screening
Weight management
Nutrition
Exercise
Support group
Eye screening
Hypertension screening
Foot care

Audience:
People with diagnosed diabetes

Year Program Established:
1979

Materials Available:
Yes

Comments:

CHAMP functions as an outreach arm of the Diabetes Care Management Program at Liberty Medical Center. The staff, including a nurse, dietitian, and assistant director, conduct community programs and health fairs at community churches. The focus is on diabetes awareness and risk reduction.

Contact:
Jeanne Charleston, R.N.
Project Director
Liberty Medical Center
2600 Liberty Heights Avenue
Baltimore, MD 21215
(301) 383–4415

Liberty Medical Center

2600 Liberty Heights Avenue
Baltimore, MD 21215

Name of Program:
Diabetes Care Management Program (DCMP)

Type of Program:
General health promotion
Diabetes education
Diabetes screening
Weight management
Nutrition
Exercise
Support group
Eye screening
Hypertension screening
Foot screening
Treatment with case management, referral, and followup
Behavior modification
Smoking cessation
Continuing education/training
Stress management

Audience:
People with diagnosed diabetes

People with hypertension
General population
Health professionals
Other adults

Year Program Established:
1987

Comments:
We have a unique interdisciplinary team. Disciplines include: Clinical nurse specialist and nurse practitioner, clinical pharmacy, dietetics, social work, internal medicine and endocrinology, and certified diabetes health educators. We also provide referral and followup to other services, as well as to our own.

Contact:
Susan Akridge, Director
Department of Gerontology and Health Education and Promotion Services
Liberty Medical Center
2600 Liberty Heights
Baltimore, MD 21215
(301) 383–4868

Massachusetts Department of Public Health
150 Tremont Street
Boston, MA 02111

Name of Program:
Massachusetts Diabetes Control Program

Type of Program:
Diabetes education
Diabetes screening
Eye screening
Hypertension screening
Foot care
Prenatal care

Audience:
People with diagnosed diabetes

Year Program Established:
1985

Materials Available:
Yes
"Blacks and Diabetes" (pamphlet)

Other Minority Groups Served:
Hispanics
Asians

Contact:
Robert Bishop, M.S.
Director
Massachusetts Diabetes Control Program
Massachusetts Department of Health
150 Tremont Street
Boston, MA 02111
(617) 727-2662

Meharry Medical College
1005 DB Todd Boulevard
Nashville, TN 37208

Name of Program:
Community Coalition for Minority Health, Diet-Smoking-Blood Pressure Control for Blacks

Type of Program:
Weight management
Hypertension
Obesity
Smoking cessation

Audience:
General population
Children and young people

Year Program Established:
1986

Materials Available:
Yes
Low-literacy awareness materials, available for duplication.

Other Minority Groups Served:
Expanding to serve poor and underserved

Comments:

The project provides an intensive health education and disease prevention program utilizing health professionals, black churches, and lay workers trained to address the disease-associated risk factors of diet, obesity, and high blood pressure. The target population is blacks in Nashville, Tennessee. The project is conducted by the Meharry Medical College. This 2-year project received one of six minority community health coalition demonstration grants funded by the Office of Minority Health in 1986.

Contact:
Dr. Margaret Hargreaves
Meharry Medical College
1005 DB Todd Boulevard
Nashville, TN 37208
(615) 327–6000

Mt. Sinai Medical Center

High Blood Pressure Council of Greater Cleveland
One Mt. Sinai Drive
Cleveland, OH 44106

Name of Program:
High Blood Pressure Council of Greater Cleveland

Sponsoring Organization:
Ohio Department of Health and the Mt. Sinai Medical Center

Type of Program:
General health promotion
Hypertension screening

Audience:
People with hypertension
General population

Year Program Established:
1979

Materials Available:
No

Comments:
We are a clearinghouse for information concerning a vast array of disease entities that affect minority populations.

Contact:
Myron Bennett

Coordinator
High Blood Pressure Council of Greater Cleveland
Mt. Sinai Medical Center
One Mt. Sinai Drive
Cleveland, OH 44106
(216) 421–6453

Newark Beth Israel Medical Center

201 Lyons Avenue
Newark, NJ 07112

Name of Program:
Diabetes-Related Lower Extremity Intervention Program

Sponsoring Organization:
New Jersey State Department of Health
Newark Beth Israel Medical Center

Type of Program:
Comprehensive diabetes management, including primary care and education. Emphasis on foot care.

Audience:
People with diagnosed diabetes (at high risk for lower extremity amputations)

Year Program Established:
1985

Materials Available:
No

Other Minority Groups Served:
Hispanics

Contact:
Carol Manchester, R.N., M.S.N., CS, CDE
Newark Beth Israel Medical Center
201 Lyons Avenue
Newark, NJ 07112
(201) 923–4149

New Jersey Commission for the Blind and Visually Impaired

1100 Raymond Boulevard
Newark, NJ 07102

Name of Program:
Diabetic Eye Disease Detection Program

Sponsoring Organization:
New Jersey State Department of Health

Type of Program:
Eye screening

Audience:
People with diagnosed diabetes

Year Program Established:
1985

Materials Available:
No

Other Minority Groups Served:
Hispanics are included in our programs

Contact:
Sunil Parikh, M.D.
Diabetic Eye Disease Detection Program
New Jersey Commission for the Blind and Visually Impaired
1100 Raymond Boulevard
Newark, NJ 07102
(201) 648–3550

North Carolina Division of Health Services

P.O. Box 2091
Raleigh, NC 27602

Name of Program:
North Carolina Diabetes Control Program

Type of Program:
Diabetes education
Diabetes screening
Weight management
Nutrition
Eye screening
Hypertension screening
Foot care
Prenatal care

Audience:
People with diagnosed diabetes
General population

Year Program Established:
1986

Materials Available:
No

Other Minority Groups Served:
Native Americans

Comments:

The North Carolina Diabetes Control Program is a state-based program funded by the Centers for Disease Control to reduce the complications and premature mortality among people with diabetes. North Carolina serves a large minority population, through a multidisciplinary approach. At the state level, the program is supported by a program coordinator and a CDC public health advisor. Consultation is also provided by a nutritionist and a health educator. Local health department programs are supported by project coordinators, nutritionists, and health educators.

Contact:
Angie Hemingway, R.N., M.P.H.
North Carolina Diabetes Control Program
P.O. Box 2091
Raleigh, NC 27602
(919) 733–7081

Osteopathic Medical Center of Philadelphia

4190 City Avenue
Rowland Hall, 4th Floor
Philadelphia, PA 19131–1696

Name of Program:
Outpatient Diabetes Teaching Center

Type of Program:
Diabetes education
Nutrition
Exercise

Audience:
People with diagnosed diabetes (including gestational diabetes)

Year Program Established:
1988

Materials Available:
Yes (contact program for more information)

Contact:
Susan Beidler-Pezdirc, CRPN, MSN, CDE
Outpatient Diabetes Education Nurse Coordinator
Osteopathic Medical Center of Philadelphia
4190 City Avenue
Rowland Hall, 4th Floor
Philadelphia, PA 19131–1696
(215) 871–1916

Settlement Health and Medical Services, Inc.

314 East 104th Street
New York, NY 10029

Name of Program:
Settlement Health and Medical Services Program

Type of Program:
Diabetes education
Diabetes screening
Weight management
Nutrition
Exercise
Primary health care services

Audience:
General population
Other

Year Program Established:
1978

Materials Available:
No (in development)

Comments:

This is a community health center providing primary health care service regardless of a patient's ability to pay. Services include prenatal, pediatric, adult, and geriatric health care and programs related to heart disease and AIDS.

Contact:
Elizabeth Benson
Executive Director
Settlement Health and Medical Services, Inc.
314 East 104th Street
New York, NY 10029
(212) 860–0401

Texas Department of Health
1100 West 49th Street
Austin, TX 78729

Name of Program:
Chronic Disease Prevention

Type of Program:
General health promotion
Diabetes education
Diabetes screening
Weight management
Nutrition
Exercise
Eye screening
Hypertension screening
Foot care
Prenatal care

Audience:
People with diagnosed diabetes
People with hypertension
General population

Materials Available:
Yes (contact program for list)

Other Minority Groups Served:
Mexican-American

Contact:
Charlene Laramey, R.N., C.S.W.
Texas Department of Health
1100 West 49th Street
Austin, TX 78729
(512) 458–7534

University of Medicine and Dentistry of New Jersey

School of Osteopathic Medicine
401 Haddon Avenue
Camden, NJ 08103–1505

Name of Program:
Diabetes and Pregnancy Program

Sponsoring Organization:
New Jersey State Department of Health

Type of Program:
Diabetes education
Diabetes screening (gestational)
Nutrition
Prenatal care

Audience:
People with diagnosed diabetes
Pregnant women

Year Program Established:
1987

Materials Available:
Yes

Other Minority Groups Served:
Hispanics

Contact:
Theresa Scholl, Ph.D., M.P.H.
University of Medicine and Dentistry of New Jersey
School of Osteopathic Medicine
401 Haddon Avenue
Camden, NJ 08103–1505
(609) 757–7735

University of Nevada Cooperative Extension

Expanded Food and Nutrition Education Program
453 East Sahara Avenue
ST&P Building, #707
Las Vegas, NV 89104

Name of Program:
Fit Ways

Type of Program:
General health promotion
Diabetes screening
Nutrition

Audience:
General population
Minority and low income families

Year Program Established:
The program has been operating for 30 years; diabetes emphasis added in 1989.

Materials Available:
Yes

Other Minority Groups Served:
Hispanic
Native American

Comments:

The Expanded Food and Nutrition Education Program is a federally funded program that provides nutrition education to low income families. The program includes screenings, referrals, and outreach.

Contact:
Linda Sleeth, R.D.
University of Nevada Cooperative Extension
453 E. Sahara Avenue
ST&P Building, #707
Las Vegas, NV 89104
(702) 731–3130

Washington Department of Health

Diabetes Program
1702 Tacoma Avenue South
Tacoma, WA 98402

Name of Program:
Community Health Care Delivery System

Type of Program:
Eye screening
Hypertension screening

Foot care
Prenatal care

Audience:
People with diagnosed diabetes
Health professionals

Year Program Established:
1989

Materials Available:
No

Contact:
Florence L. Reeves
Community Health Care Delivery System
Washington State Department of Health
Diabetes Program
1702 Tacoma Avenue South
Tacoma, WA 98402
(206) 627–8067

Recommended Readings

Access to Medical Care for Black and White Americans: A Matter of Continuing Concern. Blendon, RJ., et al. *JAMA: Journal of the American Medical Association.* 261 (2): 278–281. January 13, 1989.

A 1986 national survey of use of health services showed a significant deficit in access to health care among black compared with white Americans. This gap was experienced by all income levels of black Americans. In addition, the study pointed to significant underuse by blacks of needed medical care. Moreover, blacks compared with whites were less likely to be satisfied with the qualitative ways their physicians treat them when they are ill, more dissatisfied with the care they received when hospitalized, and more likely to believe that the duration of their hospitalizations was too short.

Are Racial Differences In the Prevalence of Diabetes in Adults Explained by Differences In Obesity? O'Brien, T.R., et al. *JAMA: Journal of the American Medical Association.* 262 (11): 1485–1488. September 15, 1989.

To determine whether the higher prevalence of diabetes found among blacks in the United States is explained by racial differences in obesity, the authors examined the prevalence of diabetes adjusted for adiposity, education, and income in a cohort of US Army veterans from the Vietnam era. Among 12,558 white men and 1,677 black men, ages 30 to 47 years, blacks were more likely than whites to have diagnosed diabetes. Within every age, adiposity, and socioeconomic stratum, blacks had a higher prevalence of diagnosed diabetes than whites. In a subgroup of veterans for whom fasting serum glucose values were measured, blacks were more likely than whites to have fasting hyperglycemia. These data provide evidence that the higher prevalence of diabetes found among blacks is not explained by differences in obesity.

Black Americans. Lipson, L.S., et al. *Diabetes Forecast.* 4 (9): 34–37. September 1988.

The growing incidence of noninsulin-dependent diabetes mellitus (NIDDM) among black Americans is discussed, noting that diabetes is the third leading cause of mortality in this population group. Other health complications in blacks with diabetes include high blood pressure and atherosclerosis. It is suggested that the current increase in diabetes among black Americans probably involves a complex combination of genetic, environmental, and nutritional factors. Guidelines for treating NIDDM and strategies for tackling problems that black Americans with diabetes face are also discussed.

Black Americans. Office of Disease Prevention and Health Promotion. In: *Disease Prevention/Health Promotion: The Facts*, p. 198–212. Palo Alto, CA: Bull Publishing Co., 1988.

Available from Bull Publishing Co., P.O. Box 208, Palo Alto, CA 94302–0208. (415) 322–2855. Price: $24.95, plus $3 shipping/handling.

This chapter presents various socioeconomic, demographic, and health-related statistics for the U.S. black population, including historical and current statistics. Data are based on U.S. Census reports, statistics compiled by the National Center for Health Statistics, and other Government surveys. Morbidity and mortality data and significant trends are provided for diabetes as well as for other major health problems in blacks, such as cancer, cardiovascular disease, infant mortality, and homicides. The chapter includes tables and references.

Black Americans: Diabetes and Obesity. *Diabetes Forecast.* p. 74–75. February 1990.

This article discusses two recent research reports relevant to the increased prevalence of diabetes and diabetes-related kidney disease in blacks. The first report discussed compared rates of diabetes and rates of obesity and educational and income levels among a group of black veterans and white veterans of the Vietnam era; the other provided data about the higher rate of diabetes-related kidney disease in the black population.

Black/White Comparisons of Premature Mortality for Public Health Program Planning: District of Columbia. Levy, M. *MMWR. Morbidity and Mortality Weekly Report.* 38 (3): 34–37. January 1989. Centers for Disease Control, U.S. Public Health Service, Department of Health and Human Services.

The District of Columbia Commission of Public Health analyzed its mortality data for 1980–1986 using measures of age-adjusted mortality, premature deaths (before age 70), and years of potential life lost before age 65 (YPLL). "Excess deaths" were calculated according to the definition of the Secretary's Task Force on Black and Minority Health of the U.S. Department of Health and Human Services. The survey found that the death rate among black residents was 37 percent higher than among whites. Diabetes-related mortality was higher in black men and women than in white men and women.

Cohort Study of Mortality in Two Clinic Populations of Patients With Diabetes Mellitus. Vander, Z.R., et al. *Diabetes Care.* 6 (4): 341–346. July-August 1983.

Mortality rates of two cohorts of patients with diabetes mellitus were estimated and compared. The Atlanta cohort was defined as all black patients receiving care at the diabetes clinic of Grady Memorial Hospital for the first time during calendar year 1971. The Memphis cohort was defined as all black patients referred from the City of Memphis Hospital outpatient clinic to a decentralized neighborhood clinic operated by the Memphis and Shelby County Health Department during September 1969 through August 1970. The Atlanta program discontinued all prescriptions of oral hypoglycemic drugs and emphasized instead an aggressive diet therapy. The Memphis program used diet therapy but also insulin and/or oral hypoglycemic agents according to current guidelines. The ratios of observed to expected deaths (standardized mortality ratios) were remarkably similar for the two cohorts. In both cohorts the standardized mortality ratios were greatest for the youngest patients and for those patients whose duration of illness was longest. Nine-year survival rates, estimated by the life-table method and adjusted for differences in frequency distributions of entry age and duration of diabetes, were also similar for the two cohorts.

Diabetes: A Dread Disease You Might Have and Not Know It. Sanders, C.L. *Ebony.* October 1985.

This article notes that black Americans, especially women, are at high risk for developing diabetes. The article explains what diabetes is, risk factors for developing the disease, symptoms, and treatment. The author notes that many people with diabetes do not realize they have the disease. The author also stresses that if diagnosed early, diabetes can be controlled, and people with diabetes can lead active, full lives.

Diabetes and Inner-City Children. Winkleman, E.A. *Diabetes Spectrum.* 3 (2): 73–78. March/April 1990.

Health professionals involved in providing diabetes services to inner-city children share their experiences in working with the children and families. The article discusses settings in which diabetic children from inner cities receive care; the type of care they receive from professionals, as well as in the home; what is or could be done to promote diabetes education in inner cities; and psychosocial problems that lead to a lack of support. A model treatment program designed to improve adherence and self-management for inner-city adolescents is examined. Featured are interviews with Allan Glasgow, M.D., of Children's Hospital in Washington, D.C.; Vinod Lala, M.D., of Lincoln Hospital in Bronx, New York; Dr. Sam Richton, of the Miami Children's Hospital; Dr. Ilene Finnoy of the Harlem Hospital Center, Elizabeth Warren-Boulton of the American Diabetes Association (ADA): and representatives from ADA affiliates in large cities.

Diabetes in Black Americans. In: *Report of the Secretary's Task Force on Black and Minority Health, Volume VII: Chemical Dependency and Diabetes*, p. 214–253. Washington, DC: U.S. Department of Health and Human Services, January 1986.

Available from the Office of Minority Health Resource Center, P.O. Box 37337, Washington, DC 20013–7337. (800) 444–6472.

This report documents the growing prevalence of diabetes in the U.S. black population since World War II. Citing statistics from surveys carried out since the early 1920's, the report notes the rise in the rate of noninsulin-dependent diabetes in blacks, particularly black women, as well as higher rates of diabetes mortality and major diabetes-related complications in the black population. The need for studies to determine the scope of the problem in blacks is emphasized, along with the need for studies on the prevalence of insulin-dependent diabetes in both white and minority populations. The report includes tables and chart.

Diabetes in Black Americans. Roseman, J.M. In: *Diabetes in America*, Chapter VIII, 1–24. Washington, DC: National Diabetes Data Group, 1985.

Available from the National Diabetes Information Clearinghouse, Box NDIC, 9000 Rockville Pike, Bethesda, MD 20892. (301) 468–2162. Price: $23.

This chapter summarizes data from population-based studies conducted between 1924 and 1983 to determine the prevalence of diabetes in U.S.

blacks. The data show that the prevalence of noninsulin-dependent diabetes (NIDDM) is greater in U.S. blacks when compared with the white population and that blacks have higher rates of diabetes-related macrovascular disease, retinopathy, renal disease, and peripheral vascular disease. Surveys also indicate that the prevalence of NIDDM and diabetes mortality rates are increasing in blacks, especially black women. Rates of insulin-dependent diabetes, however, appear to be higher in the white population of the United States. Although comparative data from Africa are scarce and of uncertain validity, the prevalence of both types of diabetes appears to be greater in U.S. blacks than in African blacks, except perhaps in urban areas. The chapter includes tables and references.

Diabetes in Minorities—Second Conference on Diabetes in Blacks Focuses on Public Awareness, Education. *Diabetes Dateline.* 11 (1): 1–2. Winter 1990.

Available from the National Diabetes Information Clearinghouse, Box NDIC, 9000 Rockville Pike, Bethesda, MD 20892. (301) 468–2162.

The second national conference focusing on the problem of diabetes in blacks centered on public and professional awareness and education. This report summarizes recommendations by conference speakers to increase professional and public awareness of diabetes as a major health problem in the black community and to promote health measures to reduce the occurrence and impact of diabetes in blacks.

Diabetes in Minorities—Soaring Prevalence of Diabetes in Blacks: A National Concern. *Diabetes Dateline.* 10 (1): 1–2. Spring 1989.

Available from the National Diabetes Information Clearinghouse, Box NDIC, 9000 Rockville Pike, Bethesda, MD 20892. (301) 468–2162.

This article summarizes major statistics on the rising prevalence of diabetes in the U.S. black population and the impact of diabetes on blacks in terms of morbidity and mortality. Findings are reported from a national conference held in 1988 to explore factors responsible for the high rate of diabetes in blacks and to identify research priorities to address the problem.

Diabetic Renal Disease in Blacks—Inevitable or Preventable? (Editorial). Rostand, S.G. *New England Journal of Medicine.* 321 (16): 1121–22. October 19, 1989.

This editorial comments on possible reasons for the higher rate of diabetic end-stage renal disease in blacks. The author cites a study by Cowie et al. that suggests that the excess rate of end-stage renal disease among blacks cannot be explained fully by age or racial differences in the prevalence of diabetes. Possible causative factors discussed in the editorial include the role and pathological features of hypertension in blacks, sodium handling in blacks, differences in changes in kidney function, and socioeconomic factors that impede access to medical care by the black population.

Diet Therapy for Minority Patients With Diabetes. Gohdes, D. *Diabetes Care.* 11 (2): 189–191. February 1988.

Diet therapy for minority diabetic patients must be directed to noninsulin-dependent diabetes (NIDDM), the most prominent form of diabetes in minority populations. Diet programs must be tailored to the cultural framework, and traditional foods with desirable characteristics can be encouraged. To teach patients about diet, educators must use educational techniques appropriate to the culture and literacy of the patient and family. Single-concept messages such as "eat less fat" or "east less food" promote learning and minimize failure. Nutrition information can be divided into sequenced manageable steps that can then be individualized to the patient's setting. No single set of exchange lists will suffice for all minority groups, nor are exchange lists themselves appropriate for all situations. To meet the needs of minority patients, nutrition educators must use a variety of tools and techniques relating to the foods of a particular ethnic group. Sound education strategies and simplified materials for NIDDM patients also should be employed.

Disparities in Incidence of Diabetic End-Stage Renal Disease According to Race and Type of Diabetes. Cowie, C.C., et al. *New England Journal of Medicine.* 321 (16): 1074–79. October 19, 1989.

This study concerned diabetic patients with end-stage renal disease (470 blacks and 861 whites) reported to the Michigan kidney registry who began treatment during 1974 through 1983. The medical records of a subpopulation of such patients (284 blacks and 310 whites) who were less than 65 years of age at the start of ESRD treatment also were reviewed to determine what type of diabetes they had. National data on the prevalence of diabetes were used in the study. The investigators found that the incidence of diabetic end-stage renal disease was 2.6-fold higher among blacks after adjustment for the higher prevalence of diabetes among blacks, with the excess risk occurring predominantly among blacks with noninsulin-dependent diabetes. Most black patients had NIDDM (7 percent), whereas most white ESRD patients had insulin-dependent diabetes (58 percent). Although the risk of diabetic end-stage renal disease was markedly greater for patients with IDDM (5.8 percent) than for those with NIDDM (0.5 percent), the results indicate an increased risk of diabetic end-stage renal disease among blacks as compared with whites, particularly blacks with NIDDM.

The Effect of Known Risk Factors on the Excess Mortality of Black Adults in the United States. Otten, Jr., M.W., et al. *JAMA: Journal* *of the American Medical Association.* 263 (6): 845–50. February 9, 1990.

The mortality rate ratios before and after adjustment for different risk factors of black vs. white adults in the National Health and Nutrition Examination Survey I Epidemiologic Followup Study were compared. For persons 35 to 54 years old, the ratio of mortality for blacks vs. whites decreased from 2.3 (unadjusted) to 1.9 when adjusted simultaneously for six well-established risk factors (smoking, systolic blood pressure, cholesterol level, body-mass index, alcohol intake, and diabetes) and decreased from 1.9 to 1.4 when adjusted for the six risk factors plus family income. Approximately 31 percent of the excess mortality can be accounted for by six well-established risk factors, a further 38 percent by family income with 31 percent unexplained. Broader social and health system changes and research targeted at the causes of the mortality gap, coupled with increased efforts aimed at modifiable risk factors, may be needed for egalitarian goals in health to be realized.

The Effective Approach and Management of Diabetes in Blacks and Other Minority Groups. Davidson, J.K In: *Report of the Secretary's Task Force on Black and Minority Health. Volume VII: Chemical Dependency and Diabetes.* p. 297–355. Washington, DC: U.S. Department of Health and Human Services, January 1986.

Available from the Office of Minority Health Resource Center, P.O. Box 37337, Washington, DC 20013–7337. (800) 444–6472.

A brief overview of diabetes, particularly as it affects minority populations in the United States, is presented. The author reviews the epidemiology and pathophysiology of diabetes, stressing implications for minority groups, and describes two ongoing, successful diabetes programs targeted to blacks in Atlanta, Georgia, and Memphis, Tennessee. The author cites experiences of the two programs and their impact on health outcomes in patients. The report includes tables, references, and charts.

A Group Approach to the Management of Diabetes in Adolescents and Young Adults. Warren-Boulton, E., et al. *Diabetes Care.* 4 (6): 620–623. November-December 1981.

An interdisciplinary team of health professionals developed a model treatment program to improve adherence, self-management, and metabolic control for five inner-city, black, young adult, diabetic women. The group met monthly for a period of 18 months. The professional approach was supportive and nonjudgmental to assist the group members in developing confidence and assuming responsibility for the successful management of their diabetes. Discussions covered the group's educational needs, insulin requirements, and psychosocial problems of adjusting to living with a chronic disease. Analysis of clinical findings showed a significant improvement in plasma glucose, hemoglobin A1c, and cholesterol levels at the end of the study.

Highlights of a Symposium, Hypertension: Treatment Factors in the Management of the Black Patient. *Journal of the National Medical Association.* 81: Supplement. April 1989.

This special issue is a compilation of papers and edited highlights of a discussion from the symposium "Treatment Factors in the Management of the Black Patient," held in Los Angeles, California, in July 1988 under the auspices of the National Medical Association. Topics addressed include epidemiologic factors, community programs to increase hypertension control, racial differences in the management of hypertension, therapeutic choices for the older patient, and recommendations of the joint national committee on hypertension as they affect blacks. Discussion topics include psychosocial stress, genetic influences, diet, renin profiling, echocardiography, various antihypertensive agents, hypertensive emergencies, and cost of care.

Maturity-Onset Diabetes of Youth in Black Americans. Winter, W.E., et al. *New England Journal of Medicine.* 316 (6): 285–291. February 5, 1987.

A study identifying an atypical form of diabetes in 12 of 129 black Americans is reported. Patients and their relatives with diabetes were included in immunologic and metabolic studies if their dependence on insulin was transient, allowing them to discontinue insulin treatment completely or for minimal periods of 1 week without developing ketoacidosis or other severe symptoms. The results of the study differentiate this type of diabetes from insulin-dependent diabetes, although it has features of noninsulin-dependent diabetes.

The Memphis and Atlanta Continuing Care Programs for Diabetes. II. Comparative Analyses of Demographic Characteristics, Treatment Methods, and Outcomes Over a 9–10 Year Follow-up Period. Davidson, J.K, et al. *Diabetes Care.* 7 (1): 25–31. January-February 1984.

The authors report followup statistics for 1,467 black patients treated at the diabetes clinics of Grady Memorial Hospital in Atlanta, Georgia, and the City of Memphis Hospital in Memphis, Tennessee. Demographic characteristics, including age, sex, duration of diabetes, and weight, are provided and compared for patients at each center, as well as initial and followup mean random blood glucose values, modes of therapy, and mortality rates. The report also provides followup data on the type of therapy in relation to glucose control and standardized mortality rates. Relative risks of mortality for each therapeutic modality were not possible to calculate.

Minority Health in Michigan: Closing the Gap. Lansing, MI: Michigan Department of Public Health. 1988. 206 p.

Available from the Office of Minority Health, Michigan Department of Public Health, 3423 North Logan/M.L. King Boulevard, P.O. Box 30195, Lansing, MI 48909. (517) 335–9287.

This comprehensive report summarizes the results of a statewide survey of minority health status, mortality, and health risks in Michigan and provides recommendations for improving minority health status in the state. The report details major causes of excess minority deaths, special problems adversely affecting health status, systemic issues, and areas for intervention. The survey found that the age-adjusted mortality rate in 1985 was 48 percent higher for minorities than for whites; major causes of excess minority deaths were heart disease, homicide, cancer, infant mortality, liver disease, stroke, diabetes, and accidents; many state residents who lack access to food and nutrition resources are members of minority groups; minorities occupy a disproportionate share of substandard homes; poor socioeconomic status leads to greater health problems and poorer access to health care for minority children and the elderly, and high school dropout rates among minorities are high, often leading to unemployment or low wage "dead-end" jobs. It was noted that there are some 45,000 migrant agricultural laborers, about 80 percent of whom are Mexican Americans. It was concluded that innovations in the policy area can contribute to improve health outcomes for minorities.

Minority Wellness Promotion: A Behavioral Self-Management Approach. Butler, F.R. *Journal of Gerontological Nursing.* 13 (8): 23–28. August 1987.

The author developed a behavioral self-management approach to maintaining health in older blacks who are essentially well and living in the community. Although the health problems of aging blacks are not racially unique, the well-established relationship between health and income in the United States ensures that elderly blacks are less healthy and more prone to health-related restriction of activities of daily living (ADL) than are whites. The primary components of community-based self-management include: (1) definition and clarification of individual goals, (2) daily self-monitoring, and (3) self-reinforcement. This self-management approach is employed in a program for elderly persons living in residential facilities established by the National Caucus and Center on Black Aging (NCBA). The program consists of health screening and preassessment, individualized planning and implementation, and evaluation. Statistics obtained during 2 years of operation on a voluntary, nonfunded basis indicate that the health status and ADL capacities of NCBA residents were significantly improved for many participants. The greatest gains were made in assisting clients to stabilize their blood pressures and to control diabetes and weight by using intensive, behavioral, self-management techniques.

Mobilizing a Minority Community to Reduce Cardiovascular Risk Factors: An Exercise-Nutrition Handbook. Community Health Assessment and Promotion Project (CHAPP). Emory University School of Medicine and Grady Hospital. Atlanta, GA.

Available from Dr. Ken Powell, Cardiovascular Health Branch, Division of Chronic Disease Prevention and Health Promotion, Centers for Disease Control, 1600 Clifton Road, Atlanta, GA 30333; (404) 639–3158. Price: Contact Dr. Powell.

This guide is based on a 3-year program conducted in Atlanta, Georgia, to document the change in modifiable risks or behaviors related to hypertension and obesity in over 400 women in a predominantly black community. The program had a 60 to 70 percent compliance rate, and significant reductions in weight and blood pressure were reported. Two additional guides also are available, *Promoting Physical Activity Among Adults* and *Physical Fitness Promotion*. The first is a handbook to assist program planners in designing interventions for community organizations and governments. It provides methods for estimating the health problems associated with a sedentary lifestyle and the number of inactive adults in the community. It also outlines types of activities that can be conducted at different sites, and it can be used to educate family practitioners about needs and issues in individual communities. *Physical Fitness Promotion* is a collection of assessment tools to evaluate the effectiveness of a program and includes samples of pretests and posttests.

Non-Insulin-Dependent Diabetes Mellitus in Black Americans: A Roundtable Discussion. Gavin, J.R., et al. Kalamazoo, MI: Upjohn Company. March 1988. 25 p.

Available from the Upjohn Company. 7000 Portage Road, Kalamazoo, MI 49001. (616) 323–4000.

This special report for health care professionals, the third in a series about noninsulin-dependent diabetes in populations at risk, concerns diabetes in black Americans. The report presents summaries, comments, recommendations, and supporting evidence developed in a roundtable discussion. Five significant themes are addressed: epidemiology, contributing factors; the role and benefit of diet and exercise; pharmacologic therapy, and patient education, awareness, and compliance. Individual comments of the professional participants are included under each theme.

Participation Rates, Weight Loss, and Blood Pressure Changes Among Obese Women in a Nutrition-Exercise Program. Lasco, R.A., et al. Public Health Reports. 104 (6): 640–647. November-December 1989.

Since 1985, a black urban community in Atlanta has planned, implemented, and evaluated a cardiovascular risk reduction project. The Community Health Assessment and Promotion Project (CHAPP) was developed to reduce the high incidence of cardiovascular risk factors in the neighborhood's predominantly black population. A community coalition designed and directed a 10-week exercise and nutrition intervention targeted to obese residents between the ages of 18 and 59 years. The program uses a wide range of strategies, including individual consultations, reminder telephone calls, incentives, rewards, and free transportation and child care, to encourage participation. Program evaluation has demonstrated high participation rates and significant reductions in weight and blood pressures both immediately after the intervention and on 4-month followup. Since completion of this evaluation study, over 400 additional community members have participated in the program.

Potential Barriers to the Translation of Scientific Knowledge Into Improved Health Care and Health for Black Persons With Diabetes. Michigan Diabetes Research and Training Center Task Force on Diabetes in the Black Population. Michigan Diabetes Research and Training Center. 1331 East Ann, Ann Arbor, MI 48109. (313) 763–5256.

A special task force established by the University of Michigan Diabetes Research and Training Center examined factors influencing diabetes care among black Americans in the State of Michigan. Barriers identified by the task force included racism, lack of knowledge, incorrect beliefs about diabetes, restricted access to care, problems in patient-provider communication, differing values and priorities, and poverty. The report also recommends basic principles to consider in addressing these barriers and possible areas for program implementation.

Prevalence of Known Diabetes Among Black Americans. Drury, T.F., and Powell, A L. *NCHS AdvanceData*. 130: 1–12. July 1987.

Available from the National Center for Health Statistics. 3700 East-West Highway, Hyattsville, MD 20782. (301) 436–8500.

This report presents statistics showing the disproportionate increase of diabetes in blacks between the years 1963 and 1985. The data presented are based on the National Health Interview Survey of the National Center for Health Statistics (NCHS). Data from earlier NCHS surveys are used to provide historical comparisons. Information is presented in chart form, broken down by demographic characteristics, age, and race. Explanations of the data are provided, as well as conclusions about the significance of the statistics.

Psychosocial Factors Influencing Inner City Black Diabetic Patients' Adherence With Insulin. Uzoma, C. U., and Feldman, R.H. *Health Education.* Special Issue. 20 (5): 29–32. December 1989.

The authors surveyed black adult diabetes patients attending an outpatient clinic in Washington D.C., to identify factors having an influence on adherence to insulin regimens. The 30-minute interview covered such factors as perceived self-efficacy, perceived barriers to treatment, perceived severity of illness, and perceived social support. Other factors such as age, duration of diabetes, income, educational level, sex, and years on insulin also were considered. The findings revealed that age and perceived self-efficacy were the strongest indicators of adherence among the patients interviewed. Female patients also more often cited barriers to treatment and support from significant others as important, while men placed less importance on barriers and tended to regard too much involvement of others in their management routine as interference.

Public Health Reports. 104 (C). November-December 1989. U.S. Public Health Service. Superintendent of Documents, U.S. Government Printing Office, Washington, DC 20402. (202) 783–3238. Price: $4.75. GPO Stock Number 717–021-00032–1.

This issue focuses on projects supported by the Public Health Service that specifically address minority health issues. Among projects described is a community weight loss intervention program for inner-city blacks (see "Participation Rates, Weight Loss, and Blood Pressure Changes Among Obese Women in a Nutrition-exercise Program"). Other articles describe programs concerned with HIV infection, cancer control, drug use, homicide, cigarette smoking, maternal and infant health, suicide, diabetes in American Indians, and tuberculosis.

Selected Minority and Disadvantaged Support Programs 1988. Office of Minority Health, Office of the Assistant Secretary for Health, DHHS. Washington, DC: Office of Minority Health. 1988.

Available from the U.S. Department of Health and Human Services, Office of Minority Health Resource Center, P.O. Box 37337, Washington, DC 20013–7337. 1–800-444–6472 or (301) 587–1938. Price: Free.

This directory provides information about funding opportunities for programs supported by private foundations and Federal Government agencies that are specifically directed to minorities or disadvantaged populations or that include minorities or the disadvantaged as special targets. Included in the directory are programs that support the training of minority health and other science professionals; support the upgrading and expansion of curricula of institutions that train professionals; and identify community efforts to improve the health status of minorities. Each program listing includes information about eligibility criteria, allowable costs and award amount, application deadlines, and review of applications. Quick reference tables assist in identifying specific types of programs.

Sociocultural Factors and Health Care-Seeking Behavior Among Black Americans. Bailey, E.J. *Journal of the National Medical Association.* 79 (4): 403–408. April 1987.

This study investigated the health care-seeking behavior of black Americans in the Detroit metropolitan area. Analyses of 176 semistructured interviews and 27 life history profiles obtained from participants, nonparticipants, clinic coordinators, community leaders, and health care professionals at local screening clinics suggest that black Americans follow a cultural specific health care-seeking pattern and that such behavior is significantly influenced by sociocultural factors. This information should be particularly useful for health care professionals and educators because it can help them plan and implement special intervention strategies for the black community.

Trends in Diabetes Mellitus Mortality. *MMWR. Morbidity and Mortality Weekly Report.* 37 (50): 769–773. December 23, 1988. Centers for Disease Control, U.S. Public Health Service, Department of Health and Human Services.

National mortality rates for 1970–1985 were analyzed to evaluate trends for diabetes as an underlying cause of death for total diabetes mellitus-related mortality using National Center for Health Statistics data. Numbers of deaths for which diabetes was listed anywhere on the death certificate were used to compute total diabetes-related mortality rates among U.S. blacks and U.S. whites, which were age adjusted by the direct method using the estimated U.S. resident population in 1980 as standard. The risk of dying from diabetes was assessed by determining mortality rates for the U.S. population known to have diabetes from prevalence estimates of diabetes in 1976, 1980, and 1984.

White Doctors and Black Patients: Influence of Race on the Doctor-Patient Relationship. Levy, D.R. *Pediatrics.* 75 (4): 639–643. April 1985.

Effective communication between doctor and patient is essential for patient satisfaction and optimal patient care. In many teaching hospitals, the doctor is commonly white and middle class, and the patient black and indigent. Racial differences, even in the absence of social class differences, may have a negative impact on the quality of the doctor-patient relationship. The impact of racism is reviewed, and recommendations to enhance the relationship between white doctors and black patients are made.

Why Us? Blacks and Diabetes. Squires, S. *American Visions.* p. 23–25. December 1988.

Reasons for the increased prevalence of noninsulin-dependent diabetes and diabetes complications in black Americans as compared with white Americans are examined. Possible causative factors may include genetics, obesity, environment, and lack of access to medical treatment. Pregnancy, as a risk factor for later development of diabetes, also is addressed.

Chapter 68

Diabetes Educational Materials in Spanish and Other Languages

Introduction

Diabetes is a major health problem among Hispanic Americans. Surveys show that the rate of diabetes in Americans of Puerto Rican, Mexican, or Cuban origin is 50 to 100 percent higher than among white Americans of non-Hispanic origin. Moreover, studies of Hispanic populations in the United States indicate that they have higher death rates from diabetes than do non-Hispanics as well as higher rates of some of the severe complications of diabetes such as kidney disease, retinopathy, and severe hyperglycemia.

Many Asian and other ethnic populations also have high rates of diabetes. To help meet the needs of educators working with non-English-speaking patients and family members, the National Diabetes Information Clearinghouse (NDIC) has prepared this listing of materials in Spanish and other languages as a resource. The materials listed include print and non-print resources about the management of diabetes, nutrition and diet, exercise, diagnosis, medications, monitoring, foot and skin care, pregnancy, and risk factors. Most of the print materials listed are written for patients and their families; the nonprint items are for use by health professionals in patient education programs. Most materials listed have been produced since 1984.

The literature search consists of three sections: the first lists print materials in Spanish and the second lists nonprint materials in Spanish. The third section lists educational materials available in other languages.

National Diabetes Information Clearinghouse. January 1993.

Each citation is presented in the following order:

- Title in Spanish (or other language) with English translation
- Physical description of audiovisual materials (if appropriate)
- Source or availability, including price when appropriate
- Abstract or description of the item

[Abbreviations used are: *LG* = language; *TI* = title; *AU* = author; *SO* = source; *CN* = corporate author; *PD* = physical description; *AV* = producer/availability; *AB* = abstract.]

Items listed are taken from the diabetes subfile of the Combined Health Information Database (CHID). The catalog, *Audiovisual Resources for Diabetes Education,* produced by the Learning Resource Center of the University of Michigan Diabetes Research and Training Center, also lists nonprint educational materials in Spanish and other languages. For additional information, contact the Learning Resource Center, University of Michigan Medical School, 1135 East Catherine Street, Ann Arbor, MI 48109–0726; telephone (313) 763–6770.

NDIC maintains the diabetes subfile on CHID, a computerized database of health education and information materials. CHID is available through BRS Online, a division of InfoPro Technologies. Many medical, university, and large public libraries subscribe to BRS service, and individuals wishing to search the database may request a search through a library. Persons with personal computers equipped with a modem also may search the database by subscribing to BRS Online. Subscription information is available from BRS, 1–800-955–0906.

No attempt has been made to assess the educational value of the items listed, and their inclusion does not imply endorsement by NDIC or the National Institute of Diabetes and Digestive and Kidney Diseases (NIDDK). The literature search is not intended to be an exhaustive listing of available materials. Rather it represents a selected listing of materials identified by NDIC staff.

The materials listed are not distributed by NDIC. Sources for items are provided in each citation. Prices and availability were verified when the listing was compiled, but readers should be aware that prices and availability are subject to change.

NDIC is a service of the National Institute of Diabetes and Digestive and Kidney Diseases, National Institutes of Health. The literature search is not subject to copyright restrictions, and individuals may feel free to duplicate any or all parts of the search.

Spanish Language Materials: Print

LG English; Spanish
TI **Americans of Latin Descent.**
AU Jewler, D.
SO Diabetes Forecast. p. 27–32. September 1988.

AB This special report addresses possible reasons for the increased incidence of noninsulin-dependent diabetes in Mexican Americans, citing evidence that it may be due to the degree of Native American ancestry. Included is a detailed discussion of the Mexican American diabetes problem, as described by a Texas medical center nurse who has specialized in the care of Mexican American diabetes patients and the provision of diabetes education programs for such patients.

LG Spanish
TI **Atencion de los Pies (Foot Care).**
SO Alexandria, VA: American Diabetes Association, Diabetes Information Service Center. April 1989. 4 p.
CN American Diabetes Association.
AV Available from American Diabetes Association, Diabetes Information Service Center, 1660 Duke Street, Alexandria, VA 22314. (800) 232–3472 or (703) 549–1500. (Also available from local Chapters). PRICE: Bulk price, single copies are free. (Also available in English).

AB Foot problems are more likely to be serious and develop quickly in patients with diabetes, underscoring the importance of daily foot care. People with diabetes may develop poor blood circulation and nerve damage (neuropathy) in their feet and legs. Feet can be protected by following a number of tips for good foot care that are listed in this brochure. These include regular visits to a physician for feet examination, washing the feet each day and keeping them dry (especially between the toes), never walking barefoot, wearing shoes that fit comfortably, changing socks daily, and checking the feet and toes each day for blisters, cuts, and scratches. This brochure also is available in English (see DMBR01690).

LG Spanish
TI **Atencion en el Dia que este Enfermo (Sick-Day Care).**
SO Alexandria, VA: American Diabetes Association, Diabetes Information Service Center. April 1989. 4 p.
CN American Diabetes Association.
AV Available from American Diabetes Association, Diabetes Information Service Center. 1660 Duke Street, Alexandria, VA 22314. (800) 232–3472 or (703) 549–1500. (Also available from local Chapters). PRICE: Bulk price, single copies are free. (Also available in English).

AB This brochure provides guidelines to help people with diabetes prepare for days when they are sick with a cold, flu, and other illnesses. The physical stress of being sick can raise blood glucose. Loss of appetite or vomiting while sick also can affect diabetes control. A sick day plan is needed, which should include instructions for blood glucose and urine ketone testing, when to call the doctor, a list of foods and fluids that can be taken, and possible medication changes. People who regularly take insulin or diabetes pills should continue to do so, even if they cannot eat. Drinking plenty of fluids during sick days is important, and if regular food cannot be consumed, sugar-containing foods or soft foods should be used in place. Since sick day medications (e.g., cough syrup containing sugar) can affect diabetes, one's doctor should always be consulted, even for non-prescription medications. This brochure also is available in English (see DMBR01687).

LG Spanish
TI **Comer Bien Para Vivir Mejor (Eat Well To Live Better).**
AU Hall, T.A.; Bertram, K.; et al.
SO Sacramento, CA: California Diabetes Control Program, Department of Health Services. 1985. 70 p.
CN Diabetes Control Program, Department of Health Services.
AV Available from California Diabetes Control Program. Department of Health Services, Continental Plaza, 601 North 7th Street, Sacramento, CA 94234–7320. (916) 323–9868. PRICE: Contact directly for details.

AB This guide for nutrition counselors is designed to assist the overweight patient with noninsulin-dependent diabetes to maintain control of his or her disease through weight loss and exercise. A calorie-controlled, high-fiber, low-fat diet is the central feature of the plan. The menus and food exchange lists are based on a daily diet that includes beans, tortillas, and other traditional Mexican foods appropriate for California's Hispanic population, and the authors advise that modification of the plan may be required to better reflect the dietary practices of Hispanic patients in the eastern United States. The professional guide is organized into four major content areas: an introduction, briefly describing the problems of diabetes among Hispanics; the high-fiber Hispanic food plan; counseling guidelines; and guidelines for exercise. Appendices include sample assessment forms and behavioral records for use in the educational program.

LG Spanish
TI **Comiendo Bien Para Mantener el Azucar Normal en Su Sangre (Eating Well To Keep Your Blood Sugar Normal).**
SO San Diego, CA: Sweet Success: California Diabetes and Pregnancy Program (CDAPP). 1990. 4 p.
CN Sweet Success: California Diabetes and Pregnancy Program.
AV Available from Education Programs Associates, Inc. 1 West Campbell Avenue, Building D, Campbell, CA 95008. (408) 374–3720. PRICE: $.35 for CDAPP members or $.50 for non-members.

AB This simple, fold-out informational booklet, designed for pregnant women with diabetes, briefly reviews the steps required to eat well and keep blood glucose levels normal. Written in clear, easy-to-understand language, the booklet emphasizes the importance of following the established food plan. Simple drawings illustrate patient care items including food exchanges, foods to avoid, and increasing fiber intake. This booklet is also available in English (See DMBR01813).

LG Spanish
TI **Como Controlar Su Diabetes (Managing Your Diabetes).**
SO Indianapolis, IN: Eli Lilly and Company. 1989. 93 p.
CN Eli Lilly and Company.
AV Available from Eli Lilly and Company. Indianapolis, IN 46285. (317) 276–2000.

AB This colorful, illustrated study guide, written in Spanish, details facts and guidelines concerning diabetes control. Characteristics of diabetes, factors associated with proper diabetes control, dietary considerations, the characteristics and use of insulin, oral hypoglycemic drugs, and self-monitoring of blood glucose are discussed. Complications (hypoglycemia, hyperglycemia and ketoacidosis) and how they can be minimized are examined. A glossary is appended. It is designed in a convenient color-coded modular format. This 14-model system can be customized to meet individual patient needs. Topics are entitled: What is Diabetes?; Taking charge of Your Diabetes; Meal Planning; Physical Activity; Insulin; Oral Hypoglycemic Medications; Self-Monitoring of Blood Glucose; Ketone Testing; Pattern Management; Complications: Hypoglycemia, Hyperglycemia, and Ketoacidosis; Long-Term Complications; and General Health Care Tips. This patient book includes a glossary of important terms. The system is useful in one-on-one or small group teaching situations as well as for larger group presentations. Also available in English (see DMDC00843).

LG Spanish
TI **Como Escoger Alimentos Saludables (How to Choose Healthy Foods).**
SO Alexandria, VA: American Diabetes Association, Inc. 1988. 4 p. (brochure/poster).
CN American Diabetes Association, Inc. American Dietetic Association.
PD Poster (11 in x 17 in), col.
AV Available from American Diabetes Association, Inc. Diabetes Information Service Center, 1660 Duke Street, Alexandria, VA 22314. (800) 232–3472 or (703) 549–1500; or American Dietetic Association. 216 West Jackson Boulevard, Suite 800, Chicago, IL 60606 (312) 899–0040. PRICE: $0.53 each.

AB This poster/brochure written in Spanish suggests guidelines on how to choose healthy foods and gives recommendations for eating foods low in fat, salt and sugar and high in fiber. What to eat on a daily basis to maintain a healthy and balanced diet is outlined. Examples of foods from different groups such as grains, meats and its substitutes, vegetables, fruits, low-fat dairy products and other fats, calories and how much to eat daily are listed.

LG Spanish
TI **Como Preparar y Administrar una Inyeccion de Insulina (Preparing and Injecting the Dose of Insulin).**
SO Indianapolis, IN: Eli Lilly and Company. 1991. 4 p.
CN Eli Lilly and Company.

AV Available from Eli Lilly and Company. Indianapolis, IN 46285. (317) 276–2000. Price: Single copy free. Order Number 60-HI-2790–0. Available to only to health professionals through Lilly sales representatives. Contact the above for referral to a local representative.

AB This brief patient information brochure describes how to prepare and administer insulin injections. Three sections cover preparing an insulin dose using one type of insulin, preparing a mixed dose of insulin, and giving the injection. Color photographs illustrate each step, from handwashing to preparation of the injection site. The brochure also details the importance of proper care of insulin to obtain quality, consistent results.

LG Spanish
TI **Como Puede Afectar, a Mi y a Mi Bebe, la Diabetes Durante el Embarazo? (What Will Diabetes in Pregnancy Do To My Baby and Me?).**
SO San Diego, CA: Sweet Success: California Diabetes and Pregnancy Program (CDAPP). 1990. 4 p.
CN Sweet Success: California Diabetes and Pregnancy-Program.
AV Available from Education Programs Associates, Inc. 1 West Campbell Avenue, Building D, Campbell, CA 95008. (408) 374–3720. PRICE: $.35 for CDAPP members or $.50 for non-members.

AB This informational booklet, designed for the woman newly diagnosed with gestational diabetes, briefly reviews the care required during and after a pregnancy complicated by gestational diabetes. Written in clear, easy-to-understand language, the brochure emphasizes the importance of working closely with the health care providers to insure a healthy pregnancy and outcome. Simple drawings illustrate patient care components, including doctor visits, support, exercise, a food plan, and blood glucose tests. This booklet is also available in English (See DMBR01811).

LG Spanish
TI **Como Usar Chemstrip bG para Medir el Nivel de Azucar en la Sangre (How to Use Chemstrip bG for Blood Glucose Testing).**
SO Indianapolis, IN: Boehringer Mannheim Corporation. 1989. 7 p.
CN Boehringer Mannheim Diagnostics.
AV Available from Boehringer Mannheim Corporation. Patient Care Systems, 9115 Hague Road, P.O. Box 50100, Indianapolis, IN

46250. (800) 858–8072. PRICE: Single copy free. Order Number 1–296-0487.

AB This Spanish-language publication presents a step-by-step guide to using Chemstrip blood glucose monitoring strips. Full-color photographs illustrate each step as it is described in the text, including pretest preparation, obtaining a blood sample, timing the test, and interpreting test results. Tips for avoiding inaccurate results are provided.

LG Spanish
TI **Como Vivir con Diabetes (How to Live with Diabetes).**
SO Austin, TX: Texas Department of Health. 1985. 70 p.
CN Texas Department of Health.
AV Available from Texas Department of Health. 1100 West 49th Street, Austin, TX 78756. (512) 458–7111. PRICE: Single copy free. Order No. 10-lOOa.

AB Diabetes is explained in simple language for Spanish-speaking people. Discussion covers causes and symptoms, explains what diabetes is, and outlines treatments including diet, exercise, oral hypoglycemic medications, and insulin. Complications such as diabetic coma, insulin reaction, problems with infections, and foot care are identified. Discussion of proper diet and nutrition includes types of foods to eat or avoid, explains calories, carbohydrates, proteins, and fats, and explains and provides a food exchange list.

LG Spanish
TI **Companeros en el control: Ayudas Para Seguir Su Plan De Diabetes (Partners in Control: Tips to Help You Stay on Your Diabetes Plan).**
AU Erica L. Labrentz, et al.
SO Indianapolis, IN: Boehringer Mannheim Diagnostics. 1985. 20 p.
AV Available from Boehringer Mannheim Diagnostics. 9115 Hague Road, P.O. Box 50100, Indianapolis, IN 46250–0100. (800) 858–8072. PRICE: Free, up to 25 copies. Order Number 1–1052-0187.

AB This booklet is designed to help people with diabetes stay on the diabetes management plans that they have set up with their health care providers. The first section describes some negative thinking habits that may keep patients from getting started on their plan. Tools for Staying on Your Plan describes several techniques to help patients learn new habits and change old ones. The third section lists suggestions for handling high-risk situations, including special occasions that may tempt one to abandon a diabetes management plan.

LG Spanish
TI **Companeros en el control: Hablemos De Diabetes (Partners in Control: Talking About Diabetes).**
AU Cook-Newell, M.
SO Indianapolis, IN: Boehringer Mannheim Diagnostics. 1985. 15 p.
AV Available from Boehringer Mannheim Diagnostics. 9115 Hague Road, P.O. Box 50100, Indianapolis, IN 46250–0100. PRICE: Free, up to 25 copies. Order number 1–1053-0187.

AB This booklet, written for people newly diagnosed with diabetes and for the general public, presents a general introduction to diabetes mellitus. The author includes information about the nature of diabetes, high-risk groups, common symptoms, types of diabetes, how diabetes affects the body, and the characteristics of high and low blood glucose. Other topics include ways to monitor the effect of diet, exercise, and insulin/diabetes pills on blood glucose. The author also gives tips on what to do if blood glucose levels become too high or too low.

LG Spanish
TI **Complicaciones del Corazon y los Vasos Sanguineos (Heart and Blood Vessel Complications).**
SO Alexandria, VA: American Diabetes Association, Diabetes Information Service Center. April 1989. 4 p.
CN American Diabetes Association.
AV Available from American Diabetes Association, Diabetes Information Service Center. 1660 Duke Street, Alexandria, VA 22314. (800) 232–3472 or (703) 549–1500. (Also available from local Chapters). PRICE: Bulk price, single copies are free. (Also available in English).

AB People with diabetes are more likely to have heart and blood vessel disease and have it at an earlier age than people without diabetes. Diabetes may damage both large and small blood vessels. The risk is further increased by high blood pressure, high cholesterol levels, and/or smoking. Damage to large blood vessels can effect the heart and legs; damage to small blood vessels can affect the eyes and kidneys. Symptoms for heart and blood vessel damage are described. Experts think that maintaining close to normal blood glucose levels helps to prevent or delay blood vessel damage. Practical health guidelines by which people with diabetes can help to prevent blood vessel damage are included. This brochure also is available in English (see DMBR01694).

LG Spanish
TI **Complicaciones de la Diabetes (Complications of Diabetes).**
SO Alexandria, VA: American Diabetes Association, Diabetes Information Service Center. April 1989. 4 p.
CN American Diabetes Association.
AV Available from American Diabetes Association, Diabetes Information Service Center. 1660 Duke Street, Alexandria, VA 22314. (800) 232–3472 or (703) 549–1500. (Also available from local Chapters). PRICE: Bulk price, single copies are free. (Also available in English).

AB Complications that occur more often in people with diabetes than in people without diabetes are discussed. These complications are often due to changes in the blood vessels or nerves. Specific complications discussed include vascular disease, which can cause heart disease or stroke; small blood vessel disease, which can lead to blindness and kidney disease; and nerve damage (neuropathy) which most often affects the feet and legs and may result in foot amputation. Good control of blood glucose and regular checkups may help delay or prevent some complications. Warning symptoms of some complications are included. This brochure also is available in English (see DMBR01688).

LG Spanish
TI **Complicaciones: Impotencia (Complications: Impotence).**
SO Alexandria, VA: American Diabetes Association, Diabetes Information Service Center. April 1989. 4 p.
CN American Diabetes Association.
AV Available from American Diabetes Association, Diabetes Information Service Center. 1660 Duke Street, Alexandria, VA 22314. (800) 232–3472 or (703) 549–1500. (Also available from local Chapters). PRICE: Bulk price, single copies are free. (Also available in English).

AB This brochure discusses impotence in men with diabetes and its causes, treatments, and prevention. Impotence related to diabetes may be caused by neuropathy, blood vessel damage, drugs, and psychological factors. Treatments include control of blood glucose levels, surgery, penile implants, and vacuum tumescence. Preventive measures include maintaining near normal blood glucose levels and avoiding heavy drinking and smoking. This brochure also is available in English (see DMBR01693).

LG Spanish
TI **Complicaciones Nerviosas (Neuropatia) (Nerve Complications (Neuropathy)).**
SO Alexandria, VA: American Diabetes Association, Diabetes Information Service Center. April 1989. 4 p.
CN American Diabetes Association.
AV Available from American Diabetes Association, Diabetes Information Service Center. 1660 Duke Street, Alexandria, VA 22314. (800) 232–3472 or (703) 549–1500. (Also available from local Chapters). PRICE: Bulk price, single copies are free. (Also available in English).

AB This brochure describes the characteristics of neuropathy (nerve damage) in diabetes, including its risk factors, symptoms, hazards, and treatment. Neuropathy can affect both people with insulin-dependent and people with noninsulin-dependent diabetes, especially those who have had diabetes for a long time. Neuropathy affects nerves that connect the spinal cord to muscles, skin, blood vessels, and organs. While it can occur in many parts of the body, it most often affects the feet and legs. Symptoms often include numbness, tingling, weakness, burning, or pain in the fingers and toes. The pain is usually worse at night and may ease in the morning. As a result of neuropathy, injuries can occur to the feet that are not noticed, which could lead to serious foot problems such as infection and gangrene. While there are, at this time, no cures for neuropathy, good foot care, loss of excess weight, and good blood glucose control may reduce the severity or risk of foot problems that are caused by their condition. This brochure also is available in English (see DMBR01692).

LG Spanish
TI **Complicaciones Renales (Nefropatia) (Kidney Complications (Nephropathy)).**
SO Alexandria, VA: American Diabetes Association, Diabetes Information Service Center. April 1989. 4 p.
CN American Diabetes Association.

AV Available from American Diabetes Association, Diabetes Information Service Center. 1660 Duke Street, Alexandria, VA 22314. (800) 232–3472 or (703) 549–1500. (Also available from local Chapters). PRICE: Bulk price, single copies are free. (Also available in English).

AB The function of the kidneys is to remove harmful wastes and chemicals from the blood. Diabetic kidney disease (diabetic nephropathy) develops over several years and may be related to high blood glucose levels that harm tiny vessels in the kidneys. Most people with diabetes who have diabetic nephropathy have had diabetes for at least 10 to 15 years. Urinary analysis for protein by a health care practitioner can indicate whether further tests are needed to check for kidney damage. Other symptoms of kidney problems are swelling of feet and ankles, feeling tired, and pale skin color. High blood pressure and frequent urinary tract infections can also affect the kidneys. If kidney damage is detected, treatment includes lowering blood pressure, reducing salt intake, and control of blood glucose levels. If kidney failure occurs, treatment requires hemodialysis, peritoneal dialysis, or a kidney transplant. This brochure also is available in English (see DMBR01691).

LG Spanish
TI **Complicaciones Visuales (Retinopatia) (Eye Complications (Retinopathy)).**
SO Alexandria, VA: American Diabetes Association, Diabetes Information Service Center. April 1989. 4 p.
CN American Diabetes Association.
AV Available from American Diabetes Association, Diabetes Information Service Center. 1660 Duke Street, Alexandria, VA 22314. (800) 232–3472 or (703) 549–1500. (Also available from local Chapters). PRICE: Bulk price, single copies are free. (Also available in English).

AB People with diabetes should visit an eye doctor regularly. Diabetic retinopathy, a complication of diabetes that affects the retina of the eye, is of two types: background retinopathy (BR) and proliferative retinopathy (PR). The former is more common, occurring in about half of all people who have had diabetes for 10 to 15 years. It is usually mild and does not affect vision; however, if it gets worse, the retina may swell (macular edema), which does affect vision. Proliferative retinopathy can cause blindness. Methods of treating and controlling diabetes-related eye problems are described, including vitrectomy, photocoagulation, and blood pressure control. Other types of eye problems in people with diabetes-include blurred vision (when diabetes is out of control), cataracts, and glaucoma. This brochure also is available in English (see DMBR01689).

LG Spanish
TI **Consejos de cuidado dental para diabeticos (Dental Tips for Diabetics).**
SO Bethesda, MD: National Institute of Dental Research. 1990. 1 p.
CN National Institute of Dental Research in cooperation with the National Institute of Diabetes and Digestive and Kidney Diseases.
AV Available from National Diabetes Information Clearinghouse. Box NDIC, Bethesda, MD 20892. (301) 468–2162. PRICE: Free.

AB This two-sided information card, written in Spanish, serves as a quick reference to the special difficulties gum infections can pose for people with diabetes. The card discusses the warning signs of oral health problems and provides information for people with diabetes on how to care for the teeth and gums. Instructions for brushing the teeth and stimulating the gums are provided. The importance of proper care for the teeth and gums for people with this disease is stressed. This information card is also available in English (see DMBR01316).

LG Spanish
TI **Cuando Uno Tiene Diabetes (When Someone Has Diabetes).**
SO Princeton, NJ: Novo Nordisk Pharmaceuticals, Inc. 1985. 25 p.
CN Novo Nordisk Pharmaceuticals, Inc.
AV Available from Novo Nordisk Pharmaceuticals, Inc. 211 Carnegie Center, Princeton, NJ 08540. (800) 727–6500; in New Jersey (609) 987–5800. PRICE: Free.

AB Information on diabetes is presented for Spanish-speaking people. Illustrations accompany the text, which encompasses subjects such as diabetes treatment, meal planning, medications, and exercise. Instructions for analyzing glucose and urine and for administering insulin are provided. READING LEVEL: 13.

LG Spanish
TI **Cuidandose Despues del Parto (Your Care After Delivery).**
SO San Diego, CA: Sweet Success: California Diabetes and Pregnancy Program (CDAPP). 1990. 4 p.

CN Sweet Success: California Diabetes and Pregnancy Program.

AV Available from Education Programs Associates, Inc. 1 West Campbell Avenue, Building D, Campbell, CA 95008. (408) 374–3720. PRICE: $0.35 for CDAPP members or $0.50 for non-members.

AB This simple, fold-out informational booklet, designed for women with diabetes who have recently had a baby, briefly reviews the steps required in diabetes management after delivery. Written in clear, easy-to-understand language, the booklet emphasizes the importance of following the established food plan. Simple drawings illustrate the topics covered, including nursing the baby, exercise, using insulin, birth control, and the importance of planning the next pregnancy. Space is included for patient notes. This booklet is also available in English (See DMBR01816).

LG Spanish

TI **Datos Sobre la Diabetes (Diabetes Fact Sheet).**

SO New York, NY: Juvenile Diabetes Foundation. 1989. 1 p.

CN Juvenile Diabetes Foundation.

AV Available from Juvenile Diabetes Foundation. JDF World Headquarters. 432 Park Avenue South, New York, NY 10016. (212) 889–7575 or (800) JDF-CURE or (800) 533–2873.

AB This Spanish-language factsheet briefly describes diabetes mellitus as a chronic metabolic disorder that adversely affects the body's ability to manufacture and utilize insulin, a hormone necessary for the conversion of food into energy. The factsheet includes statistics about the incidence of diabetes and its complications in the United States. Topics noted include number of fatalities; heart disease and stroke; kidney disease; blindness; amputations; and the cost of diabetes to the nation. The last part of the factsheet provides information on the Juvenile Diabetes Foundation (JDF) International, an organization founded in 1970 by parents of children with diabetes. Brief statistics about the JDF International and its financial support of diabetes research are noted. The factsheet is also available in English (accession number DMDC00902).

LG English; Spanish

TI **Diabetes.**

SO Los Angeles, CA: National Association for Hispanic Elderly. 1990. 15 p.

CN National Association for Hispanic Elderly.

AV Available from Asosiacion Nacional Pro Personas Mayores. 3325 Wilshire Boulevard, Suite 800, Los Angeles, CA 90010. (213) 487–1922. PRICE: $1.50 for set of 5 brochures on various health topics.

AB This brochure, part of a series of health brochures, is targeted to elderly Hispanics and the health professionals who work with this population. The brochure is bilingual to assist both the non-English speaking patient and the non-Spanish speaking practitioner. Topics covered in the brochure include tips for weight loss; the risk factors for diabetes; increasing one's level of exercise; the importance of quitting smoking; ways to follow a lower sodium diet; and the importance of limiting the consumption of alcohol. Numerous colorful line drawings illustrate each point.

LG Spanish
TI **La Diabetes: Una Enfermedad Que Nos Puede Afectar a Todos Sin Excepcion (Diabetes: An Equal Opportunity Disease).**
AU Davidson, J. A.
SO Diabetes Forecast. p. 25. September 1988.

AB This editorial, written both in English and Spanish, stresses that diabetes does not discriminate on the basis of race. Problems experienced by minority diabetes patients include difficulty in comprehending the doctor's advice, lack of money for health care, difficulty in taking time from work to see a doctor, and low exposure to or opportunity to use information on diet and exercise for diabetes management. Also available in English (see DMJA03192).

LG English; Spanish
TI **Diabetes: Good Hygiene/La Buena Higiene. Rev ed.**
AU anon.
SO Austin: Texas Department of Health; n.d. 4p.
AV Texas Department of Health. Chronic Disease Prevention Diabetes Program, 1100 West 49th Street; Austin, TX 78756. (512) 458–7534, ext. 6474. PRICE: Free.

AB This illustrated Spanish/English brochure outlines the health care precautions people with diabetes should practice.

LG Spanish
TI **Diabetes Gravidica: Un Embarazo Feliz y Saludable (Gestational Diabetes: A Healthy Happy Pregnancy).**

AU Jornsay, D.L., et al.
SO Indianapolis, IN: Boehringer Mannheim Diagnostics. 1988. 41 p.
AV Available from Boehringer Mannheim Diagnostics. 9115 Hague Road, P.O. Box 50100, Indianapolis, IN 46250–0100. PRICE: Free up to 25 copies. Order number 01128700–1288.

AB This patient education brochure, written in Spanish, reviews gestational diabetes and encourages the pregnant woman to become a vital member of her own health care team. The authors define gestational diabetes; describe the potential effects on the baby's health; delineate the roles of various health care team members; and discuss testing blood glucose, proper nutrition, exercise, insulin, and what happens to the mother after the baby is born. A brief glossary is included. The brochure is also available in English (see DMBR00777).

LG English; Spanish
TI **Diabetes and Pregnancy: A Fact Sheet.**
SO San Diego, CA: San Diego and Imperial Counties Diabetes and Pregnancy Program. l99x. 2 p.
CN San Diego and Imperial Counties Diabetes and Pregnancy Program.
AV Available from Regional Perinatal System. 225 Dickinson Street, H-410, San Diego, CA 92103. (619) 294–6142. PRICE: $.20 each or 50 for $6.00.

AB This brief factsheet lists basic information about diabetes and pregnancy. Written in question-and-answer format, the factsheet covers pregnancy planning, the importance of good blood glucose control, how to improve blood glucose control, and how to best utilize the health care team to maximize the chances for a healthy pregnancy and a healthy baby. A questionnaire designed to gather demographic information is included. Also included is a form to request further information about diabetes and pregnancy.

LG English; Spanish
TI **Diabetic Retinopathy.**
SO San Francisco, CA: American Academy of Ophthalmology. 1987. 2 p.
CN American Academy of Ophthalmology.
AV Available from the American Academy of Ophthalmology. P.O. Box 7424, San Francisco, CA 94120. (415) 561–8500. PRICE: Free.

AB This factsheet for primary care physicians, discusses the prevalence, types, and treatment of diabetic retinopathy. The factsheet defines the two types of diabetic retinopathy as nonproliferative or background retinopathy and proliferative diabetic retinopathy. Treatment options discussed include laser photocoagulation and vitreous surgery (vitrectomy). The factsheet stresses the importance of referral to an ophthalmologist upon diagnosis of diabetes mellitus and thereafter for periodic ophthalmic examinations. One chart summarizes the information presented. The factsheet is also available in Spanish.

LG English; Spanish
TI **La Dieta Diabetica (The Diabetic Diet in Spanish). 3rd ed.**
SO Santa Monica: California Dietetic Association. 1989. 34 p.
CN Los Angeles District of the California Dietetic Association, Publications Advisory Committee.
AV Available from California Dietetic Association. Los Angeles District, P. O. Box 3506, Santa Monica, CA 90403. PRICE: $4.00 each for 1–24 copies; 25–49 copies, $3.50 each; 50 or more copies, $3.00 each.

AB This bilingual version of the new Exchange Lists for Meal Planning lists a wide variety of foods used in U.S. Spanish-speaking communities and describes how the foods fit into the exchange lists. The meat list is simplified to facilitate both teaching and translating into Spanish. Carbohydrate, protein, fat, and calorie contents are provided for 14 Spanish recipes. A short bibliography is included.

LG English; Spanish
TI **Eating for Your Health: Recipes for People with Diabetes, Their Families and Everyone Else!**
AU Spilker, R.H., ed.
SO Toledo, OH: Toledo Family Health Center, Inc. 1989. 50 p.
CN Toledo Family Health Center.
AV Available from Toledo Family Health Center, Inc. 117 Main Street, Toledo, OH 43605. (419) 697–2704. PRICE: $2.50.

AB This bilingual (English and Spanish) cookbook features traditional Mexican recipes, donated by residents of Toledo, Ohio, and modified to reduce the amount of sugar, fat and calories. The serving size, exchange values, and calorie levels are included with each recipe. Sections include recipes for sauces and appetizers, side dishes, entrees, desserts, and beverages.

LG Spanish
TI **En que Consiste el Analisis de Sangre? (What is Blood Testing?)**
SO Alexandria, VA: American Diabetes Association, Diabetes Information Service Center. December 1988. 4 p.
CN American Diabetes Association.
AV Available from American Diabetes Association, Diabetes Information Service Center. 1660 Duke Street, Alexandria, VA 22314. (800) 232–3472 or (703) 549–1500. (Also available from local Chapters). PRICE: Bulk price, single copies are free. (Also available in English).

AB This brochure discusses and emphasizes the importance of blood testing for people with diabetes as one of the main tools for keeping diabetes in control. The goal is to keep blood glucose levels as near to normal as possible by properly balancing diet, exercise, and insulin or oral medicines. Procedures for testing blood glucose using visually read strips or a meter are discussed. This brochure also is available in English (see DMBR01681).

LG Spanish
TI **Enfermedad periodontal en los diabeticos: guia para los pacientes (Periodontal Disease and Diabetes: A Guide for Patients).**
SO Bethesda, MD: National Institutes of Health, National Institute of Dental Research. 1990. 10 p.
CN National Institute of Dental Research (NIH 87–2946).
AV Available from National Diabetes Information Clearinghouse, Box NDIC, Bethesda, MD 20892. (301) 468–2162. PRICE: Free.

AB This Spanish language brochure provides guidelines for the prevention of periodontal disease in patients with diabetes. Susceptibility to gum diseases, particularly among people with diabetes, may result from thickening of blood vessels, bacteria, or poor diabetes control. A discussion of how gum disease develops describes gingivitis, periodontitis, and tooth loss. Treatment information includes plaque removal and periodontal surgery, and addresses special treatment considerations for patients with diabetes. The booklet also provides practical information for preventing the periodontal complications of diabetes and illustrates step-by-step brushing and flossing techniques. Dental caries, thrush and dry mouth are other oral complications associated with diabetes. Proper brushing and flossing on a daily basis, in conjunction with regular dental checkups, are the best preventive measures for these oral diseases. This publication is also available in English (see DMBR01479).

LG Spanish
TI **Equilibrar: Alimento, Ejercicio, Medicamentos (Balance: Food, Exercise, Medicines).**
SO Alexandria, VA: American Diabetes Association, Diabetes Information Service Center. December 1988. 4 p.
CN American Diabetes Association.
AV Available from American Diabetes Association, Diabetes Information Service Center. 1660 Duke Street, Alexandria, VA 22314. (800) 232–3472 or (703) 549–1500. (Also available from local Chapters). PRICE: Bulk price, single copies are free. (Also available in English).

AB This pamphlet describes the roles of diet, exercise, and medication in good diabetes control. All three affect the blood glucose level of people with diabetes, and too much or too little of any of these factors can disrupt diabetes control. Food raises the blood glucose level, so it is important to watch how much food is eaten and when it is eaten. This can be done with a meal plan. Exercise lowers blood glucose and is helpful for losing weight (important in noninsulin-dependent diabetes), but should not be overdone. Insulin and oral drugs lower blood glucose. People taking insulin must be especially careful to time their insulin injections to coincide with mealtimes and exercise schedules. This brochure also is available in English (see DMBR01683).

LG Spanish
TI **Estiramientos Y Flexiones (Flex and Stretch).**
SO Somerville, NY: Hoechst-Roussel Pharmaceuticals. 1989. 4 p.
CN Hoechst-Roussel Pharmaceuticals.
AV Available from Hoechst-Roussel Pharmaceuticals. Somerville, NJ 08876. (908) 231–4600. PRICE: Single copy free. Order Number Q69331.

AB This brief patient education brochure illustrates flexing and stretching exercises in simple line drawings. A blank chart is provided in which to record daily exercise and pulse rate activity. A list of aerobic activities and the suggested objective for each are included. The addresses of two resources for additional information are also included.

LG Spanish
TI **Examen de Orina para Quetonas (Urine Testing for Ketones).**

SO Alexandria, VA: American Diabetes Association, Diabetes Information Service Center. April 1989. 4 p.
CN American Diabetes Association.
AV Available from American Diabetes Association, Diabetes Information Service Center. 1660 Duke Street, Alexandria, VA 22314. (800) 232–3472 or (703) 549–1500. (Also available from local Chapters). PRICE: Bulk price, single copies are free. (Also available in English).

AB This brochure discusses the characteristics of urinary ketones in diabetes, why urine testing is important in diabetes management, how such testing is done, and what to do if ketones are present. Ketones may appear in the urine when the body doesn't have sufficient insulin, when blood glucose levels fall too low, or during illness. Directions for when to test for ketones, how to perform the test, and when to call the doctor are provided. Moderate or large amounts of ketones are dangerous and upset the chemical balance of the blood, poisoning the body. This brochure also is available in English (see DMBR01684).

LG Spanish
TI **Examenes Durante el Embarazo (Tests in Pregnancy).**
SO San Diego, CA: Sweet Success: California Diabetes and Pregnancy Program (CDAPP). 1990. 4 p.
CN Sweet Success: California Diabetes and Pregnancy Program.
AV Available from Education Programs Associates, Inc. 1 West Campbell Avenue, Building D, Campbell, CA 95008. (408) 374–3720. PRICE: $.35 for CDAPP members or $.50 for non-members.

AB This simple, fold-out informational booklet briefly reviews the diagnostic and other tests that may be performed during pregnancy. Written in clear, easy-to-understand language, the booklet discusses the alfa fetoprotein (AFP) test, ultrasound, nonstress test, contraction stress test, and monitoring of the baby's movements. Simple drawings illustrate the topics covered. Space is included for patient notes. This booklet is also available in English (See DMBR01817).

LG Spanish
TI **Examenes Para La Diabetes (Tests For Diabetes).**
SO San Diego, CA: Sweet Success: California Diabetes and Pregnancy Program (CDAPP). 1990. 4 p.
CN Sweet Success: California Diabetes and Pregnancy Program.

AV Available from Education Programs Associates, Inc. 1 West Campbell Avenue, Building D, Campbell, CA 95008. (408) 374–3720. PRICE: $.35 for CDAPP members or $.50 for non-members.

AB This simple, fold-out informational booklet briefly reviews the diagnostic test for gestational diabetes that may be performed during pregnancy. Written in clear, easy-to-understand language, the booklet outlines the procedures followed during the 3-hour glucose tolerance test. Simple drawings illustrate the topics covered. Space is included for patient notes. This booklet is also available in English (See DMBR01819).

LG Spanish
TI **La Gordura No Dura! (The Fat Person Does Not Last!).**
SO Santa Fe, NM: Hispanic Marketing Consultants. 1987. 10 p.
CN Diabetes Research and Education Foundation.
AV Available from Hispanic Marketing Consultants. 33 Camarada Road, Santa Fe, NM 87505. (505) 986–8817. PRICE: 50 for $25.00.

AB This Spanish language brochure presents the story of one family's experiences when a family member is diagnosed with noninsulin-dependent diabetes mellitus (NIDDM). Told through the use of photographs with conversational captioning, the story focuses on the control of NIDDM through diet modification and weight loss. After a diagnosis by the family doctor, a dietitian is consulted. The dietitian explains more about diabetes, emphasizes the importance of eating a balanced diet and achieving a desirable weight, and points out the dangers of some of the complications that can occur. The inside front cover of the brochure provides a simple definition of diabetes and describes the risk factors of heredity, obesity, and age. A table lists common symptoms for severe and mild cases of diabetes. The inside back cover presents tips for getting one's diet off to a good start.

LG Spanish
TI **Guia de Comida: Diabetes Antes y Durante el Embarazo (Food Guide: Diabetes Before and During Pregnancy).**
SO San Diego, CA: Sweet Success: California Diabetes and Pregnancy Program. 1988. (poster).
CN Sweet Success (California Diabetes and Pregnancy Program.
PD Poster (11 in × 17 in), col.

AV Available from Education Programs Associates, Inc. 1 West Campbell Avenue, Building D, Campbell, CA 95008. (408) 374–3720. PRICE: $0.10 each plus shipping and handling.

AB This glossy, color-coded Spanish-language poster presents an overview of meal planning before and during pregnancy for women with diabetes. Foods are grouped into eight categories: milk, starch, vegetables, fruits, protein, fats, free foods, and foods to avoid. Each category includes simple line drawings of the foods described to assist those with limited reading skills. Measurements are also indicated in both words and pictures. Space is included for the woman to write down her own sample meal plan. This poster is also available in English (see DMAV01715)

LG Spanish

TI **Guia de Nutricion: Diabetes Antes y Durante el Embarazo (Nutrition Guide: Diabetes Before and During Pregnancy).**

AU Gunderson, E.P., et al.

SO San Diego, CA: Sweet Success: California Diabetes and Pregnancy Program. 1988. 36p.

AV Available from Education Programs Associates, Inc. Distribution Department, 1 West Campbell Avenue, Building D, Campbell, CA 95008. (408) 374–3720. PRICE: $1.65 for CDAPP members or $2.50 for non-members.

AB This booklet reviews nutritional recommendations before and during pregnancy for women with diabetes. Written in clear, easy-to-understand language, the booklet outlines basic principles for a food plan and categorizes foods into seven groups: milk products, dried beans and peas, protein foods, vegetables, fruits, grains and starches, and fats and oils. The author also discusses weight gain during pregnancy; how to treat low blood glucose; sources of simple sugars; the fat and sodium levels in cheese, crackers and snacks, and the combinations of food groups used to prepare meals. Illustrations and food examples use traditional foods from the Hispanic culture. Simple drawings illustrate the topics covered. This booklet is also available in English (See DMBR01821).

LG Spanish

TI **Hechos Sobre la Diabetes.**

SO Downsview, Ontario: Multicultural Health Coalition; 1985. 6p.

CN Multicultural Health Coalition.

AV MHC/CSM; Suite 407; 1017 Wilson Ave.; Downsview, Ontario M3K 1Z1; Canada. (416) 630–8835. PRICE: $0.10; minimum order of 50 plus $2.50 shipping and handling (U.S. Funds).

AB This pamphlet presents basic information about diabetes, including its treatment, symptoms, how it develops, and the risk factors that can increase a person's chances for developing diabetes. The components of a treatment plan, the importance of diabetes education, and examples of foods from the six major food groups are included. The pamphlet also is available in English, French, Chinese, Portuguese, Italian, Ukrainian, Polish, Hindi, Russian, Vietnamese, Finnish, Punjabi, and Greek. READING LEVEL: 10.

LG Spanish
TI **Hiperglicemia: Exceso de Azucar in la Sangre (Hyperglycemia: High Blood Sugar).**
SO Princeton, NJ: Novo Nordisk Pharmaceuticals, Inc. 1992. (poster).
CN Novo Nordisk Pharmaceuticals, Inc.
PD Poster (8 1/2 in x 11 in), b/w.
AV Available from Novo Nordisk Pharmaceuticals, Inc. 100 Overlook Center, Suite 200, Princeton, NJ 08450–7810. (800) 727–6500. PRICE: Single copy free.

AB This poster reviews the symptoms of and treatment for hyperglycemia (high blood sugar). Line drawings illustrate the symptoms of extreme thirst, frequent urination, dry skin, hunger, blurred vision, drowsiness, and nausea. Brief textual information lists the causes of hyperglycemia and target and problem blood glucose levels. Two panels remind the reader to test blood glucose levels and to contact a health care provider if results are over 250 mg/dl at repeated testing. This poster is also available in English (see DMAV01742).

LG Spanish
TI **Hiperlipemia (Altos niveles de grasa en la sangre) (Hyperlipidemia (High Blood-Fat Levels)).**
SO Alexandria, VA: American Diabetes Association, Diabetes Information Service Center. April 1989. 4 p.
CN American Diabetes Association.
AV Available from American Diabetes Association, Diabetes Information Service Center. 1660 Duke Street, Alexandria, VA 22314. (800) 232–3472 or (703) 549–1500. (Also available from

local Chapters). PRICE: Bulk price, single copies are free. (Also available in English).

AB High blood fat levels (hyperlipidemia) produce an increased risk for heart and blood vessel disease by causing arterial buildup of fat (hardening of the arteries). This results in narrowing or cutting off blood flow, which can result in a heart attack or stroke. Such problems can be caused by too much cholesterol in the diet and by saturated fats which give rise to cholesterol. Dietary guidelines are included for reducing cholesterol, saturated fat, and total fat intakes. It also is advised to exercise at least three times a week and not to smoke. This brochure also is available in English (see DMBR01695).

LG Spanish

TI **Hipertension (Alta Tension Arterial) (Hypertension (High Blood Pressure)).**

SO 50 Alexandria, VA: American Diabetes Association, Diabetes Information Service Center. April 1989. 4 p.

CN American Diabetes Association.

AV Available from American Diabetes Association, Diabetes Information Service Center. 1660 Duke Street, Alexandria, VA 22314. (800) 232–3472 or (703) 549–1500. (Also available from local Chapters). PRICE: Bulk price, single copies are free. (Also available in English).

AB People with diabetes are more likely to have high blood pressure (hypertension) than people without diabetes, and people with non-insulin-dependent diabetes are more likely to have high blood pressure than people with insulin-dependent diabetes. This brochure discussed how blood pressure is measured, why high blood pressure is dangerous, how people can know if their blood pressure is high, and how high blood pressure can be treated and prevented. High blood pressure can damage blood vessels leading to the heart, brain, and kidneys; if this occurs, heart attack, stroke, and kidney disease may result. Weight loss, limiting salt and alcohol intakes, regular exercise, stress reduction, and quitting smoking may reduce blood pressure in some people. Others may need prescribed medications to lower their blood pressure. This brochure also is available in English (see DMBR01696).

LG Spanish

TI **Hipoglicemia: Bajo Nivel de Azucar en la Sangre (Hypoglycemia: Low Blood Sugar).**

SO Princeton, NJ: Novo Nordisk Pharmaceuticals, Inc. 1992. (poster).

CN Novo Nordisk Pharmaceuticals, Inc.

PD Poster (8 1/2 in × 11 in), b/w.

AV Available from Novo Nordisk Pharmaceuticals, Inc. 100 Overlook Center, Suite 200, Princeton. NJ 08450–7810. (800) 727–6500. PRICE: Single copy free.

AB This poster reviews the symptoms of and treatment for hypoglycemia (low blood sugar). Line drawings illustrate the symptoms of shaking, fast heartbeat, sweating, anxiety, dizziness, hunger, impaired vision, weakness and fatigue, headache, and irritability. Brief textual information lists the causes of hypoglycemia and target and problem blood glucose levels. Three panels remind the reader to test blood glucose levels, drink juice or eat hard candies to treat a hypoglycemic reaction, and to eat a snack within 30 minutes after symptoms go away. This poster is also available in English (see DMAV01744).

LG English; Spanish

TI **Joslin Procedure Guides.**

SO Indianapolis, IN: Boehringer Mannheim Corporation. 1986. (illustrated procedure guides).

CN Boehringer Mannheim Corporation.

PD Illustrated procedure guides

AV Available from Boehringer Mannheim Corporation. 9115 Hague Road, P.O. Box 50100, Indianapolis, IN 46250. (800) 858–8072.

AB Developed in conjunction with the Joslin Diabetes Center, these illustrated guides teach and reinforce the correct techniques and procedures for self-monitoring of blood glucose with Boehringer Mannheim Diagnostics products. There are four guides available: How to Use Chemstrip bG (in English or Spanish); How to Use Accu-Chek bG and Chemstrip bG; and How to Use Accu-Chek II and Chemstrip bG. (AA).

LG Spanish

TI **Lo que Todo el Mundo Deberia Saber Sobre la Diabetes (What Everyone Should Know About Diabetes).**

SO South Deerfield, MA: Channing L. Bete Company, Inc. 1991. 15 p.

CN Channing L. Bete Company, Inc.

AV Available from Channing L. Bete Company, Inc. 200 State Road, South Deerfield, MA 01373–0200. (413) 665–7611 or (800) 628–7733. Order Number 37127.

AB This booklet, written in Spanish, contains information about diabetes in a question and answer format. The disease process of diabetes, who gets diabetes, its symptoms, diagnosis, and treatment are all examined. Definitions of insulin dependent (IDDM) and non-insulin dependent diabetes mellitus (NIDDM) are provided. Insulin administration, insulin reaction and diabetic coma are also discussed. Complications such as arteriosclerosis, vision problems, foot gangrene, and psychological effects are examined. Other concerns to people with diabetes are addressed and include work, life insurance, marriage and children, travel and other activities of daily living.

LG English; Spanish

TI **Meal Planning for People with Diabetes/Planificacion de Comidas para Personas con Diabetes.**

AU Bauer, C.E.; Moralez, V.; Freeburn, K.

SO Austin, TX: National Migrant Resource Program, Inc. 1990. 72 p.

CN Migrant and Rural Community Health Association (Bangor, MI).

AV Available from National Migrant Resource Program, Inc. 2512 South IH-35, Suite 220, Austin, TX 78704. (512) 447–0770, (800) 531–5120. PRICE: $3.50 ($2.50 to PHS 329/330-funded projects).

AB This illustrated booklet, written in both English and Spanish, provides information on meal planning and nutrition for people with diabetes. The information is organized into four sections which cover diabetes characteristics and diabetic diets; food exchange lists for each food group and their nutritional value; suggestions for using the exchange lists for dietetic and common Mexican foods; and guidelines for living with diabetes (medications, diet, exercise, special occasions, sick days). English and Spanish versions are replicated on opposite pages throughout the booklet.

LG Spanish

TI **Mezclando Insulinas (Mixing Insulins).**

SO Franklin Lakes, NJ: Becton Dickinson. 1985. 8 p.

AV Available from Becton Dickinson and Company. Consumer Products Division, One Becton Drive, Franklin Lakes, NJ 07417. (800) 526–4650. PRICE: Free.

AB A technique for filling a syringe with a mixed dose of regular and NPH insulins is illustrated in color photographs. This brochure is also available in English (see DMBR00733).

LG Spanish
TI **Mi Plan De Comidas (My Food Plan).**
SO San Diego, CA: Sweet Success: California Diabetes and Pregnancy Program (CDAPP). 1990. (chart).
CN Sweet Success: California Diabetes and Pregnancy Program.
PD Chart (8 1/2 in × 11 in).
AV Available from Education Programs Associates, Inc. 1 West Campbell Avenue, Building D, Campbell, CA 95008. (408) 374–3720. PRICE: $.05 for CDAPP members or $.10 for non-members.

AB This one-page chart provides a form to fill in with a diabetes meal plan. Spaces are provided to write in the times of meals, the number of choices for each meal from the seven food groups listed, and menu ideas for each meal. Space is also included on the form for the name and telephone number of the nutritionist and the recommended intake levels of calories, cholesterol, protein and fat. Food groups listed are milk, dried beans, protein foods, vegetables, fruits, grains and starches, and fats and oils. This chart also is available in English (See DMAV01723).

LG English; Spanish
TI **Nutrition Guide: Diabetes Before and During Pregnancy (Professional Statement).**
AV Gunderson, E.P.
SO San Diego, CA: Sweet Success: California Diabetes and Pregnancy Program. July 1988. 15 p.
AV Available from Education Programs Associates, Inc. 1 West Campbell Avenue, Building D, Campbell, CA 95008. (408) 374–3720. PRICE: $.35 for CDAPP members or $.50 for non-members.

AB This professional statement reviews some of the educational materials available through the California Diabetes and Pregnancy Program. Items discussed include the Nutrition Guide to Diabetes Before and During Pregnancy (9th grade reading level) and the Food Guide to Diabetes Before and During Pregnancy (low literacy). The author describes each booklet in detail, including why each section was included and how each section can benefit the women for which it was written. The statement is available in English and Spanish.

LG Spanish
TI **100,000 Tienen Diabetes y No lo Saben: Usted Puede Ser Uno de Ellos! (100,000 People Have Diabetes: You May be One of Them!).**
SO Carolina, PR: Pfizer Pharmaceuticals. 19xx. 1 p.
CN Pfizer Pharmaceuticals.
AV Available from Pfizer Pharmaceuticals. P.O. Box 1859, Carolina, PR 00628–1859. (809) 257–5000. PRICE: Free.

AB The symptoms of noninsulin-dependent diabetes are described. Diagnosis and treatment are briefly explained. READING LEVEL: 8. This fact sheet is also available in English (see DMDC00603).

LG Spanish
TI **Planificacion de Comidas con Alimentos Mexicanoamericanos (Meal Planning with Mexican-American Foods).**
SO Alexandria, VA: American Diabetes Association. 1989. 8 p.
CN American Dietetic Association. American Diabetes Association.
AV Available from American Diabetes Association. Diabetes Information Service Center, 1660 Duke Street, Alexandria, VA 22314. (800) 232–3472 or (703) 549–1500. PRICE: $0.60 each or $15.00 for 25 copies, plus shipping and handling. Order Number 1/90–20M.

AB This brochure, written in Spanish, is a guide to adapting traditional Hispanic cooking to conform with recommended dietary guidelines for people with diabetes. Tips for healthier preparation of traditional foods are provided, with an emphasis on lowering fat content. Modifications for meal planning and specific items are included. Exchange list information for traditional Mexican food items is given. Four recipes and a glossary of terms are also included. This brochure is also available in English.

LG Spanish
TI **Por Favor, Digame Que Puedo Comer (Please Tell Me What I Can Eat).**
SO Princeton, NJ: Novo Nordisk Pharmaceuticals, Inc. 1991. (chart).
CN Novo Nordisk Pharmaceuticals, Inc.
PD Chart (8 1/2 in × 13 3/4 in), col.

AV Available from Novo Nordisk Pharmaceuticals, Inc. 100 Overlook Center, Suite 200, Princeton, NJ 08450–7810. (800) 727–6500. PRICE: Single copy free.

AB This Spanish language chart, designed for people with diabetes, reviews dietary guidelines. One side of the chart provides six suggestions for reducing fat, watching out for sugar and sodium, and drinking plenty of liquids. The verso of the chart reviews food exchanges (bread, meat, vegetable, fruit, milk, and fat) and how they should be combined for a healthy daily diet. Each concept is presented through illustration, with only simple headings for text. The chart is also available in English (see DMAV01738).

LG Spanish
TI **Pruebas con Resultados Visuales (Visual Reading of Blood Glucose Test Results).**
SO Indianapolis, IN: Boehringer Mannheim Diagnostics. 1989. 15 p.
CN Boehringer Mannheim Corporation.
AV Available from Boehringer Mannheim Diagnostics. Patient Care Systems. 9115 Hague Road, P.O. Box 50100, Indianapolis, IN 46250. (800) 858–8072. PRICE: Single copy free. Order Number 011313001–0289.

AB This Spanish-language publication presents a step-by-step guide to using Chemstrip blood glucose monitoring strips and the Match-Maker blood glucose monitor. Full-color photographs illustrate each step as it is described in the text, including pretest preparation, obtaining a sample, timing the test, reading and interpreting test results, and recording test timing and results. Tips for obtaining better test results are provided.

LG Spanish
TI **Que es la Diabetes Dependiente de la Insulina? (Diabetes tipo I) (What is Insulin-Dependent Diabetes? (Type I Diabetes)).**
SO Alexandria, VA: American Diabetes Association, Diabetes Information Service Center. April 1989. 4 p.
CN American Diabetes Association.
AV Available from American Diabetes Association, Diabetes Information Service Center. 1660 Duke Street, Alexandria, VA 22314. (800) 232–3472 or (703) 549–1500. (Also available from local Chapters). PRICE: Bulk price, single copies are free. (Also available in English).

AB This brochure discusses the nature of insulin-dependent diabetes and its prevalence, why insulin must be administered by injection rather than orally, and the signs and symptoms of insulin-dependent diabetes. It is not known exactly what causes diabetes, but genetic influences and other factors appear to be involved. Guidelines are outlined for living with diabetes, including the roles of insulin administration, meal planning, exercise, and blood and urine testing in diabetes management. Finally, three key problems that may arise in insulin-dependent diabetes are described: hypoglycemia, hyperglycemia, and ketoacidosis. This brochure also is available in English (see DMBR01677).

LG Spanish
TI **Que es la Diabetes no Dependiente de la Insulina? (Diabetes tipo II) (What is Non-Insulin-Dependent Diabetes? (Type II Diabetes)).**
SO Alexandria, VA: American Diabetes Association, Diabetes Information Service Center. April 1989. 4 p.
CN American Diabetes Association.
AV Available from American Diabetes Association, Diabetes Information Service Center. 1660 Duke Street, Alexandria, VA 22314. (800) 232–3472 or (703) 549–1500. (Also available from local Chapters). PRICE: Bulk price, single copies are free. (Also available in English).

AB This brochure discusses the nature, prevalence, and symptoms of non-insulin-dependent diabetes. This type of diabetes often develops slowly, with symptoms that can be so mild that they are not noticed. Half of all Americans with this type of diabetes may not know it. Guidelines are outlined for living with diabetes, emphasizing a healthy diet and regular exercise; for people with this type of diabetes, losing weight is important for normalizing blood glucose levels. Adverse complications that can develop without proper treatment are cited; however, it is believed that these problems can be prevented with good blood glucose control. Guidelines are listed for good diabetes control. This brochure also is available in English (see DMBR01678).

LG Spanish
TI **Que es la Hiperglicemia? (What is Hyperglycemia? (High Blood Sugar)).**

SO Alexandria, VA: American Diabetes Association, Diabetes Information Service Center. December 1988. 4 p.

CN American Diabetes Association.

AV Available from American Diabetes Association, Diabetes Information Service Center. 1660 Duke Street, Alexandria, VA 22314. (800) 232–3472 or (703) 549–1500. (Also available from local Chapters). PRICE: Bulk price, single copies are free. (Also available in English).

AB This brochure discusses the causes and symptoms of hyperglycemia (high blood glucose), and describes how patients can determine when their blood glucose is too high and how it can be lowered. This complication occurs when the body has insufficient insulin or cannot use insulin properly, resulting in high blood glucose levels. For people with diabetes, self-monitoring of blood glucose can determine whether blood glucose levels are elevated. It is important that hyperglycemia be treated as soon as it is detected; failure to treat it can lead to diabetic coma (ketoacidosis). Exercise can lower blood glucose levels, but a person should not exercise if ketones are present in the urine. Methods for controlling hyperglycemia under a doctor's supervision are discussed. This brochure also is available in English (see DMBR01679).

LG Spanish

TI **Que es la Hipoglicemia? (What is Hypoglycemia? (Low Blood Sugar)).**

SO Alexandria, VA: American Diabetes Association, Diabetes Information Service Center. December 1988. 4 p.

CN American Diabetes Association.

AV Available from American Diabetes Association, Diabetes Information Service Center. 1660 Duke Street, Alexandria, VA 22314. (800) 232–3472 or (703) 549–1500. (Also available from local Chapters). PRICE: Bulk price, single copies are free. (Also available in English).

AB This brochure discusses the causes and symptoms of hypoglycemia (low blood glucose), and describes how patients can determine when their blood glucose is too low and how it can be raised. This complication often is called an insulin reaction, caused by taking too much insulin, eating too little food, not eating on time, or exercising too much. Symptoms include shakiness, dizziness, sweating, hunger, headache, pale skin color, clumsy/jerky movements, and tingling sensations around the mouth. Self-monitoring of blood glucose can determine whether blood glucose levels are too low or falling. Suggestions for treating hypoglycemia, including hypoglycemia resulting in loss of consciousness are provided. This brochure also is available in English (see DMBR01680).

LG Spanish
TI **Quetoacidosis (Ketoacidosis).**
SO Alexandria, VA: American Diabetes Association, Diabetes Information Service Center. April 1989. 4 p.
CN American Diabetes Association.
AV Available from American Diabetes Association, Diabetes Information Service Center. 1660 Duke Street, Alexandria, VA 22314. (800) 232–3472 or (703) 549–1500. (Also available from local Chapters). PRICE: Bulk price, single copies are free. (Also available in English).

AB This brochure describes the characteristics, warning signs, causes, and treatment of ketoacidosis, a serious condition that can lead to diabetic coma and possibly death. Ketoacidosis may happen to people with insulin-dependent diabetes; it does not occur in people with noninsulin-dependent diabetes. Ketoacidosis means the presence of dangerously high levels of ketones that build up in the blood and appear in the urine when the body does not have sufficient insulin. It is an emergency condition and requires hospitalization. It can be prevented by learning its warning signs (thirst/dry mouth, frequent urination, high blood glucose and urinary ketone levels, tiredness, dry/flushed skin, fruity odor on breath, confusion, nausea) and by regular testing of urine and blood. This brochure also is available in English (see DMBR01685).

LG Spanish
TI **Recetas para Diabeticos (Recipes for Diabetics).**
SO Austin, TX: Texas Department of Health. 1989. 31 p.
CN Texas Department of Agriculture.
AV Available from the Texas Department of Health. Chronic Disease Prevention Program, 1100 West 49th Street, Austin, TX 78756. (512) 458–7534. This publication is out of print. However, a photocopy of the publication will be sent upon request; it can be photocopied freely. PRICE: Single copy free.

AB This Spanish-language booklet presents exchange list information and recipes for some traditional Mexican dishes. One section gives guidelines for understanding nutritional labeling on food items, and an extensive chart lists herbs and spices and notes the foods that they complement best.

LG Spanish
TI **Recomendaciones Para Los Pies: Para un Mejor Cuidado de la Diabetes. (Foot Notes: For Better Diabetic Care).**
AU Suren, J.
SO Franklin Lakes, NJ: Becton Dickinson. 19xx. 12 p.
AV Available from Becton Dickinson and Company. Consumer Products Division, One Becton Drive, Franklin Lakes, NJ 07417. (800) 526–4650. PRICE: Free.

AB Foot hygiene rules for people with diabetes are listed in a large-print, illustrated text. Consideration is given to shoes, skin dryness and cracking, bathing, and nail trimming. Sources of information about diabetes are listed. Written in Spanish.

LG Spanish
TI **Si Usted Obtiene 'C' en esta Simple Prueba, Cuidado!: Es un Candidato a la 'D'iabetes (If You Get 'C' on this Simple Test, You May Be at Risk for Diabetes).**
SO Carolina, PR: Pfizer Pharmaceuticals. 19xx. 1 p.
CN Pfizer Pharmaceuticals.
AV Available from Pfizer Pharmaceuticals. P.O. Box 1859, Carolina, PR 00628–1859. (809) 257–5000. PRICE: Free.

AB This fact sheet poses four questions aimed at determining a person's risk of developing diabetes. It describes what diabetes is, how a doctor will diagnose and treat it, and the importance of following doctor's orders. The fact sheet is also available in English (see DMDC00604).

LG English; Spanish
TI **Signs and Symptoms of Diabetes: Add Up Your Scores (Senales y Sintomas de Diabetes: Sume los Puntos Suyos).**
SO Princeton, NJ: Novo Nordisk Pharmaceuticals, Inc. 1991. (poster).
CN Novo Nordisk Pharmaceuticals, Inc.
PD Poster (15 in × 20 in), col, Spanish and English.
AV Available from Novo Nordisk Pharmaceuticals, Inc. 100 Overlook Center, Suite 200, Princeton, NJ 08450–7810. (800) 727–6500. PRICE: Single copy free.

AB This poster presents an easy to use guide to the signs and symptoms of diabetes. Each of 13 symptoms is illustrated and assigned a point value. The poster urges people with a certain score to see their health care provider for testing. Symptoms covered are frequent urination, constant hunger, craving extra liquids, unexplained weight loss, sores that won't heal, vaginal infections, sexual dysfunction (impotence), blood glucose above 140 mg/dl, family member with diabetes, being overweight, numbness and tingling of feet, blurred vision, and constantly feeling tired. The poster is in English on one side and in Spanish on the other.

LG Spanish
TI **El Stress y la Diabetes (Stress and Diabetes).**
SO Alexandria, VA: American Diabetes Association, Diabetes Information Service Center. April 1989. 4 p.
CN American Diabetes Association.
AV Available from American Diabetes Association, Diabetes Information Service Center. 1660 Duke Street, Alexandria, VA 22314. (800) 232–3472 or (703) 549–1500. (Also available from local Chapters). PRICE: Bulk price, single copies are free. (Also available in English).

AB Everyday living with diabetes can be stressful, and stress and emotions can affect control of blood glucose. Illness also can cause stress. The best way to prevent a minor illness from becoming a major problem is for people with diabetes to have a plan for sick days, which should include guidelines for blood glucose and urinary ketone testing. Methods for reducing stress include determining and eliminating the cause of stress, stress relaxation techniques, regular exercise. It is argued that the better stress is controlled, the more one's diabetes will be under control. This brochure also is available in English (see DMBR01697).

LG Spanish; English
TI **Su Plan de Comida (Your Food Plan).**
AU anon.
SO Jacksonville, FL: Paramount Miller Graphics, Inc. 1992. 5p.
AV Available from Paramount Miller Graphics, Inc. 5299 St. Augustine Road, Jacksonville, FL 32207. (904) 448–1700. PRICE: \$0.50 each/1–500; \$0.45 each/500–1000.

AB Foods within each exchange group are illustrated in this full-color, fold-out chart. All foods are labeled in Spanish and English. Space is provided to list food selections and the number of portions for each food group at each meal.

LG English; Spanish
TI **Sweet Success: Diabetes and Pregnancy Program of San Diego and Imperial Counties.**
SO San Diego, CA: San Diego and Imperial Counties Diabetes and Pregnancy Program. 199x. 4 p.
CN San Diego and Imperial Counties Diabetes and Pregnancy Program.
AV Available from Regional Perinatal System. 225 Dickinson Street, H-410, San Diego, CA 92103. (619) 294–6142. PRICE: $.25 each or 10 for $2.00.

AB This bilingual brochure briefly reviews diabetes and pregnancy and introduces the services available through the Sweet Success Program in San Diego and Imperial Counties, California. The brochure stresses that the best way to have a healthy pregnancy and baby is to achieve and maintain good blood glucose control before the pregnancy begins. Other topics covered include diabetes control, community services offered through the Sweet Success program, and guidelines as to who can use these services. Contact information is included.

LG English; Spanish
TI **Sweet Success: Gestational Diabetes Fact Sheet Set.**
SO San Diego, CA: San Diego and Imperial Counties Diabetes and Pregnancy Program. 199x. 13 p.
CN San Diego and Imperial Counties Diabetes and Pregnancy Program.
AV Available from Regional Perinatal System. 225 Dickinson Street, H-410, San Diego, CA 92103. (619) 294–6142. PRICE: $1.00 each.

AB This set of 13 factsheets presents information about gestational diabetes in a clear, easy-to-read format. Among topics covered in the factsheets are an overview of gestational diabetes (GDM), diagnostic tests used to determine GDM, a checklist of health care behaviors for the woman with GDM, suggested meal plans for women with GDM both during and after pregnancy, exercise during pregnancy, blood glucose testing, kick counts (monitoring the fetal activity), other tests to check on the status of the fetus, a checklist of possible problems and suggestions for stress-reducing activities, a case example of one woman's experience with GDM, and checklists of postnatal care for both mother and baby.

LG Spanish
TI **Tratamiento de las Reacciones a la Insulina (Treating Insulin Reactions).**
SO Alexandria, VA: American Diabetes Association, Diabetes Information Service Center. April 1989. 4 p.
CN American Diabetes Association.
AV Available from American Diabetes Association, Diabetes Information Service Center. 1660 Duke Street, Alexandria, VA 22314. (800) 232–3472 or (703) 549–1500. (Also available from local Chapters). PRICE: Bulk price, single copies are free. (Also available in English).

AB This brochure discusses the symptoms and treatment of insulin reactions, also known as hypoglycemia (low blood glucose). The condition can be caused by taking too much insulin, eating too little food (or not eating on time), or by exercising too much. Symptoms include shakiness, dizziness, sweating, hunger, headache, or sudden mood changes. Suggestions for treating reactions are provided, including the administration of glucagon if a person loses consciousness. This brochure also is available in English (see DMBR01686).

LG Spanish
TI **1,200 Calorias (1,200 Calories).**
SO Indianapolis, IN: Eli Lilly and Company. 1988. 6 p.
CN Eli Lilly and Company.
AV Available from Eli Lilly and Company. Indianapolis, IN 46285. (317) 276–2010. PRICE: Single copy free.

AB This Spanish-language chart presents recommended exchange lists and sample menus for a 1,200 calorie diet suitable for people with diabetes. Food selections are drawn from traditional Hispanic foods. Instructions and tips for following a daily meal plan are provided, including measuring portions, selecting and preparing foods, and adjusting the meal plan where needed.

LG Spanish
TI **Usted: El ingredient mas importante de exito evando se vive con diabetes (You: the most important ingredient for success in living with diabetes).**
SO New York, NY: Roering/Pfizer Pharmaceuticals. 1992. 18p.

AV Available from Medcom/Trainex. P.O. Box 3225, Garden Grove, CA 92642. (800) 877–1443. PRICE: $165.00. Order Number 959TP.

SO Garden Grove, CA: Medcom/Trainex. 1983. (videocassette).

PD 1 cassette; 15 min; sd; col; 1/2 in. Also available in 3/4 in videocassette and sound filmstrip.

AB Emphasizing that exercise and a well-balanced, low-calorie diet may be all that is needed for people with noninsulin-dependent diabetes to control their disease, this videotape discusses choosing an exercise program and getting started. The videotape is also available in Spanish. (DA-M).

LG English; Spanish

TI **Home Monitoring: Blood Glucose and Ketones.**

AV Available from Medcom/Trainex. P.O. Box 3225, Garden Grove, CA 92642. (800) 877–1443. PRICE: $165.00. Order Number 955TP.

SO Garden Grove, CA: Medcom/Trainex. 1983. (videocassette).

PD 1 cassette; 19 min; sd; col; 1/2 in. Also available in 3/4 in videocassette, sound filmstrip, slide-tape, LaBelle or Audiscan cartridge.

AB Home blood glucose monitoring is described as an accurate and immediate method of determining blood sugar to provide better control in the daily balancing of diet, exercise, and medication. The program describes how home blood glucose monitoring is performed, both visually and with a meter, and it explains a method for testing for ketones in the urine. This item is also available in Spanish.

LG English; Spanish

TI **Home Monitoring: Urine and Ketones.**

AV Available from Medcom/Trainex. P.O. Box 3225, Garden Grove, CA 92642. (800) 877–1443. PRICE: $165.00. Order Number 956TP.

SO Garden Grove, CA: Medcom/Trainex. 1983. (videocassette).

PD 1 cassette; 20 min; sd; col; 1/2 in; also available in 3/4-in videocassette, sound filmstrip, slide-tape, LaBelle or Audiscan cartridge.

AB Various techniques for testing urine for the presence of glucose and ketones are described and illustrated. Basic terminology is explained, and factors that can affect test readings are discussed. This item is also available in Spanish.

LG English; Spanish
TI **In Balance: In Control. 4 Module Set (diabetes management).**
SO Indianapolis, IN: Boehringer Mannheim Corporation. 1987. (videocassette, looseleaf binder).
CN Boehringer Mannheim Corporation.
PD 1/2 in VHS or 3/4 in videocassette, with module guides, 52 p.
AV Available from Diabetes Customer Service, Boehringer Mannheim Corporation. 9115 Hague Road, P.O. Box 50100, Indianapolis, IN 46250–0100. (800) 858–8072. PRICE: $199.80 (1/2 in VHS videocassettes or 3/4 in videocassettes; either set includes a professional guide and a set of 10 patient guides for each module. Order Number 00608 for VHS, or 00607 for 3/4 inch format.

AB This instructional program is designed both for physicians caring for patients with diabetes and the patients themselves. The program includes four separate modules on videocassette, each accompanied by a professional guide and a patient guide. Module I, 'Understanding Your Diabetes,' explains diabetes; the role of diet, medication and exercise in blood glucose control; and the importance of self blood glucose monitoring. Module II, 'Food Facts of Diabetes,' introduces the six food groups; describes the relationship of the meal plan, medication and exercise; and emphasizes that people with diabetes can develop a meal plan they can live with and enjoy. Module III, 'Diabetes Medication as Directed,' explains how medication works; why insulin is prescribed for some and hypoglycemic agents for others; handling and administering medication; and potential side effects. Module IV, 'When Control Gets Out of Balance,' covers symptoms, causes, prevention, and treatment of hypoglycemia and hyperglycemia; ketoacidosis and urine testing for ketones; and sick day guidelines. The program is also available in Spanish.

LG English; Spanish
TI **Insulin Therapy.**
SO Calhoun, KY: NIMCO, Inc. 1988. (videocassette).
CN NIMCO, Inc.
PD VHS videocassette (24 min), col.
AV Available from NIMCO, Inc. 117 Highway 815, P.O. Box 9, Calhoun, KY 42327–0009. (800) 962–6662. FAX: (502) 273–5844.

PRICE: $99.95. Order No. NIM-MF024-V for English version, NIM-MF024-S for Spanish version.

AB This patient education videotape describes and explains insulin therapy. The program explains how insulin works; describes various types of insulin available and their actions; presents in detail how insulin should be used; and addresses the care of insulin, traveling, measurement, injection techniques, and possible complications. The videotape is intended to teach people with diabetes how to identify, protect, and use insulin properly; to provide a knowledge base upon which the diabetes educator can build; and to serve as a refresher for people who have used insulin previously. (AA-M).

LG Spanish
TI **Manual de Instrucciones Glucometer II (Instruction Manual: Glucometer II) .**
SO Elkhart, IN: Miles Laboratories. 1986. (audiocassette and instruction booklet).
CN Miles Laboratories.
PD audiocassette; instruction booklet, 29 p.
AV Available from Miles Laboratories, Inc. Ames Division, P.O. Box 70, Elkhart, IN 46515. (800) 348–8100. PRICE: Single copy free.

AB This audiocassette and instruction booklet, usually accompanying the Glucometer II blood glucose monitor, provide instructions for the proper use of the monitor. Numerous pictures in the booklet present a step-by-step guide to obtaining the blood sample, using the test strips, setting and reading the monitor, and interpreting the results. Instructions for changing the batteries are included. One section gives suggestions for trouble-shooting problems and how to proceed if the monitor needs repair or replacement. The warranty of the product, plus the names, addresses, and telephone numbers of Miles Laboratories divisions worldwide are appended. The audiocassette contains the same instructional information in an audio format, particularly useful for people with limited reading skills.

LG English; Spanish
TI **Overweight: What Can I Do About It?**
SO Timonium, MD: Milner-Fenwick, Inc. 1987. (videocassette).
CN Milner-Fenwick, Inc.
PD Videocassette (13 min).

AV Available from Milner-Fenwick, Inc. 2125 Greenspring Drive, Timonium, MD 21093–9989. (800) 638–8652 or (301) 252–1700. PRICE: $250.00. Order Number: WC-02.

AB This videocassette provides people with diabetes with practical guidelines for losing weight and keeping it off. The need to establish a daily calorie limit and make nutritious lower calorie food selections is emphasized. Techniques to modify eating behavior and increase activity level are also discussed. The videocassette is also available in Spanish. (AA-M).

LG English; Spanish
TI **Self-Monitoring of the Blood Glucose.**
AV Available from Nimco, Inc. P.O. Box 9, 117 Highway 815, Calhoun, KY 42327. (800) 962–6662. PRICE: $59.95 plus $6.00 shipping and handling, for slide/tape or videocassette or filmstrip. No charge for preview.
CN Nimco, Inc.
SO Calhoun, KY: Nimco, Inc. 1982. (slide/tape program).
PD Slides with Audiotape (15 min). Also available in videocassette and filmstrip formats, col.

AB In this patient education videotape, available in either English or Spanish, the problems of abnormal blood glucose levels and the effects of insulin on glucose metabolism are explained. Methods for keeping levels in the normal range are discussed, and use of an insulin pump is briefly noted. The disadvantages of urine testing and the advantages of blood glucose monitoring are summarized. The program is also available in slide/tape or filmstrip formats. (AA-M).

LG English; Spanish
TI **Taking Care of Your Body.**
AV Available from Medcom/Trainex. P.O. Box 3225, Garden Grove, CA 92642. (800) 877–1443. PRICE $165.00. Order Number 962TP.
SO Garden Grove, CA: Medcom/Trainex. 1983. (videocassette).
PD 1 cassette; 18 min; sd; col; 1/2 in; also available in 3/4-in videocassette, sound filmstrip, slide-tape, LaBelle or Audiscan cartridge.

AB Since diabetes causes the affected individual to be more prone to infection, the program stresses a daily routine of careful examination of the skin, teeth, feet, and legs as an important component of good personal hygiene. Daily precautions against possible injury and damage to the feet and legs are presented. Early recognition and treatment of cuts, bruises, and other injuries are emphasized as important factors in good diabetes care. The program also provides guidelines for sick-day care. The program is also available in Spanish.

LG English; Spanish
TI **Taking Charge: A Focus on Diabetes and Pregnancy.**
SO Washington, DC: Universal Health Associates, Inc. 1988. (videocassette).
CN Canadian Diabetes Association and Oracle Film and Video.
PD 1/2 in VHS or Beta videocassette (10 min 25 sec), col.
AV Available from Universal Health Associates, Inc. P.O. Box 65465, Washington, DC 20035. (202) 429–9506. PRICE: $79.00 (Preview $35.00) plus shipping $4.50. Order No. TCP200.

AB This instructional videotape presents the facts that every woman should know regarding diabetes and pregnancy. It emphasizes the importance of constant communication between the woman with diabetes and her health care team. Gestational diabetes is discussed along with the possibility of insulin treatment, factors describing high risk groups, and the importance of strict control, exercise and communication. Specific topics include adjusting meal plans, exercise, and insulin; appropriate weight gain; tips on monitoring and acceptable levels of blood glucose; and reducing complications. (AA-M).

LG English; Spanish
TI **Taking Charge: Living with Diabetes.**
SO Washington, DC: Universal Health Associates, Inc. 1990. (videocassette series).
CN Oracle Film and Video; Canadian Diabetes Association.
PD 8 VHS or Beta 1/2 in or 3/4 in videocassettes (8–12 min each), col.
AV Available from Universal Health Associates, Inc. P.O. Box 65465, Washington, DC 20035. (202) 429–9506. PRICE: $95.00. Order No. DS540.

AB This series of eight audiovisual programs is designed to help people with diabetes understand and control their condition. The presentations include an introductory videotape produced from a multi-image, sound-slide presentation, plus seven single-projector, slide-tape programs. The eight programs cover an introduction, meal planning, exercise, insulin, monitoring, noninsulin-dependent diabetes mellitus (NIDDM), pregnancy, and complications. The videos are assigned to provide information to help people with diabetes become self-sufficient, without overwhelming medical details and terminology. The series is also available in Spanish. (AA-M).

LG English; Spanish
TI **What is Diabetes?**
SO Timonium, MD: Milner-Fenwick, Inc. (videocassette).
CN Milner-Fenwick, Inc.
PD 1/2 in VHS or BETA or 3/4 in U-Matic videocassette; or 16 mm film, col.
AV Available from Milner-Fenwick, Inc. 2125 Greenspring Drive, Timonium, MD 21093. (800) 638–8652 or (301) 252–1700 (in Maryland, collect). PRICE: $250.00 (video formats) or $295.00 (16 mm film) per program.

AB This series of award-winning videocassettes addresses the wide variety of concerns confronting persons with insulin-dependent or noninsulin-dependent diabetes. Topics covered include skin and foot care, blood glucose monitoring, diet and exercise, insulin administration and management, how to avoid diabetic complications, diabetic retinopathy, overweight control, and gestational diabetes. Each program requires only a minimum of supervision, and is authoritatively prepared and designed to complement the ongoing education efforts of professionals treating diabetic patients.

Other Language Materials: Print

LG French
TI **Bien Manger = Bonne Sante.**
SO Toronto: Canadian Diabetes Association; 1986. 223p.
CN Canadian Diabetes Association.
AV Canadian Diabetes Association; 78 Bond Street; Toronto, Ontario M5B 2J8. (416) 362–4440. PRICE: $12.95.

AB A variety of recipes for people with diabetes are given. Information about meal planning is provided using the Food Group System of the Canadian Diabetes Association. Sample menus are provided. READING LEVEL: 10.

LG Polish

TI **Cukrzyca Fakty.**

SO Downsview, Ontario: Multicultural Health Coalition; 1985. 6p.

CN Multicultural Health Coalition.

AV MHC/CSM; Suite 407; 1017 Wilson Ave.; Downsview, Ontario M3K 1Z1; Canada. (416) 630–8835. PRICE: $0.10, minimum order 50 plus $2.50 shipping and handling (U.S. Funds).

AB This pamphlet presents basic information about diabetes, including its treatment, symptoms, how it develops, and the risk-factors that can increase a person's chances for developing diabetes. The components of a treatment plan, the importance of diabetes education, and examples of foods from the six major food groups are included. The pamphlet also is available in English, French, Chinese, Portuguese, Italian, Ukrainian, Hindi, Russian, Spanish, Vietnamese, Finnish, Punjabi, and Greek. READING LEVEL: 10.

LG French

TI **Le Diabete Apres Soixante Ans: Idees de Bons Repas (Diabetes Over 60: Meals To Serve You Well).**

SO Toronto, ONT: Canadian Diabetes Association; 1986. 28p.

CN National Nutrition Committee, Canadian Diabetes Association.

AV Canadian Diabetes Association; 78 Bond Street; Toronto, ONT M5B 2J8. (416) 362–4440. PRICE: Free in Canada: $0.25 elsewhere.

AB This booklet was developed to help older people with diabetes prepare satisfying and interesting meals. It contains sample menu suggestions, recipes for one or two servings, shopping and food storage ideas, tips on food preparation, and hints for "pepping up" meals. Foods to keep on an "emergency shelf" are listed, and precautions with respect to sugar, sodium, and cholesterol are spelled out. The booklet is also available in English.

LG English; French

TI **Diabetes Complications: Are You at Risk?.**

AU Hanna, P.A.

SO Diabetes Dialogue. 36(2): 7–12. Spring 1989.

AB Although many of the complications of diabetes may result from high blood glucose levels, several other risk factors are known to contribute to the occurrence and more rapid progression of these complications. This article, written for the person with diabetes, reviews the complications of diabetes and the risk factors for developing them. Topics addressed include hypertension, high cholesterol levels, cigarette smoking, and obesity.

LG English; French
TI **Diabetes and Employment: What Are Your Rights?.**
AU Skippen, J.D.
SO Diabetes Dialogue. 37(2): 11–13. Summer 1990.

AB This article discusses employment situations in which the legal rights of people with diabetes may have been violated. After a brief discussion of the Canadian Human Rights Code in general, the author explains how the laws affect individual work place situations for the person with diabetes. The author encourages any person who believes that he or she has experienced employment discrimination to consult a union representative, a lawyer, or the relevant Human Rights Commission.

LG French
TI **Le Diabetes et les Gens Ages (Diabetes and Seniors).**
AU anon.
SO Toronto: Canadian Diabetes Association; 1985. 12p.
CN National Education Committee, Canadian Diabetes Association.
AV Canadian Diabetes Association; 78 Bond Street; Toronto, Ontario, Canada M5B2J8. (416) 362–4440. PRICE: Single copy free in Canada; $0.25 elsewhere.

AB Written to help French-speaking older people manage their diabetes, this booklet presents risk factors associated with the disease and focuses on weight reduction and control. Suggestions for meal planning on a limited budget, overcoming the temptation to overeat, and exercise are provided. Because many elderly people take several medications in addition to insulin or hypoglycemic agents, suggestions for keeping track of the various medicines and avoiding undesirable interactions are presented. Urine and blood testing are briefly explained. Other topics are dealing with stress, prevention of complications, foot care, and fitting diabetes into one's social life. The causes, symptoms, and treatment of hypoglycemia and hyperglycemia are explained. The booklet is also available in English.

LG Russian; English
TI **Diabetes Handbook.**
AU Schulhoff, J.M.; Lichtman, T., eds.

SO Chicago, IL: Jewish Federation of Metropolitan Chicago. 1988. 95 p.

AV Available from Jewish Federation of Metropolitan Chicago. 1 South Franklin Street, Chicago, IL 60606. (312) 346–6700. PRICE: Single copy free. ATTN: Debra Liebow.

AB This bilingual patient education handout, written for persons newly diagnosed with diabetes mellitus, is intended to answer many of the initial questions about diabetes. The text, in both Russian and English, addresses the types of diabetes, signs and symptoms of diabetes, complications, food and diabetes, food exchange lists, meal planning, information about cholesterol and saturated fats, oral antidiabetic therapy, insulin therapy, urine testing, exercise, foot care, skin care, dental care, hypoglycemia, hyperglycemia, and lifestyle changes. Line drawings, charts, and diagrams illustrate many of the concepts presented.

LG Chinese

TI **Facts on Diabetes (Chinese).**

SO Downsview, Ontario: Multicultural Health Coalition; 1985. 6p.

CN Multicultural Health Coalition.

AV MHC/CSM; Suite 407; 1017 Wilson Ave.; Downsview, Ontario M3K 1Z1; Canada. (416) 630–8835. PRICE: $0.10, minimum order of 50 plus $2.50 shipping and handling (U.S. Funds).

AB This pamphlet presents basic information about diabetes, including its treatment, symptoms, how it develops, and the risk factors that can increase a persons chances for developing diabetes. The components of a treatment plan, the importance of diabetes education, and examples of foods from the six major food groups are included. The pamphlet also is available in English, French, Portuguese, Italian, Ukrainian, Polish, Hindi, Russian, Spanish, Vietnamese, Finnish, Punjabi, and Greek. READING LEVEL: 10.

LG Greek

TI **Facts on Diabetes (Greek).**

SO Downsview, Ontario: Multicultural Health Coalition; 1985. 6p.

CN Multicultural Health Coalition.

AV MHC/CSM; Suite 407; 1017 Wilson Ave.; Downsview, Ontario M3K 1Z1; Canada. (416) 630–8835. PRICE: $0.10, minimum order of 50 plus $2.50 shipping and handling (U.S. Funds).

AB This pamphlet presents basic information about diabetes, including its treatment, symptoms, how it develops, and the risk factors that can increase a person's chances for developing diabetes. The components of a treatment plan, the importance of diabetes education, and examples of foods from the six major food groups are included. The pamphlet also is available in English, French, Chinese, Portuguese, Italian, Ukrainian, Polish, Hindi, Russian, Spanish, Vietnamese, Finnish, and Punjabi. READING LEVEL: 10.

LG Russian
TI **Facts on Diabetes (Russian).**
SO Downsview, Ontario: Multicultural Health Coalition; 1985. 6p.
CN Multicultural Health Coalition.
AV MHC/CSM; Suite 407; 1017 Wilson Ave.; Downsview, Ontario M3K 1Z1; Canada. (416) 630–8835. PRICE: $0.10, minimum order of 50 plus $2.50 shipping and handling (U.S. Funds).

AB This pamphlet, written in Russian, presents basic information about diabetes, including its treatment, symptoms, how it develops, and the risk factors that can increase a person's chances for developing diabetes. The components of a treatment plan, the importance of diabetes education, and examples of foods from the six major food groups are included. The pamphlet also is available in English, French, Chinese, Portuguese, Ukrainian, Polish, Hindi, Spanish, Vietnamese, Finnish, Punjabi, and Greek. READING LEVEL: 10.

LG Italian
TI **Fatti Sul Diabete.**
SO Downsview, Ontario: Multicultural Health Coalition; 1985. 6p.
CN Multicultural Health Coalition.
AV MHC/CSM; Suite 407; 1017 Wilson Ave.; Downsview, Ontario M3K 1Z1; Canada. (416) 630–8835. PRICE: $0.10, minimum order of 50 plus $2.50 shipping and handling (U.S. Funds).

AB This pamphlet presents basic information about diabetes, including its treatment, symptoms, how it develops, and the risk factors that can increase a person's chances for developing diabetes. The components of a treatment plan, the importance of diabetes education, and examples of foods from the six major food groups are included. The pamphlet also is available in English, French, Chinese, Portuguese, Ukrainian, Polish, Hindi, Russian, Spanish, Vietnamese, Finnish, Punjabi, and Greek. READING LEVEL: 10.

LG Chinese; English
TI **Food and Diabetes.**
SO Seattle, WA: American Diabetes Association, Washington Affiliate; 1985. 16p.
CN American Diabetes Association, Washington Affiliate. International District Community Health Center.
AV American Diabetes Association, Washington Affiliate. 557 Roy Street, Lower Level, Seattle, WA 98109. (800) 628–8808 (in Washington state only) or (206) 282–4616. PRICE: $2.00; plus for shipping and handling: $1.75 (to $5.00), $3.00 (to $10.00), $4.50 (to $25.00).

AB Synchronous Chinese and English texts explain glucose metabolism; describe foods in the carbohydrate, protein, and fat categories; and list food types and portions recommended for maintenance of normal blood glucose. Two sample meal plans are offered. The symptoms and treatment of hypoglycemia are briefly described. The pamphlet also is available in English, Vietnamese, Spanish, Chinese, and Pagalog (Phillipine). READING LEVEL (English): 8.

LG Portuguese
TI **Manual Para Diabeticos. (Manual for Diabetics).**
SO Cambridge, MA: Visiting Nurse Association of Cambridge; 1985. 12p.
CN Associacao Das Enfermeiras Visitantes De Cambridge (Visiting Nurse Association of Cambridge).
AV Visiting Nursing Association of Cambridge; P.O. Box 262; 35 Bigelow Street; Cambridge, MA 02139. (617) 547–2620. PRICE: $0.50 each.

AB This pamphlet, written for the Portuguese-speaking person with diabetes, emphasizes management of diabetes by strict adherence to the recommended guidelines and methods of self care and also provides a basic background for understanding the disease and facilitating its control. Special considerations include detailed foot care, footwear, exercise, and dietary principles and guidelines, as well as lists of food by category.

LG Portuguese
TI **O Que Voce Deve Saber Acerca Dos Diabetes.**
SO Downsview, Ontario: Multicultural Health Coalition; 1985. 6p.
CN Multicultural Health Coalition.

AV MHC/CSM; Suite 407; 1017 Wilson Ave.; Downsview, Ontario M3K 1Z1; Canada. (416) 630–8835. PRICE: $0.10, minimum order of 50 plus $2.50 shipping and handling (U.S. Funds).

AB This pamphlet presents basic information about diabetes, including its treatment, symptoms, how it develops, and the risk factors that can increase a person's chances for developing diabetes. The components of a treatment plan, the importance of diabetes education, and examples of foods from the six major food groups are included. The pamphlet also is available in English, French, Chinese, Italian, Ukrainian, Polish, Hindi, Russian, Spanish, Vietnamese, Finnish, Punjabi, and Greek. READING LEVEL: 10.

LG Italian
TI **Un Programma Di Informazione Per I Diabetici: Principi, Mezzi, Verifica. (A Program For Diabetics Education: Principles, Means and Evaluation).**
AU Bruni, B.; Barbero, P.L.; et al.
SO Torino, Italy: Centor di Diabetologia Karen Bruni; n.d. 24p.
AV Dr Prof B. Bruni; Centro di Diabetologia Karen Bruni; Ospedale Maria Vittoria; Via Cibrario n. 72; 10144 - Torino (Italy). PRICE: Contact directly for details.

AB This patient education handbook, in Italian, presents a patient information program as a primary treatment tool for diabetes. Phase I, Basic Information, consists of an individual checklist of 20 items to be completed, responsibility for which is shared between the professional and the patient; several video-sound slide shows and films; and an information booklet. Phase II, Advanced Information, continually up-dates the diabetic's knowledge through periodic discussion meetings and a magazine covering new techniques and investigations.

LG French
TI **Renseignements sur le Diabete.**
SO Downsview, Ontario: Multicultural Health Coalition; 1985. 6p.
CN Multicultural Health Coalition.
AV MHC/CSM; Suite 407; 1017 Wilson Ave.; Downsview, Ontario M3K 1Z1; Canada. (416) 630–8835. PRICE: $0.10, minimum order of 50 plus $2.50 shipping and handling (U.S. Funds).

AB This pamphlet presents basic information about diabetes, including its treatment, symptoms, how it develops, and the risk factors that can increase a person's chances for developing diabetes. The components of a treatment plan, the importance of diabetes education, and examples of foods from the six major food groups are included. The pamphlet also is available in English, Chinese, Portuguese, Italian, Ukrainian, Polish, Hindi, Russian, Spanish, Vietnamese, Finnish, Punjabi, and Greek. READING LEVEL: 10.

LG French
TI **Savoir Choisir: Pour Bien Vivre (Choose: A Healthy Lifestyle).**
SO Toronto, Ontario. Canadian Diabetes Association. 1990. 4 p.
CN Canadian Diabetes Association.
AV Available from Canadian Diabetes Association, 78 Bond Street, Toronto, Ontario M5B 2J8, CANADA. (416) 362–4440. PRICE: Single copy free.

AB This brochure encourages the general reader to enjoy a healthy lifestyle and thereby lower the risk of developing diabetes, heart disease, or other related health problems. Written in a format that presents a variety of health and nutrition facts and tips, the brochure discusses recommended dietary levels of fat, fiber, and salt; regular exercise; alcohol; skipping meals; and snacking. Also included is information about the Canadian Diabetes Association's cookbook that emphasizes healthy cooking. The brochure concludes with a checklist of changes to make for a healthy lifestyle and encourages the reader to make a commitment to start regular exercise and improve eating habits. This brochure is also available in English (reference DMBR01753).

LG Chinese
TI **Some Facts About Oral Diabetes Medications (Orinase, Diabinese, Tolinase, Dymelor). (Chinese translation).**
SO San Francisco, CA: SRx Regional Program. 1988. 1 p.
CN SRx Regional Program (Medication Education for Seniors).
AV Available from SRx Regional Program. 1182 Market Street, Suite 204, San Francisco, CA 94102.

AB This fact sheet for Chinese-speaking persons with diabetes provides information and guidelines concerning oral diabetic drugs. Information is provided on their importance to diabetes management, how they work, and how they should be taken. Specific health hints and cautions are included. This fact sheet also is available in English, Vietnamese, and Spanish (see DMDC00851, DMDC00853 and DMDC00854).

LG French
TI **Vive la Sante!: Vive la Bonne Alimentation! (Good Health Eating Guide). (large print).**
SO Toronto, Ontario. Canadian Diabetes Association. 1990. 2 p.
CN Canadian Diabetes Association.
AV Available from Canadian Diabetes Association, 78 Bond Street, Toronto, Ontario M5B 2J8, CANADA. (416) 362–4440. PRICE: Single copy free.

AB This eating guide presents food exchange lists; an eating plan chart; common household measures and their metric equivalents; and tips for meal planning, shopping, and cooking for the person with diabetes. Foods are grouped into the following categories: proteins; starch; milk; fruits and vegetables; fats and oils; and extras. For each group, detailed suggestions for purchase and preparation are included. Additional information on points for good health; dietetic foods; alcohol; and what to do when the patient is too sick to eat regular meals is included. The guide is presented as a colorful, easy-to-use chart and utilizes a large-print format. It is also available in English (reference DMBR01750).

LG Laotian, English
TI **You and Diabetes.**
SO Des Moines, IA: Department of Human Services. 198x. 25 p.
CN Bureau of Refugee Services.
AV Available from Department of Human Services. Dena Raske, Bureau of Refugee Services, 1200 University Avenue, Suite D, Des Moines, IA 50314. (515) 283–7903. PRICE: Single copy free.

AB This bilingual document, written in both English and Laotian, presents a broad overview of the care and management of diabetes mellitus. Topics covered include the signs and symptoms of diabetes, the etiology and epidemiology of the disease, meal planning and weight control, medications used to manage diabetes, urine testing, exercise, skin and foot care, insulin, high and low blood glucose, and doctor-patient relationships. Simple line drawings illustrate the main concepts presented.

Other Language Materials: Audiovisuals

LG English; French
TI **Walking in Balance/Vivre en Harmonie.**

SO Scarborough, Ontario: City Communications. 1985. (videocassette).

CN Canadian Diabetes Association.

PD 3/4 in or 1/2 Beta or 1/2 VHS videocassette (25 min), col.

AV Available from City Communications. 3011 Markham Road, Unit #60, Scarborough, Ontario M1X1L7, Canada. (416) 321–1056. PRICE: $95.00 (3/4 in), $80.00 (1/2 in Beta) and $80.00 (1/2 in VHS). Retail sales tax (7 percent) extra to non-exempt Ontario purchasers.

AB This color videotape addresses diabetes and diabetes education among the Native Canadian population. Several Canadian researchers express their views about the possible cause of the increasing incidence of diabetes among the natives. Diabetes educators discuss appropriate teaching methods, and individuals with diabetes discuss the problems they experience in having diabetes. (AA).

Index to Diabetes Sourcebook